Manual of
MIDWIFERY
and Gynecological Nursing

AF070458

Manual of
MIDWIFERY
and Gynecological Nursing

FOURTH EDITION

Annamma Jacob MSc (N)
Former Principal, Bhagwan Mahaveer Jain College of Nursing
Bengaluru, Karnataka, India

Formerly
Professor, St Philomena's College of Nursing
Bengaluru, Karnataka, India
Principal, BNE, SIB, CMAI, Cunningham Road
Bengaluru, Karnataka, India
Nurse Supervisor, Suburban Medical Center
Paramount, Southern California, USA
Assistant Director of Nursing, Al Sabah Hospital
Ministry of Public Health, Kuwait
Sister Tutor, LT College of Nursing, SNDT Women's University
Mumbai, Maharashtra, India
Junior Tutor, College of Nursing
CMC Hospital, Vellore, Tamil Nadu, India

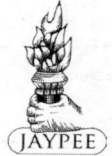

JAYPEE BROTHERS MEDICAL PUBLISHERS
The Health Sciences Publisher
New Delhi | London

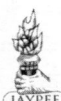

Jaypee Brothers Medical Publishers (P) Ltd

Headquarters
Jaypee Brothers Medical Publishers (P) Ltd
EMCA House, 23/23-B
Ansari Road, Daryaganj
New Delhi 110 002, India
Landline: +91-11-23272143, +91-11-23272703
+91-11-23282021, +91-11-23245672
Email: jaypee@jaypeebrothers.com

Corporate Office
Jaypee Brothers Medical Publishers (P) Ltd
4838/24, Ansari Road, Daryaganj
New Delhi 110 002, India
Phone: +91-11-43574357
Fax: +91-11-43574314
Email: jaypee@jaypeebrothers.com

Overseas Office
J.P. Medical Ltd
83 Victoria Street, London
SW1H 0HW (UK)
Phone: +44 20 3170 8910
Fax: +44 (0)20 3008 6180
Email: info@jpmedpub.com

Website: www.jaypeebrothers.com
Website: www.jaypeedigital.com

© 2023, Jaypee Brothers Medical Publishers

The views and opinions expressed in this book are solely those of the original contributor(s)/author(s) and do not necessarily represent those of editor(s) and publisher of the book.

All rights reserved. No part of this publication may be reproduced, stored or transmitted in any form or by any means, electronic, mechanical, photocopying, recording or otherwise, without the prior permission in writing of the publishers.

All brand names and product names used in this book are trade names, service marks, trademarks or registered trademarks of their respective owners. The publisher is not associated with any product or vendor mentioned in this book.

Medical knowledge and practice change constantly. This book is designed to provide accurate, authoritative information about the subject matter in question. However, readers are advised to check the most current information available on procedures included and check information from the manufacturer of each product to be administered, to verify the recommended dose, formula, method and duration of administration, adverse effects and contraindications. It is the responsibility of the practitioner to take all appropriate safety precautions. Neither the publisher nor the author(s)/editor(s) assume any liability for any injury and/or damage to persons or property arising from or related to use of material in this book.

This book is sold on the understanding that the publisher is not engaged in providing professional medical services. If such advice or services are required, the services of a competent medical professional should be sought.

Every effort has been made where necessary to contact holders of copyright to obtain permission to reproduce copyright material. If any have been inadvertently overlooked, the publisher will be pleased to make the necessary arrangements at the first opportunity.

Inquiries for bulk sales may be solicited at: jaypee@jaypeebrothers.com

Manual of Midwifery and Gynecological Nursing

First Edition: 2009
Second Edition: 2012
Third Edition: 2017
Fourth Edition: **2023**

ISBN: 978-93-5696-159-3

Printed at Rajkamal Electric Press, Kundli, Haryana.

Preface to the Fourth Edition

Manual of Midwifery and Gynecological Nursing, 4th edition is written at an unusual time for the country and world. Across countries, cultures and beliefs, the world is for once united facing a common threat, the corona pandemic. In healthcare professions, all we have strived for in providing ethical care to patients has broken down in the current pandemic period.

There has been significant loss of autonomy, shared decision making and confidentiality in doctor-patient and nurse-patient interactions. There is complete loss of rapport building mechanisms, communication methods and ways to reassure patients. Medical isolation of patients to protect others has meant that patients go through the illness entirely alone and sometimes die alone without the family by their side. COVID-19 patients cannot even see the faces of their healthcare providers which dehumanizes the patient, increasing their anxiety, distrust and sorrow. It is our hope and prayer that this difficult time will soon pass and care of the sick will return to earlier standards for all, including maternal and newborn care. As the manual is ready for printing in early 2023 the author feels great relief as we have almost recovered from the pandemic in the country through great efforts implemented by the governments at the union and state levels and health workers countrywide. Very few cases only are reported presently, and people have returned to normal life.

Several midwifery and gynecological nursing topics are added in this edition as it is being revised after a period of four years. It is my hope and desire that the subjects and topics included now will make the book more comprehensive, contributing to knowledge of the subject—obstetric and gynecological nursing for all student nurses who use this hand-book. Suggestions and recommendations from users will help improve and hence such encouragement is always welcome. Big thanks and gratitude go the officials and concerned staff personnel of Jaypee Brothers Medical Publishers in Delhi and Bengaluru offices for their support and encouragement.

Annamma Jacob

Preface to the First Edition

Delivering safe, sensitive and thoughtful care, to patients and their families, is a goal of every nurse. To this end, *Manual of Midwifery* includes special features to help nurses acquire knowledge, master skills and gain competence, when caring for their patients.

It is a comprehensive, yet concise clinical reference designed for use by midwifery students and nurses. The manual presents all need-to-know information about mothers in prenatal, intranatal and postnatal periods, and babies in the neonatal period. Problems commonly encountered by mothers during pregnancy, delivery and immediate postpartum periods, and babies in the neonatal period are included. Each entry is formatted consistently for quick access to important information.

Nursing care plans are included with selected topics, and a list of NANDA (North American Nursing Diagnosis Association) approved Nursing Diagnoses is given as Appendix for use in different situations in the care of mothers and babies.

The contents of the book are arranged in alphabetical sequence for quick reference and study in the clinical area, at home or in the community as well. Nursing considerations including health education are highlighted in every topic.

The book is pocket-sized, yet contains all aspects of childbearing and newborn period. I hope, it will be of immense value to the students and nurses in their learning and practice of midwifery.

Annamma Jacob

Acknowledgments

First and foremost, I express my deep sense of gratitude to God Almighty for the physical and emotional strength and circumstances given to me during the period of my work on this book.

The concept of writing a *Manual of Midwifery and Gynecological Nursing* was brought to me by Mr Venugopal (Branch Manager) of M/s Jaypee Brothers Medical Publishers (P) Ltd, Bengaluru Branch. I am very grateful to the whole team of M/s Jaypee Brothers Medical Publishers (P) Ltd, New Delhi, India, who helped and guided me, Shri Jitendar P Vij (Group Chairman), Mr Ankit Vij (Managing Director), Mr MS Mani (Group President), Dr Madhu Choudhary (Director–Educational Publishing), Ms Pooja Bhandari (Production Head), Ms Sunita Katla (Executive Assistant to Group Chairman and Publishing Manager), Ms Samina Khan (Executive Assistant to Director–Educational Publishing), Ms Alisha Talwar (Development Editor), Mr Rajesh Sharma (Production Coordinator), Ms Seema Dogra (Cover Visualizer), Mr Narsingh Kumar (Proofreader), Mr Om Prakash Mishra (Typesetter), Mr Satender Singh (Graphic Designer) and their team members, for all their support to work in this project and make it a success. Without their cooperation, I could not have completed this project. I thank them very sincerely for being my motivation.

My special thanks are due to my talented and committed colleagues, Ms Jessy Jacob, Ms Jadhav Sonali Tarachand and Ms Malliga Christeena who offered timely assistance and directions which resulted in the completion of this project.

I thank my students of midwifery, both present and past who have challenged and taught me and guided me in the direction for this book.

I thank my family members especially my husband, Mr AJ Jacob who supported me and provided continuous assistance in preparing this manual.

Contents

CONTENTS

A

1. Abdominal Examination 1
2. ABO Incompatibility 4
3. Abnormal Uterine Action 5
4. Abnormal Uterine Bleeding 13
5. Abortion 19
6. Adenomyosis 33
7. Adoption 34
8. AIDS in Pregnancy 40
9. Amniocentesis 47
10. Amniotic Fluid Embolism 49
11. Anemia in Pregnancy 50
12. Antenatal Assessment 61
13. Antepartum Hemorrhage 65
14. Assisted Reproductive Technology 83

B

15. Basic Life Support/Cardiopulmonary Resuscitation 88
16. Biophysical Profile 93
17. Birth Injuries in Newborns 95
18. Breastfeeding 104
19. Breast Cancer 108
20. Breast Infection in Puerperium 143
21. Breech Presentation 145
22. Brow Presentation 153

C

23. Cesarean Section 155
24. Carcinoma Cervix 163
25. Cancer Uterus 166
26. Cardiac Disease in Pregnancy 169
27. Cephalopelvic Disproportion 181
28. Chromosome Abnormalities in Newborns 184
29. Congenital Uterine Anomalies/Abnormalities 190

Manual of Midwifery and Gynecological Nursing

30. Congenital Anomalies in Newborns 195
31. Contracted Pelvis 215
32. Contraction Stress Test 217
33. Contraception 219
34. Convulsions in Newborns 236
35. Cordocentesis (Percutaneous Umbilical Blood Sampling) 238
36. Cord Presentation 240
37. Cord Prolapse 241

D

38. Diabetes in Pregnancy 243
39. Diagnosis of Pregnancy 257
40. Diagnostic Procedures in Gynecology and Obstetrics 263
41. Diarrhea in Newborns 297
42. Disseminated Intravascular Coagulation 299
43. Drugs in Obstetrics 302
44. Dysmenorrhea 317
45. Dyspareunia 318

E

46. Eclampsia 319
47. Ectopic Pregnancy 322
48. Endometriosis 327
49. Endoscopic Surgery in Gynecological Patients 332
50. Episiotomy 335
51. External Cephalic Version 338

F

52. Face Presentation 340
53. Fetal Circulation 345
54. Fetal Distress 347
55. Fetal Heart Rate Monitoring Cardiotocography (CTG) 348
56. Fetal Imaging 353
57. Fetal Skull 356
58. Fibroid Tumors in Uterus 363
59. Forceps Delivery 374

G

60. Gene Disorders, Genetic Screening and Genetic Counseling 378
61. Gynecological Disorders in Pregnancy 392

H

62. Hyaline Membrane Disease/Respiratory Distress Syndrome 406
63. Hydatidiform Mole/Vesicular Mole 408
64. Hydramnios/Polyhydramnios 411
65. Hyperemesis Gravidarum 416
66. Hysterectomy 419
67. Hysterosalpingography 421

I

68. Immediate Care of the Newborn 422
69. Immunization 425
70. Induction of Labor 429
71. Infections in Newborns 437
72. Infectious Conditions of Pelvic Organs 441
73. Infections in Pregnancy 446
74. Infertility 449
75. Instruments in Obstetrics and Gynecology 456
76. Intrauterine Growth Restriction (Retardation) 488
77. Intrauterine Tamponade Using Bakri Balloon 491
78. Inversion of Uterus 495

J

79. Jaundice in Neonate 498

L

80. Labor—Stage I 501
81. Labor—Stage II 508
82. Labor—Stage III 515
83. Lactation 520
84. Low Birth Weight Baby 525

M

85. Maternal Pelvis 526
86. Meconium Aspiration Syndrome 531
87. Medical Termination of Pregnancy 533
88. Menopause 535
89. Minor Disorders of Pregnancy 540
90. Minor Disorders of Newborn 544
91. Minor Surgeries in Gynecological Patients 550
92. Multifetal Pregnancy 557

xiv Manual of Midwifery and Gynecological Nursing

N

93. National Family Welfare Programs 563
94. Neonatal Intensive Care Unit 576
95. Newborn Assessment 593
96. Newborn Care 596
97. Non-stress Test 605
98. Nursing Diagnosis 606
99. Nursing Care of Newborn in Incubator/Isolette 619

O

100. Obstructed Labor 621
101. Occipitoposterior Position 625
102. Oxytocin Challenge Test 627

P

103. Partograph 628
104. Pelvic Inflammatory Disease 633
105. Physiological Changes in Pregnancy 637
106. Physical Examination of Newborn 644
107. Polycystic Ovary Syndrome 651
108. Postpartum Care 654
109. Postdated Pregnancy/Post-term Pregnancy 667
110. Postnatal Assessment (Postdelivery Assessment) 670
111. Precipitate Labor 674
112. Pregnancy-induced Hypertension 676
113. Premature Rupture of Membranes 686
114. Premenstrual Syndrome 687
115. Preterm Baby 689
116. Preterm Labor 692
117. Prolonged Labor 695
118. Psychiatric Disorders during Pregnancy 697
119. Psychiatric Disorders in Puerperium 701
120. Puberty 704
121. Puerperal Sepsis 707

R

122. Rectovaginal Fistula 710
123. Respiratory Distress in Newborns 712
124. Respiratory Distress Syndrome 713

Contents

125. Resuscitation of the Newborns	715
126. Retained Placenta	722
127. Retroversion of Uterus	723
128. Rhesus Incompatibility	724
129. Rupture of Uterus	726

S

130. Shock in Obstetrics	729
131. Shoulder Dystocia	733
132. Sexually Transmitted Diseases	735
133. Sexual Violence	744
134. Single Parent	747
135. Stillbirth	750

T

136. Teenage Pregnancy and Adolescent Pregnancy	753

U

137. Ultrasonics in Obstetrics	755
138. Unwed Mother	759
139. Uterine Prolapse	763
140. Urinary Tract Infections	767

V

141. Vasa Previa	771
142. Vasectomy Operation/Male Sterilization	772
143. Vesicovaginal Fistula	775
144. Ventouse Delivery (Vacuum-assisted Birth)	778
145. Vomiting in Newborns	780

Study Questions	*782*
Bibliography	*799*
Index	*803*

INC Syllabus

GNM SYLLABUS

Midwifery and Gynecological Nursing: Practical

Placement: Third Year (Part – I) **Time: 560 hours**
Internship: 384 hours

Area	Duration	Objectives	Skills	Assignment	Assessment methods
Antenatal clinic/ward	3 weeks	• Assessment of pregnant women • Counselling of a antenatal mothers	• Diagnose pregnancy using pregnancy detection kit (preg-card) • Antenatal history taking • Physical examination • Antenatal examination – abdomen and breast • Recording weight and BP • Hemoglobin estimation	• Conduct antenatal examinations –20 • Health talk – 1 • Case study – 1	• Verification of the findings of antenatal examinations • Assessment of skills using checklist

Area	Duration	Objectives	Skills	Assignment	Assessment methods
			- Urine testing for sugar and albumin - Immunization - Assessment of risk status - Antenatal counselling - Maintenance of antenatal records - SBA module		
Labor room	6 weeks	- Assess the woman in labor - Carry out per vaginal (PV) examinations - Monitor women in labor - Conduct normal deliveries	- Assessment of woman in labor - Vaginal examinations (PV) and their interpretation - Monitoring women in labor using the partograph - Caring for women in labor - Setting up of the labor unit including the newborn corner	- Perform per vaginal examinations – 5 - Conduct normal deliveries – 20 - Perform and suture episiotomies – 5 - Resuscitate newborns – 5	- Assessment of clinical performance with rating scale - Assessment of each skill with checklist - Practical examination

Area	Duration	Objectives	Skills	Assignment	Assessment methods
		• Perform episiotomy and suture it • Resuscitate newborns	• Conduct normal delivery including active management of third stage of labor (AMTSL) • Provide essential newborn care • Immediate newborn assessment • Resuscitation of the newborn • Assessment of the risk status of the newborn • Episiotomy and suturing • Administration of uterotonic drugs – oxytocin, misoprostol • Administration of magnesium sulphate • Maintenance of labor and birth records • SBA module	• Witnessing abnormal deliveries - 5 • Case book recording	

Area	Duration	Objectives	Skills	Assignment	Assessment methods
Operation theatre	2 weeks	Prepare and assist with cesarean section, MTP, tubectomy and other surgical procedures	• Preparation for cesarean section and other surgical procedures • Assist in cesarean section • Prepare and assist in MTP procedures • Prepare and assist for tubectomy	• Assist with cesarean section – 2 • Case book recording	Assessment of skill with checklist
Postnatal ward	5 weeks	• Provide nursing care to postnatal mother and the baby • Counsel and teach mother and family for parenthood	• Examination and assessment of mother and the baby • Identification of deviations • Care of postnatal mothers and baby • Perineal care • Breast care	• Provide postnatal care to mothers and babies – 20 • Health talks – 1 • Case study – 1 • Case presentation – 1	• Assessment of clinical performance with rating scale • Assessment of each skill with checklist • Practical examination

Area	Duration	Objectives	Skills	Assignment	Assessment methods
			• Lactation management • Breastfeeding • Kangaroo mother care (KMC) • Immunization • Teaching postnatal mother on mother craft, postnatal care, exercise, immunization		
NICU	4 weeks	Provide nursing care to newborns at risk	• Newborn assessment • Admission of neonates • Feeding of high-risk newborn—katori spoon, paladai, tube feeding, total parenteral nutrition • Thermal management of newborns—kangaroo mother care, care of baby in radiant warmer and incubator	• Case study - 1 • NSSK module	• Assessment of clinical performance with rating scale • Assessment of each skill with checklist • Practical examination

Area	Duration	Objectives	Skills	Assignment	Assessment methods
			• Monitoring and care of neonates • Administration of medications • Intravenous therapy • Assisting in diagnostic procedures • Assist in exchange transfusion • Care of baby in ventilator, phototherapy, • Practice infection control protocols • Health education and counselling of parents • Maintenance of records and reports		

Area	Duration	Objectives	Skills	Assignment	Assessment methods
Family welfare clinic	2 week	Counsel for and provide family welfare services	• Family planning counselling techniques • Insertion of IUCD • Teaching by demonstration on the use of different family planning methods • Arrange for and assist with family planning operations • Maintenance of records and reports	• IUCD insertion – 5 • Family planning counselling – 2	Assessment of clinical performance with rating scale • Assessment of each skill with checklist • Practical examination
Gynecology ward	2 weeks	• Provide care for patients with gynecological disorders	• Assist with gynecological examination • Assist and perform diagnostic and therapeutic procedures • Teach women on breast self examination (BSE)	• Provide care to assigned patients • Nursing care plan-1 • Menopause counseling – 1	• Assess each skill with checklist • Assess performance with rating scale

Area	Duration	Objectives	Skills	Assignment	Assessment methods
		• Counsel and educate patient and families	• Health education on perineal hygiene and prevention of sexually transmitted infections • Pre and postoperative care of women undergoing gynecological surgeries • Menopause counseling		• Evaluation of care plan

BSC NURSING

Practicum

Placement: VI and VII Semester

Semester: Midwifery/Obstetrics and Gynecology (OBG) Nursing-I

Skill Lab and Clinical: Skill Lab – 1 Credit (40 hours); Clinical – 3 Credits (240 hours)

Practice Competencies: On completion of the course, the students will be able to:
- Counsel women and their families on pre-conception care
- Demonstrate lab tests, e.g., urine pregnancy test
- Perform antenatal assessment of pregnant women
- Assess and care for normal antenatal mothers
- Assist and perform specific investigations for antenatal mothers
- Counsel mothers and their families on antenatal care and preparation for parenthood
- Conduct childbirth education classes
- Organize labor room
- Prepare and provide respectful maternity care for mothers in labor
- Perform pervaginal examination for a woman in labor if indicated
- Conduct normal childbirth with essential newborn care
- Demonstrate skills in resuscitating the newborn
- Assist women in the transition to motherhood
- Perform postnatal and newborn assessment
- Provide care for postnatal mothers and their newborn
- Counsel mothers on postnatal and newborn care
- Perform PPIUCD insertion and removal

- Counsel women on family planning and participate in family welfare services
- Provide youth friendly health services
- Identify, assess, care and refer women affected with gender based violence

Skill Lab: Procedures/skills for demonstration and return demonstration:
- Urine pregnancy test
- Calculation of EDD, obstetrical score, gestational weeks
- Antenatal assessment
- Counseling antenatal mothers
- Micro birth planning
- PV examination
- Monitoring during first stage of labor—plotting and interpretation of partograph
- Preparation for delivery—setting up labor room, articles, equipment
- Mechanism of labor—normal
- Conduction of normal childbirth with essential newborn care
- Active management of third stage of labour
- Placental examination
- Newborn resuscitation
- Monitoring during fourth stage of labour
- Postnatal assessment
- Newborn assessment
- Kangaroo mother care
- Family planning counseling
- PPIUCD insertion and removal

CLINICAL POSTINGS (6 weeks × 40 hours per week = 240 hours)

Clinical area	Duration (weeks)	Clinical learning outcomes	Procedural competencies/ clinical skills	Clinical requirements	Assessment methods
Antenatal OPD and antenatal ward	1 week	• Perform antenatal assessment • Perform laboratory tests for antenatal women and assist in selected antenatal diagnostic procedures • Counsel antenatal women	• History collection • Physical examination • Obstetric examination • Pregnancy confirmation test • Urine testing • Blood testing for hemoglobin, grouping and typing • Blood test for malaria • Kick chart • USG/NST • Antenatal counseling • Preparation for childbirth • Birth preparedness and complication readiness	• Antenatal palpation • Health talk • Case study	• OSCE • Case presentation

Clinical area	Duration (weeks)	Clinical learning outcomes	Procedural competencies/ clinical skills	Clinical requirements	Assessment methods
Labor room	3 weeks	• Monitor labor using partograph • Provide care to women during labor • Conduct normal childbirth, provide care to mother and immediate care of newborn	• Assessment of woman in labor • Partograph • Per vaginal examination when indicated • Care during first stage of labor • Pain management techniques • Upright and alternative positions in labor • Preparation for labor—articles, physical, psychological • Conduction of normal childbirth • Essential newborn care • Newborn resuscitation • Active management of third stage of labor • Monitoring and care during fourth stage of labor	• Partograph recording • PV examination • Assisting/conduction of normal childbirth • Case study • Case presentation • Episiotomy and suturing if indicated • Newborn resuscitation	• Assignment case study • Case presentation • OSCE

Clinical area	Duration (weeks)	Clinical learning outcomes	Procedural competencies/ clinical skills	Clinical requirements	Assessment methods
Post-partum clinic and postnatal ward including FP unit	2 weeks	• Perform postnatal assessment • Provide care to normal postnatal mothers and newborn	• Postnatal assessment • Care of postnatal mothers—normal • Care of normal newborn • Lactation management	• Postnatal assessment • Newborn assessment • Case study	• Assignment • Case study • Case presentation
		• Provide postnatal counseling • Provide family welfare services	• Postnatal counseling • Health teaching on postnatal and newborn care • Family welfare counseling	• Case presentation • PPIUCD insertion and removal	

Note: Partial completion of SBA module during VI semester.

VII SEMESTER

Midwifery/Obstetrics and Gynecology (OBG) Nursing–II Practicum

Skill Lab and Clinical: Skill Lab – 1 Credit (40 hours); Clinical – 4 Credits (320 hours)

Practice Competencies: On completion of the course, the students will be able to:
- Identify, stabilize and refer antenatal women with complications
- Provide care to antenatal women with complications
- Provide post abortion care and counselling
- Assist in the conduction of abnormal vaginal deliveries and cesarean section
- Demonstrate skills in resuscitating the newborn
- Assist and manage complications during labor
- Identify postnatal and neonatal complications, stabilize and refer them
- Provide care for high risk antenatal, intranatal and postnatal women and their families using nursing process approach
- Provide care for high risk newborn
- Assist in advanced clinical procedures in midwifery and obstetric nursing
- Provide care for women during their non childbearing period
- Assess and care for women with gynecological disorders
- Demonstrate skills in performing and assisting in specific gynecological procedures
- Counsel and care for couples with infertility

Skill Lab: Procedures/skills for demonstration and return demonstration:
- Antenatal assessment and identification of complications
- Post abortion care and counseling
- Counseling antenatal women for complication readiness
- Mechanism of labor—abnormal
- Assisting in the conduction of abnormal vaginal deliveries and caesarean section
- Management of complications during pregnancy/labor/post-partum (case studies/simulated scenarios)
- Administration of Inj. magnesium sulphate
- Starting and maintaining an oxytocin drip for PPH
- Management of PPH: Bimanual compression of uterus
- Management of PPH: Balloon tamponade
- Instruments used in obstetrics and gynecology
- Visual inspection of cervix with acetic acid
- Cervical biopsy
- Breast examination
- Counseling of infertile couples.

Clinical Postings (8 weeks × 40 hours per week = 320 hours)

Clinical areas	Duration (weeks)	Learning outcomes	Procedural competencies/clinical skills	Clinical requirements	Assessment methods
Antenatal OPD/ infertility clinics/ reproductive medicine and antenatal ward	2 weeks	• Perform/assist in selected advanced antenatal diagnostic procedures • Provide antenatal care for women with complications of pregnancy • Counsel antenatal mothers • Provide post abortion care and postnatal counseling	• Kick chart, DFMC • Assist in NST/CTG/USG • Assisting in advanced diagnostic procedures • Care of antenatal women with complications in pregnancy • Antenatal counseling • Preparation for childbirth, birth preparedness and complication readiness • Post-abortion care	• Antenatal palpation • Health talk • Case study	• Simulation • Case presentation • OSCE

Clinical areas	Duration (weeks)	Learning outcomes	Procedural competencies/clinical skills	Clinical requirements	Assessment methods
			• Post-abortion counseling • Counseling infertile couples		
Labor room	2 weeks	• Conduction of normal childbirth • Conduct/assist in abnormal deliveries • Monitor labor using partograph • Identify and manage complications during labor	• Assessment of woman in labor • Partograph • Per vaginal examination if indicated • Obstetric examination • Care during first stage of labor • Pain management techniques • Upright and alternative positions in labor	• Partograph recording • Pain management during labor • Conduction of normal childbirth • Assisting in abnormal deliveries • Managing complication during labor • Case study	• Assignment • Case study • Case presentation • Simulation • OSCE

Provide counseling and support to infertile couples

Clinical areas	Duration (weeks)	Learning outcomes	Procedural competencies/ clinical skills	Clinical requirements	Assessment methods
			• Preparation for labor—articles, physical, psychological • Conduction of normal childbirth • Essential newborn care • Newborn resuscitation • Active management of third stage of labor • Monitoring and care during fourth stage of labor	• Case presentation	

Clinical areas	Duration (weeks)	Learning outcomes	Procedural competencies/clinical skills	Clinical requirements	Assessment methods
			• Identification, stabilization, referal and assisting in management of prolonged labor, cervical dystocia, CPD, contracted pelvis • Assist in the management of abnormal deliveries—posterior position, breech deliveries, twin deliveries, vacuum extraction, forceps delivery, shoulder dystocia		

Clinical areas	Duration (weeks)	Learning outcomes	Procedural competencies/ clinical skills	Clinical requirements	Assessment methods
			- Assist in cervical encerclage procedures, D&C, D&E - Identify, assist and manage trauma to the birth canal, retained placenta, postpartum hemorrhage, uterine atony - Management of obstetric shock		
Postnatal ward	1 week	- Perform postnatal assessment and identify postnatal complications - Provide postnatal care - Provide family welfare services	- Postnatal history collection and physical examination - Identify postnatal complications	- Health talk - Postnatal assessment	- Role play - Assignment

INC Syllabus

Clinical areas	Duration (weeks)	Learning outcomes	Procedural competencies/ clinical skills	Clinical requirements	Assessment methods
			• Care of postnatal mothers—abnormal deliveries, cesarean section • Care of normal newborn • Lactation management • Postnatal counselling • Health teaching on postnatal and newborn care • Family welfare counseling	• Newborn assessment • Case studies • Case presentation • PPIUCD insertion and removal	• Case study • Case presentation • Simulation • Vignettes • OSCE
• Neonatal intensive care unit	1 week	• Perform assessment of newborn and identify complications/ congenital anomalies	• Neonatal assessment—identification of complication, congenital anomalies • Observation of newborn • Neonatal resuscitation	• Case study • Case presentation • Assignments • Simulated practice	• Case presentation • Care study • Care plan • Simulation • Vignettes • OSCE

Clinical areas	Duration (weeks)	Learning outcomes	Procedural competencies/ clinical skills	Clinical requirements	Assessment methods
		• Perform neonatal resuscitation • Care of high risk newborn • Provide care for newborns in ventilator, incubator, etc. • Assist/perform special neonatal procedures	• Phototherapy and management of jaundice in newborn • Assist in exchange transfusion • Neonatal feeding—spoon and katori, paladai, NG tube • Care of baby in incubator, ventilator, warmer • Infection control in the nursery • Neonatal medications • Starting IV line for newborn, drug calculation		

Clinical areas	Duration (weeks)	Learning outcomes	Procedural competencies/clinical skills	Clinical requirements	Assessment methods
Obstetric/gyne operation theatre and gynecology ward	2 weeks	• Assist in gynecological and obstetric surgeries • Care for women with gynecological disorders	• Observe/assist in cesarean section • Management of retained placenta • Gynecological surgeries • Hysterectomy • Uterine rupture • Care of women with gynecological conditions • Health education	• Assisting in obstetric and gynecological surgery • Tray set-up for cesarean section • Care plan	• Assignment • Tray set-up for obstetric and gynecological surgeries • Case presentation • Simulation • Vignettes

1. ABDOMINAL EXAMINATION

An abdominal examination followed by a physical examination is done for every pregnant woman at each clinic visit. Abdominal examination includes inspection, measurements, palpation and auscultation.

INSPECTION

- Visual assessment of the abdomen helps to know the size, shape, and contour of the abdominal wall and to note skin changes of pregnancy and scars
- Measuring fundal height provides information regarding the progressive growth of the fetus in relation to presumed gestational age by dates
- Palpation using Leopold's maneuvers gives information about the lie, presentation, position and variety of the fetus
- Auscultation of the fetal heartbeats confirms the presence a live fetus and aids to add to the information gathered about the position, presentation and lie of the fetus.

PROCEDURE OF PERFORMING AN ABDOMINAL EXAMINATION AND PALPATION (Figs. 1.1A to D)

- Explain to woman what will be done and how she may co-operate
- Instruct the woman to empty her bladder
- Draw curtains around the bed.

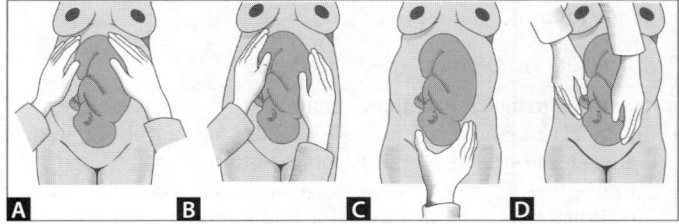

Figs. 1.1A to D: Abdominal palpation (Leopold's maneuvers). **A.** First maneuver (fundal palpation); **B.** Second maneuver (lateral palpation); **C.** Third maneuver (Pawlik's grip); **D.** Fourth maneuver (pelvic palpation).

Inspection and Measurements

- Position the woman for examination with a pillow under head and upper shoulders, arms by side, and abdomen exposed from below the breasts to the symphysis pubis
- Inspect the abdomen for scars, hernia, linea nigra, striae gravidarum, and state of umbilicus, skin condition and contour
- Determine the fundal height using the ulnar side of the palm
- Measure fundal height using measuring tape or pelvimeter
- Measure abdominal girth by encircling the woman's abdomen with a tape, measure at the level of the umbilicus.

Palpation

- Instruct the woman to relax her abdominal muscles by bending her knees slightly and doing relaxation breathing
- Be sure your hands are warm before beginning to palpate, rest your hands lightly on the mother's abdomen, while giving explanation about the procedure
- Keeping fingers of hands together, apply smooth deep pressure as firm as is necessary to obtain accurate findings (for palpation, use the flat palmar surface of fingers and not finger tips).

Perform Fundal Palpation (First Maneuver)

- Face the woman's head
- Place your hands on the sides of the fundus and curve the fingers around the top of the uterus
- Palpate for size, shape, consistency and mobility of the fetal part in the fundus.

Perform Lateral Palpation (Second Maneuver)

- Continue to face the woman's head
- Place your hands on the sides of the uterus about midway between the symphysis pubis and the fundus
- Apply pressure with one hand against the side of the uterus pushing the fetus to the other side and stabilizing it there
- Palpate the other side of the abdomen with the examining finger from the midline to the lateral side, and from the fundus

to the symphysis pubis using smooth pressure and rotatory movements
- Palpate both sides of the abdomen.

Pawlik's Grip (Third Maneuver)

- Continue to face the woman's head and make sure the woman has her knees slightly bent
- Grasp the portion of the lower abdomen immediately above the symphysis pubis between thumb and middle finger (If the head is above the brim it will be readily movable and ballotable. If not movable, it is indicative of an engaged head).

Pelvic Palpation (Fourth Maneuver)

- Turn and face the woman's feet, make sure her knees are slightly bent
- Place your hands on the sides of the uterus, with the palm of your hands just below the level of umbilicus and your fingers directed towards the symphysis pubis
- Press deeply with your fingertips into the lower abdomen and move them towards the pelvic inlet
- The hands converge around the presenting part when the head is not engaged
- The hands will diverge away from the presenting part and there will be no give or mobility if the presenting part is engaged
- In order to ascertain the attitude, the occipital and sincipital prominences are located:
  - If the head is well flexed, the sinciput will be felt on the opposite side from the back and higher than the occiput
  - If the head is deflexed the prominences are on the same level
  - If the head is extended as in a face presentation, the bulk of the head is felt on the same side as the back.
- This maneuver helps ascertain the presenting part (by palpating the cephalic prominences); the attitude of the head (from the position of the sinciput and occiput) and engagement by noting whether there is convergence or divergence of the finger tips.

Auscultation

- Place fetoscope or stethoscope over the convex portion of the fetal back closest to the anterior uterine wall (left scapular region) and listen to fetal heart sounds
- Inform the mother of your findings, make her comfortable

Location of the Maximum Intensity of Fetal Heart Tones

- **Cephalic presentation:** Midway between umbilicus and level of anterior superior iliac spine
- **Breech presentation:** At level with or above umbilicus
- **Transverse lie:** In lateral abdominal area
- **Anterior variety:** Close to the abdominal midline
- **Posterior variety:** In the flank area.

2. ABO INCOMPATIBILITY

The mother with blood group O has naturally occurring anti-A and anti-B antibodies. The antibodies are usually of immunoglobulin M (IgM) class and are too large to cross the placenta. However, some women produce antibodies of immunoglobulin G (IgG) class, which are smaller than IgM and can cross the placenta. Once in fetal circulation the IgG anti-A and anti-B antibodies attach to the red cells of fetuses with blood group A or B and cause variable amount of hemolysis due to antigen-antibody reaction. Although 20% of babies have ABO blood group incompatibility, only in 5%, hemolysis occurs and in affected babies jaundice appears within 24 hours. Both first and subsequent babies are at risk. The diagnosis is made only after birth and the baby is either blood group A or B, while the mother is group O.

The management of ABO isoimmunization depends on the severity of the hemolysis. In most cases, hemolysis is mild and no treatment is required. Adequate hydration is maintained and sepsis is avoided. Phototherapy may be required in few cases.

ABO incompatibility protects the fetus from rhesus incompatibility because the mother's anti-A and anti-B antibodies will destroy any fetal cells leaking into maternal circulation.

3. ABNORMAL UTERINE ACTION

Any deviation of the normal pattern of uterine contractions affecting the course of labor is designated as abnormal or disordered uterine action.

ASSOCIATED CLINICAL CONDITIONS

- First pregnancy in older women
- Prolonged pregnancy
- Over distension of the uterus due to twins and/or hydramnios
- Contracted pelvis
- Malpresentation and deflexed head
- Full bladder and loaded rectum
- Injudicious administration of sedatives, analgesics and oxytocics
- Premature attempt at vaginal delivery or attempted instrumental delivery.

TYPES OF ABNORMAL UTERINE ACTION

- Excessive contraction:
  - Precipitate labor if no obstruction
  - Tonic uterine contraction and retraction ring (Bandl's ring) in presence of obstruction.
- Uterine inertia:
  - Spastic lower segment
  - Constriction ring
  - Generalized tonic contraction
  - Cervical dystocia.

Precipitate Labor

The total duration of labor is less than two hours. Rapid expulsion of fetus occurs due to hyperactive uterine contractions associated with diminished soft tissue resistance.

Risks

Maternal
- Excessive laceration of cervix, vagina and perineum
- Postpartum hemorrhage

- Inversion of uterus
- Infection.

Fetal
- Intracranial hemorrhage
- Bleeding from torn cord
- Injury to skull and other hazards if delivery occurs in standing position.

Obstetrical Management

- Hospitalization prior to delivery of women with history of previous precipitate delivery
- Suppression of contraction during labor
- Elective induction of labor by low rupture of membranes
- Controlled delivery of head with liberal episiotomy.

Tonic Uterine Contraction and Retraction

Gradual increase in intensity, duration and frequency of uterine contraction occurs. The relaxation phase becomes less and less, leading to a state of tonic contraction. Retraction continues and lower segment elongates and becomes progressively thinner to accommodate the fetus. A circular groove encircling the uterus is formed between the active upper segment and the distended lower segment called the retraction ring or Bandl's ring.

Clinical Features

- Patient is restless from continuous pain and discomfort
- Features of exhaustion and ketoacidosis
- Hard, convex and tender, upper segment and distended, tender lower segment
- Pathological retraction ring felt obliquely between the umbilicus and symphysis pubis
- Fetal parts may not be well defined
- Fetal heart sound (FHS) usually is absent
- Dry, hot vagina with offensive discharge
- Cervix fully dilated and membranes absent.

Abnormal Uterine Action

Obstetrical Management

Supportive therapy
- Morphine intramuscularly
- Intravenous (IV) infusion with 5% Dextrose and Ringers lactate
- Prophylactic antibiotic.

Definitive therapy
- Forceps or Ventouse delivery if the pelvic outlet is adequate
- Cesarean section if there is evidence of cephalopelvic disproportion (CPD).

Spastic Lower Segment

A state in which there is lack of fundal dominance, inadequate relaxation between contractions and raised basal tone of contractions.

Clinical Features

- Severe pain referred to the back with evidence of dehydration and ketoacidosis
- Distended bladder and stomach
- Premature attempts to bear down
- Uterus tense and tender even after contraction passes of
- Evidence of fetal distress
- Thick edematous cervix, which is not well applied to presenting part
- Inappropriate dilatation of cervix, absence of membranes and meconium stained liquor.

Obstetrical Management

- Correction of dehydration and ketoacidosis with IV infusion
- Sedation, nutrition by IV and careful watch of fetal condition
- Cesarean section in the presence of complicating factors such as contracted pelvis, malpresentation or maternal or fetal distress.

Constriction Ring

One form of incoordinate uterine action where there is localized spastic contraction of a ring of circular muscle fibers of the uterus.

It is usually formed at the junction of the upper and lower segments around a constricted part of the fetus, usually around the neck in cephalic presentation. It is usually reversible and maternal condition is not much affected.

Associated factors for Occurrence

- Injudicious administration of oxytocics
- Premature rupture of membranes
- Premature attempt at instrumental delivery.

Diagnosis

Constriction ring may develop in all stages of labor. Failure of the presenting part to advance even with effective contractions with the cervix lying loose is suspicious.

It is diagnosed during cesarean section in the first stage, during forceps application in the second stage and during manual removal of placenta in the third stage.

Obstetrical Management

- **First stage:** The ring may have to be cut vertically during cesarean section to deliver the baby
- **Second stage:** Cesarean section, if the baby is in good condition Forceps delivery after administering medications to relax the ring, e.g. adrenaline hydrochloride and amyl nitrate inhalation alternatively
- **Third stage:** Manual removal of placenta under anesthesia.

Generalized Tonic Contraction (Uterine Tetany)

Pronounced retraction occurs involving whole of the uterus up to the internal os. There is no physiological differentiation of the active upper segment and the passive lower segment of the uterus. The uterine contraction ceases and the whole uterus undergoes tonic muscular spasm holding the fetus inside.

Causes

- Injudicious administration of oxytocin
- Repeated unsuccessful attempt at artificial delivery
- Powerful contractions of the uterus in an attempt to overcome the obstruction.

Clinical Features

- Prolonged labor with severe and continuous pain
- Dehydration and ketoacidosis
- Uterus tense, tender and smaller in size
- Fetal parts not well-defined and FHS not audible
- Jammed fetal head with big caput
- Dry, edematous vagina.

Obstetrical Management

- Deep sedation
- Correction of dehydration and ketoacidosis
- Administration of antibiotics
- In active management spontaneous delivery after the abnormal action passes off, if no obstruction. In the presence of obstruction, destructive operation followed by exploration of uterus.

Cervical Dystocia

The normal pattern of uterine contraction is maintained, but the external os fails to dilate. Cervical dystocia is common during the first stage of labor.

Management

- Ventouse extraction
- Cesarean section if vaginal delivery is unsafe.

NURSING PROCESS

Assessment

- Obstetric history, note history of precipitous labor
- Nature of uterine contractions; duration, intensity and interval

- Length of labor and status of membranes
- Fetal heart sounds
- Maternal health and psychological status
- Progress of labor as per vaginal examination.

Nursing Diagnosis

- Risk for maternal injury
- Risk for fetal injury
- Risk for deficient fluid volume
- Ineffective coping.

Expected Outcomes

The client will:
- Accomplish cervical dilation up to at least 1.2 cm/hour for primipara, 1.5 cm/hour for multipara in active phase, with fetal descent at least 1 cm/hour for primipara and 2 cm/hour for multipara
- Display fetal heart rate (FHR) within normal limits, with good variability and no decelerations noted
- Maintain fluid balance as evidenced by moist mucous membranes, appropriate urine output and palpable pulses
- Verbalize understanding of what is happening (identify and use) and effective coping techniques.

Nursing Interventions

1. **Accomplishing cervical dilation and fetal descend:**
   - Review history of labor, onset and duration
   - Note timing and type of medications. Avoid administration of narcotics or of epidural block anesthetics until cervix is 4 cm dilated
   - Assess uterine contractile pattern manually or electronically via external or internal monitor with internal uterine pressure catheter
   - Note condition of cervix. Monitor signs of amnionitis such as elevated temperature, white blood cell (WBC), odor and color of vaginal discharge

- Note effacement, fetal station and fetal presentation
- Place client in lateral recumbent position and encourage bed rest or sitting position/ambulation, as tolerated
- Encourage client to void every 1 to 2 hours. Assess for bladder fullness over symphysis pubis
- Assess degree of hydration (note amount and type of intake)
- Review bowel habits and regularity of evacuation
- Remain with client if possible and provide quiet environment as indicated
- Have emergency delivery kit available when precipitate labor is suspected
- Palpate abdomen of thin client for presence of pathological retraction ring between segments
- Investigate reports of severe abdominal pain. Note signs of fetal distress, cessation of contractions and presence of vaginal bleeding
- Prepare client for amniotomy and assist with the procedure, when cervix is 3–4 cm dilated
- Initiate infusion of oxytocin (pitocin) or prostaglandins as ordered
- Administer narcotic or sedative as ordered
- Prepare for forceps delivery as necessary
- Assist with preparation for cesarean delivery as indicated.

2. **Maintaining fetal heart rate within normal limits:**
   - Assess FHR manually or electronically
   - Note uterine pressures during resting and contractile phases via intrauterine pressure catheter
   - Identify maternal factors such as dehydration, acidosis, anxiety or vena caval syndrome
   - Note frequency of uterine contractions. Notify physician if frequency is 2 minutes or less
   - Assess for fetal malpositioning, using Leopold's maneuvers and findings on internal examination. Review results of ultrasonography
   - Monitor fetal descent in birth canal in relation to ischial spines
   - Prepare client for the most expedient method of delivery if fetus is in brow or face presentation

- Assess for deep transverse arrest of the fetal head
- Have client assume hands-and-knees position, or lateral Sim's position on side opposite that to which fetal occiput is directed, if fetus is in occiput posterior (OP) position
- Note color and amount of amniotic fluid when membranes rupture
- Observe for visible cord prolapse when membranes rupture, and occult cord prolapse as indicated by variable decelerations on monitor strip, especially if fetus is in breech presentation
- Note odor and change in color of amniotic fluid with prolonged rupture of membranes
- Administer antibiotic to client as indicated
- If fetus fails to rotate from OP to occiput anterior (OA) position, prepare for delivery in posterior position with vacuum extractor
- Prepare for cesarean delivery of breech presentation, if fetus fails to descend, labor progress ceases or CPD is identified.

3. **Maintaining fluid balance:**
   - Keep accurate record of intake and output, test urine for ketones and assess breath for fruity odor
   - Monitor vital signs. Note reports of dizziness with change of position
   - Assess lips and oral mucous membranes and degree of salivation
   - Note abnormal FHR response
   - Encourage oral fluids as appropriate
   - Review laboratory data, e.g. hemoglobin, hematocrit, serum electrolytes and serum glucose
   - Administer fluids intravenously.

4. **Improving coping behaviors:**
   - Determine progress of labor. Assess degree of pain in relation to dilation and effacement
   - Acknowledge reality of client's reports of pain/discomfort
   - Determine anxiety level of client and partner. Note manifestations of frustration
   - Provide comfort measures and reposition client, encourage ambulation as appropriate

- Demonstrate and encourage use of relaxation techniques, including patterned breathing
- Provide encouragement to client/couple for efforts taken
- Give factual information about what is happening.

4. ABNORMAL UTERINE BLEEDING

Bleeding from the uterus may be irregular acyclic, prolonged, scanty or excessive related to various causes **(Box 4.1)**.

MENORRHAGIA (HYPERMENORRHEA)

Excessively prolonged or profuse menses.

Causes

Local

- Pelvic pathology
- Fibroid uterus
- Adenomyosis
- Pelvic endometriosis
- Intrauterine contraceptive device (IUCD) in utero
- Chronic tubo-ovarian mass
- Tubercular endometritis
- Retroverted uterus
- Granulosa cell tumor of the ovary.

Systemic

- Severe hypertension
- Congestive cardiac failure.
- Hypothyroidism

Box 4.1: Common types of bleeding.

Menorrhagia (Hypermenorrhea)
Polymenorrhea (Epimenorrhea)
Metrorrhagia (Irregular bleeding between periods)
Oligomenorrhea (Scanty menstruation)
Hypomenorrhea (Shorter duration and amount of menstrual flow)
Dysfunctional uterine bleeding (DUB)

- Leukemia
- von Willebrand's disease
- Idiopathic thrombocytopenic purpura
- Emotional upset
- Dysfunctional uterine bleeding.

Diagnosis

- Long duration of flow
- Passage of clots
- Excessive bleeding
- Pallor.

Treatment

Definitive treatment is appropriate to the cause.

POLYMENORRHEA (EPIMENORRHEA)

Definition

Polymenorrhea is occurrence of menstrual cycles of greater than usual frequency (too frequent menstruation). It is cyclic bleeding where the cycle is reduced to an arbitrary limit of less than 21 days and remains constant. If the cycle is associated with excessive or prolonged bleeding it is called epimenorrhea.

Causes

- Hyperstimulation of the ovary by the pituitary hormones. Seen during adolescence, preceding menopause and following delivery and abortion
- Ovarian hyperemia as in pelvic inflammatory disease (PID) or ovarian endometriosis.

Treatment

Medical

- Hormones:
  - Progestin
  - Estrogen

- Progestogen
- Danazol
- Mifepristone (RU 486)
- Gonadotropin-releasing hormone (GnRH) agonists.
- Antifibrinolytic agents:
  - Tranexamic acid
  - Ethamsylate.

Surgical Management

- Uterine curettage
- Endometrial ablation/resection
- Hysterectomy.

METRORRHAGIA

Irregular acyclic bleeding from the uterus between periods.

Causes

- Dysfunctional bleeding during adolescence, following childbirth and abortion, and preceding menopause
- Submucous fibroid
- Uterine polyp
- Endometrial carcinoma
- Breakthrough bleeding in pill users
- IUCD in uterus.

Treatment

Treatment is directed to the underlying pathology.

OLIGOMENORRHEA

Menstrual bleeding occurring more than 35 days apart and which remains constant at that frequency with minimal quantity of blood loss.

Causes

- Age related: During adolescence and premenopausal period
- Weight related: Obesity

- Stress and exercise related
- Endocrine disorders: Polycystic ovarian disorder, hyperprolactinemia, hyperthyroidism
- Androgen producing tumors: Ovarian, adrenal
- Tubercular endometritis.

Management

Directed to the specific cause.

HYPOMENORRHEA

Scanty menstruation that lasts for less than 2 days.

Causes

- Endometrial tuberculosis
- Uterine synechiae (adhesions)
- Hormonal: Use of oral contraceptives
- Thyroid dysfunction
- Premenopausal period
- Malnutrition.

Management

Cause related.

DYSFUNCTIONAL UTERINE BLEEDING

Dysfunctional uterine bleeding (DUB) is a state of abnormal uterine bleeding without any clinically detectable organic, systemic or iatrogenic cause. Bleeding occurs following anovulation due to dysfunction of hypothalamopituitary-ovarian axis.

Types of Dysfunctional Uterine Bleeding

- Ovular bleeding:
  - Polymenorrhea
  - Oligomenorrhea
  - Functional menorrhagia.

- Anovular bleeding:
  - Menorrhagia.

Ovular Bleeding

- Polymenorrhea usually occurs following childbirth and abortion during adolescence, premenopausal period and in PIDs
- Oligomenorrhea occurs in adolescence and preceding menopause and is rare
- Functional menorrhagia is quite uncommon and is due to irregular shedding of the endometrium or irregular ripening of the endometrium. The condition occurs in extremes of reproductive period.

Possible causes
- Incomplete withdrawal of luteinizing hormone (LH), incomplete atrophy of the corpus luteum and persistent secretion of progesterone
- Inhibition of follicle-stimulating hormone (FSH) that suppresses ripening of the follicle in the next cycle
- Variation of the endometrial receptors, which are sensitive to the influence of estrogen and progesterone.

These hormonal factors contribute to poor formation and inadequate function of the corpus luteum. Secretion of estrogen and progesterone is inadequate to support the endometrial growth.

Anovular Bleeding

Menorrhagia

In anovular type, bleeding is usually excessive. Endometrial growth is under the influence of estrogen throughout the cycle. The endometrium is fragile due to inadequate structural and stromal support, and the endometrium remains fragile with the withdrawal estrogen, due to negative feedback action of FSH, the endometrial shedding continues for longer period.

Metropathia hemorrhagica (cystic glandular hyperplasia)

This type of abnormal bleeding occurs in premenopausal women due to disturbance of the rhythmic secretion of gonadotropins. As there is no ovulation, the endometrium is under the influence of estrogen without the negative feedback inhibition of FSH. After a variable period, however, the estrogen level falls resulting in endometrial shedding with heavy bleeding. Bleeding also occurs when the endometrial growth have outgrown their blood supply. Due to increased endometrial thickness, tissue breakdown continues for a long time. Bleeding is heavy as there is no vasoconstrictor effect of Prostaglandin F2alpha ($PGF_{2\alpha}$). Bleeding is prolonged until the endometrium and blood vessels regenerate to control it.

Investigations

- Assessment of bleeding:
  - History of number of perineal pads used per day, passage of clots, duration of bleeding, use of contraceptives, emotional status.
- Blood tests:
  - Hemoglobin, platelet count, prothrombin time, bleeding time, partial thromboplastin time, serum thyroid-stimulating hormone (TSH), T3 and T4 in suspected cases.
- Dilation and curettage (D and C)
- Internal examination:
  - Vaginal examination including speculum examination.
- Ultrasound and color Doppler:
  - Transvaginal sonography (TVS)
  - Saline Infusion sonography (SIS).
- Hysteroscopy:
  - For evaluation of endometrial lesion and to take biopsy from offending lesion.
- Laparoscopy:
  - To exclude unsuspected pathology such as endometriosis, PID or ovarian tumor.
- Hysterography:
  - To exclude fibroid polyp or congenital malformation of uterus.

Management

- Pubertal menorrhagia; age less than 20 years:
  - Rest
    Adequate explanation, reassurance and psychological support
  - Correction of anemia
  - Hematinics and blood transfusion if needed
  - Progestogen therapy: e.g. equine conjugated estrogen 20–40 mg, IV for 6–8 hours followed by combined oral pills.

- Reproductive period (20–40 years):
  - Rest during bleeding phase
  - Correction of anemia with diet, hematinics and if needed blood transfusion
  - Investigations and treatment for any systemic or endocrinal abnormalities
  - Hormone therapy; combined oral pills for three consecutive cycles in ovular type of bleeding. Cyclic progestogen in anovular type of bleeding
  - Intrauterine progestin: Levonorgestrel intrauterine system (LNG IUS)
  - Depot progestin preparations: Depot medroxyprogesterone acetate (DMPA)
  - Danazol: Gestrinone, Mifepristone (RU 486)
  - Nonhormonal management: Antifibrinolytic agents
  - Surgical management; uterine curettage, endometrial ablation/resection, hysterectomy.
- Postmenopausal bleeding:
  - Treatment of cause if found
  - Hysterectomy with bilateral Salpingo oophorectomy for recurrent or continued bleeding.

5. ABORTION

Expulsion of an embryo or fetus from the uterus prior to the stage of viability, which is 20 weeks gestation, or fetal weight less than 500 grams. Different types of abortion are listed in **Box 5.1**.

Box 5.1: Classification/Clinical types of abortion.

Spontaneous/isolated:
- Threatened
- Inevitable
- Complete
- Incomplete
- Missed

Induced:
- Legal [medical termination of pregnancy (MTP)]
- Illegal (criminal)
- Septic (infection present)

Recurrent abortion

SPONTANEOUS/ISOLATED ABORTION

Threatened Abortion

A clinical entity where the choriodecidual hemorrhage (the process of abortion) has begun, but not progressed to the stage of irreversibility. The cervix is not open and the products of conception are not expelled **(Fig. 5.1)**.

Investigations

- Hemoglobin estimation
- Urine pregnancy test
- Serum human chorionic gonadotropin (hCG).

Clinical Features

- History of amenorrhea for more than 6 weeks
- Bleeding which is fresh and scanty
- Mild uterine cramps and back ache (sometimes painless bleeding)
- Signs of early pregnancy

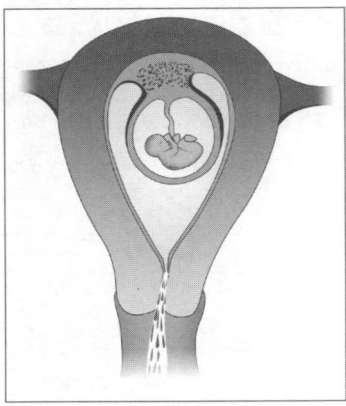

Fig. 5.1: Threatened abortion

- Cervix soft with os closed
- Uterus soft.

Obstetrical Management

- Hospitalization and complete bed rest until bleeding stops
- Hormonal supportive therapy up to 14–16 weeks
- Hematinics, laxatives and sedatives if required.

Inevitable Abortion

In this type of abortion, the process of abortion has begun and progressed to such an extent that expulsion of the products of conception seems inevitable **(Fig. 5.2)**.

Clinical Features

- History of amenorrhea
- Vaginal bleeding with passage of fresh blood and clots
- Pain due to uterine contractions and cervical dilation
- Pallor
- Cold, clammy extremities
- Tachycardia

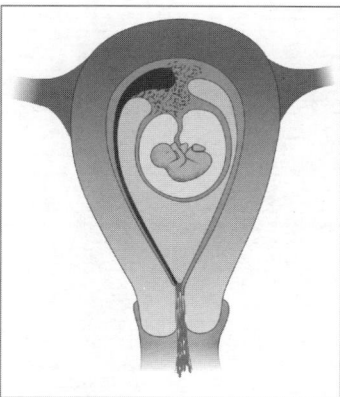

Fig. 5.2: Inevitable abortion.

- Hypotension
- Cervix soft to firm and bulky, corresponding to the period of gestation.

Investigations

- Blood group and cross matching
- Hemoglobin
- White blood cell (WBC); total and differential
- Ultrasonography.

Management

- Resuscitation with intravenous (IV) fluids and blood if patient is in shock
- Dilatation and suction curettage to evacuate uterus
- Antibiotics
- Tetanus toxoid and anti-D for Rh-negative mother.

Complete Abortion

In complete abortion the products of conception are expelled completely (en mass) from the uterus and the uterine cavity is empty **(Fig. 5.3)**.

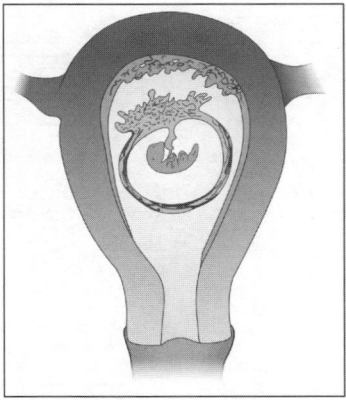

Fig. 5.3: Complete abortion.

Clinical Features

- History of:
  - Variable period of amenorrhea
  - Lower abdominal pain and vaginal bleeding with passage of a fleshy mass
  - Decrease in bleeding and pain following expulsion of products of conception
  - Vaginal bleeding minimal
- On examination:
  - Uterus is smaller than the period of gestation on internal examination
  - Cervical os is closed
  - Expelled mass may be seen intact.

Investigation

Ultrasonography: Uterine cavity found empty.

Management

- Sedatives
- Hematinics if blood loss was significant
- Tetanus toxoid
- Anti-D for Rh-negative mothers
- Rarely curettage may be necessary if bleeding continues or ultrasonography reveals products in the uterine cavity.

Incomplete Abortion

The entire products of conception are not expelled and a part of it is left inside the uterine cavity **(Fig. 5.4)**.

Clinical Features

- History of:
  - Variable period of amenorrhea
  - Vaginal bleeding; continuous or recurrent
  - Passage of fleshy mass per vagina
  - Lower abdominal pain of colicky nature.

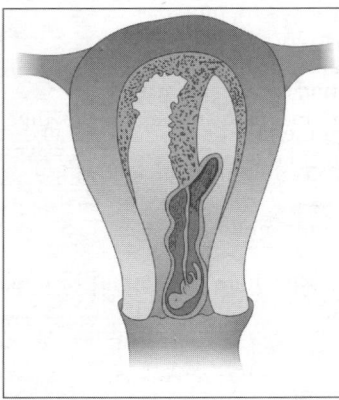

Fig. 5.4: Incomplete abortion.

- On vaginal examination:
  - Uterus smaller than the period of amenorrhea
  - Internal os open and uterus soft
  - Expelled mass may be found incomplete.

Investigations

- Blood group and cross matching
- Hemoglobin
- WBC
- Ultrasonography.

Management

Resuscitation if patient is in shock with IV fluids and blood.
- In recent cases:
  - Dilatation and curettage to empty the uterus using blunt curette under general anesthesia.
- In old cases:
  - Suction curettage under antibiotic cover
  - Tetanus toxoid

Missed Abortion

In missed abortion the fetus is dead and retained inside the uterus for a variable period of time.

Clinical Features

- History of:
  - Variable period of amenorrhea followed by vaginal bleeding or brownish discharge and spotting
  - Subsidence of pregnancy symptoms.
- On examination:
  - Uterine size smaller than the period of amenorrhea
  - Cervix soft with internal os closed
  - Retrogression of breast changes.

Investigations

- Pregnancy test becomes negative
- Ultrasonography
- Doppler examination reveals absence of fetal hydantoin syndrome (FHS)
- Immunological test for pregnancy: Negative
- Serum fibrin degradation products (FDP), bleeding and clotting times, and platelet count if disseminated intravascular coagulation (DIC) is suspected.

Management

- Uterus less than 12 weeks:
  - Dilatation and suction evacuation.
- Uterus more than 12 weeks:
  - Ripening of the cervix with prostaglandin gel and then 2 hourly injections of prostidin.
- Postabortion:
  - Examine expelled products to ensure completeness

- Anti-D to Rh-negative mother
- Hematinics to correct anemia.

- Tetanus toxoid and anti-D where indicated
- Antibiotics and hematinics as prescribed.

INDUCED ABORTION

Legal Abortion/Medical Termination of Pregnancy

Medical termination of pregnancy (MTP) is deliberate termination of pregnancy prior to viability of the fetus. In India abortion laws were liberalized in 1971. The act came into force in 1972.

First Trimester MTP

- Medical methods using:
    - Mifepristone (RU 486) with misoprostol
    - Methotrexate with misoprostol
    - Tamoxifen with misoprostol.
- Surgical methods:
    - Menstrual regulation; aspiration of endometrial cavity using a 5–7 mm polythene cannula attached to a 50 mL syringe
    - Manual vacuum aspiration
    - Suction evacuation.

Second Trimester MTP (13–20 Weeks)

- Medical methods:
    - Extraovular instillation of drugs/abortifacients e.g. Ethacridine 0.1% $PGF_{2\alpha}$, Hypertonic saline (20%).
- Surgical methods:
    - Dilatation and evacuation (D and E)
    - Hysterotomy.

Termination 16–20 Weeks

- Intra-amniotic instillation of abortifacient drugs
- Extra-amniotic instillation of ethacridine lactate
- Prostaglandins.

Septic Abortion

A type of abortion associated with sepsis of the products of conception. There is increased association of sepsis in illegal induced abortion because of:
- Improper antiseptic and aseptic measures
- Incomplete abortion
- Inadvertent injury to the genital organs and adjacent organs.

Clinical Features

- History of recent termination of pregnancy (by an unauthorized person)
- Variable period of amenorrhea along with high fever, chills and rigors
- Vomiting, diarrhea and diffuse abdominal pain
- Foul smelling vaginal discharge, which is often purulent, accompanied by vaginal bleeding and history of passage of products of conception per vagina
- Pain in abdomen of varying degrees
- A rising pulse rate of 100–120/min or more and decreased blood pressure
- Tender uterus with a boggy feel
- Pallor and sweating
- Delirium and features of toxemia
- Abdominal distension, ileus
- Cervix soft, os may be open
- Fornices may feel tender and boggy if a pelvic abscess has formed
- There may be evidence of trauma to the genital tract/uterus.

Investigations

- Complete blood count and urinalysis
- Blood urea, creatinine and serum electrolytes
- High vaginal swab
- Blood culture when septicemia is suspected
- Blood gas analysis in severe cases

- Serum fibrin degradation products to facilitate the early detection and treatment of DIC
- Pelvic ultrasonography
- Radiography of chest.

Management

- Shock is to be treated aggressively
- An indwelling catheter to be introduced and urine output closely monitored as guide to IV therapy
- In mild cases: Antibiotics and evacuation of uterus under anesthesia
- In severe cases:
  - Oxygen 6–8 L/min
  - IV crystalloids and plasma expanders
  - Blood transfusion
  - Central venous pressure (CVP) monitoring
  - Prophylactic anti-tetanus and anti-gasgangrene serum intramuscular (IM)
  - Analgesics and sedatives as required.

Illegal Abortion/Criminal Abortion (Unsafe Abortion)

This is defined as the procedure of termination of unwanted pregnancy either by persons lacking the necessary skills or in an environment lacking the minimal standards or both [World Health Organization (WHO), 1992].

RECURRENT ABORTION/HABITUAL ABORTION

Spontaneous and recurrent abortion occurring consecutively on three or more occasions is called recurrent or habitual abortion. It may be primary or secondary, if it occurs after the birth of a viable baby.

Etiology

- Systemic maternal disorders such as syphilis, diabetes mellitus, chronic nephritis, essential hypertension and rhesus (Rh) incompatibility

- Hormonal problems, e.g. progesterone deficiency, polycystic ovarian disease (PCOD) and thyroid dysfunction
- Cervical incompetence
- Developmental abnormalities of uterus such as bicornuate uterus and septate uterus
- Chromosomal defects in the fetus
- Idiopathic causes.

Investigations

- Blood group and Rh typing
- Hemoglobin and complete blood count (CBC)
- Karyotyping
- Urine routine and culture
- Glucose tolerance test
- Liver, renal and thyroid function tests
- TORCH titer estimation
- Hysterosalpingogram
- Cervical swab culture
- Hormone assays as indicated.

Management

Interconceptional Period

- Counseling of the couple to alleviate anxiety
- Surgical correction of uterine abnormality
- Genetic counseling as indicated
- Hormonal therapy for those with hormone deficiency
- Treatment for genital tract infections.

During Pregnancy

- Reassurance
- Rest for a period of at least 2 weeks beyond the expected time of abortion (as known from history)
- Avoidance of strenuous activities, intercourse and traveling
- Hormonal therapy to sustain pregnancy, e.g. progesterone, human chorionic gonadotropin (HCG)
- Cerclage operation for incompetent os.

NURSING PROCESS

Assessment

- History of associated medical conditions such as essential hypertension, vascular disease, ABO incompatibility
- Pregnancy if wanted or not
- Nutritional status
- Pelvic cramping or backache
- Exposure to toxic or teratogenic agents
- History of pelvic inflammatory disease, sexually transmitted disease or TORCH infections
- Vaginal bleeding
- Dilation of cervix
- Uterine abnormalities
- Estimated date of delivery
- Genetic conditions in the family.

Nursing Diagnoses

- High-risk for maternal injury
- High-risk for spiritual distress
- Knowledge deficit regarding cause of abortion, selfcare, contraception/future pregnancy
- High-risk for altered sexuality
- Knowledge deficit regarding reproduction, self-care and Rh factor
- Anxiety
- Pain/Discomfort.

Expected Outcomes

The client will:
- Report any bleeding and be free of negative effects of termination
- Express feelings of self-worth and her values and beliefs
- Explain proper use of desired contraceptive methods
- Resume sexual activity and use contraception if desired/needed
- Verbalise accurate information about the reproductive system
- Report anxiety reduced to manageable level
- Report pain/discomfort minimized and/or controlled.

Nursing Interventions

1. **Managing bleeding:**
   - Assess vital signs and urine output
   - Note skin color and temperature
   - Estimate blood loss using pad count/weight
   - Assess for and review signs and symptoms of DIC
   - Provide IV/oral fluids as appropriate
   - Administer volume expander/blood products as indicated
   - Assist with necessary therapeutic procedures, e.g. dilatation and curettage (D and C), labor induction with oxytocin or prostaglandin
   - Provide reassurance to client/couple.

2. **Enhancing feelings of self worth and spirituality:**
   - Determine client's/couple's religious preferences
   - Ascertain specific needs of client, i.e. baptising products of conception, performing pooja and/or formal burial
   - Provide information in non-judgmental manner
   - Encourage being aware of own beliefs about events that are occurring
   - Provide opportunity for expression of anger or concern
   - Note expressions of hopelessness and/or helplessness
   - Encourage participation in treatment plan and care
   - Encourage and assist in obtaining counseling and support from clergy/poojari as desired
   - Explain grief response that may occur
   - Stress the importance of follow-up visits.

3. **Enhancing knowledge about abortion and contraception:**
   - Provide/review information about the cause of abortion when known, e.g. genetic anomalies, infection, Rh incompatibility
   - Discuss alternative methods of contraception where indicated
   - Identify signs and symptoms to be reported to physician/health care workers
   - Review need for Rh immunoglobulin G (IgG) depending on client's Rh status
   - Encourage interaction with couples who have experienced similar occurrence, when possible
   - Refer for genetic counseling as appropriate.

4. **Planning to resume sexual activity and use contraception if needed:**
   - Encourage open discussion about sexual activities and future pregnancies
   - Discuss resuming sexual activity, including alternative means of gratification, as indicated
   - Determine past methods of contraception, if any
   - Provide specific information about contraceptive methods chosen
   - Let client/couple know it is all right to feel what they are feeling and be where they are
   - Discuss concerns/expectations about future plan, including pregnancies and feelings about self in this situation.

5. **Enhancing knowledge about reproduction and post abortion care:**
   - Assess level of client's knowledge and provide information about reproduction
   - Reinforce postabortion instructions concerning the use of sanitary pads and resumption of sexual activity
   - Provide information about the implications of Rh (D)-negative blood and the need for Rh IgG administration
   - Identify signs and symptoms to be reported to the physician
   - Verify Rh-negative status and administer Rh IgG if indicated.

6. **Dealing with anxiety:**
   - Acknowledge the client's anxiety and encourage ventilation of feelings
   - Be empathetic and nonjudgmental
   - Provide instructions in breathing and relaxation techniques
   - Explain procedures before they are performed and stay with the client to provide concurrent feedback
   - Have a support person remain with the client, particularly, if she is undergoing a second-trimester procedure requiring induction of labor.

7. **Controlling pain/discomfort:**
   - Explain to client the nature of discomfort experienced/expected
   - Determine the extent and location of discomfort
   - Provide instructions in relaxation and breathing techniques

- Administer narcotic/non-narcotic analgesics, sedatives and antiemetics as indicated
- Provide information about the use of prescription or nonprescription analgesics.

6. ADENOMYOSIS

A condition where there is ingrowth of the glandular and stromal components of the endometrium directly into the myometrium.

PROBABLE CAUSES

- Repeated childbirths
- Vigorous curettage
- Excess of estrogen, which causes hyperplasia of endometrium
- Pelvic endometriosis.

CLINICAL FEATURES

- Patient is usually parous with age about 40 years
- Hypogastric mass occupying the midline
- Menorrhagia (excessive bleeding) in about 70%
- Dysmenorrhea/increased colicky pain during menstruation
- Dyspareunia (painful coitus)
- Frequency of urination
- Uniform enlargement of the uterus on pelvic examination
- Ultrasound findings: Heterogeneous echogenecity, multiple cysts in the myometrium and increased vascularity within the myometrium
- Magnetic resonance imaging (MRI): Thickened junctional zone.

Characteristics

- Diffuse, symmetrical enlargement of the uterus
- Posterior uterine wall more thickened than anterior wall
- Size of uterus about 12–14 weeks pregnant uterus or large size orange
- Absence of capsule surrounding the growth.

TREATMENT

- Conservative surgery: Partial resection of the adenomyomata
- Hysterectomy with or without salpingo-oophorectomy for parous women
- Hormone therapy for dysmenorrhea and menorrhagia:
  - Intrauterine levonorgestrel system (LNG IUS)
  - Cyclic estrogen and progesterone treatment.

7. ADOPTION

DEFINITION

Adoption is the legal process through which the adopted child becomes the lawful child of the adoptive parents with all the rights, privileges and responsibilities that are attached to a biological child.

CHILD ADOPTION IN INDIA

Children are believed to be a cluster of hoy and the future of the country depends on them. Generally, children born in India are compared, taken care of and given all necessities for their all-round development, whereas on the other hand there are over 60,000 children being abandoned per year in India. It is very state that in some cases, these children become victims of human trafficking and sexual violence. In many fortunate cases, children are taken to an adoption agency where they may hope for a better life while waiting to get adopted. According to the central adoption agency Central Adoption Resource Authority (CARA), from April 2020 to March 2021, there were 3142 in-country adoptions and 412 inter-country adoptions. In the previous year, 2019-2020, 3351 in-country and 394 inter-country adoptions in India. This indicates that more adoptions are within the country and mostly between related individuals such as step parent adoption where the new partner of a parent may legally adopt a child from the parents' previous relationship. Inter-family adoptions also occur through surrender, as a result of parental death or when the child cannot otherwise be cared for and a family member agrees to take over.

Reasons for Adoption

- Infertility is the main reason, parents seek to adopt children they are not related to.
- Divorce or death of one parent:
  Compassion motivated by religious or philosophical conviction to avoid contributing to perceived overpopulation and the belief that they are more responsible to care for otherwise parentless children than to reproduce.
- To insure that inheritable diseases such as sickle-cell anemia are not passed on and health concerns relating to pregnancy and child birth.
- Genuine love for the child or baby.
- Couple with 3 or more children of same sex.
- Persons having carrier status of certain diseases.
- Single parents who want to experience parenthood.

ADOPTION LAWS IN INDIA

Adoption in India was regulated by Governmental Acts from early time. These were: (1) The Guardian and Wards Act of 1890 (GWA), (2) Hindu Adoption and Maintenance Act of 1956 (HAMA) and (3) the Juvenile Justice Act of 2000, amended in 2006 (JJA).

1. The Guardian and Wards Act of 1890 (GWA).
   This was the first secular law that allowed for a child to be adopted in India. The salient features of this Act were:
   - The parent adopting is a 'guardian' and the child adoptee is 'a ward', meaning the same rights of a biological child aren't inherent;
   - Anyone under the age of 18 years can be a ward;
   - The guardianship can be revoked by courts or by guardian;
   - A will is required for any property/goods to be bequeathed to the child;
   - This will be legally contested by 'blood' relatives;
   - Both spouses can legally be guardians where the man adopts with the consent of his wife.
   - Single persons can adopt without any age difference restrictions.

2. **Hindu Adoption and Maintenance Act, 1956 (HAMA)**
   The Act covers Hindus, Buddhists, Jains and Sikhs. Some relevant parts of the Act are:
   - Married couples or single adults can adopt;
   - Legally the man adopts with the consent of his wife;
   - A single man or woman can adopt;
   - If a biological child already exists in the family, a child of the opposite sex has to be adopted;
   - Children adopted under this act get the same legal rights as a biological child might;
   - Children under the age of 15 years can be adopted;
   - A single man adopting a girl should be at least 21 years older than child;
   - A single woman adopting a boy should be at least 21 years older than the child; and
   - Adoption under this Act is irrevocable.
3. **The Juvenile Justice (Care and Protection) Act of 2000 amended in 2006 (JJ Act)**
   The JJ Act is meant mainly for the care and rehabilitation of children in conflict with the law. There was the need for a law that would allow children the same rights, whether they were biological or adopted. There was also the need for a law that delinked adoption from the religion of the adoptive parent(s). The JJ Act filled this space and a tiny section was added on for adoption. The Amendment Act of 2006 has since expanded the provisions. The main strengths of this Act are:
   - Any Indian citizen can adopt a child who is legally free for adoption;
   - The adoptee gets the same rights that a biological child might;
   - The religion of the adoptive parent(s) is not relevant;
   - Single persons can adopt;
   - The adoption is irrevocable;
   - Some time limits have been set to ensure that children are considered legally free for adoption earlier; and
   - The trust is on the best interest of the child.

Section 3 (a. a) of the Act defines adoption as "the process through which the adopted child is permanently separated from his biological parents and becomes the legitimate child of adoptive parents with all rights, privileges and responsibilities that are attached to the relationship". While the Act covers all of India, it is only possible to adopt under this Act in areas where JJ Boards (provided under the Act) have been constituted. This is an ongoing process with majority of states issuing notifications constituting these boards. Indian Citizens, non-resident Indians and non-Indians residing outside India can adopt a child from India. While these adoptions are also legalized under the Acts mentioned above, the rules related to these adoptions can be different. These are dependent on the regulations of the countries in which the adoptive families reside and the relevant immigration laws.

Adoption means a legal process that allows someone to become the parent of a child, even though the parent and child are not related by blood. But in every other way, adoptive parents are the child's parents.

In India the Central Adoption Resource Authority (CARA) is a statutory body of the Ministry for Women and Child Development, Government of India. It functions as the nodal body for adoption of Indian Children and is mandated to monitor and regulate in-country and inter-country adoptions. CARA is designated as the Central Authority to deal with inter-country adoptions in accordance with the provisions of the Hague Convention on inter-country Adoption, 1993 ratified by Government of India in 2003. CARA primarily deals with adoption of orphan, abandoned and surrendered children through its associated/recognized adoption agencies.

Eligibility Criteria for Prospective Adoptive Parents

1. The prospective adoptive parents shall be physically, mentally and emotionally stable, financially capable and shall not have any life threatening medical condition.
2. Any prospective adoptive parents, irrespective of his/her marital status and whether or not he/she has biological son or daughter, can adopt a child subject to following conditions:
a. The consent of both the spouses for the adoption shall be required in case of married couple.
b. A single female can adopt a child of any gender.
c. A single male shall not be eligible to adopt a girl child.

3. No child shall be given in adoption to a couple unless they have at least two years of stable marital relationship and both should agree for the adoption
4. The age of prospective adoptive parents, as on the date of registration shall be counted for deciding the eligibility, and the eligibility of prospective adoptive parents to apply for children of different age groups shall be as under:

Age of child	Maximum composite age of prospective adoptive parents (couple)	Maximum age of single prospective adoptive parent
Up to 4 years	90 years	45 years
Above 4 and up to 8 years	100 years	50 years
Above 8 and up to 18 years	110 years	55 years

5. In case of couple, the composite age of prospective adoptive parents shall be counted.
6. The minimum age difference between the child and either of the prospective adoptive parent shall not be less than 25 years.
7. The age criteria for prospective adoptive parents shall not be applicable in case of relative adoption by step parent.
8. Couples with three or more children shall not be considered for adoption except in case of special need children, hard to place children and in case of relative adoption and adoption by step parent.

Eligibility of a Child to be Adopted

- Any orphan, surrendered or abandoned child is legally declared free for adoption by child welfare as per the guidelines of the Central Government of India.
- A child without a legal parent or guardian or the parents are not capable of taking care of the child.
- A child deserted or unaccompanied by parents or guardian and the child welfare committee (CWC) has declared the child as abandoned.

- A child renounced on account of physical and emotional factors that are beyond the control of parents or guardian, he/she is considered a surrendered child as declared by the CWC.
- A child considered legally free for adoption if, even after trying their level best, the police fails to find the real parent or guardian of the child.

Steps to Adopt a Child in India

1. **Register on the CARA website**
   The Central Adoption Resource Authority has a centralized system for adoption across India. Irrespective of the village, town, city or state a person lives in, if he/she wishes to adopt a child, she needs to register on the online portal named "Carings" on the CARA website. Once the login is done, the person/persons waiting to adopt a child will fill out a few questions related to their adoption preferences and upload certain documents to prove their identity. This is just a short online form and document upload. They will then get their registration number and their spot in the queue. Then they become officially the prospective adoptive parents (PAP).

2. **Complete the home study**
   After registration on the "Carings" portal, a social worker from the adoption agency nearest to their address will conduct a home study. The purpose of the home study is to verify the information submitted during registration, to guide them about any gaps, to answer any questions they may have, and to ensure that the environment of the family is conducive for the child. The social worker will also give them a form to fill out, where they will explain their desire to adopt a child and show their readiness to do so. A sum of INR 6000 is payable by cheque to the adoption agency towards the home study expenses. The adoption agency will approve and upload their home study report into the "Carings" system. The prospective parents are then eligible to receive referral for a child.

3. **Bring the child home under a foster care agreement**
   When the "Carings" system matches the prospective parents with a child, they will be notified along with all the relevant

information about the child. They will have about 48 hours to say yes or no to the child. If the answer is yes, they can visit the child care institution within two weeks to bring the child home. The adoption agency will prepare the foster care documents and schedule a court date so you can get approval to take the child with you. At this stage, they will have to pay a one-time fee of INR 40,000. This fee is for all the administrative and legal costs of completing the adoption process.

4. **Show up for the court date**
   After sending the child home with his/her adoptive parents, the adoption agency will work on getting a court date to get the adoption formally approved by a judge. When the date is set, the adoptive parents will appear at the court along with their child in the district where the agency is located. When the judge approves the adoption, the child becomes theirs.

5. **Completing the Adoption Procedure**
   The adoption agency will receive the courts formal order, based on which they will procure the birth certificate and mail to parents. The child becomes officially the child of adoptive parents.

8. AIDS IN PREGNANCY

Acquired immune deficiency syndrome (AIDS) is the most severe form of a continuum of illnesses associated with human immunodeficiency virus known as retroviruses. These viruses carry their genetic material in the form of ribonucleic acid (RNA) rather than deoxyribonucleic acid (DNA). Infection with HIV occurs when it enters the host CD4 (T) cell and causes this cell to replicate viral RNA and viral proteins, which in turn invade other CD4 cells.

The stage of HIV decease is based on clinical history, physical examination, laboratory evidence of immune dysfunction, signs and symptoms, infections and malignancies. The stage of primary infection is acute and spans the time from infection to antibody development. Four categories of infected states have been denoted:
- Primary infection (CDC Category A)
- Asymptomatic HIV (CDC Category B)
- Symptomatic HIV (CDC Category C)
- AIDS (CDC Category D).

RISK FACTORS

Human immunodeficiency virus (HIV) is transmitted through bodily fluids by high-risk behaviors such as heterosexual intercourse with HIV infected partner, injection, drug use and male homosexual behaviors. Also at risk are people who received transfusions of blood or blood products contaminated by HIV, children born to mothers with HIV infection, breastfed infants of HIV infected mothers and health care workers exposed to needle-stick injuries associated with an infected patient.

CLINICAL FEATURES

Symptoms are widespread and may affect any organ system. Manifestations range from mild abnormalities in immune response without overt signs and symptoms to profound immune suppression, life-threatening infection, malignancy and the direct effect of HIV on body tissues.

Respiratory

- Shortness of breath, dyspnea, cough, chest pain, and fever are associated with opportunistic infections including pneumocystis carinii pneumonia (PCP), tuberculosis, legionella and cytomegalovirus (CMV) infections
- HIV-associated tuberculosis occurs early in the course of HIV infection, often preceding a diagnosis of AIDS.

Gastrointestinal

- Loss of appetite, nausea, vomiting
- Oral and esophageal candidiasis
- Chronic diarrhea with devastating effects, e.g. weight loss, fluid and electrolyte imbalances, perianal skin excoriation and weakness.

Wasting Syndrome (Cachexia)

- Multifactorial protein-energy malnutrition
- Profound weight loss
- Intermittent or constant fever with no concurrent illness.

Neurologic

- HIV encephalopathy
- HIV-related neuropathy
- Central and peripheral neuropathies.

Integumentary

- Kaposi's sarcoma, herpes simplex and herpes zoster and various forms of dermatitis
- Folliculitis, eczema or psoriasis.

Reproductive

- Persistent/recurrent vaginal candidiasis
- Ulcerative sexually transmitted diseases
- Venereal warts and cervical cancer
- Pelvic inflammatory disease.

Hematologic and Lymphatic

- Non-Hodgkin's lymphoma—Mostly in the brain, bone marrow and gastrointestinal (GI) tract.

DIAGNOSIS

- Initial screening test for specific antibodies using enzyme-linked immunosorbent assay (ELISA). Positive tests are confirmed by western blot. The median time between HIV infection and AIDS is about 10 years
- Evaluation of CD4 cell counts:
    - At CD4 counts of more than 500/mL, there is no evidence of immunosuppression
    - At CD4 counts 200–500/mL, there is greater likelihood of developing symptoms
    - At CD4 counts less than 200/mL, patients suffering from persistent thrush and temperature more than 38°C for 2 or more weeks are at risk of developing complications of the disease.

MANAGEMENT

- Prenatal HIV counseling to all pregnant women
- HIV screening for women with tuberculosis, pneumonia, thrush and other opportunistic infections
- Prenatal care to include:
  - Monitoring of immune status
  - Prophylaxis of opportunistic infections
  - Assessment for presence of other sexually transmitted diseases (STDs).
- Strategies to prevent vertical transmission:
  - Decrease fetal exposure by preventing chorioamnionitis, shortening the duration of labor and preventing vaginitis
  - Elective cesarean section at term/onset of labor, to prevent exposure of fetus to infectious secretions in the birth canal
  - Prophylactic regime of zidovudine to all HIV-infected pregnant women after appropriate counseling.
- Assessment of progression of the disease by regular CD4 lymphocyte count.

Universal Precautions and Other Measures to Protect Health Team Workers

General Precautions

- Frequent hand washing freely with soap and water
- Limiting the attending staff to a minimum
- Avoiding any staff member with skin conditions or injuries from attending to infected patient
- Cuts and abrasions should be covered with waterproof dressings.

Universal Precautions

- All attending staff must wear disposable sterile gowns over plastic aprons, waterproof shoe covers, gloves and goggles to protect eyes.

Obstetric Precautions

- Limit vaginal examinations to a minimum
- Avoid using scalp electrodes or intrauterine monitoring catheters

Manual of Midwifery and Gynecological Nursing

- All linen should be disinfected in hypochlorite solution
- All cotton swabs, dressing pads, mops, etc. must be discarded in a container with hypochlorite solution
- All needles, syringes and sharp blades must be collected and disposed off with due precautions (in puncture proof containers)
- After delivery, the floor must be cleaned with antiseptic solution observing all precautions
- Fumigate the labor room/operation room
- Autoclave all instruments after proper washing and cleaning.

Intrapartum Therapy

- Administer zidovudine during labor as ordered (2.0 mg/kg IV in first hour, thereafter 1.0 mg/kg/hour throughout labor)
- Avoid artificial rupture of membranes, use of scalp electrodes or intrauterine pressure catheters
- After delivery, administer zidovudine oral syrup to new born in the dose of 2.0 mg/kg body weight for 6 weeks postpartum.

NURSING PROCESS

Assessment

- Risk factors including sexual practices, history of IV drug use
- Psychological status
- Nutritional status: Factors that may interfere with oral intake such as vomiting, pain and difficulty swallowing as well as monitor weight, serum protein and albumin
- Skin and mucous membranes:
  - Redness, ulcerations and creamy-white patches in oral cavity
  - Excoriation and infection in perianal area
  - Breakdown, ulceration and infection of skin.
- Respiratory status:
  - Cough, sputum production, shortness of breath, orthopnea, tachypnea, and chest pain
  - Pulmonary function using chest X-ray and arterial blood gases.

- Neurologic status:
  - Sensory deficits such as visual changes
  - Numbness, tingling in the extremities, altered gait, paresis or seizure activity.
- Fluid and electrolyte status:
  - Skin turgor and dryness, urine output, specific gravity and blood pressure, serum electrolytes and mental status.
- Level of knowledge and reaction to diagnosis.

Nursing Diagnoses

- Risk for infection related to immunodeficiency
- Activity intolerance related to weakness and fatigue
- Impaired nutrition: Less than body requirements
- Deficient knowledge related to selfcare and preventing HIV transmission
- Social isolation related stigma of the disease
- Anticipatory grieving related to change in lifestyle and unfavorable prognosis.

Expected Outcomes

The client will:
- Develops no opportunistic infection
- Tolerates regular home care and self-care activities
- Maintains optimal nutritional status during prenatal period
- Evidences increased knowledge of disease prevention and care during pregnancy
- Demonstrates improved socialization
- Expresses grief reactions and appears relaxed.

Nursing Interventions

1. **Preventing infection:**
   - Instruct client and family to monitor for signs and symptoms of infection
   - Recommend strategies to prevent infection

- Monitor laboratory values that indicate the presence of infection such as white cell count and differential
- Strongly urge patient and spouse to avoid exposure to body fluids and to use condoms for sexual activities
- Maintain strict aseptic precautions for invasive procedures
- Instruct patient to take precautions to protect her from getting opportunistic infections from others.

2. **Improving activity tolerance:**
   - Monitor ability to perform daily activities (self-care and home care)
   - Assist in planning daily routines to maintain balance between activity and rest
   - Instruct client in energy conservation techniques, e.g. sitting while washing or preparing meals
   - Instruct to use measures such as relaxation and guided imagery to reduce fatigue
   - Discuss and plan to improve dietary plan to meet energy needs.

3. **Improving nutritional status:**
   - Assess weight, dietary intake, serum albumin, serum protein and blood urea nitrogen
   - Instruct patient about ways to supplement nutritional value of meals
   - Determine nutritional needs during pregnancy and explain the need for consuming adequate calories.

4. **Improving knowledge:**
   - Explain measures to manage self-care activities to the extent possible
   - Explain the nature of disease (HIV) and mode of transmission
   - Discuss the methods of management
   - Discuss measures to prevent spread of infection to fetus and others
   - Discuss precautions to be taken to prevent developing additional infections.

5. **Decreasing sense of social isolation:**
   - Provide an atmosphere of acceptance and understanding of patient, spouse and family

- Assess patient's level of social interaction to provide a baseline for monitoring changes in behavior
- Encourage patient to express feelings of isolation and aloneness Assure patient that these feelings are not abnormal
- Assure patient, spouse and family that AIDS does not spread through casual contact.

6. **Coping with grief:**
   - Help to explore and identify resources for support and mechanisms for coping
   - Encourage to maintain contact with family, friends and co-workers and to continue usual activities whenever/as much as possible
   - Encourage using any support group if available.

9. AMNIOCENTESIS

Amniocentesis is a deliberate puncture of amniotic sac per abdomen for withdrawal of a sample of amniotic fluid surrounding an embryo in the uterus. It is generally done between 14–16 weeks by inserting a 20–22 gauge spinal needle and a syringe to withdraw about 10–20 mL of amniotic fluid. The procedure is performed under continuous ultrasonographic guidance.

INDICATIONS

- Antenatal diagnosis of chromosomal and genetic disorders such as cystic fibrosis, inborn errors of metabolism, neural tube defects
- Rhesus isoimmunization of the mother
- Maternal illness, which may affect the fetus, e.g. toxoplasmosis
- Induction of abortion by instillation of hypertonic saline, urea or prostaglandins
- Decompression of the uterus in acute hydramnios (in later months)
- To give amnioinfusion in oligohydramnios (in second half)
- For assessment of fetal maturity by estimating the lecithin-sphingomyelin ratio (in second half)
- In fetal distress, to detect meconium staining of liquor (in later months)
- For performing amniography or fetography (in second half).

PROCEDURE

- After emptying the bladder, the patient is made to lie in dorsal position
- The abdominal wall is prepared aseptically and draped
- The proposed site is infiltrated with 2 mL of 1% lignocaine
- An ultrasound examination is done and the placenta localized and a pool of liquor is found
- The physician inserts a needle about 4" in length through the abdominal wall into the uterus under direct ultrasonic guidance
- The stilette is withdrawn and a few drops of liquor are discarded
- About 10–20 mL amniotic fluid is withdrawn for diagnostic purposes or a smaller amount if the amniocentesis is performed in the first trimester.

AFTERCARE

- Following the procedure, the fetal heart must be auscultated
- The woman must be given clear instructions about when to expect the results of the test and about activities in the next few days
- If the mother has Rh-negative blood group, anti-D immunoglobulin to be administered if indicated.

RISKS OF AMNIOCENTESIS

Maternal

- Infection
- Hematoma
- Antepartum hemorrhage
- Rhesus isoimmunization
- Premature rupture of membranes and premature labor.

Fetal

- Death
- Feto-maternal hemorrhage
- Abortion
- Preterm labor
- Amniotic fluid leakage
- Respiratory distress
- Talipes.

10. AMNIOTIC FLUID EMBOLISM

This is a rare, but potentially catastrophic condition that occurs when amniotic fluid enters the maternal circulation via the uterus or placental site. The body responds in two phases. The initial phase is pulmonary vasospasm causing hypoxia, hypotension and cardiovascular collapse. The second phase is the development of left ventricular failure, with hemorrhage and coagulation disorder followed by pulmonary edema.

TIMING OF OCCURRENCE

- Following procedures such as artificial rupture of membranes and insertion of intrauterine catheter
- In labor, after spontaneous rupture of membranes associated with strong uterine contractions (hypertonic contractions)
- Perforated or ruptured uterus
- Trauma during intrauterine manipulation such as internal podalic version
- Cesarean section.

CLINICAL SIGNS AND SYMPTOMS

- Generalized pruritus, bronchospasm, hypotension and tachycardia occurring within few minutes
- Sudden onset of maternal respiratory distress, cyanosis and retrosternal pain
- Fetal distress in response to uterine hypoxia
- Cardiopulmonary arrest follows quickly in few minutes
- Convulsions may occur followed by acute collapse and shock
- Blood coagulopathy following the initial collapse
- Death within one hour occurs in about 50%.

MEASURES OF MANAGEMENT/INTERVENTION

Diagnosis

- Amniotic fluid embolism should be considered in all cases of unexplained collapse
- Clinical picture as described

- Blood coagulation studies
- Postmortem.

Treatment

Immediate resuscitation consisting of:
- Oxygenation and ventilation
- Hydrocortisone in large doses
- Aminophylline IV for respiratory distress
- Correction of blood loss and coagulation defects if indicated.

Prognosis

- Mortality rate is very high about 50% within one hour from onset
- Mothers who survive are likely to suffer a degree if neurological impairment.

COMPLICATIONS

- Disseminated intravascular coagulation (DIC)
- Acute renal failure
- Fetal demise.

11. ANEMIA IN PREGNANCY

Anemia is a reduction in the oxygen-carrying capacity of the blood, which may be due to reduced number of red blood cells (RBCs), a low concentration of hemoglobin or a combination of both **(Box 11.1)**.

Box 11.1: Classification of anemia.

Nutritional anemia:
- Iron deficiency
- Folate deficiency
- Vitamin B_{12} deficiency

Anemia due to increased blood loss:
- Hookworm infestation

Anemia due to hemolysis:
- Hemoglobinopathies
- Malaria
- Sickle cell anemia

Bone marrow insufficiency:
- Aplastic anemia due to radiation or drugs
- Severe infection

IRON DEFICIENCY ANEMIA

Inadequate food intake is the most common cause for iron deficiency in the tropics. In a healthy individual, a daily intake of dietary iron of 15 mg can replenish the daily loss of 1.5 mg. In the tropical countries, especially with low socioeconomic group, the daily requirement is likely to be more due to:
- Faulty dietary habit (chiefly cereals and pulses)
- Faulty absorption mechanism (intestinal worm infestation, hypochlorhydria)
- Iron loss (repeated pregnancies, menstruation).

Clinical Features

Clinical features depend on the degree of anemia. In early stages, patient may not show any symptoms and features develop slowly:
- Lassitude and feeling of weakness
- Anorexia and indigestion
- Palpitation caused by ectopic beats
- Dyspnea, giddiness and swelling of legs
- Glossitis, stomatitis and koilonychia
- Crepitations may be heard at the base of the lungs due to congestion.

Investigations

- Hemoglobin (8–10 g% mild, 6.5–8 g% moderate less than 6.5 g% severe)
- Total RBC count
- Packed cell volume
- Peripheral blood smear
- Serum iron below 30 µg/100 mL
- Total iron binding capacity > 400 µg/100 mL
- Serum ferritin below 10 µg/L
- Percentage of saturation 10% or less
- Examination of stool to detect helminthic infestation, specifically in tropics
- Urine for routine and culture examination.

Treatment

- Prophylaxis: Avoidance of frequent childbirths; minimum interval between pregnancies to be at least 2 years
- Supplementary iron therapy: Daily administration of 200 mg ferrous sulfate with 1 mg folic acid to start in the second trimester (soon after nausea of pregnancy subsides)
- Dietary prescription: A realistic balanced diet, rich in iron and protein which is affordable by patient to be advised, e.g. liver, meat, egg, green vegetables, green peas, beans, whole wheat, green bananas, onion stalks, and jaggery to be included in diet
- Adequate treatment to eradicate the cause of anemia, e.g. hookworm infestation, dysentery, bleeding piles, urinary tract infection
- Antibiotic therapy to treat any infection if present
- Parenteral iron therapy if oral therapy is contraindicated (intolerance to oral iron or if the mother is seen for the first time during the last 8–10 weeks with severe anemia).

Complications of Severe Anemia

During Pregnancy

- Pre-eclampsia may be related to malnutrition
- Occurrence of infections due to diminished resistance causing bone marrow depression
- Heart failure at 30–32 weeks of pregnancy
- Preterm labor.

During Labor

- Uterine inertia
- Hemorrhage
- Cardiac failure
- Shock.

Puerperium

- Puerperal sepsis
- Subinvolution
- Failing lactation

- Puerperal venous thrombosis
- Pulmonary embolism.

Effects on Baby

- Increased incidence of low birth weight babies
- Intrauterine death.

FOLATE AND B$_{12}$ DEFICIENCY

Causes

Folic acid deficiency during pregnancy is caused by:
- Increased demand due to increased RBC volume in pregnancy and developing fetus
- Diminished absorption related to intestinal malabsorption syndrome
- Abnormal demand in cases of twins, infection and hemorrhagic states during pregnancy
- Failure of utilisation when client has infection or on anticonvulsant drugs
- Diminished storage associated with hepatic disorders and vitamin C deficiency
- Inadequate intake due to nausea, vomiting and loss of appetite and dietary insufficiency. The main sources of folic acid are green vegetables, cauliflower, spinach, liver and kidney. Excessive cooking destroys much of the folate in food.

Clinical Features

- The onset is usually insidious and is first revealed in the last trimester or in early puerperium
- Anorexia or protracted vomiting
- Occasional diarrhea
- Constitutional symptoms like unexplained fever
- Pallor of varying degree
- Ulceration of mouth and tongue
- Hemorrhagic patches under the skin and conjunctiva
- Enlarged liver and spleen
- Features of pre-eclampsia.

Diagnosis

- Acute onset especially in last trimester and early puerperium
- Typical blood picture and bone marrow biopsy
- Serum folate less than 3 mg/mL
- Anemia fails to respond to iron therapy
- The association of megaloblastic bone marrow with higher serum iron.

Treatment

- Prophylactic folic acid therapy (indicated in all pregnant women)
- Specific therapy includes daily administration of folic acid 5 mg orally for at least four weeks following delivery
- Supplementary intramuscular vitamin B_{12} 100 µg daily or on alternate days
- Ascorbic acid 100 mg orally three times a day to enhance the action of folic acid.

RARE FORMS OF ANEMIA

Sickle Cell Disease

Sickle cell disease is characterized by a hemoglobinopathy in which defective genes produce abnormal hemoglobin beta chains; the resulting hemoglobin is called HbS. In sickle cell anemia (HbS) abnormal genes have been inherited from both parents. While in sickle cell trait (HbAS), only one abnormal gene has been inherited.

Character of Red Blood Cells

HbS in oxygenated state behaves normally, but in the deoxygenated state (psychological stress, cold climate and extreme temperature changes, strenuous physical exertion and fatigue, infection, hypoxia, dehydration and pregnancy); it aggregates, polymerizes and distorts the RBCs. These sickle shaped cells block the microcirculation due to their rigid structure. The cells have shorter life span and are more fragile. Increased destruction leads to hemolysis, anemia and jaundice.

Diagnosis

- Identification by sickling test
- Persistent reticulocytosis
- High fasting serum iron level
- Identification by hemoglobin electrophoresis.

Effects on Pregnancy

- Increased incidence of pre-eclampsia, postpartum hemorrhage and infections
- Intrauterine growth retardation (IUGR) and fetal loss
- Increased maternal morbidity and mortality due to pulmonary infarction, congestive heart failure and embolism.

Effects on Disease

- Hemolytic crisis: Hemolysis with rapidly developing anemia and jaundice associated with leukocytosis and fever
- Painful crisis: Due to vascular occlusion of various organs by capillary thrombosis resulting in infarction. Abdominal pain, vomiting, chest pain, hemoptysis or hematuria occur depending on the site of vascular occlusion.

Treatment

- Preconceptional counseling
- Early termination of pregnancy, if parents desire
- Careful antenatal supervision
- Avoidance of air traveling
- Prophylactic folic acid 5 mg daily
- Regular blood transfusion at 6 weeks interval to keep hematocrit (Hct) value above 25% and HbS under 50%
- Prompt treatment of infections or unusual symptoms
- Oxygen therapy during labor and delivery
- Adequate fluid therapy to avoid dehydration
- Prophylactic antibiotics in puerperium.

Contraception

Women with sickle cell anemia are generally subfertile. Those who become pregnant need close supervision and further pregnancies to be avoided.
- Barrier method of contraception is ideal
- Sterilization may be considered because of the short life span of the patient
- Oral pills and intrauterine device are contraindicated as it may aggravate the risk of thromboembolism and infection.

Thalassemia

Thalassemia is a hemoglobinopathy. The disease is characterized by diminished synthesis of hemoglobin beta chains (globin chains). As a result, the red cells are formed with inadequate hemoglobin content. These patients have a microcytic, hypochromic anemia with hemoglobin levels ranging from 8–10 gm/dL.

Clinical Features

The syndromes are of two types: The alpha and beta thalassemia depending on whether the alpha or the beta globin chain synthesis of the adult hemoglobin is depressed.

In women with alpha thalassemia major, if pregnancy occurs, the end result is usually prematurity and nonimmune hydrops. For women with alpha thalassemia trait, iron and folic acid supplementation is required. Parenteral iron should not be given because the patient may develop hemosiderosis from iron overload.

Beta thalassemia major is a genetic defect where the red cell survival time is reduced. Severe anemia usually develops in childhood. There is progressive hepatosplenomegaly, impaired growth, anemia, congestive cardiac failure and intercurrent infections. Chances of survival beyond teens are uncommon.

Patients with beta thalassemia minor (thalassemia trait) have an outcome similar to patients with normal hemoglobin and they do not require iron supplementation during pregnancy unless there is evidence of iron deficiency. If hemoglobin is low, blood transfusion is better and parenteral iron should not be given.

Management

Blood of the husband should be tested for any abnormality. If the hemoglobin is found abnormal, the couple is counseled of the potential risks to the offspring. Amniotic fluid fibroblasts obtained by amniocentesis, trophoblasts obtained by chorion-villus biopsy and fetal blood obtained by cordocentesis could be used for prenatal diagnosis.

Other Rare Inherited Anemias

- Glucose-6-phosphate dehydrogenase (G6PD) deficiency. This condition is inherited through an X-linked gene and is therefore seen predominantly in males. G6PD is an enzyme necessary for the survival of the RBC. When it is deficient, RBCs are destroyed in the presence of certain substances. These substances include sulfonamides, Vitamin K analogues, salicylates and camphor (found in products such as Vicks vapoRub). Clinically G6PD takes two forms:
  - Jaundice in the neonatal period
  - Acute self-limiting hemolysis precipitated by contact with the substances listed above.
- Spherocytosis: In this condition, the red cells are spherical instead of biconcave and are easily destroyed. It may cause haemolytic jaundice in the neonate.

NURSING PROCESS

Assessment

- Fatigue, weakness, general malaise
- Tachycardia/tachypnea; dyspnea on exertion
- Lethargy, apathy, lassitude and lack of interest in surroundings
- Muscle weakness and decreased strength
- Increased systolic with stable diastolic pressure
- Throbbing carotid pulsations
- History of chronic blood loss, e.g. heavy menses, gastrointestinal (GI) bleeding

- Pallor of skin and mucous membranes
- Delayed capillary refill
- Brittle, spoon shaped nails
- Decreased dietary intake, low intake of animal protein and high intake of cereal
- Stomatitis and glossitis
- Beefy red/smooth appearance of tongue (folic acid/vitamin B_{12} deficiencies).

Diagnostic Studies

- Complete blood count:
  - Hemoglobin and hematocrit (Hb/Hct)
  - Erythrocyte count
  - Stained RBC examination
  - Reticulocyte count
  - White Blood Cells
  - Erythrocyte sedimentation rate.
- Hemoglobin electrophoresis
- Serum folate and Vitamin B_{12}
- Serum ferritin and total iron binding capacity
- Guaiac test (occult blood in stools)
- Bone marrow aspiration.

Nursing Diagnoses

- Activity intolerance
- Risk for infection
- Deficient knowledge regarding condition, prognosis, treatment and selfcare
- Imbalanced nutrition: Less than body requirements.

Expected Outcomes

The client will:

- Report increase in activity tolerance; demonstrate a decrease in physiological signs of intolerance, e.g. pulse, blood pressure (BP) and respirations remain within normal range
- Be free of signs of infection

Anemia in Pregnancy

- Verbalize understanding of the nature of disease process, diagnostic procedures and potential complications
- Demonstrate progressive weight gain; experience no signs of malnutrition.

Nursing Interventions

1. **Increasing activity tolerance:**
   - Assess client's ability to perform normal tasks/activities of daily living, noting reports of weakness, fatigue and difficulty accomplishing tasks
   - Note changes in balance/gait disturbance and muscle weakness
   - Monitor BP, pulse and respirations during and after activity, e.g. increased heart rate, dizziness dyspnea, tachypnea and cyanosis
   - Recommend quiet atmosphere and bedrest if indicated
   - Suggest client to change position slowly, monitor for dizziness
   - Assist client to prioritize ADL/desired activities. Alternate rest periods with activity periods
   - Provide or recommend assistance with activities, allowing client to do as much as possible
   - Plan activity progression with client. Increase activity levels as tolerated
   - Identify/implement energy-saving techniques, e.g. sitting to perform tasks, using shower chair
   - Instruct client to stop activity if palpitations, chest pain, shortness of breath, weakness or dizziness occur
   - Monitor laboratory studies, e.g. Hb/Hct and RBC count, arterial blood gases
   - Provide supplemental oxygen as indicated
   - Collaborative interventions: Administer whole blood/packed RBCs, blood products as indicated. Monitor closely for transfusion reactions.

2. **Reducing risk of infection:**
   - Promote meticulous hand washing by caregivers and client
   - Maintain strict aseptic techniques with procedures

- Provide/instruct in meticulous skin, oral and perineal care
- Promote adequate fluid intake
- Observe for erythema/drainage if any wound is present
- Obtain specimens for culture/sensitivity as indicated
- Collaborative interventions: Administer topical antiseptics and systemic antibiotics as prescribed.

3. **Improving knowledge regarding condition (anemia), prognosis, treatment and selfcare:**
   - Provide information about specific anemia and explain that therapy depends on the type and severity of anemia and stage of pregnancy
   - Review purposes and preparations for diagnostic studies
   - Explain that blood taken for laboratory studies will not worsen anemia
   - Review required diet alterations to meet specific dietary needs (determined by type of anemia/deficiency)
   - Discuss foods to avoid (e.g. coffee, tea, egg yolk, milk, fiber and soy protein) at the time when client is eating high iron foods
   - Provide information about purpose, dosage, schedule, precautions, and potential side effects, interactions and adverse reactions to all prescribed medications
   - Stress importance of regular prenatal check-ups and reporting signs of fatigue, weakness, paresthesias, irritability and impaired memory
   - Advise taking iron preparations with meals or immediately after meals
   - Review good oral hygiene and necessity for regular dental care
   - Instruct to avoid aspirin products
   - Refer to appropriate community centers for iron, folic acid and food supplements.

4. **Improving nutritional status:**
   - Review nutritional history, including food preferences
   - Observe and record client's food intake
   - Weigh periodically as appropriate

- Recommend small, frequent meals, and/or between meal nourishment
- Suggest bland diet, avoiding hot, spicy or very acidic foods as indicated
- Have client record and report occurrence of nausea/vomiting, flatus and other related symptoms such as irritability or impaired memory
- Encourage/assist with good oral hygiene before and after meals, use soft-bristled toothbrush for gentle brushing
- Collaborative interventions: As follows:
  - Arrange consultation with dietitian
  - Monitor laboratory studies, e.g. Hb/Hct, blood urea nitrogen (BUN), albumin, protein, serum iron, vitamin B_{12}, folic acid and total iron-binding capacity
  - Administer medications as indicated, e.g. vitamin and mineral supplements (vitamin B_{12}, folic acid, ascorbic acid, ferrous sulfate and ferrous gluconate).

12. ANTENATAL ASSESSMENT

Assessment of the antenatal mother is done when she visits the clinic. The initial assessment is best done as soon as possible after pregnancy has been confirmed.

INITIAL ASSESSMENT

Objectives

- To obtain a detailed health history and to carry out screening tests as appropriate
- To ascertain baseline recordings of weight, height, blood pressure (BP) and hemoglobin level
- To identify risk factors by taking accurate details of past and present medical and obstetric history
- To give advice on matters pertaining to pregnancy, health of mother and fetus and care to be taken in the prenatal period
- To help allay anxiety and fear associated with pregnancy.

Components

- Health history
- Obstetric history
- Physical and pelvic examinations
- Laboratory tests
- Health education.

Health History

Health history of the pregnant client includes:
- Identifying information such as name, age and address
- Chief complaints in her own words: Some of the medical conditions that require special attention are urinary tract infection, essential hypertension, asthma, epilepsy, diabetes and cardiac conditions
- Family history: History of conditions that are genetic, familial or have racial characteristics such as:
    - Diabetes in first-degree relatives
    - Hypertension
    - Multiple pregnancies
    - Conditions like sickle cell anemia and thalassemia.
- Menstrual history: Age at menarche, history, duration and amount of menstrual flow, disfunctional menstrual bleeding, and premenstrual spotting.

Obstetric History

- Past pregnancies: This includes determining:
    - Obstetrical score (gravidity, parity, number of living children and abortions)
    - Rh and ABO blood type
    - Medical problems during pregnancy
    - Obstetrical problems during pregnancy, labor and delivery
    - Status of newborn at birth
    - Genetic abnormalities or neonatal problems.
- Present pregnancy: Determining with the mother:
    - The date of last menstrual period (LMP)
    - The expected date of delivery (EDD)
    - Present weeks of gestation

Antenatal Assessment

- Presence of disorders of pregnancy
- Manifestations of any associated medical problem
- Manifestations of obstetrical problems such as pregnancy induced hypertension, gestational diabetes and emotional status (acceptance of pregnancy).

Physical Examination

A complete screening physical examination is done during the initial prenatal visit.

- Physical measurements, i.e. temperature, pulse, respirations and BP, height, weight
- General observations and client's own evaluation of physical and emotional state
- Review of all body systems
- Abdominal examination:
  - Observation of the size and shape of uterus
  - The contour of abdomen and skin changes of pregnancy
  - Determination of the lie, presentation, position and variety of the fetus
  - Measurement of fundal height **(Table 12.1 and Fig. 12.1)** and abdominal girth
  - Auscultation of fetal heart tones **(Table 12.2)**.

Table 12.1: Measurement of the fundal height.

Weeks of gestation	Approximate expected location of fundal height
12	Level of the symphysis pubis Wee
16	Half way between symphysis pubis and umbilicus
20	1–2 finger breadths below the umbilicus
24	Level of the umbilicus
28–30	One-third of the way between umbilicus and xiphoid process (3 finger breadths above the umbilicus)
32	Two-third of the way between umbilicus and xiphoid process (3–4 finger breadths below the xiphoid process)
38	Level of the xiphoid process
40	2–3 finger breadths below the xiphoid process if lightening occurs

Table 12.2: Location of fetal heart tones in various fetal presentations and positional varieties.

Presentations and Positional varieties	Location
Cephalic	Midway between umbilicus and level of anterior superior iliac spine
Breech	At the level or above umbilicus
Anterior positions	Close to abdominal midline
Transverse	In lateral abdominal area
Posterior	In flank area on the same side

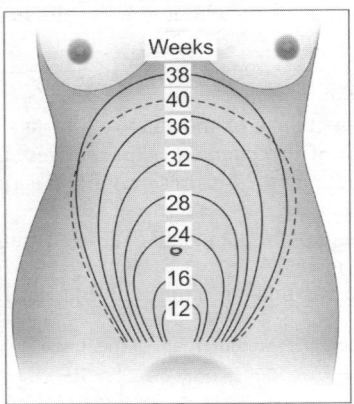

Fig. 12.1: Approximate height of the fundus as the uterus enlarges.

Pelvic Examination

A pelvic examination includes speculum examination, bimanual and retrovaginal examination as well as evaluation of the bony pelvis for assessment of pelvic capacity.

Laboratory Tests

- ABO blood group and Rh factor
- Hemoglobin and hematocrit

- Venereal disease research laboratory (VDRL) test
- Human immunodeficiency virus (HIV) tests
- Rubella immune status
- Blood glucose
- Urinalysis.

Health Education

- Anatomy and physiology as they relate to pregnancy, labor and birth
- Care during prenatal period such as nutrition, exercises, posture and body mechanics
- Stages and phases of labor and woman's physical responses
- Breathing techniques for different stages of labor
- Care of newborn.

13. ANTEPARTUM HEMORRHAGE

It is defined as bleeding that occurs from or into the genital sac after the stage of viability that is 28 weeks of pregnancy, but before the birth of the baby.

Box 13.1: Classification of antepartum hemorrhage.

Placental site bleeding
- Abruptio placentae or accidental hemorrhage
- Placenta previa

These two types are based on the site of attachment of the placenta

Extra placental bleeding
- Local causes:
    - Cervical polyps
    - Vulval varicosities
    - Cervical erosions
    - Cervical carcinoma
    - Trauma
- Other causes or unexplained causes:
    - Coagulopathies
    - Idiopathic bleeding
- Unexpected or indeterminate causes.

GENERAL MANAGEMENT OF ANTEPARTUM HEMORRHAGE

When the patient is first seen with an antepartum hemorrhage (APH), the cause of bleeding or the diagnosis is not obvious in many cases. An initial protocol of general management of cases is essential:

- If the woman is first seen at home, it is desirable to do a minimum of examination and send her to the hospital immediately
- Assessment to see if the patient needs immediate resuscitation is the first priority on arrival at the hospital
- Resuscitative measures like intravenous (IV) infusion and sedation may be indicated in some cases
- Vaginal examination, which can result in dangerous bleeding, should not be performed
- Clinical assessment may then be done to determine the underlying cause
- If bleeding persists and is of an alarming proportion or if the fetus is beyond 37 weeks or patient is in labor, then an active plan to terminate the pregnancy may be made
- If not, an expectant treatment is carried out with the aim of continuing the pregnancy till the fetus has gained acceptable level of maturity. It is essential to be prepared to change to an active policy if need arises.

ABRUPTIO PLACENTAE (ACCIDENTAL HEMORRHAGE)

Definition

A condition characterized by premature separation of a normally situated placenta.

Incidence

It is seen in 1–3% deliveries and occurs in the last trimester of pregnancy with the incidence increasing as the term approaches. Recurrence rates are about 5–17% after the first episode and about 25% after the second. Each successive episode is usually more severe than the last.

Etiology

The exact cause of separation of a normally situated placenta remains obscure in majority of cases. The prevalence is seen more in association with:
- High parity and advancing age of mother
- Trauma like a kick on the abdomen or a fall
- Maternal drug abuse, notably cocaine
- Malnutrition, especially folic acid deficiency
- Smoking
- Pre-eclampsia, chronic hypertension and nephritis
- Sudden reduction in the size of the uterus by rupture of membranes in hydramnios, or delivery of the first baby of twins
- Short cord, either relative or absolute.

Pathogenesis

Rarely the entire placenta may get separated from the placental wall. Separation of only a portion of the placenta is however, sufficient to cause severe bleeding. If abruption occurs due to mechanical causes such as trauma or sudden decompression of the uterus, it leads to marginal separation of the placenta. The bleeding is from the torn uterine sinuses and the blood tracks downwards between the membranes and uterine wall to be revealed outside. In cases associated with preeclampsia, chronic hypertension or chronic nephritis, degeneration and necrosis of the decidua basalis occurs with formation of decidual hematoma. The hematoma leads to separation of the placenta. The retroplacental hematoma is evident only after placental separation.

If a major spiral artery is involved, a big hematoma is formed. As the uterus remains distended with the fetus it fails to contract and compress the bleeding points. The blood may accumulate behind the placenta, dissect downwards in between the membranes and the uterine wall or may gain access into the amniotic cavity after rupturing through the membranes.

Classification of the Hemorrhage

- **Revealed or external hemorrhage:** The effused blood escapes under the placental margin and makes its way between the membranes and the uterine wall down to the internal os from where it passes through the cervix into the vagina.

- **Concealed hemorrhage:** Almost the whole amount of effused blood is retained due to loss of tone or excitability of the uterine musculature. Sometimes bleeding takes place into the amniotic sac. There is usually a little external bleeding in concealed accidental hemorrhage.

    Couvelaire uterus or uteroplacental apoplexy: In case of concealed accidental bleeding, intramuscular hemorrhage and subperitoneal ecchymosis are found in the uterine wall, more commonly in the region of the placental site. Bleeding may also occur into the broad ligaments. The condition can only be diagnosed on laparotomy.

- **Mixed type of hemorrhage:** In this type the bleeding is partly external and partly concealed. The clinical features of different types of accidental hemorrhages are compared in **Table 13.1**.

Table 13.1: Comparison of clinical features in different types of accidental hemorrhage.

Symptoms	Revealed	Mixed
Abdominal pain	Abdominal discomfort or pain followed by vaginal bleeding—usually slight	Acute, intense pain in abdomen followed by slight vaginal bleeding. Pain becomes continuous
Character of bleeding	Continuous, dark color and amount slight to moderate	Continuous, dark color (usually slight) or blood stained serous discharge
General condition	Proportionate to the visible blood loss. Shock is usually absent	Shock is pronounced, which is out of proportion to the visible blood loss
Pallor	Related to the visible blood loss	Pallor is usually severe and out of proportion to the visible bleeding
Features of pre-eclampsia	May be absent	Pre-existing pre-eclamptic toxemia (PET) or may appear

Contd...

Contd...

Symptoms	Revealed	Mixed
Uterine height	Proportionate to the period of gestation	May be disproportionate, enlarged and globular
Uterine feel	Normal feel with localized tenderness	Uterus is tense, tender and rigid
Fetal parts	Can be identified easily	Difficult to make out
Fetal heart tones (FHR)	Usually present	Usually absent
Urine output	Normal	Usually diminished
Blood hemoglobin	Low value, proportionate to the blood loss	Markedly lower, out of proportion to the visible blood loss
Coagulation profile	Usually undisturbed	Variable disturbance: • Clotting time increased • Fibrinogen level low • Platelet level low • Fibrin degradation product (FDP) increased

Clinical Manifestations

Concealed Variety

Concealed accidental hemorrhage is a serious complication of pregnancy. In severe cases, the signs and symptoms are due to loss of blood, uterine inertia and overdistension of the uterus.

- **Signs and symptoms of circulatory collapse are:**
  - Skin surface cold and slightly moist from sweating
  - Breathing shallow and labored
  - Deep pallor and subnormal temperature
  - Rapid pulse of 120–160 per minute and low blood pressure
  - Initial restlessness
  - Loss of consciousness (constitutional symptoms are disproportionate to the amount of blood lost).
- **On examination per abdomen:**
  - Uterus is unduly large and very tender
  - Uterus tense and feels almost wooden in consistency

- Uterine size larger than expected period of gestation due to accumulation of blood within the uterus
- No uterine contractions
- Fetal parts cannot be felt easily
- There may be evidence of fetal distress and fetal tachycardia in the milder cases. Fetal heart sounds (FHS) are often absent in severe cases.
- **On vaginal examination:**
  - A little bleeding from the uterus will usually be detected, although in rare cases there is none.

Revealed Variety

- Bleeding per vagina accompanied by pain and tenderness
- The head-brim relationship is not disturbed
- Labor is often premature with increased necessity for operative interference
- Presence of retroplacental clot/hematoma on ultrasound examination
- Uterine feel normal with localized tenderness
- FHS usually present and fetal parts can be identified easily.

Investigations

- Ultrasonography
- Hemoglobin
- Coagulation profile
- Urine for protein.

Management

All, but mild cases are dangerous and surgical treatment may be required. The fundamental objectives of treatment are:
- Immediate resuscitation
- Relief of pain
- Detection and correction of coagulation failure
- Prevention of renal failure
- Rapid delivery.

Resuscitation

Initial treatment should be restorative, consisting of rest, warmth, sedation, and transfusion of as much blood as is necessary to overcome shock and re-establish a good circulation with the minimum of delay.

- Grouping and cross matching of patient's blood against available blood
- Monitoring pulse and blood pressure (BP) every 30 minutes or more frequently if needed
- Measure fundal height and abdominal girth at intervals and note any increase in size of the uterus denoting progressive bleeding (in concealed type)
- Transfuse blood sufficiently rapidly to restore the circulation and BP to normal levels
- Ensure adequacy of transfusion by monitoring central venous pressure (CVP).

Relief of Pain

Administration of pethidine 50–100 mg or injection morphine 10–15 mg at intervals until pain is alleviated and restlessness is controlled.

Detection and Correction of Coagulation

Fibrinogen level should be estimated first. If it is below 100 mg/mL (normal level 250–400 mg%), there may be coagulation failure and bleeding can be uncontrollable. Transfusion of fresh whole blood or triple strength plasma or dried fibrinogen reconstituted in distilled water is administered.

Prevention of Renal Failure

Prompt delivery and avoidance of hypotension are the best ways of preventing renal failure.

Rapid Delivery

Uterine activity is, in fact the best means of controlling hemorrhage. The measures followed are:
- Artificial rupture of membranes
- Oxytocin infusion.

Rupturing the membranes is effective as it increases the uterine tone compresses the separating placenta between the fetal bulk and the uterine wall.

Intravenous oxytocin drip started 2 hours after the rupture of membranes usually helps control hemorrhage and bring about spontaneous delivery.

Vaginal delivery is preferred when the mother is in good condition and the presenting part is lying well in the pelvis. Cesarean delivery is indicated in the following cases:
- Severe concealed accidental hemorrhage with a mature live or distressed fetus
- Continued vaginal bleeding and absence of uterine activity
- Uterus remains inactive, BP difficult to maintain, pulse rate rises and general condition deteriorates. Cesarean section or cesarean hysterectomy may be done to control bleeding
- Abdominal hysterectomy may be necessary if uncontrollable postpartum hemorrhage (PPH) occurs from uterine atony (couvelaire uterus) occurs.

Complications of Placental Abruption

- Disseminated intravascular coagulation with moderate to severe placental abruption
- Postpartum hemorrhage may occur as a result of couvelaire uterus or disseminated intravascular coagulation (DIC) or both
- Air embolism, an occasional occurrence when the sinuses in the placental bed have been broken
- Fetal hypoxia and its sequelae due to placental separation
- Fetal death depending on gestation and blood loss
- Renal failure as a result of hypovolemia
- Pituitary necrosis as a consequence of prolonged and severe hypotension.

PLACENTA PREVIA

Definition

When the placenta is situated wholly or partially in the lower uterine segment, it is called placenta previa.

Incidence

The overall incidence is about 1:300 deliveries.

Etiology

The exact cause of placenta previa is not known. Certain conditions are known to predispose to a low-lying placenta with a greater frequency. These are:
- Grand multiparity
- Multiple pregnancies
- Previous lower segment cesarean section or myomectomy causing defective blood circulation in the region of the scar
- Uterine anomalies may predispose to low implantation as well as malpresentations
- Defective decidua results in spreading of the chorionic villi over a wide area of uterine wall to get nourishment
- Big surface area of the placenta as in twins may encroach onto the lower segment.

Classification

There are four types of placenta previa depending upon the degree of extension of placenta to the lower segment (**Fig. 13.1**).

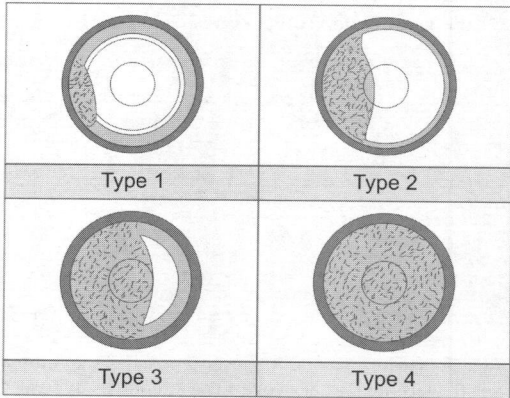

Fig. 13.1: Relationship of placenta previa to cervical os.

Type I—Lateral Placenta Previa

The major part of the placenta is attached to the upper segment and only the lower margin of the placenta reaches into the upper portion of the lower uterine segment. These patients have the lowest risk of antepartum bleeding.

Type II—Marginal Placenta Previa

In this case, the edge of the placenta reaches the margin of the internal os, but does not cover it. Depending on the position of the placenta, this can be of two types:
- Type II Anterior
- Type II Posterior.

The posterior variety is likely to get compressed between the fetal head and the sacral promontory during labor causing interruption in the fetal blood supply, leading to fetal distress.

Type III—Incomplete Central Placenta Previa

Here, the placenta covers the internal os when it is closed, but only partially covers it when it is fully dilated.

Type IV—Central Placenta Previa

The placenta completely covers the internal os at all times (even after it is fully dilated). This is the most dangerous variety as there is high-risk of torrential vaginal bleeding **(Figs. 13.2A to D)**.

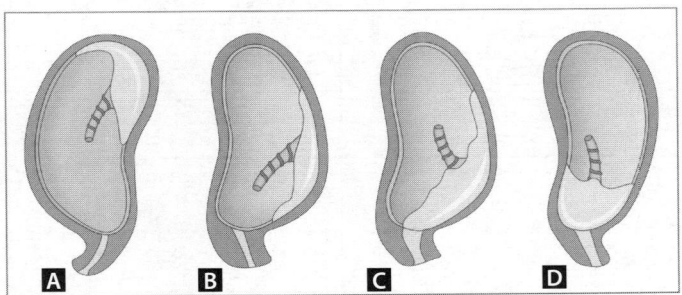

Figs. 13.2A to D: Placenta previa. **A.** Placenta reaches the internal os when closed, Type II; **B.** Placenta partially covers the internal os, Type III; **C.** Placenta covers the internal os when it is closed, Type IV; **D.** Placenta completely covers the internal os at all times.

Cause of Hemorrhage

As the placental growth slows down in later months and the lower segment progressively dilates, the inelastic placenta is sheared off the wall of the lower segment. This leads to opening up of utero-placental vessels and leads to an episode of bleeding. As it is a physiological phenomenon, which leads to separation of the placenta, the bleeding is said to be inevitable. The separation of the placenta may be provoked by trauma such as vaginal examination, coital act, external version or rupture of membranes. The blood is almost always maternal.

Clinical Features

- Revealed hemorrhage: Painless and recurrent bouts of hemorrhage are characteristic:
    - The classical features of bleeding in placenta previa are sudden onset, painless, apparently causeless and recurrent
    - In about one-third of cases there is usually a history of 'warning hemorrhage,' which is slight. Subsequent bouts may be heavier than the previous one due to separation of fresh areas of placenta
    - In majority of cases, bleeding occurs before 38 weeks and earlier bleeding is more likely to occur in major degrees
    - There may not be any bleeding in central placenta previa until labor begins.

    The clinical features of placenta previa and abruptio are compared in **Table 13.2**.

Table 13.2: Features of placenta previa and abruptio placentae.

Clinical features	Placenta previa	Abruptio placentae
Nature of bleeding	Painless, apparently causeless and recurrent Bleeding is always revealed	Painful, often attributable to pre-eclampsia, or trauma and continuous
Character of blood	Bright red	Dark colored
General condition and anemia	Proportionate to visible blood loss	Out of proportion to visible blood loss
Height of fundus	Proportionate to gestation period	May be disproportionately enlarged in concealed type

Contd...

Clinical features	Placenta previa	Abruptio placentae
Feel of uterus	Soft and relaxed	May be tense, tender and rigid
Malpresentation	Malpresentation is common. The head is high floating	Unrelated, the head may be engaged
Fetal heart sound (FHS)	Usually present	Usually absent, specially in concealed type
Ultrasonography	Placenta in lower segment	Placenta in upper segment
Vaginal examination	Placenta is felt in the lower segment	Placenta is not felt in lower segment

- Deterioration of general condition and anemia are proportionate to the visible blood loss
- On abdominal examination:
  - Size of the uterus is proportionate to the period of gestation
  - The uterus feels relaxed, soft and elastic without any area of tenderness
  - Persistence of malpresentation such as breech or transverse or unstable lie
  - Floating fetal head: The fetal head cannot be pushed down into the pelvis
  - Fetal heart sounds are usually present unless there is major separation of placenta.
- Vaginal inspection: The blood is bright red as the bleeding occurs from the separated utero-placental sinuses close to the cervical opening and escapes out immediately
- Vaginal examination should not be done outside of the operation theater in the hospital as it can provoke torrential bleeding and may be fatal. To be done in the operation theater under anesthesia with everything ready for cesarean section
- Ultrasonography: This is the most accurate method today for localization of the placenta.

Management

The first step in the management is hospitalization. Once hospitalized, the patient is resuscitated if in shock with IV fluids and blood transfusion. Subsequent management depends upon the duration of gestation and the severity of her condition. Accordingly management can be conservative or immediate delivery.

Expectant Management

The expectant care comprises judicious noninterference and intensive monitoring; and is called the Johnson and Macafee protocol.
- The prerequisites for inclusion into expectant management:
    - Gestational age less than 37 weeks duration
    - Initial bout of bleeding less than 600 mL
    - Patient not in labor
    - Maternal and fetal condition not in jeopardy
    - Cessation of bleeding should extend for more than one week to call it successful.
- The expectant management consists of the following measures:
    - Complete bed rest until 2–3 days after bleeding stops
    - Blood to be grouped, cross-matched and reserved for the patient at all times
    - Iron, vitamin and calcium supplements are continued. Laxatives may be given to avoid straining at stools
    - Hemoglobin is estimated at regular intervals
    - The patient's pulse rate, BP and fetal heart sounds are monitored till her condition is stable
    - Approximately 3 days after all bleeding has ceased; a gentle speculum (Cusco's speculum) examination should be performed to rule out any local cause of bleeding
    - Ultrasound examination is performed for placental localization
    - Minimal ambulation after bleeding stops and to keep (admitted) in hospital until delivery.

Definitive Management

The definitive management comprises prompt delivery. This is considered whenever:
- The patient has first bout of bleeding after 37 completed weeks
- Successful conservative treatment brings the patient up to 37 weeks

- If the initial or subsequent bout of bleeding is very severe
- Patient is in labor
- Evidence of maternal or fetal jeopardy
- Intrauterine fetal death

The definitive management consists of the following:

Vaginal examination

A vaginal examination is gently performed in operation theater keeping all the necessary articles ready for cesarean section. This way the diagnosis is confirmed and the degree of placenta previa is ascertained. Vaginal examination is not done if major degree of placenta previa is confirmed by ultrasonography.

Amniotomy/Artificial rupture of membranes (ARM)

Low rupture of membranes is done using a long Kocher's forceps, in vertex presentation and when placenta previa is of Grade I or Grade II anterior variety, the bleeding is slight and the labor is already in progress.

Benefits of amniotomy

- Free escape of amniotic fluid permits the presenting part to descend completely into the lower uterine segment and fill it so as to compress the placental site
- At the same time an oxytocin drip is started to augment labor, if not contraindicated.

These steps help to check further separation of the placenta.

Precautions during delivery

- Blood volume to be restored
- Ergometrine should be given IV with the delivery of anterior shoulder to prevent PPH
- Cervix must be examined soon after delivery to detect any tear
- Hemoglobin level of newborn to be checked.

Cesarean section

Lower segment cesarean section is the treatment of choice in:
- Placenta previa of Grade II posterior, Grade III and Grade IV even where the baby is dead

- Lesser degree of placenta previa where amniotomy fails to stop bleeding or fetal distress appears
- Complicating factors associated with lesser degrees of placenta previa where vaginal delivery is anticipated to be unsafe.

Prognosis

The prognosis varies with the type of placenta previa, the method of treatment and the condition of the patient on arrival in the hospital.

Perinatal mortality occurs due to intrapartum asphyxia resulting from placental separation, the hazards of delivery in malpresentations, prematurity and congenital malformations.

NURSING PROCESS

Assessment

- Blood pressure: High if mother has pregnancy-induced hypertension (PIH), low with hemorrhage
- Bleeding: Dark, bright or concealed
- Abdomen: Soft in placenta previa, hard, board like and tense with abruptio placentae
- Uterine fundus: Rising with abruptio placentae
- Progressive decrease of relaxation of uterus between contractions
- Hyperactive fetus
- Fetal bradycardia or tachycardia
- Urine output: Decreased, specific gravity increased
- Pain: May have pain with retroplacental hemorrhage. Sudden onset, constant and localized. No pain for placenta previa.

Diagnostic Studies

- Elevated white blood cell (WBC) count, lowered hemoglobin and hematocrit levels
- Coagulation time prolonged [prothrombin time (PT), partial thromboplastin time (PTT), and activated partial thromboplastin time (APTT)]
- Amniocentesis to determine lecithin/sphingomyelin (L/S) ratio in placenta previa

- Kleihauer-Betke test on maternal serum and amniotic fluid for presence of fetal blood
- Ultrasonography findings.

Nursing Diagnoses

- Deficient fluid volume (isotonic)
- Ineffective uteroplacental tissue perfusion
- Fear
- Risk for maternal injury
- Acute pain
- Deficient knowledge regarding reason for hemorrhage, prognosis and treatment needs.

Expected Outcomes

The client will:
- Demonstrate stabilization in fluid balance
- Demonstrate adequate perfusion as evidenced by FHR and activity
- Discuss fears regarding self, fetus and future pregnancies, and demonstrate problem solving and effective use of resources
- Display normal blood profile and urine output
- Report pain/discomfort relieved/controlled
- Participate in learning process and verbalize in simple terms information about the clinical situation.

Nursing Interventions

1. **Stabilizing/improving fluid balance:**
    - Evaluate, report and record amount and nature of blood loss. Initiate pad count, weigh pads/underpads
    - Institute bedrest. Instruct to avoid Valsalva's maneuver
    - Position client appropriately, either supine with hips elevated or semi-Fowler's position for placenta previa
    - Note vital signs, capillary refill of nail beds, color of mucous membranes/skin and temperature. Measure CVP if available
    - Monitor uterine activity, fetal status and any abdominal tenderness

- Avoid rectal or vaginal examination
- Record intake and output, obtain hourly urine samples; measure specific gravity
- Auscultate breath sounds
- Collaborative interventions: As follows:
  - Obtain/review stat blood work; complete blood count (CBC), type and cross match, rhesus (Rh) titer, fibrinogen levels, platelet count, APTT and PT
  - Insert indwelling urinary catheter
  - Administer IV solutions, plasma expanders, whole blood or packed cells as indicated
  - Prepare for cesarean delivery if any of the following are diagnosed: severe abruptio placentae DIC and placenta previa when fetus is mature; vaginal delivery is not feasible and bleeding is excessive.

2. **Enhancing uteroplacental tissue perfusion:**
   - Note maternal circulatory status and blood volume
   - Auscultate and report FHR, note bradycardia or tachycardia. Note change in fetal activity (hyperactivity or hypoactivity)
   - Record maternal blood loss and any uterine contractions
   - Encourage bedrest in lateral position
   - Collaborative interventions: As follows:
     - Administer supplemental oxygen to client
     - Carry out or repeat nonstress test (NST), as indicated
     - Replace maternal fluid/blood losses
     - Assist with ultrasonography and amniocentesis as indicated and explain procedures
     - Obtain specimens of maternal blood, urine and amniotic fluid for tests
     - Prepare client for appropriate surgical intervention as indicated.

3. **Helping to deal with fears regarding self, fetus and future pregnancies:**
   - Discuss situation and understanding of situation with client and spouse
   - Monitor client's/couple's verbal and nonverbal responses
   - Listen actively to client's concerns

- Provide opportunity for client to ask questions. Answer questions honestly
- Involve client in planning and participating in care as much as possible
- Collaborative interventions: As follows:
  - Explain procedures and their importance
  - Contact spiritual advisor as appropriate.

4. **Reducing chances of maternal injury:**
   - Assess amount of blood loss. Monitor for signs and symptoms of shock
   - Note temperature, WBC count and odor and color of vaginal discharge, obtain culture if appropriate
   - Record intake and output. Note urine specific gravity
   - Monitor for adverse response to administration of blood products, such as allergic or hemolytic reaction, treat per protocol
   - Inspect client for petechiae or for bleeding from gums/mucous membranes or IV site
   - Collaborative interventions: As follows:
     - Obtain blood type and cross match
     - Administer IV fluids for replacement
     - Monitor coagulation studies, e.g. APTT, platelet count and fibrinogen levels, fibrin split product (FSP)/fibrin degradation product (FDP)
     - Administer cryoprecipitate and fresh frozen plasma, as indicated. Avoid administration of platelets if consumption is still occurring; i.e. if platelet level is dropping
     - Administer heparin if indicated
     - Administer antibiotic parenterally
     - Treat underlying problem, e.g. surgery for abruptio placentae, bed-rest for placenta previa.

5. **Relieving or controlling pain/discomfort:**
   - Determine nature, severity (using 0–10 scale), location and duration of pain
   - Assess client's/couple's psychological stress and emotional response to event

- Provide quiet environment and diversional activities. Instruct client in relaxation methods, e.g. deep breathing, visualization, distraction
- Explain procedures, answer questions honestly, encourage expression of feelings/concerns
- Collaborative interventions: As follows:
  - Administer narcotics or sedatives as appropriate
  - Prepare for surgical procedure; administer preoperative medications, if indicated.

6. **Enhancing learning about the condition and management:**
   - Explain prescribed treatment and rationale for the hemorrhagic condition. Reinforce information provided by other health care providers
   - Allow client opportunity to ask questions and verbalize misconceptions
   - Discuss possible short-term maternal/fetal implications of bleeding episode
   - Review long-term implications of situations requiring follow-up and additional treatment.

14. ASSISTED REPRODUCTIVE TECHNOLOGY

Assisted reproductive technology (ART) is a general term referring to methods used to achieve pregnancy by artificial or partially artificial means. It is reproductory technology used in infertility treatment. In reproductive technology, the process of intercourse is bypassed either by insemination, e.g. intrauterine insemination (IUI) or fertilization of the oocytes in the laboratory environment, i.e. in in vitro fertilization (IVF) **(Box 14.1)**.

Box 14.1: Different techniques of assisted reproductive technology (ART).

Intrauterine insemination (IUI)
In vitro fertilization and embryo transfer (IVF-ET)
Gamete intrafallopian transfer (GIFT)
Zygote intrafallopian transfer (ZIFT)
Intracytoplasmic sperm injection (ICSI)

INTRAUTERINE INSEMINATION

Intrauterine insemination involves placing increased concentration of motile sperms close to the fallopian tubes bypassing the endocervical canal, which is abnormal. IUI may be either artificial insemination by husband (AIH) or artificial insemination by donor (AID).

Indications

- Hostile cervical mucus
- Cervical stenosis
- Oligospermia or asthenospermia
- Immune factor (male or female)
- Male factor impotency or anatomical defect (hypospadias), but normal ejaculate can be obtained
- Unexplained infertility.

Technique

About 0.3 mL of washed and concentrated sperms are injected through a flexible polyethylene catheter within the uterine cavity around the time of ovulation. The processed motile sperms for insemination should atleast be 1 million. Fertilizing capacity of spermatozoa is 24–48 hours. The procedure may be repeated 2–3 times over a period of 2–3 days. Generally 4–6 cycles of insemination with or without superovulation are advised.

When large volumes of washed and processed sperms are placed within the uterine cavity, around the time of ovulation, it causes perfusion of the fallopian tubes with spermatozoa. Hence this method is known as fallopian tube sperm perfusion. In conjunction with ovulation induction, pregnancy rate is 25–30% per cycle.

Artificial Insemination by Donor

When the semen of a donor is used for insemination, it is called AID. The indications are untreatable azoospermia, athenospermia, genetic disease, and Rh-negative donor insemination for a woman with Rh-sensitisation.

Indications

- Azoospermia
- Immunological factors, which are not correctable
- Genetic disease in the husband.

The donor should be healthy and serologically and bacteriologically free from venereal diseases, AIDS and hepatitis. The recipient and donor must be matched for blood grouping and Rh typing. Either fresh or frozen semen is used.

A total of 3–6 cycles may have to be used for success. Insemination when combined with superovulation enhances success rate. Two inseminations, 18 and 42 hours after human chorionic gonadotropin (hCG) administration give higher result when compared to single insemination after 36 hours.

Artificial Insemination Husband

An AIH semen is done for 4 cycles. The results are better if combined with ovulation induction for multiple ovulation. It is indicated in:

- Oligospermia after sperm washout
- Impotency
- Premature ejaculation, retrograde ejaculation
- Hypospadias
- Antispermal antibodies in the cervical mucus
- Unexplained infertility
- X-Y fractionation of sperms for sex selection, in genetic and chromosomal abnormalities.

Egg Donor

Egg donors are resources for women with no eggs due to surgery, chemotherapy, genetic causes, poor egg quality, previously unsuccessful IVF cycles or advanced age. In the egg donor process, eggs are retrieved from a donor's ovaries, fertilized in the laboratory with the sperm from the recipient's spouse/partner and the resulting healthy embryos are returned to the recipient's uterus.

IN VITRO FERTILIZATION AND EMBRYO TRANSFER

In vitro fertilization and embryo transfer (IVF-ET) fertilization of an ovum outside the body, a technique used when a woman has blocked fallopian tubes or some other impediment to the union of sperm and ovum in the reproductive tract. The woman is given hormone therapy causing a number of ova to mature at the same time (superovulation) several of them are then removed from the ovary through a laparoscope.

The ova are mixed with spermatozoa from her spouse and incubated in a culture medium until the blastocyst is formed. The blastocyst is then implanted in the mother's uterus and the pregnancy allowed to continue normally.

Indications

- Tubal disease
- Endometriosis
- Cervical hostility
- Unexplained infertility
- Male factor infertility
- Failed ovulation induction.

Patient Selection

- Age less than 35 years
- Presence of at least one functioning ovary
- Normal seminogram for husband
- Couple negative for human immunodeficiency virus (HIV) and hepatitis.

Steps

- Induction of superovulation using drugs such as clomiphene citrate and Gonadotropin releasing hormone (GnRH).
- Monitoring of follicular growth: This is done by cervical mucus study, sonographic measurement of the follicle and serum estriol estimation.

- Ovum retrieval: This is done through vaginal route. A small needle is inserted through the back of the vagina and guided via ultrasound into the ovarian follicles to collect the fluid that contains the ova about 36 hours after hCG administration, but before ovulation occurs.
- Fertilization (in vitro): The sperm used for insemination in vitro is prepared by the wash and swim up technique. Approximately 50,000–100,000 sperms are placed into the culture media containing the oocyte within 4–6 hours of retrieval. The semen is collected just prior to ovum retrieval. Sperm density and motility are most important criteria for successful IVF.
- Embryo transfer: The fertilized ova at the 4–8 cell stage are placed into the uterine cavity close to the fundus about 48–72 hours later through a fine flexible tube transcervically. Not more than three embryos are transferred per cycle to minimize multiple pregnancy.

GAMETE INTRA FALLOPIAN TRANSFER

In this procedure, both the sperm and the unfertilized oocyte are transferred into the fallopian tubes using laparoscopy following transvaginal ovum retrieval. Fertilization is then achieved *in vivo*.

The prerequisite for gamete intra fallopian transfer (GIFT) procedure is to have normal uterine tubes. The result is poor in male factor abnormality. Superovulation is done as in IVF. Two hours prior to ovum retrieval, semen specimen is obtained. The semen is washed by a technique called 'swim up', the most fertile fraction of the sperm is obtained and used for transfer.

ZYGOTE INTRA FALLOPIAN TRANSFER

In zygote intra fallopian transfer (ZIFT), egg cells are removed from the woman's ovaries and fertilized in the laboratory; the resulting zygote is then placed into the fallopian tube through laparoscope or through uterine opening under ultrasonic guidance. The technique is a suitable alternative of GIFT when defect lies in male factor or in case of failed GIFT. GIFT or ZIFT are avoided when tubal factors of infertility are present.

Intracytoplasmic Sperm Injection

Intracytoplasmic sperm injection (ICSI) method is beneficial in the case of male factor infertility where the sperm counts are very low or failed fertilization with previous IVF attempts. The ICSI procedure involves a single sperm carefully injected into the center of an egg using a micro needle.

Sperm is retrieved from the ejaculate or by testicular sperm extraction (TESE) or by microsurgical epididymal sperm aspiration (MESA). Indications are azoospermia, severe oligospermia, sperm antibodies, and obstruction of afferent duct system and failure of IVF.

PROGNOSIS OF ARTIFICIAL REPRODUCTIVE METHODS

The pregnancy rate within two years after the start of investigation ranges between 30 and 40%. The rate is higher if AID cases are included. However, if pregnancy occurs, there is two-fold increased chance of abortion, five times of ectopic and the perinatal mortality rate doubles.

15. BASIC LIFE SUPPORT/ CARDIOPULMONARY RESUSCITATION

Basic life support (BLS) is the emergency treatment of a victim of cardiac or respiratory arrest through cardiopulmonary resuscitation (CPR) and emergency cardiac care until more definitive medical treatment is available. CPR is an emergency procedure in which the heart and lungs are forced to work by manually compressing the chest overlying the heart and forcing air into the lungs. CPR is often used to maintain circulation and respiration when the heart or lung has stopped functioning.

The objective is to ensure oxygenation of the brain, heart and other vital organs until appropriate definite medical treatment (advanced life support) can restore normal circulatory and respiratory actions.

SEQUENCE OF BASIC LIFE SUPPORT (Box 15.1)

The new guidelines by [American Heart Association (AHA), 2010] have changed the sequence of CPR from A-B-C (Airway-Breathing-Circulation) to C-A-B (Chest Compressions-Airway-Breathing):

- **Determine unresponsiveness (Figs. 15.1A to C):** If a mother is found collapsed, her level of consciousness is to be determined by gently shaking a shoulder and enquiring "are you alright"
- **Determine pulselessness (Fig. 15.2):** Check for carotid pulse on one side of neck for not more than 5 seconds

Box 15.1: Summary of the sequence of basic life support (BLS).

Determine unresponsiveness
Determine pulselessness
Call for help
Position the victim
Rescuer position
Perform chest compressions
Open the airway
Perform rescue breathing

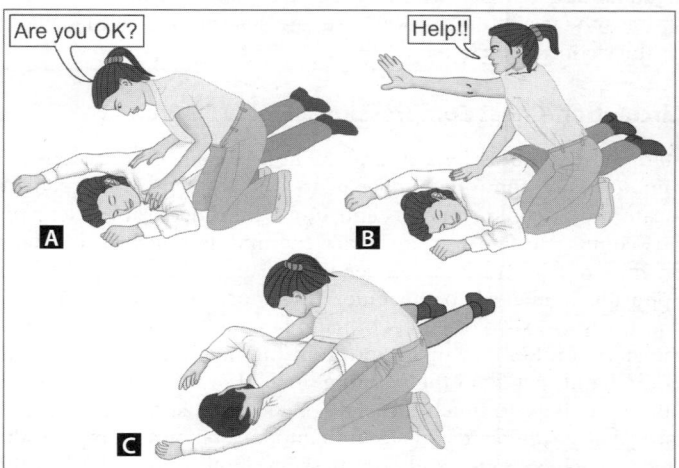

Figs. 15.1A to C: Determining unresponsiveness. **A.** Ensuring victim's status of consciousness; **B.** Calling for assistance; **C.** Positioning victim for further steps.

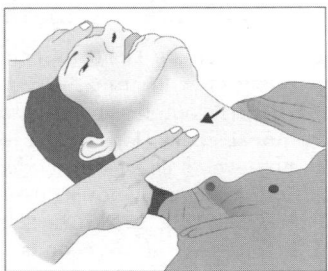

Fig. 15.2: Checking for carotid pulse.

- **Call for help:** If no response, call for help and request someone to get an automated external defibrillator (AED) if available; do not leave the patient to get help
- **Position the victim (mother):** Position the patient on an arrest board or on a flat firm surface on her back; remove pillows and place victim's arms alongside the body
- **Rescuer position (midwife):** To provide BLS, the midwife must stand at a suitable height by the victim's side near her chest or have the victim on the floor and kneel at the side, at the level of the victim's shoulders.

Circulation/Chest Compressions (Figs. 15.3A and B)

Start chest compressions at a rate of at least 100 compressions per minute. Using the index finger nearest to the legs of the patient, locate the lower rib margin and move the fingers up where the ribs connect to the sternum. Place the middle finger of this hand on the notch and index finger next to it. Place the heel of the opposite hand next to the index finger on the sternum. Ensure that the long axis of the heel of hand is parallel to the long axis of the sternum. Remove first hand from the notch and place on top of the hand that is on the sternum. Extend or interlace fingers, do not allow them to touch the chest. Keep arms straight, shoulders directly over the hands on sternum and lock elbows. Compress the chest 2 inches (5 cm) and compression depth of one-third of the chest.

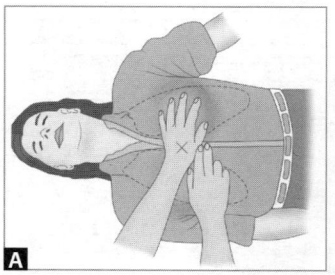 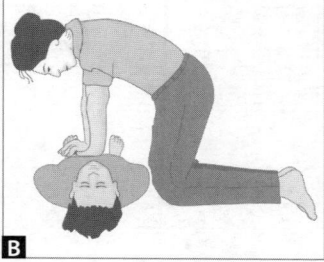

Figs. 15.3A and B: Chest compressions. **A.** Positioning hands for chest compressions; **B.** Positioning of rescuer during cardiac compressions.

Release the external chest compression completely and allow the chest to return to its normal position after each compression. The time allowed for release should be equal to the time required for compression. Do not lift hands off the chest. The rate of compressions should be 30 compressions to 2 ventilations. Re-evaluate the patient after four cycles 'use the mnemonic 1 and 2 and 3...' to keep rhythm and timing. For CPR performed by one or two rescuers the compression rate is 100 per minute.

Airway (Fig. 15.4)

Open the victim's airway by using one of the following maneuvers.

Head Tilt-chin Lift Maneuver

Place one hand on the victim's forehead and apply firm backward pressure with the palm to tilt the head back. Then place the fingers of the other hand under the bony part of the lower jaw near the chin and lift up to bring the jaw forward.

Jaw Thrust Maneuver

Grasp the angles of the patient's lower jaw and lift with both hands, one on each side, displacing the mandible forward.

Mouth to Mouth Maneuver

Provide mouth to mouth respiration, place an airway if available.

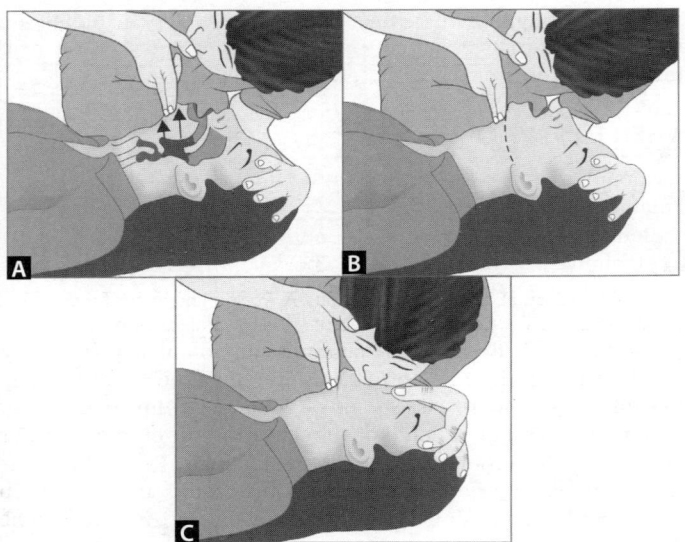

Figs. 15.4A to C: Airway. **A.** Head tilt-chin lift maneuver; **B.** Jaw thrust maneuver; **C.** Providing mouth to mouth respiration.

Breathing

Occlude nostrils with thumb and index finger of the hand on the forehead that is tilting the head back. Form a tight seal over the patient's mouth or place an appropriate respiratory arrest device (Ambu bag and mask) and give two full breaths of approximately 0.5–2 seconds allowing time for both inspiration and expiration.

Observe for rise and fall of chest. Perform two rescue breathing after 30 compressions (the ratio remains the same for single or two person rescuers).

Using Special Resuscitation Equipment (Automated External Defibrillator)

While resuscitation proceeds, simultaneous efforts must be made to obtain and use special resuscitation equipment to manage breathing and circulation, and to provide definitive care. Definitive care includes defibrillation, pharmacotherapy for dysrhythmias and acid-base disturbances, and ongoing monitoring and skilled care in an intensive care unit.

WHEN TO STOP CPR?

Cardiopulmonary resuscitation can be stopped when the following situations occur:
- Return of spontaneous circulation as evidenced by the rescuer obtaining a palpable pulse in the victim or the victim has a normal rhythm in the monitor
- Arrival of code team or medical help
- Exhaustion of rescuer
- When victim is pronounced dead.

16. BIOPHYSICAL PROFILE

The biophysical profile (BPP) is a noninvasive dynamic assessment of the fetus and fetal environment.

PARAMETERS

The BPP consists of five parameters **(Table 16.1)**:
- Fetal heart rate reactivity
- Fetal breathing movements
- Gross body movements
- Fetal tone
- Amniotic fluid volume.

Each area receives a score of '0' (absent) or 2 (present) based on established criteria. Therefore, BPP evaluates fetal status using a methodology modeled after the Apgar score, a numerical expression of the condition of newborn.

TIMING AND INDICATIONS

The decision to perform a BPP is usually taken after a non-reassuring finding on a non-stress test. In response to systemic hypoxia, the fetus demonstrates alterations in movement, muscular tone and heart rate pattern. Normal biophysical activities indicate a functional central nervous system (CNS).

Table 16.1: Biophysical profile variables and scoring criteria.

Variable	Normal score = 2	Abnormal score = 0
Fetal breathing movements	One or more episodes of 30 sec duration during the 30 min testing period	Absent or breathing movement of < 30 sec duration
Gross body movement	A minimum of three discrete body or limb movements during the 30 min test period	Less than 3 fetal movements during the test period
Fetal tone	One or more episodes of active extension with return to flexion of fetal limbs or trunk or opening and closing of the hand	Slow extension with return to flexion, movement of limb in full extension or absence of movement
Amniotic fluid volume index	One or more pockets of amniotic fluid measuring ≥ 1 cm in two perpendicular planes	Pockets of amniotic fluid are < 1 cm or absent
Non-stress test	Reactive	Nonreactive

Note: Adapted from 'Dynamic ultrasound-Based Fetal Assessment: The fetal biophysical profile score' by Manning F.A. Clinical Obstetrics and gynecology. 1995:38;26-34.

PATIENT PREPARATION

The BPP is indicated as a result of a non-reassuring finding from a previous fetal surveillance test. Therefore a primary area of client preparation is emotional support, education and counseling in the face of a potential pregnancy crisis.

PROCEDURE

Level-II or comprehensive ultrasonography is used to examine the variables of the test. A nonstress test (NST) is completed before the ultrasound examination.

A BPP score of 8–10 is normal, a score of 6 is equivocal (inconclusive) and a score of 4 or less indicates fetal compromise.

The biophysical activities of the fetus provide a reflexion of CNS activity because the CNS is among the tissues most sensitive to altered oxygen supply.

Progressive fetal hypoxia is manifested as loss of biophysical functions. The multiple-variable input of the BPP scoring system improves the specificity and sensitivity of the technique compared with the use of single variable surveillance techniques. Thus BPP is an accurate indicator of impending fetal crisis.

Follow-up

When the BPP score is low, induced labor is considered. When the BPP score is normal, intervention is indicated only for specific obstetrical or maternal factors.

17. BIRTH INJURIES IN NEWBORNS

Birth injuries/trauma in newborns are described under the headings listed in **Box 17.1**:

INJURIES TO HEAD

Cephalhematoma

A cephalhematoma is an effusion of blood under the periosteum, which covers the skull bones. During vaginal birth if there is friction between the fetal skull and the bones of the maternal pelvis, the periosteum is torn from the bone causing bleeding underneath **(Fig. 17.1)**.

Box 17.1: Birth injuries in newborns.

Injuries to the head
Injuries to skin and superficial tissues
Injuries to muscle
Nerve injuries
Fractures

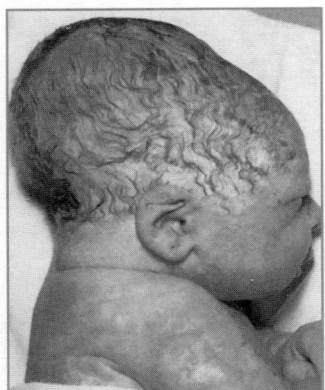

Fig. 17.1: Cephalhematoma.

Predisposing Circumstances

- Cephalopelvic disproportion
- Precipitate labor.

Presentation

- Unilateral: Confined to one bone
- Bilateral/double hematoma: On both sides.

The swelling appears after 12 hours, grows larger over subsequent few days and may persist for weeks. The swelling is circumscribed, does not pit on pressure and does not cross a suture line.

Management

No treatment is required. The blood is absorbed and swelling subsides. Hyperbilirubinemia may occur when the blood gets absorbed.

Subaponeurotic Hemorrhage

Under the scalp, the epicranial aponeurosis is pulled away from the periosteum of the skull bones and bleeding occurs between the two with a resultant swelling **(Fig. 17.2)**.

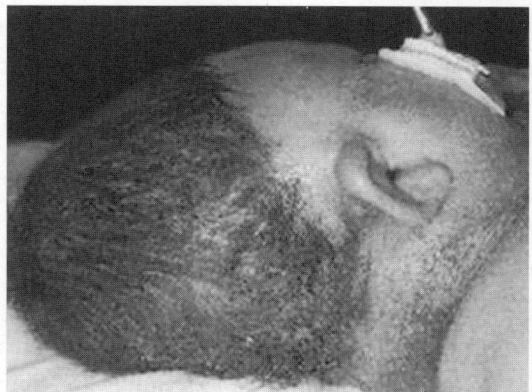

Fig. 17.2: Subaponeurotic hemorrhage.

Predisposing Circumstances

- Vacuum extraction
- Normal vaginal birth.

Presentation

The swelling is seen at birth, increases in size, and is a firm, fluctuant mass. It can cross suture lines and the swelling can extend into the subcutaneous tissue of neck and eyelids. Bruising may be seen for days and weeks. Blood gets reabsorbed and the swelling subsides in 2–3 weeks.

Management

No treatment is required. Hyperbilirubinemia may complicate the recovery.

Note: If the bleeding is severe, the baby will show signs of shock and require supportive care.

Subdural Hemorrhage

When there is trauma to the fetal head involving excessive compression, abnormal stretching and eventually tearing of the dura occurs

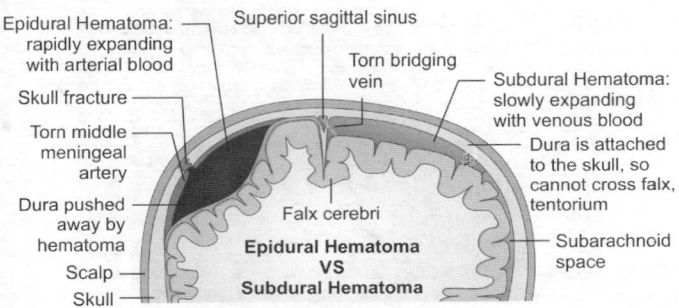

Fig. 17.3: Epidural and Subdural hematoma.

leading to rupture of the venous sinuses and the development of subdural hemorrhage **(Fig. 17.3).**

Predisposing Circumstances

- Rapid, abnormal or excessive molding such as in precipitate labor or rapid birth
- Malpositions and malpresentations
- Cephalopelvic disproportion
- Undue compression during forceps application.

Presentation

- The baby with a large subdural hemorrhage is likely to have severe asphyxia
- As the blood accumulates, the baby develops cerebral irritation, cerebral edema and raised intracranial pressure
- Vomiting, non-response, a bulging anterior fontanelle, abnormal eye movements, apnea, bradycardia and convulsions are likely to occur.

Management

- Supportive treatment for controlling the consequences of asphyxia and intracranial pressure

- Subdural taps to drain large collections of blood
- This type of hemorrhage can be fetal.

Scalp Injuries

Minor Injuries

Minor injuries of the scalp such as abrasions caused by forceps, incised wound inflicted during cesarean section or episiotomy occur occasionally. The incised wound may bleed and require stitches on occasion. The wound should be dressed with antiseptics.

Fracture Skull

Fracture of the vault of the skull (frontal or parietal bone) as a fissure or depression may occur following wrong application of forceps and delivery through a flat pelvis with projected sacral promontory.

The fracture may be associated with cephalhematoma, extradural or subdural hemorrhage or a hematoma. Fissure fracture if uncomplicated is symptomless. With depressed fracture, neurological symptoms may occur later. Treatment is conservative in symptomless cases. In presence of symptoms, the depressed bone has to be elevated or the hematoma to be aspirated or excised surgically.

INJURIES TO SKIN AND SUPERFICIAL TISSUES

Skin Injuries

Forceps blades usually cause bruises and lacerations on the face. These are treated with antiseptics (cleaning). These heal well without leaving behind any trace of injury.

Bruise and Edema of Scalp

Bruise and edema of scalp (caput succedaneum) occur if the head remains on the perineum for a long period. In breech presentation this occurs on buttocks and in face presentation eyelids, lips or nose become edematous and congested. No treatment is required **(Fig. 17.4)**.

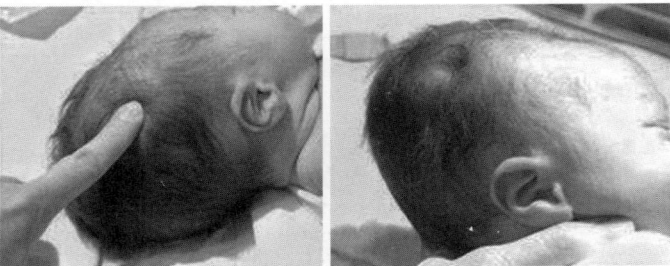

Fig. 17.4: Caput succedaneum.

INJURIES TO MUSCLES

Sternomastoid Hematoma

Appears about 7–10 days after birth and is usually situated at the junction of upper and middle third of the muscle. It is caused by rupture of the muscle fibers and blood vessels causing hematoma.

It is associated with difficult breech delivery or excessive lateral flexion of the neck during normal delivery. There is transient torticollis. Gentle movements with stretching of neck muscles after feeds are helpful. Massaging should be avoided. The swelling disappears by 6 months of age.

Necrosis of the Subcutaneous Tissue

It may occur with superficial skin remaining intact. Small, hard, subcutaneous nodule appears few days after birth. It is the result of fat necrosis due to pressure and takes several weeks to disappear. No treatment is required.

NERVE INJURIES

Facial Palsy (Fig. 17.5)

Damage of the facial nerve usually results from its compression against the ramus of the mandible by a forceps blade, resulting in a unilateral facial palsy.

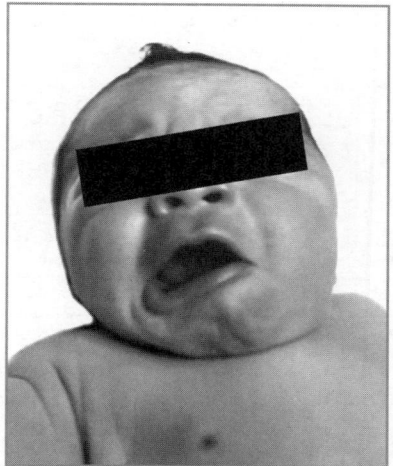

Fig. 17.5: Facial palsy (mouth drawn over to the normal side).

There is unilateral facial weakness with the eyelid of the affected side remaining open and the mouth drawn over to the normal side. There is no specific treatment. If the eyelid remains open, it is protected with antiseptic ointment. Feeding difficulties are overcome with the baby's own adaptation. Spontaneous resolution occurs in 7–10 days.

Brachial Palsy

Trauma to the nerve roots or trunk of the brachial plexus is involved. This results from excessive lateral flexion, rotation or traction of the head and neck during a birth by breech or when shoulder dystocia occurs. This can lead to three main injuries.

Erb's Palsy (Fig. 17.6)

There is damage to the upper brachial plexus involving 5th and 6th cervical nerve roots. The baby's affected arm is inwardly rotated, the

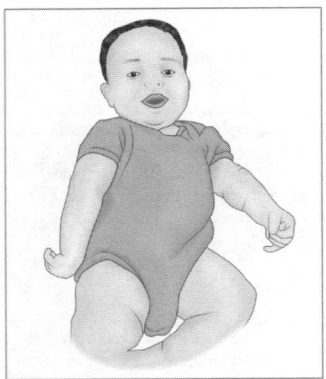

Fig. 17.6: Erb's palsy (affected arm rotated inwardly).

elbow is extended, the wrist is pronated and flexed and the hand is partially closed (waiter's tip position). Moro reflex and biceps jerks are absent on the affected side. Massage and passive movements are advocated. Full recovery takes weeks or months. Severe injury may produce permanent disability.

Klumpke's Palsy

There is damage to the lower brachial plexus involving the 7th and 8th cervical and the first thoracic nerve roots. The upper arm has normal movement, but the lower arm, wrist and hand are affected. There is wrist drop and flaccid paralysis of the hand with no grasp reflex. Treatment consists of splinting the arm with the forearm pronated and the fingers extended.

Total Brachial Plexus Palsy

There is damage to all the brachial plexus nerve roots. There is complete paralysis of the arm and hand, with a lack of sensation and circulatory problems. If there is bilateral paralysis, spinal injury should be suspected. X-ray and/or ultrasound examination of the clavicle, arm, chest and cervical spine, and assessment of the joints are to be done. Passive movements of joints and limb should be initiated under the direction of a physiotherapist.

FRACTURES

Types

Skull Bone Fractures

These fractures are already described in 'Injuries to Head' topic.

Clavicle

Fracture of clavicle can occur if there is shoulder dystocia or during a birth by breech. The affected bone is usually the one which is nearest the maternal symphysis pubis. It is possible to feel a distortion in the bone and crepitus or callus formation during an examination.

Humerus

Mid-shaft fracture can occur with shoulder dystocia or during birth of baby by the breech when the extended arm is brought down and born. Considerable deformity is evident on examination and the baby will be reluctant to move the arm owing to pain.

Femur

Mid-shaft fractures can occur during a birth by the breech when the extended legs are brought down and born. Considerable deformity is evident on examination and the baby will be reluctant to move the leg owing to pain.

Management and Care

In case of suspected fractures, an X-ray examination can confirm the diagnosis. The baby is likely to experience pain; therefore careful handling, cleansing and changing of dress are required.

Positioning on the affected side or back is more comfortable for the baby. Mild analgesia may also be appropriate. Fracture of clavicle requires no specific treatment. Bandaging using a splint is done for fracture of femur. Splinting the arm to the chest with a bandage is done for fracture of humerus. Stable union of a fractured clavicle usually occurs in 7–10 days, while the humerus and the femur take 2–3 weeks.

18. BREASTFEEDING

Breast care and preparation for breastfeeding begin in the antepartal period.

BREAST CARE MEASURES

Breast care measures for continuing lactation and preventing engorgement are as follows:
- Begin breastfeeding as soon as possible after delivery (within one hour of delivery)
- Nurse the baby every 2–3 hours without missing any feeding or using any supplements
- Use both breasts at each feeding. Start on the breast used last during the previous feeding allowing each breast to get emptied
- Allow the baby to suck on each breast for 5–10 minutes to start with and then build up to complete emptying of one breast (about 20 minutes) before switching on to the other to finish the feeding
- Apply warmth to breasts, especially prior to each breastfeeding, using warm clothes, or warm shower, to promote milk flow
- If there is areolar enlargement, do manual expression of the milk to soften the areola prior to nursing the baby
- Use manual expression of milk to empty the breasts after the baby has nursed if they are still uncomfortable, full and engorged after the feeding
- Maintain good support to the breasts without any pressure points.

Care of Breast and Nipple

- Wash only with water (especially the nipples) and no soap, alcohol or drying agents as they can cause cracking of the nipples
- Expose nipples to air for 15–20 minutes after a feeding

- Following exposure, rub in a nipple cream, A and D ointment or hydrous lanolin
- If nipples become tender:
  - Enhance the letdown before feeding, with warmth
  - Nurse on the less sore nipple first until there is letdown, then switch the baby to the sore nipple. Finish the feeding with the less sore nipple
  - Breastfeed more frequently for shorter periods of time
  - Change the baby's position for feeding, which will change the pressure points on the nipple, e.g. shifting from an arm hold to a football hold.
- Be sure to break the suction before removing the baby from the breast.

PREPARATION BEFORE BREASTFEEDING

For Mother

The mother should be prepared for each breastfeeding by taking the following measures:
- Be in a comfortable position, which allows for proper positioning of her baby; this can be accomplished in a side lying, reclining, or sitting position with generous use of pillows **(Figs. 18.1A to E)**
- Take measures to be free of after-birth pains or episiotomy or laceration repair pain
- Have the bladder emptied prior to feeding
- Be rested and relaxed
- Wash hands and clean the nipples by gently wiping them off with plain water.

For Baby

Preparation of the baby for breastfeeding includes the following steps:
- Have a clean, dry diaper on the baby; If swaddle wrapping is used, have it loose enough to permit freedom of legs
- Hold the baby with the head and body well supported

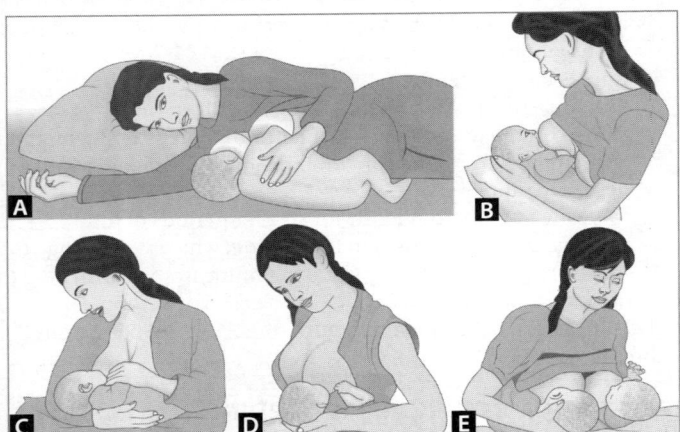

Figs. 18.1A to E: Breast feeding positions. **A.** Feeding in lying down position; **B.** Holding the baby across the lap; **C.** Holding the baby across the lap supporting with the arm; **D.** Holding the baby underarm, sitting on edge of bed; **E.** Positioning twin babies underarm.

- Hold the breast and shape it in a way that facilitates the baby's grasping it and let the baby find the breast and grasp the nipple. Touch the baby's cheek with the nipple and the baby will turn towards the breast (use of the rooting reflex)
- Express a few drops of milk so that they are on the surface of the nipple; this provides the baby with instant gratification
- Guide the baby to grasp more than just the nipple; the baby must compress the areola with his gums in order to obtain colostrum or milk (Mother would feel the rhythmic movements of compression, sucking and swallowing and a steady pull as the feeding continues)
- Babies usually will suck a bit, rest a bit and then suck some more, maintaining their hold on the nipple
- Suction must be broken by slipping a finger into the corner of the baby's mouth and between the baby's gums to avoid injury to the nipple from pulling the baby off
- Once removed from the breast, the baby must be burped before putting on other breast and at the end of feeding **(Figs. 18.2A to C)**.

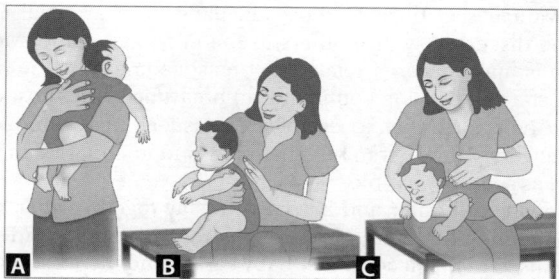

Figs. 18.2A to C: Burping positions. **A.** Upright position on mother's shoulder; **B.** Sitting position on mother's lap; **C.** Prone position on mother's lap.

BABY-FRIENDLY HOSPITAL INITIATIVE

In 1989, World Health Organization (WHO) and United Nations Children's Fund (UNICEF) issued a joint statement to protect, promote and support breastfeeding during maternity services. Based on this statement, 'ten steps' to breastfeeding were formulated. These ten steps are the basic of Baby-Friendly Hospital initiative. Every hospital providing maternity services and care of the newborns should:

- Have a written breastfeeding policy, which is communicated to all health care staff
- Train all health care staff in skills necessary to implement this policy
- Inform all pregnant women about benefits and management of breastfeeding
- Help mothers initiate breastfeeding within half an hour of birth
- Show mothers how to breastfeed and maintain lactation even when they are separated from their infants
- Give newborns no food or drink other than breastmilk unless medically indicated
- Practice rooming-in; allow mothers and newborns to remain together 24 hours a day
- Encourage breastfeeding on demand
- Give no artificial teats or pacifiers
- Foster establishment of breastfeeding support groups.

Advantages of breastfeeding and dangers of artificial feeding must be discussed with mothers in the antenatal clinic. Mother's questions and concerns related to breastfeeding must be cleared so that she will develop confidence to breastfeed. The most crucial time to help a mother to establish breastfeeding is immediately after delivery. Allow her to hold her baby and to initiate skin to skin contact as soon as possible.

Allowing a mother and her baby to stay together after birth is called rooming-in. This practice helps the mother to understand and get used to the needs of her baby earlier and increases bonding between her and her baby. Rooming-in enables a mother to breastfeed her baby on demand.

A baby should get feeds whenever he wants throughout the day and night and not just during specified timings only. A mother does not have to wait for a baby to cry. She can learn to respond to signs such as rooting, which show that her baby is ready for feeding. A baby should feed for as long as he wants.

19. BREAST CANCER

Breast cancer is malignant tumor that starts in the cells of the breast. A malignant tumor is a group of cancer cells that can grow into (invade) surrounding tissues or spread (metastasize) to a distant area of the body. The disease occurs most entirely in women, but men can also get it.

Breast cancer is the second most prevalent cancer in women. The chance of developing breast cancer for an average 40-year-old woman is 1 in 1000. The risk increases as women get older. There is increase of new cases in the recent years, which were attributed in part to the earlier detection of breast cancer through increased use of breast self-examination (BSE), clinical breast examination and diagnostic screenings, including mammography. Statistical evidence indicates that over an entire life time, a woman's risk for developing breast cancer is 1 in 8. When broken by age the risk by age 39 years is 1 in 209, and it increases to 1 in 24 by age 59. Approximately 80% of breast cancers are diagnosed after 50 years of age (Jemal A, Siegel R, Ward E. 2006).

NORMAL BREAST

The female breast is made up mainly of lobules, which are milk producing glands, ducts that are tiny tubes that carry the milk from the lobules to the nipple and stroma that contain fatty tissue and connective tissue, surrounding the ducts and lobules, as well as blood vessels and lymphatic vessels.

Lymphatic System of Breast (Fig. 19.1)

The lymph system is one way breast cancers can spread. This system has several parts. Lymph nodes are small bean-shaped collections of immune system cells (cells that are important in fighting infections) that are connected by lymphatic vessels. Lymphatic vessels carry clear fluid called lymph away from the breast. Breast cancer cells can enter lymphatic vessels and begin to grow in lymph nodes. Most lymphatic vessels connect to lymph nodes under the arm (axillary lymph nodes) and those above or below the collar bones (supraclavicular or infraclavicular) nodes.

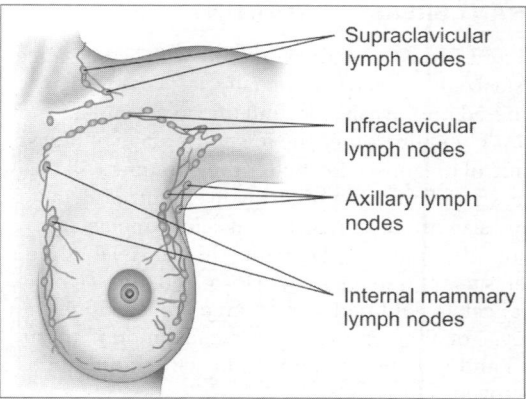

Fig. 19.1: Lymph nodes in relation to breast.

RISK FACTORS OF BREAST CANCER

The risk of breast cancer rises as women age, most notably after the age of 40 years. Risk factors for breast cancer include:
- Family history of breast cancer (first-degree relative, i.e. mother, sister, daughter)
- Biopsy confirmed atypical hyperplasia
- Early menarche (before age of 12 years)
- Late menopause (after age of 55 years)
- Recent use of contraceptives or postmenopausal use of estrogen therapy
- Never having children or having the first child after age of 30 years
- High socioeconomic status and high level of education
- Alcohol consumption of more than 2–5 drinks per day
- Presence of breast cancer (BRCA)-1 or BRCA-2 (genes on chromosome-17) is responsible for majority of inherited breast cancers
- Obesity and high-fat intake (controversial)
- Exposure to chemical carcinogens
- Poor diet and lack of exercise (life-style changes).

MALIGNANT BREAST CONDITIONS

- **Localized breast cancer** is one, in which the cancer has not metastasized (spread), is usually less than 2 cm in size, is considered noninvasive beyond the breast and has potential for the best client outcome. The lower the stage of breast cancer at the time of diagnosis, the better the outcome will be. According to the size of tumor, nodal involvement, and metastasis the Tumor size, node involvement, and metastasis, the TNM (Tumor size, Node involvement, Metastasis) method of staging cancer is used. Management of localized breast cancer, in which the cancer is confined to one area, can include lumpectomy (removal of the tumor and a small amount of surrounding tissue) and radiation therapy. Adjacent lymph nodes may also be removed.
- **Invasive breast cancer** is that which has extended beyond the local epithelium and has the potential to spread from the breast

to other areas of the body. Invasive cancer meets TNM criteria for stage 2 and 3.

- **Metastatic breast cancer** is breast cancer that has spread to other parts of the body. It meets the criterion for TNM stage 4, which is a metastasized tumor of any size. Once metastasis occurs, there is no cure and life expectancy is short. Thus, therapeutic intervention is primarily supportive in nature.

STAGING OF BREAST CANCER

A staging system is a standardized way for cancer care team to summarize the information about how far the tumor has spread. The most common system used to describe the stages of breast cancer is the American Joint Committee on Cancer (AJCC) TNM system. Staging involves classifying the cancer by the extent of disease. Clinical staging involves the physician's estimate of the size of the breast tumor (T), the extent of axillary lymph node involvement (N) and metastasis to distant organs (M). The staging is determined by physical examination and imaging studies.

Stage 0: A precancer state of the breast; Ductal carcinoma in situ (DCIS) and Paget disease of the nipple with no invasion are precancer states of the breast.

Stage 1A: The tumor is 2 cm or less and has not spread to lymph nodes or to distant sites.

Stage 1B: The tumor is 2 cm or less with micrometastasis in 1–3 axillary lymph nodes.

Stage 2A: The tumor is 2 cm or less. Has spread to 1–3 axillary lymph nodes with the tumor in lymph nodes larger than 2 cm or less (sentinel, axillary or mammary lymph nodes).

Stage 2B: The tumor is larger than 2 cm, but less than 5cm. It has spread to 1–3 axillary lymph nodes.

Stage 3A: The tumor is not more than 5 cm. It has spread to 4–9 axillary lymph nodes and no spread to distant sites.

Stage 3B: The tumor has grown into the chest wall or skin. It has spread to 1–3 axillary lymph nodes or it has enlarged the internal mammary glands.

Stage 3C: The tumor is of any size with spread to 10 or more axillary lymph nodes.

Stage 4: The cancer is of any size. It has spread to distant organs or to lymph nodes far from the breast. The most common sites are bone, liver, lung and brain.

CLINICAL MANIFESTATIONS

Breast cancers can occur anywhere in the breast, but are usually found in the upper outer quadrant, where the most breast tissue is located. Generally the lesions are nontender, fixed rather than mobile and hard with irregular borders. With the increased use of mammography more women are seeking treatment at earlier stages of illness. These women often have no signs or symptoms other than a mammography abnormality. Women who ignore symptoms in early stages show up with signs of dimpling, nipple retraction or skin ulceration. Nipple thickening, pain and discharge are seen in patients with Paget disease.

DIAGNOSIS OF BREAST CANCER

Breast Self-examination (Figs. 19.2 and 19.3)

By regularly examining her own breast, a woman is likely to notice any changes that occur. The best time for breast self-examination (BSE) is about a week after periods, when the breasts are not tender or swollen. If the periods are not regular , BSE is best done on the same day of every month. It may be done either in standing position, in front of a mirror or in lying down (supine) position.

Examination in Standing and Supine Positions

Step 1: Stand in front of a mirror with both hands down:
- Standing in front of the mirror, check both breasts for anything unusual. Check for any change in contour of your breasts. Check the upper and outer part of your breast (towards the armpit). This is where half of all breast cancers are found.

Step 2: Standing in front of the mirror, both hands clasped behind head:

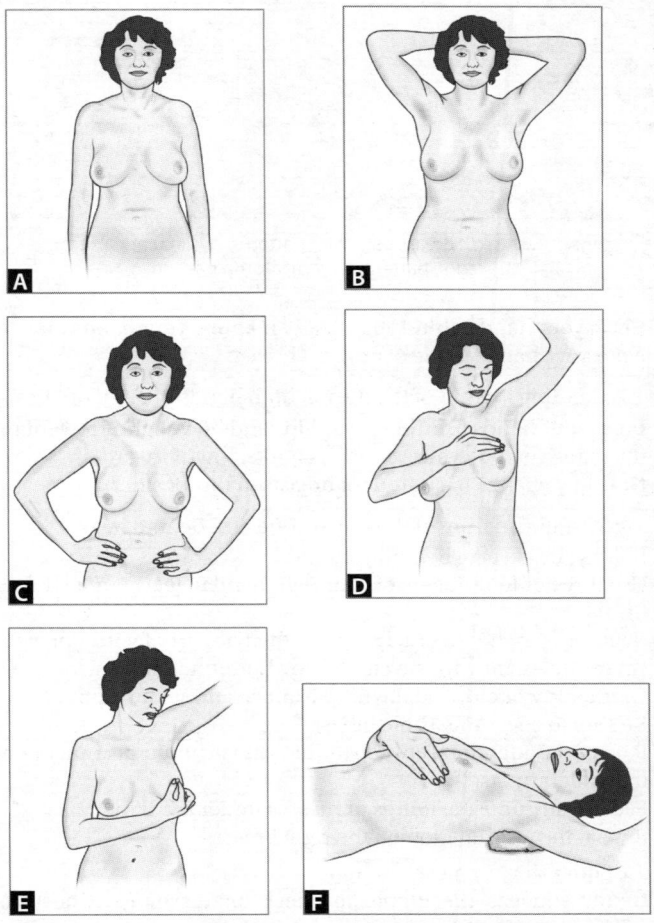

Figs. 19.2A to F: Breast self-examination steps. **A.** Step 1: Standing infront of mirror, both hands down; **B.** Step 2: Infront of mirror hands clasped behind head; **C.** Step 3: Hands pressed on hips; **D.** Step 4: One arm behind head; **E.** Step 5: Squeezing nipple to check for discharge; **F.** Step 6: Examination lying down.

114 Manual of Midwifery and Gynecological Nursing

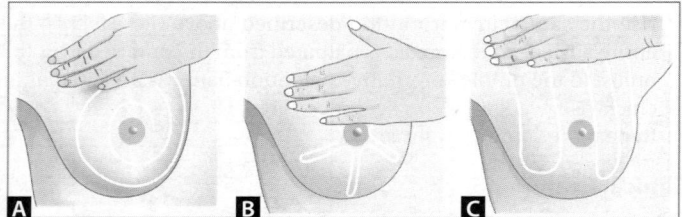

Figs. 19.3A to C: Breast palpation patterns. **A.** Circular pattern; **B.** Wedge pattern; **C.** Vertical strip pattern.

- Clasp your hand behind your head and press your hands forward
- Note any change in the contour of breasts.

Step 3: Standing in front of the mirror, both hands pressed on hips:
- Press your hands firmly on your hips and bow slightly toward the mirror as you pull your shoulders and elbows forward
- Note any change in contour of breasts in this position.

Step 4: Standing in front of the mirror, one arm behind head:
- Raise your left arm behind your head
- Use three or four fingers of your right hand to feel your left breast firmly
- Beginning at the outer edge, press the flat part of your fingers in small circles, moving the circles slowly around the breast
- Gradually work toward the nipple and examine the nipple
- Be sure to cover the whole breast
- Pay special attention between the breasts and underarm, including the underarm itself
- Feel for any unusual lumps or masses under the skin
- Repeat the examination on the right breast.

Step 5: Squeezing nipples:
- Gently squeeze the nipple to check for discharge. Check for puckering, dimpling or scaling of the skin.

Step 6: Examination in lying down position:
- Lie flat on your back with your left arm over head and a pillow or folded towel under your left shoulder; this position flattens the breast and makes it easier to check)

- Use the same circular motion described above (i.e. Step 4); the entire surface of the breast is palpated from the outer edge of the breast to the nipple; alternative palpation patterns are circular or clockwise, wedge and vertical strip **(Figs. 19.3A to C)**
- Repeat the same on right breast.

Clinical Examination

Physical Assessment

When a patient presents with breast problem, the health care personnel conducts a general health assessment including history of cancer, obstetric history, present medications and use of hormonal contraceptives, hormonal therapy or fertility treatment.

Inspection of Breasts

The breasts are inspected for size and symmetry. The skin is inspected for color, thickening or edema. Erythema (redness) may indicate benign local inflammation or a superficial lymphatic invasion by a neoplasm. To identify dimpling or retraction, the patient is instructed to raise both arms overhead as well as place her hands on her waist and push in. Changes seen during these suggest underlying mass.

Palpation

The breasts are examined with the patient sitting up (upright) and lying down (supine). The entire surface of the breast and axillary tail is systematically palpated using the pads of 2nd, 3rd and 4th fingers held together making small circles. The axillary lymph nodes are examined for size, location, mobility and consistency.

Mammography (Fig. 19.4)

Mammography is a breast-imaging technique, which can detect non-palpable lesions and assist in diagnosing palpable masses. The breast is mechanically compressed from top to bottom (craniocaudal view) and side to side (medio-lateral and oblique view) for obtaining pictures. Women may experience some fleeting discomfort because maximum compression is necessary for proper

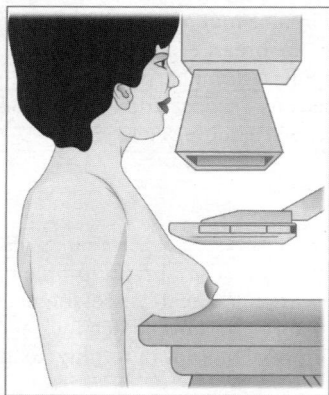

Fig. 19.4: Mammography examination.

visualization. Mammography may detect a breast tumor before it is clinically palpable, i.e. smaller than 1 cm.

Ultrasonography

Ultrasonography (ultrasound) is used as a diagnostic adjunct to mammography to help distinguish fluid-filled cysts from other lesions. A thin coating of lubricating jelly is spread over the area to be imaged. A transducer is then placed on the breast. The transducer transmits high-frequency sound waves through the skin toward the area of concern. The technique diagnoses cysts with accuracy, but cannot rule out definitively the presence of malignant lesions.

Magnetic Resonance Imaging (Fig. 19.5)

Magnetic resonance imaging (MRI) is a highly sensitive and useful diagnostic adjunct to mammography. An intravenous (IV) injection of gadolinium, a contrast dye is given to improve visibility. The patient lies face down and the breast is placed through a depression in the table. A coil is placed around the breast and the patient is placed inside the MRI machine. The procedure takes about 30–40 minutes.

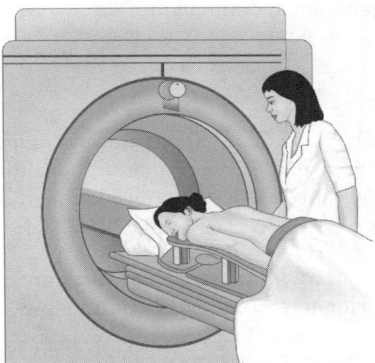

Fig. 19.5: Magnetic resonance imaging (MRI) of breast.

Percutaneous Biopsy

Fine needle aspiration (FNA) is a noninvasive biopsy technique that is generally well-tolerated by most women. For palpable masses, a surgeon performs this procedure. A small gauge needle (25 or 22G) attached to a syringe is inserted into the mass or area of nodularity. Suction is applied to the syringe and multiple passes are made through the mass. Any cellular material obtained in the hub of the needle is spread on a glass slide or placed in a preservative and sent to the laboratory for analysis.

Core Needle Biopsy

This procedure is similar to FNA except a larger gauge needle is used (usually 14G). A local anesthetic is applied and tissue cores are removed via a spring loaded device. The procedure allows more definitive diagnosis than FNA, because actual tissue and not just cells are removed. It is often performed for relatively large tumors that are close to the skin. Ultrasound guided core biopsy and MRI guided core biopsy are newer diagnostic techniques.

Surgical Biopsy

Surgical biopsy is usually performed using local anesthesia and IV sedation. After an incision is made, the lesion is excised an sent to a laboratory for pathologic examination. Two types of surgical biopsy are excision and incision.

Excision Biopsy

Excision biopsy is the standard procedure for complete pathological assessment of a palpable breast mass. The entire mass, plus a margin of surrounding tissue is removed. This may be referred to as a lumpectomy. A frozen section analysis of the specimen may be performed at the time of biopsy by the pathologist who does an immediate reading intraoperatively and provides a provisional diagnosis for a patient who had no previous tissue analysis.

Incision Biopsy

Incision biopsy surgically removes a portion of a mass. This is done to confirm a diagnosis and to conduct special studies. This is often performed on women with locally advanced breast cancer or on women with suspected recurrence, whose treatment may depend on the results of special studies. This procedure is less common as core needle biopsy may give the same information.

TYPES OF BREAST CANCER

Ductal Carcinoma In Situ

Ductal carcinoma is a type of cancer that is characterized by the proliferation of malignant cells inside the milk ducts without invasion into the surrounding tissues. Therefore, it is a non-invasive form of cancer and is also called as intraductal carcinoma. Ductal carcinoma in situ (DCIS) is frequently manifested on mammogram with the appearance of calcifications and it is considered breast cancer stage '0'. If DCIS is left untreated there is an increased likelihood that it will progress to invasive cancer. The most traditional treatment is total or simple mastectomy (removal of breast only) with a cure rate of 98–99%. Addition of the medication tamoxifen (Nolvadex) significantly reduced local recurrence rates after surgery and radiation. The medication is usually prescribed for 5 years.

Invasive Cancer

Infiltrating ductal carcinoma: This is the most common histological type of breast cancer and accounts for 75% of all cases. The tumors arise from the duct system and invade the surrounding tissues. They often form a solid irregular mass in the breast **(Fig. 19.6)**.

Infiltrating lobular carcinoma: This type of carcinoma accounts for about 5–10% of breast cancers, The tumors arise from the lobular epithelium and typically occur as an area of ill-defined thickening in the breast. The are often multicentric and can be bilateral.

Medullary carcinoma: This accounts for about 5% of breast cancers, and it tends to be diagnosed more often in women less than 50 years. The tumors grow in a capsule inside a duct. They can become large and may be mistaken for a fibroadenoma. The prognosis is often favorable.

Mucinous carcinoma: This accounts for about 3% of breast cancers and often presents in postmenopausal women 75 years and older. A mucin producer, the tumor is also slow growing and thus the prognosis is more favorable than in many other types.

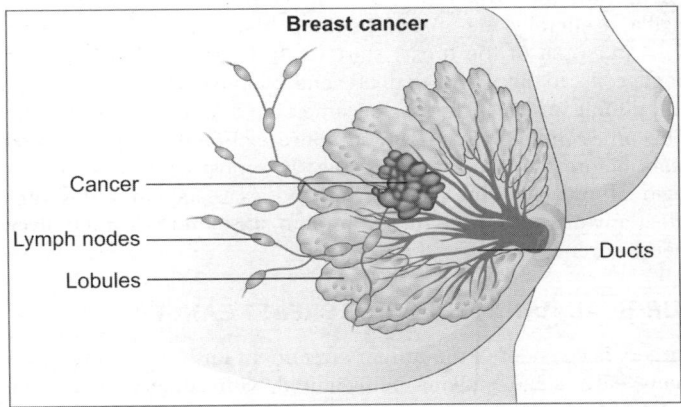

Fig. 19.6: Breast cancer.

Tubular ductal carcinoma: This type of carcinoma accounts for about 2% of breast cancers. Because axillary metastases are uncommon with this histology, prognosis is usually excellent.

Inflammatory carcinoma: This is rear (1-2%) and aggressive type that has unique symptoms. The cancer is characterized by diffuse edema and brawny erythema of the skin, resembling an orange peel. This is due to malignant cells blocking the lymph channels in the skin. An associated mass may or may not be present. The disease can spread to other parts of the body rapidly. Chemotherapy is usually given to control the disease progression, but radiation and surgery may also be useful.

Paget disease of breast: This accounts for 1% of diagnosed breast cancer cases. Symptoms typically include a scaly, erythematous, pruritic lesion of the nipple. Paget disease often represents DCIS of the nipple, but may have an invasive component.

PROGNOSIS

The two most important factors considered, while determining the prognosis of patient with breast cancer are: The tumor size and whether the tumor has spread to the lymph nodes under the arm (axilla). Generally, the smaller the tumor, the better is the prognosis.

Carcinoma of the breast starts with a genetic alteration in a single cell and takes time to divide and double in size. A carcinoma may double in size 30 times to became 1 cm or larger, at which point it becomes clinically apparent. Tumors are often present for several years before they become palpable. The most common route of regional spread is to the axillary lymph nodes. Distant metastasis can affect any organ, but the most common sites are bone, lung, liver, pleura adrenals, skin and brain.

SURGICAL MANAGEMENT OF BREAST CANCER

Surgery is considered the primary treatment for breast cancer with many early stage patients being cured with surgery alone. The goals of breast cancer surgery include the complete resection of the primary tumor, with negative margins to reduce the risk of local recurrences, and pathologic staging of the tumor and axillary lymph nodes to provide necessary prognostic information. Several different types of surgeries are available for the treatment of breast cancer.

Different types of surgeries are available for treatment of breast cancer. Surgical removal of breast is termed mastectomy.

MASTECTOMY

Mastectomy is a surgery to remove the breast. Sometimes other tissues near the breast, such as lymph nodes, are also removed. Surgery is most often used to treat breast cancer. In some cases, a mastectomy is done to help prevent breast cancer for those who have a high risk for it. This includes women with genes linked to breast cancer, such as $BRCA_1$ or $BRCA_2$ gene.

Types of Mastectomy Procedures

- Total (simple) mastectomy.
  This method removes the whole breast, including the nipple, areola and most of the overlying skin.
- Modified radical mastectomy.
  This includes the nipple, the areola, the overlying skin, and the lining over the chest muscles. Some of the lymph nodes under the arm are also removed. In some cases part of the chest wall muscle is also removed.
- Radical mastectomy
  The entire breast is removed including the nipple, the areola, the overlying skin, and the lymph nodes under the arm and the chest muscles under the breast. This method is advised when breast cancer has spread to the chest muscles **(Fig. 19.7)**.
- Skin sparing and nipple sparing mastectomies are done when breast reconstruction is done right after mastectomy

Risks of Mastectomy

Some possible complications of mastectomy include:
- Short-term breast swelling.
- Breast soreness.
- Hardness due to scar tissue that can form at the site of the incision.
- Wound infection or bleeding.

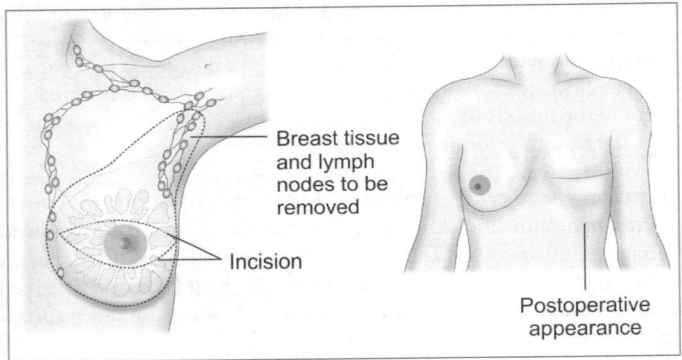

Fig. 19.7: Modified radical mastectomy.

- Lymph edema of the arm if lymph nodes were removed.
- Phantom breast pain.
  This may be helped with medicine, exercise and massage.
- A clear fluid (seroma) is often found in the breast after mastectomy. It can be drained in the surgeon's office. It can then be treated with compression.
- A pulling feeling near or under the arm after surgery.
- Depression and feelings of loss of sexual identity may occur after a mastectomy.

Problems after Lymph Node Removal

- Problems with lymphatic drainage can cause swelling (Lymphedema) in the affected arm.
- There is greater risk for infection from injury to the arm.
- There is a higher risk for blood clots in the armpit veins after surgery to the area.

Safety Steps Include

- No needlesticks or IVs placed in the affected arm.
- No blood pressure measurements in the affected arm.
- Follow instructions about arm exercises carefully.

- Avoid injuries such as scratches or splinters to the affected arm.
- Elevate the arm, with your hand above your elbow periodically, to help drain lymphatic fluid.
- Wear gloves when doing activities where there is a chance to get a cut in the fingers or hands and when using strong chemicals such as detergents or household cleaners.
- Avoid wearing any tight items on the affected arm such as elastic cuffs, tight wrist-watch, etc.
- Use the unaffected arm or both arms to carry heavy packages or bags.
- Avoid insect bites or stings by using insect repellents or wearing long sleeves.

Radiation Therapy

Radiation therapy is used to decrease the chance of a local recurrence in the breast by irradiating residual microscopic cancer cells. Breast conservation treatment followed by radiation therapy for Stage I and II breast cancer results in a survival rate equal to that of modified radical mastectomy (Fisher et al, 2002).

External beam radiation is the most common type, which begins about six weeks after breast surgery. If systemic chemotherapy is indicated, radiation therapy usually begins after its completion. External beam radiation, which delivers high energy photons from a linear accelerator, is administered to the entire region. Each treatment lasts only a few minutes and generally given 5 days a week for 5-6 weeks.

Another approach is intraoperative radiation therapy (IORT) in which a single intense dose of radiation is delivered to surgical site in the operating room immediately following the lumpectomy. This method of radiation is indicated for women at high-risk for cancer recurrence, i.e. chest wall involvement, four or more positive nodes and tumors larger than 5 cm.

Generally, radiation therapy is well-tolerated. Acute side effects consist of mild to moderate erythema, breast edema and fatigue. Occasionally skin breakdown may occur. These side effects usually dissolve within a few weeks to a few months.

Self-care instructions: This instructions are given for patients receiving radiation include:

- Use mild soap with minimal rubbing
- Avoid deodorants and perfumed soaps
- Use hydrophilic lotions (water dissolving) such as Eucerin, Lubriderm or Aquaphor
- Avoid tight clothes, excessive temperatures and ultraviolet light
- Use nondrying soap if pruritus occurs.

Sun exposure to the treated area to be minimized and use of sunscreen lotion with 15 or above SPF is advised. Momentary sharp or shooting pain of minor degrees are normal after radiation.

Chemotherapy (Systemic)

Chemotherapy as an adjuvant therapy and involves the use of anti-cancer agents in addition to other treatments (i.e. surgery, radiation) to delay or prevent recurrence of breast cancer. It is considered for patients who have positive lymph nodes or invasive tumors.

Chemotherapy regimen combines several agents (polychemotherapy)P generally administered over a period of 3–6 months. A regimen of cyclophosphamide, methotrexate and fluorouracil is usually given to patients who are at a low-risk of recurrence. A combination of cyclophosphamide, doxorubicin (Adriamycin) and fluorouracil (CAF) is a combination regimen administered to high-risk patents. Common physical side effects of chemotherapy for breast cancer may include nausea, vomiting, bone marrow suppression, taste changes, alopecia, mucositis, skin changes and fatigue. A weight gain of more than 5 kg occurs in about half of all patients, the cause is unknown.

Hormonal Therapy

The use of adjuvant hormonal therapy, with or without the addition of chemotherapy, is considered in women who have hormone receptor-positive tumors. Its use can be determined by the results of an estrogen and progesterone receptor assay. About two-thirds of breast cancers are found to be estrogen receptor positive. Hormone therapy involves the use of medications that compete with estrogen by binding to the receptor sites or by blocking estrogen production [Selective estrogen receptor modulators (SERMs)]. Premenopausal and perimenopausal women are more likely to have non-hormonal dependent lesions, whereas postmenopausal women are more likely to have hormone-dependent lesions.

Tamoxifen has been the primary hormonal agent used in the treatment of premenopausal and postmenopausal breast cancers. Tamoxifen has estrogen antagonistic (estrogen-blocking) effects on certain tissues. Its effects in the breast prevent estrogen from binding to the receptor sites thus preventing tumor growth. Tamoxifen can also stop the growth and even shrink tumors in women with metastatic breast cancer. It can also be used to reduce the risk of developing breast cancer in women at high-risk.

Side effects of adjuvant hormonal therapy include hot flashes, vaginal dryness, nausea and vomiting, risk of thromboembolic events and risk of osteoporosis. Patients need to be instructed to take measures for prevention and management of such conditions.

TARGETED THERAPY (FOR BREAST CANCER)

Targeted therapy is a cancer treatment that uses drugs to target specific genes and proteins that are involved in the growth and survival of cancer cells. Targeted therapy affects the tissue environment that helps a cancer grow and survive or it can target cells related to cancer growth, like blood vessel cells. Doctors often use targeted therapy along with chemotherapy and other treatments.

How does Targeted Therapy Work?

Targeted therapies can do different things to the cancer cells they target.
- Block or turn off signals that tell cancer cells to grow and divide.
- Prevent the cells from living longer than normal.
- Destroy cancer cells.

Types of Targeted Therapy

The most common types are:
- Monoclonal antibodies.
- Monoclonal antibodies block a specific target on the outside of cancer cells. These can also send toxic substances right to cancer

cells. For example, they can help chemotherapy and radiation therapy reach cancer cells better. Monoclonal antibodies are also a type of immunotherapy.
- Small molecule drugs.
- These can block the processes that help cancer cells multiply and spread. Angiogenesis inhibitors are examples for this. Angiogenesis inhibitors block nutrients reaching the cell.

Some types of targeted therapies are specific to a type of cancer. Others are known as tumor-agonistic or site-agonistic treatments. They treat tumors anywhere in the body by focusing on the specific genetic change. About 20 to 25% of breast cancers have too much protein called 'human epidermal growth factor receptor' (HER_2). This protein makes tumor cells grow. If the cancer is "HER_2 positive", targeted therapy is an option.

Limitations of Targeted Therapy

- A targeted treatment will not work if the tumor does not have a target.
- Having the target does not mean the tumor will respond to the drug.
- The response to the treatment may not last over time.
- These drugs may cause serious side effects such as skin, hair, nail or eye problems.

Most people with cancer also need surgery, chemotherapy, radiation therapy or hormone therapy.

Breast Reconstruction After Surgery

Breast reconstruction can provide a significant psychological benefit for women who are struggling with the emotional distress of losing a breast. Consultation with a plastic surgeon can help the patient understand the procedures for which she is a candidate. Factors to consider include body size and shape, physical health and personal habits. Realistic explanation can help the patient avoid unrealistic expectations. Once reconstruction is complete, the opposite breast may require augmentation, reduction or mastopexy to achieve symmetry on both sides.

Prosthetics

Breast prosthesis, an external form, which simulates the breast is another option. Most prosthesis is made of silicone. They can be placed inside a pocket in a bra or can adhere directly to the chest wall. Until the surgical incision is well-healed, i.e. 4–6 weeks, temporary lightweight cotton-filled form can be used. Breast prosthesis can provide a psychological benefit and assist the woman in resuming proper posture, because it helps balance the weight of the remaining breast.

PREVENTION STRATEGIES IN THE HIGH-RISK PATIENTS

American Cancer Society (ACS) recommend following prevention strategies.

Long-term surveillance

This includes clinical breast examination twice a year starting as early as 25 years of age:
- Mammograms from age of 25 years
- Breast self-examination from age of 25 years
- MRI and ultrasound of breasts in addition to screening test. MRI is more sensitive than mammography in BRCA-1 and BRCA-2 carriers (Warner et al, 2004).

Chemoprevention

Chemorprevention is a primary prevention modality that aims at prevention of the disease before it starts. The drug tamoxifen was found to be an effective chemotherapeutic agent (Finsher et al, 1998).

Raloxifene (Evista) is another medication found effective in reducing breast cancer risk with fewer side effects.

Prophylactic Mastectomy

Prophylactic mastectomy is another therapeutic modality found effective in reducing the risk of cancer by 90% (Rebecca et al, 2004). Possible candidates include women with a strong family history of breast cancer, a diagnosis of atypical hyperplasia, BRCA gene mutation and previous cancer in one breast.

NURSING MANAGEMENT

The diagnosis of cancer or its recurrence causes great anxiety in patients about their future and long-term survival. Some patients are more likely than others to experience side effects of certain therapies such as vomiting after chemotherapy and edema after radiation therapy. This allows nurses to reduce their discomforts and teach about appropriate management strategies. The nurse must understand that patients who undergo mastectomy and lymph node dissection may experience problems such as lymphedema, decreased arm mobility and seroma formation (collection of serous fluid) in the axilla and neuropathic sensations with resulting distress. Psychological needs of the patient needs to be addressed also.

Nursing Assessment

Assessment for patients with breast conditions involve careful medical and gynecologic history taking with special emphasis on breast history including symptoms specially suspected of breast conditions, laboratory test results and biopsy reports.

Nursing Diagnoses

Preoperative

Based on the health history and other assessment data, major preoperative nursing diagnoses may include the following:
- Deficient knowledge about the planned surgical treatments
- Anxiety related to the diagnosis of cancer
- Fear related to specific treatments and body image changes
- Risk for ineffective coping (individual or family) related to diagnosis of breast cancer and related treatment options
- Decisional conflict related to treatment options.

Postoperative

Major postoperative nursing diagnoses may include the following:
- Pain and discomfort related to surgical procedure
- Disturbed sensory perception related to nerve irritation in affected arm, breast or chest wall

- Disturbed body image related to loss or alteration of the breast
- Risk for impaired adjustment related to the diagnosis of cancer and surgical treatment
- Self-care deficit related to partial immobility of upper extremity on affected side
- Risk for sexual dysfunction related to loss of body part, change in self-image and fear of partner's responses
- Deficient knowledge regarding drain management following surgery
- Deficient knowledge regarding arm exercises to regain mobility of affected extremity
- Deficient knowledge regarding hand and arm care after an axillary lymph node dissection (ALND).

Expected Outcomes

The major goals of nursing care may include increased knowledge about the disease and its treatment, reduction of preoperative and postoperative fear, anxiety and emotional stress; improvement of decision making ability; pain management; improvement in coping abilities; improvement of sexual function and the absence of complications. Plans for nursing interventions should include specific actions that the client completes to achieve the highest level of wellness possible or to achieve peace regarding the diagnosis.

Nursing Interventions

Nursing interventions should be planned and implemented to achieve the goals listed above in the pre and postoperative periods. Adequate health educations to be provided to enable the patient go home without undue fear and anxiety when discharged from the hospital. Interventions involve educating the clients regarding the diagnosis, consequence, specific procedures, counseling regarding expected outcomes, providing emotional support as well as reducing anxiety, fear and stress. It is important to educate about strategies for promotion of good health, disease prevention and recommendations for regular exercise, healthy eating and scheduling necessary assessments and screening (medical check-ups).

1. Manage pain and promote comfort
   - Assess pain and stiffness of the affected arm and administer narcotics or analgesics as ordered.
   - Consider normality of phantom pain, acknowledge patient's anxiety and provide support.
   - Assist the patient to find position of comfort.
     - Reposition on unaffected side and back.
     - Splint or support chest during coughing and deep breathing exercise.
   - Encourage early ambulation
   - Provide regular wound care and drain care
   - Administer antibiotics as required
   - Encourage patient to use affected arm for personal hygiene such as combing care, washing face and eating.
2. Patient education for hand and arm care after axillary lymph node dissection
   - Avoid obtaining blood pressure reading, injections and blood draws in the affected extremity.
   - Use sunscreen (higher than 15.SPF) for extended exposure to sun
   - Apply insect repellent to avoid insect bites
   - Wear gloves for gardening
   - Wear cooking mitten or a hot pot holder for removing vessels from stove or cook tops.
   - Avoid cutting cuticles and nails too short
   - Use electric razor for shaving arm pits
   - Avoid lifting objects greater than 2 – 4 kg
   - If a trauma or break in the skin occurs, wash the area with soap and water and apply an antibacterial ointment (bacitracin or Neosporin). Observe the area and extremity for 24 hours, if redness, swelling or fever occur, contact physician
3. Encourage to perform hand exercises to maintain movements of the affected arm, to avoid/reduce lymph edema and joint stiffness. Postoperative hand excises are to begin in the first 24 hours in accordance with medical advice and as the patient can tolerate. Hand exercises are to be continued after the patient goes home and she can chose those that are suitable and comfortable for her from the several exercises explained below."

Patient Instructions

1. Begin exercises like deep breathing the day after surgery as appropriate and advised by the doctor.
2. Plan to take pain medications 20 to 30 minutes before starting exercises.
3. Do the exercises three times a day, every day, until you have regained full range of motion in your arm(s).
4. Try to do the exercise daily at the same time as far as possible, for example, before breakfast, lunch and dinner.
5. Wear comfortable, loose clothing.
6. Exercise after a warm shower, whenever possible, when the muscles are warm and relaxed.
7. Breathe deeply and often as you do each exercise.
8. Do the exercise until you feel a slight stretch and no pain.
9. Do not exercise too much in the early weeks following surgery.
10. If you have more pain or discomfort than before, you may be doing too much exercise.

General Guidelines for Exercises

Start the following exercises 3 to 7 days after surgery when your doctor says it is alright.

- Use the hand on your affected side to comb hair, bath, get dressed and eat.
- With your arm raised, open and close your hand 15 – 20 times.
  - Bend and straighten your elbow several times.
  - Bend your elbow and touch your opposite shoulder a few times.
  - Raise your arm up to shoulder height or whatever is tolerable without putting strain on your drains. Repeat 3 to 4 times.
- Practice deep breathing exercise at least six times a day.
  This exercise will help maintain normal movement of chest making it easier for your lungs to work. Further exercise can be started a week or more after surgery after your doctor says it is alright.
- Wear comfortable loose clothing when doing the exercise.
- Do the exercise slowly until you feel a gentle stretch and hold each stretch till the end of the motion and slowly count to five.

- Do each exercise 5 – 7 times and try to do the exercise correctly.
- Do the exercise twice a day until you get back to your normal flexibility. Continuing to do some exercises during the months after surgery can help you keep good mobility of your hand.
- Be sure to take deep breaths, in and out as you do each exercise.
- The exercises are set up so that you start them lying down, move to sitting and finish them standing up.

a. Stage 1 Exercise

These are exercises that can be taken while the drains are still in place.

1. **Pump it up**

   This exercise helps reduce swelling after surgery by using the muscles as a pump to improve the circulation in the affected arm **(Fig. 19.8)**.

   Steps:
   - Patient to lie on the unaffected side with the affected arm straight out, resting on top of a pillow.
   - Slowly bend the elbow while making a fist at the same time.
   - Next, slowly straighten your elbow while opening the fist at the same time.
   - Repeat this pumping motion 15 to 25 times.

2. **Shoulder circles/shoulder rolls**

   This exercise can be done sitting or standing. This can help relieve tension in the shoulders **(Fig. 19.9)**.
   - Lift both shoulders up toward your ears, keeping the chin tucked in slightly.
   - Gently rotate both shoulders forward, arm slowly down and back making a circle.

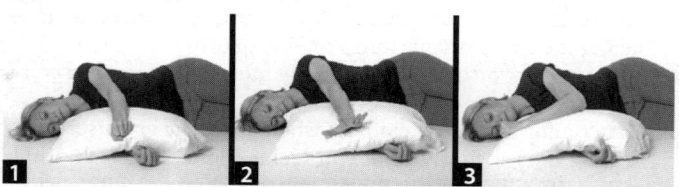

Fig. 19.8: Pump it up exercise.

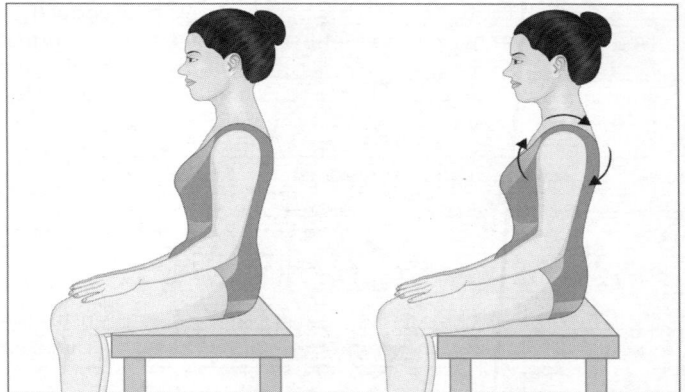

Fig. 19.9: Shoulder circles or shoulder rolls exercise.

- Make five slow circles in one direction, then switch and make five slow circles in the opposite direction.

3. **Arm lifts**

   This exercise can be done sitting or standing, it helps improve movement in shoulders **(Fig. 19.10)**.
   - Clasp the hands together in front of chest. Point the elbows out.
   - Slowly lift the arms upwards until you feel a gentle stretch, but no pain.
   - Hold for 5 to 10 seconds and then slowly return to the start position.
   - Repeat 5 to 10 times.

4. **Shoulder blade squeeze**

   This exercise helps increase your shoulder blade movement **(Fig. 19.11)**.

   This can be done sitting (without resting the back on the chair) or standing.
   - Hold the arms at the side, against body with elbows bent.
   - Slowly bring the elbows straight backwards, while squeezing the shoulder blades together to feel a gentle stretch.
   - Hold this position for 5 to 10 seconds and then slowly return to the start position.

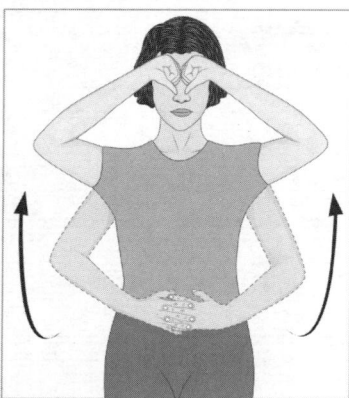

Fig. 19.10: Arm lift exercise.

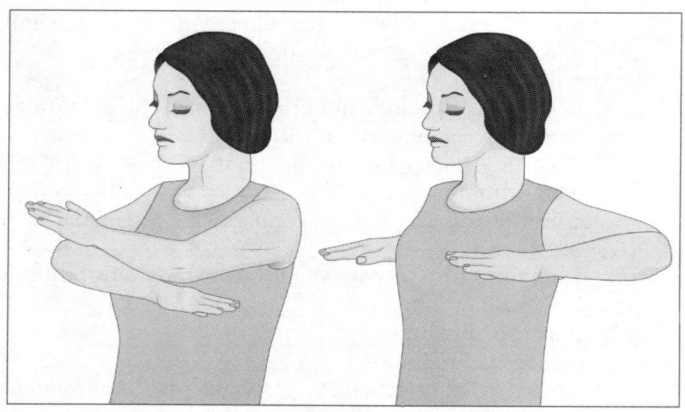

Fig. 19.11: Shoulder blade squeeze exercise.

- Relax your arm(s) and repeat 5-7 times.
- Remember to keep breathing throughout the stretch.

5. **Ball squeezing exercise**

   A rubber ball or a crumpled newspaper is squeezed in the hand of the involved side.

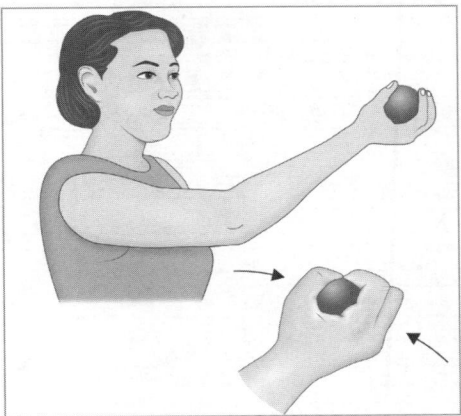

Fig. 19.12: Ball squeezing exercise.

These exercises are to be done after the drain(s) have been removed **(Fig. 19.12)**.
- Hold the ball and squeeze it as hard as possible with thumb and fingers.
- Squeeze for 3 to 5 seconds and then release.
- Perform ten repetitions before doing it with the other hand (if needed).

b. **Stage 2 Exercises**

These exercises are to be done after the drain(s) have been removed.

6. **Wand exercises (external rotation)**

This exercise helps increase your ability to move your shoulders forward **(Fig. 19.13)**.

To do this exercise, a wand (cane) is required – try a broom handle, rod or stick.
- Lie on your back with knees bend. Hold the wand/rod in hands. The hands should be as wide apart as shoulders.
- Lift the wand over the head as far as you can until you feels a stretch. The unaffected arm can be used to lift the wand higher.

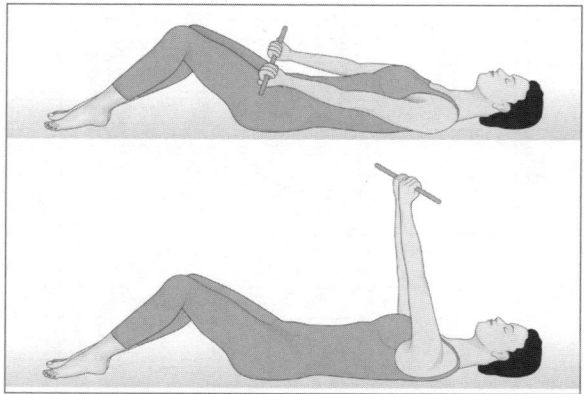

Fig. 19.13: Wand exercise.

- Hold for five seconds, then gently lower arms.
- Repeat 5 to 10 times.

7. **Elbow spread exercise (Winging it exercise)**
   This exercise helps to stretch the front of chest and shoulders. Do the exercise on a bed or floor **(Fig. 19.14)**.
   - Lie on the back with the knees bend.
   - With the fingers touch the ears with the elbows pointed to the ceiling.
   - Move the elbows apart until a stretch is felt, but no pain.
   - Hold this position for 5 to 10 seconds, and then slowly return to the start position.
   - Remember to keep breathing throughout the stretch.

8. **Wall climbing (wall crawling)**
   This exercise help increase movements in shoulders. Try to reach a little higher on the wall each day. This exercise is done in two positions: **[Fig. 19.15(i) and Fig. 19.15(ii)]**:
   1. Facing the wall
   2. With the affected side to the wall (Sidewall stretch).
   a. Facing the wall
      - Stand facing the wall.
      - Place the palm of the hand of affected arm flat on the wall.

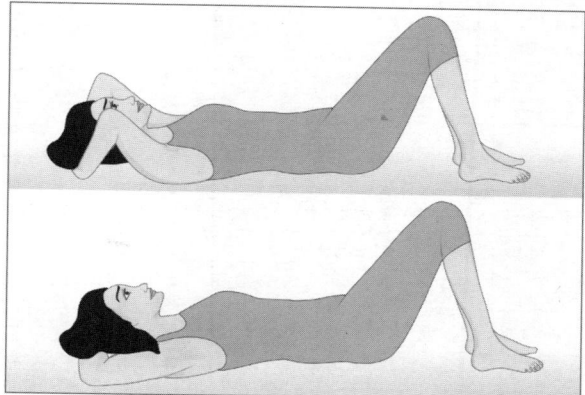

Fig. 19.14: Elbow spread exercise.

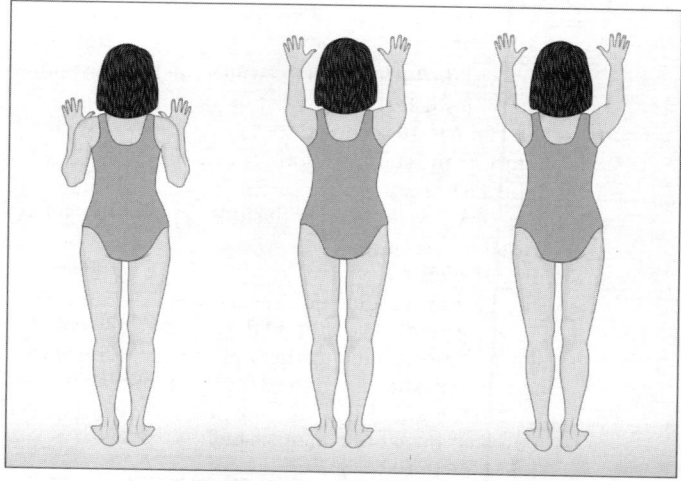

Fig. 19.15(i): Wall climbing facing the wall.

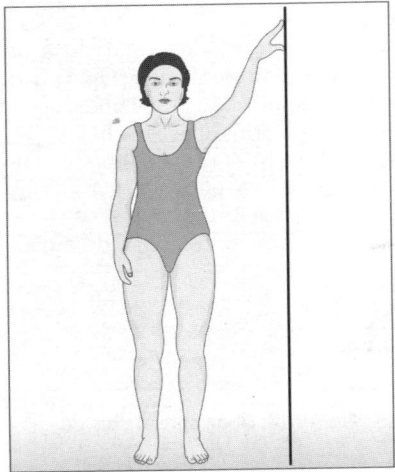

Fig. 19.15(ii): Wall climbing exercise: sidewall stretch.

- Slowly slide the hand up the wall as high as the patient can until she feels a stretch, but no pain.
- Hold for 5 to 10 seconds.
- Return to the start position.
- Repeat 5 to 10 times.
  If surgery was done on both sides, repeat this exercise with the other arm.
b. Sidewall stretch
  - Stand with your affected side to the wall.
  - Place the palm of your hand flat against the wall.
  - Slowly slide the hand up the wall, as high as the patient can go until she feels a stretch. Do not rotate the body toward the wall. Keep the body facing forward even if it means you cannot go up as high.
  - Hold for 5 to 10 seconds.
  - Return to start position.
  - Repeat 5 to 10 times.

9. **Side bends**

 This exercise is more advanced and can be performed once a day when the patient feels ready **(Fig. 19.16)**.
 - Sit on a chair and clasp both hands together in the lap.
 - Slowly lift both arms above the head.
 - Bend at the waist to move the body to the right. Use the right hand to gently pull the left arm a little further to the right. Keep sitting firmly on the chair.
 - Hold this position for five seconds and then slowly return to the start position.
 - Repeat this stretch to the left side using the left hand to pull the right arm further.
 - Repeat 5 to 10 times.

10. **Arm swinging/Pendulum exercise**

 Pendulum exercise is to prevent shoulder joint stiffness **(Fig. 19.17)**.
 - Lean over with your arm supported on a table or chair.
 - Relax the arm of the affected side, letting it hang straight down.

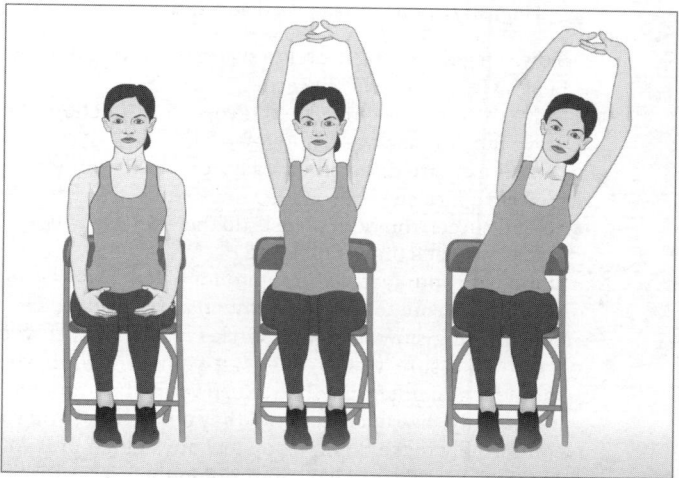

Fig. 19.16: Side bends exercise.

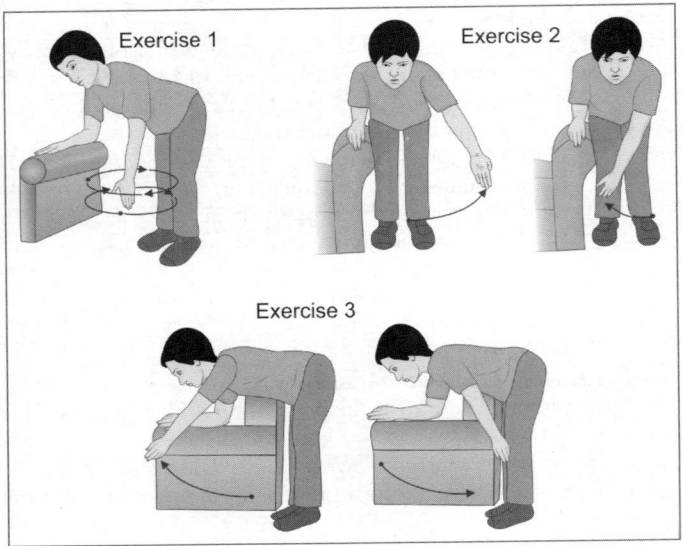

Fig. 19.17: Arm swinging/Pendulum exercise.

- Slowly begin to swing the relaxed arm by moving the body.
- Let gravity gently sway the arm.
- Move the arm in a circle, then reverse the direction. Next move the arm backward and forward.
- Do this exercise three times a day, for 5 to 10 minutes

11. **Arm circle exercise**

    If you had surgery on both breasts do this exercise with both arms, one arm at a time **(Fig. 19.18)**.
    - Stand with your feet slightly apart for balance. Raise your affected arm out to the side as much as you can.
    - Start making slow backward circles in the air with your arm. Make sure you are moving your arm from your shoulder and not from elbow. Keep your elbow straight.
    - Increase the size of circles until they are as big as you can comfortably make them. If you feel any aching or if your arm is tired, take a break. Start doing the exercise when you feel better.

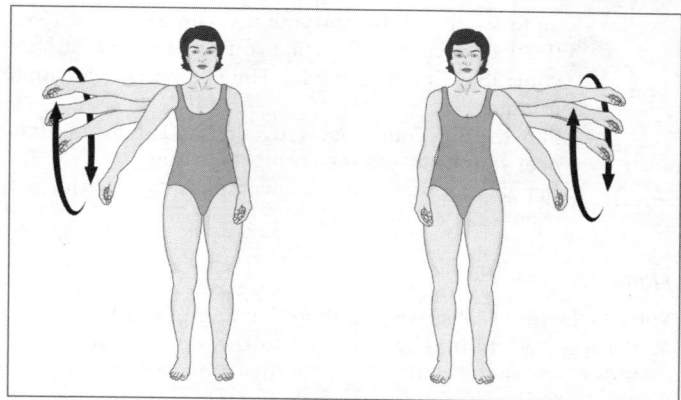

Fig. 19.18: Arm circle exercise.

12. Hands behind head exercise

This exercise can be done while sitting or standing **(Fig. 19.19)**.
- Clasp your hands together on your lap if sitting, and clasp the extended hands in front at hip level if standing
- Slowly raise the clasped hands towards the head, up to forehead level. Do not bend your head forward

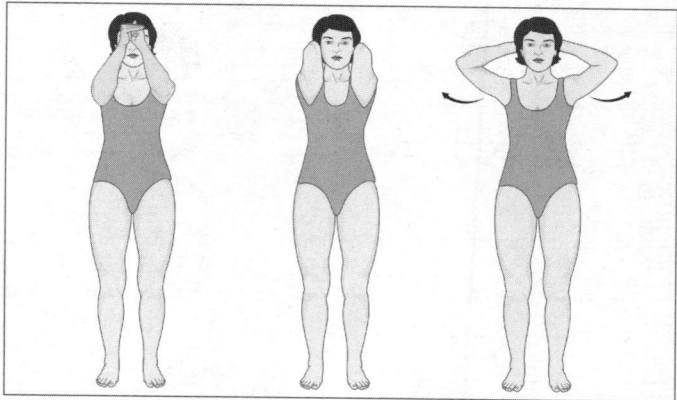

Fig. 19.19: Hands behind head exercise.

- Slide your hands behind your head until you reach well at the back of your neck. When you get to this point, spread your elbows out to the sides. Hold in this position for one minute.
- Slowly bring your elbows together and slide your hands over your head and then bring them down.
- Repeat the steps at a slower pace and perform the exercise."

Figure "W" Exercise

You can do this exercise while sitting or standing **(Fig. 19.20)**.

- Form a "W" with your arms out to the side and arms facing forwards. Try to bring your up so they are even with your face. Then bring them to the highest comfortable position.
- Pinch your shoulder blades together as if you are squeezing a pencil between them.
- Hold the furthest position that does not cause discomfort. Squeeze your shoulder blades together and downward for five seconds.
- Slowly bring your arms back down to the starting position. Repeat the movement 10 times.

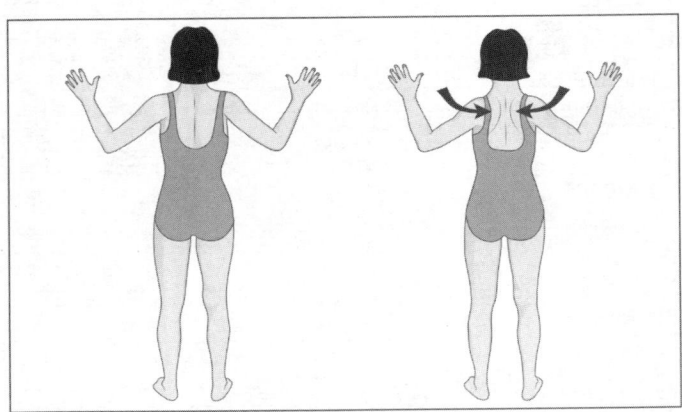

Fig.19.20: Figure "W" exercise.

Precautions to be Taken

- If any shortness of breath, pain or tightness in the chest is felt, stop exercising immediately. Inform the doctor to develop a plan of movement right for the patient.
- If changes are noticed in the arm, hand, trunk or shoulder including swelling stop doing upper body exercises and inform doctor.

Special Considerations

1. Proper assessment should be done before and after exercise to prevent complications.
2. Inform the treating physician for any untoward complications noted. Early detection can lessen the extent of damage that might happen.
3. It may take 6 to 8 weeks to regain full movement of arm(s). If difficulties in regaining full movement in arms after this time, the surgeon may make a referral to physiotherapy.

20. BREAST INFECTION IN PUERPERIUM

Inflammation or infection of breast is called mastitis.

INFECTION: MODES/CAUSES/ONSET

Modes of Infection

- Infection of the breast tissue following cracked nipple
- Infection gaining access through the lactiferous duct leading to development of primary mammary adenitis.

Organisms

- *Staphylococcus aureus* from the nasopharynx of the baby
- *Candida albicans*.

Onset

- Bacterial infection is acute during the late first week of puerperium
- In mammary adenitis, the onset is insidious and usually occurs near the end of second week

- *Candida* infection has sudden onset and generally after the first week
- Acute mastitis may occur even several weeks after delivery.

CLINICAL FEATURES

- Generalized malaise and headache
- Temperature 102°F or above with chills
- Swelling on one side of the breast with severe pain
- Hot, flushed skin, which feels tense and tender
- Pus discharge from nipple in breast abscess.

TREATMENT

Prophylactic

- Antenatal care of breasts such as washing of the nipples to keep the patency of the duct during last months of pregnancy and teaching the patient manual expression and clearance of colostrum from 36th week
- Prevention of breast engorgement
- Isolation of the infected baby.

Curative

- Isolation of mother and baby
- Manual expression of milk and suspension of feeding on affected breast
- Antibiotic therapy
- Analgesics and sedatives as required.
- Suppression of lactation using bromocriptine (parlodel)
- Fungicidal treatment with nystatin for both mother and baby in *Candida* infection
- If an abscess has formed, it needs to be drained under general anesthesia.

Health Education

- Prenatal education on preparation of nipples for feeding
- Measures to prevent engorgement of breasts

- Prevention of cracking of nipples and care of nipples if cracks develop
- Cleaning of nipples with water prior to feeding and following feeding
- Care of breasts and feeding methods with flat or depressed nipples.

21. BREECH PRESENTATION

In breech presentation, the fetus lies longitudinally with the buttocks in the lower pole of the uterus. The presenting diameter is bitrochanteric 10 cm and the denominator is sacrum.

TYPES OF BREECH PRESENTATION

Complete/Incomplete Types

There are two types of breech presentation (**Figs. 20.1A to D**).

Complete Breech or Flexed Breech (Fig. 20.1B)

The fetus is in normal attitude of full flexion. The thighs are flexed at the hips and the legs are flexed at knees. The presenting part consists of two buttocks, external genitalia and two feet. It is commonly present in multiparae.

Incomplete Breech

This is due to varying degrees of extension of thighs or legs at the podalic pole. There are three varieties in this:
- Breech with extended legs or Frank breech (**Fig. 20.1A**)
  In this type, the thighs are flexed on the abdomen and the legs are extended at the knee joints. The presenting part consists of the two buttocks and external genitalia only. It is commonly present in primigravidae.
- Footling presentation (**Fig. 20.1C**)
  One or both feet present because neither hips nor knees are fully flexed. The feet are lower than the buttocks, which distinguish it from complete breech.
- Knee presentation (**Fig. 20.1D**)
  Thighs are extended, but knees are flexed, bringing the knees down to present at the brim. This is very rare.

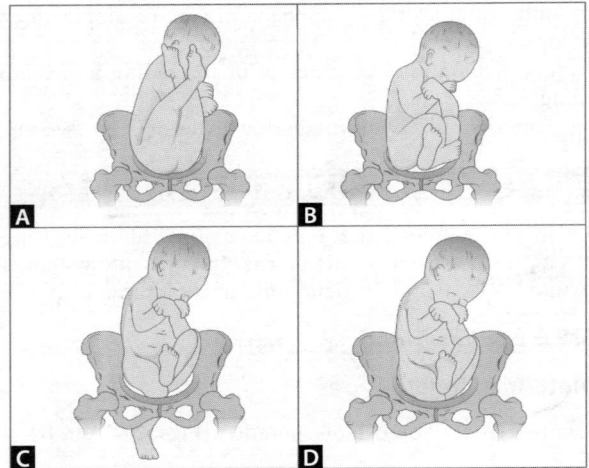

Figs. 20.1A to D: Types of breech presentation.

Spontaneous/Assisted Types

- **Spontaneous breech delivery:** The delivery occurs with little assistance from the attendant.
- **Assisted breech delivery:** The buttocks are born spontaneously, but some assistance is necessary for delivery of extended legs or arms and the head.
- **Breech extraction:** Manipulative delivery carried out to hasten the process in an emergency situation such as fetal distress.

CAUSES OF BREECH PRESENTATION

No definite cause is identified, but the following circumstances favor breech presentation:
- Prematurity: This is the most common cause
- Extended legs: Spontaneous cephalic version may be prevented if the fetus lies with extended legs, splinting the back
- Multiple pregnancy: This limits the space available for each fetus to turn and thus one or both fetuses may present by breech

- Polyhydramnios or oligohydramnios: Distension of the uterine cavity by excessive fluid or inadequate fluid may cause this
- Hydrocephaly: The increased size of the fetal head is accommodated in the fundus
- Uterine abnormalities such as septate uterus and bicornuate uterus
- Placenta previa
- Pelvic tumors
- Multiparity
- Cornual implantation of the placenta.

DIAGNOSIS

Antenatal

Palpation

- On palpation the lie is longitudinal, with soft, irregular breech occupying the lower pole of the uterus
- Head in fundus as hard mass movable independently of the neck
- Irregular small parts of the feet by the side of head in frank breech.

Auscultation

Usually located at a higher level around the umbilicus in complete breech and at a lower level in the midline due to engagement in frank breech.

Ultrasound Examination

Confirms the clinical diagnosis.

X-ray Examination

Confirms clinical diagnosis and permits pelvimetry.

Positions

The sacrum is the denominator in breech. There are four positions:

- Left sacroanterior (LSA)—the most common
- Right sacroanterior (RSA)
- Right sacroposterior (RSP)
- Left sacroposterior (LSP).

Diagnosis During Labor

Breech presentation may be diagnosed on admission in labor.

Vaginal Examination

The breech feels soft and irregular, with no sutures palpable. The anus may be felt and fresh meconium on the examining finger is usually diagnostic. If the legs are extended the external genitalia are very evident, but it may be edematous. An edematous vulva may be mistaken for a scrotum.

If a foot is felt, it must be differentiated from a hand (The foot is at right angles to the leg and the heel has no equivalent in the hand). Presentation may be confirmed by ultrasound scan or X-ray.

MANAGEMENT

Antenatal Management

Identification of associated abnormalities such as fetal malformation or placenta previa if suspected should be carried out. Ultrasound examination is very useful in the diagnosis of fetal abnormalities as well as localization of placenta.

External Cephalic Version

This is done between 32 and 35 weeks of pregnancy depending on the parity and individual assessment of the case. Primigravidae with a frank breech are more likely to need it earlier than a multipara with flabby uterine and abdominal muscles. If the version is not successful, another attempt after one week is done.

Contraindications
- Preeclampsia or hypertension because of the increased risk of placental abruption

- Multiple pregnancy
- Oligohydramnios
- Ruptured membranes
- A hydrocephalic fetus
- Any condition, which would require delivery by cesarean section.

Complications

- Knotting of the umbilical cord: This should be suspected if bradycardia occurs and persists. The fetus is immediately turned back to a breech presentation. The woman is admitted and if necessary, cesarean section is done
- Separation of placenta: Pain or vaginal bleeding during and after the procedure indicates this
- Rupture of the membranes: If this occurs, the cord may prolapse because neither the head nor the breech is engaged.

SPONTANEOUS BREECH DELIVERY

Left Sacroanterior Position

- Lie is longitudinal
- The attitude is one of complete flexion
- The presentation is breech
- The position is left sacroanterior
- The denominator is the sacrum
- The presenting part is the anterior buttock (left)
- The bitrochanteric diameter 10 cm, enters the pelvis in the left oblique diameter of the brim
- The sacrum points to the left iliopectineal eminence.

Mechanism

- **Compaction:** Descent takes place with increasing compaction, owing to increased flexion of the limbs.
- **Internal rotation of the buttocks:** The anterior buttock reaches the pelvic floor first and rotates 45° or one-eighth of a circle along the right side of the pelvis to lie underneath the symphysis pubis. The bitrochanteric diameter comes in the anteroposterior diameter of the outlet.

- **Lateral flexion of the body:** The anterior buttock escapes under the symphysis pubis, the posterior buttock sweeps the perineum and the buttocks are born by a movement of lateral flexion.
- **Restitution of the buttocks:** The anterior buttock turns slightly to the mother's right side.
- **Internal rotation of the shoulders:** The shoulders enter the pelvis in the same oblique diameter as the buttocks—the left oblique. The anterior shoulder rotates forwards one-eighth of a circle along the right side of the pelvis and escapes under the symphysis pubis, the posterior shoulder sweeps the perineum and the shoulders are born.
- **Internal rotation of the head:** The head enters the pelvis with sagittal suture in the transverse diameter of the brim. The occiput rotates forwards along the left side and the suboccipital region impinges on the undersurface of the symphysis pubis.
- **External rotation of the body:** At the same time the body turns so that the back is uppermost.
- **Birth of the head:** The chin, face and sinciput sweep, the perineum and the head is born in a flexed attitude.

ASSISTED BREECH DELIVERY

Assisted breech delivery requires a high degree of skill and is best conducted by experienced obstetricians.

Conditions

- Careful pelvic assessment early in labor
- Vaginal examination when membranes rupture to exclude cord prolapse
- Adequate sedation and analgesia in the first stage
- Confirm full dilatation of cervix vaginally before conducting second stage of labor
- Plan to conduct delivery under pudendal block
- Have a pediatrician ready to attend to the baby.

Procedure

- Second stage is allowed to continue as long as descend of presenting part is uninterrupted and there are no signs of fetal or

maternal distress. When breech reaches the pelvic floor, an episiotomy is performed.
- In complete breech, the feet and legs present and as they appear, they are eased out with digital pressure.
- If legs are extended, the anterior buttock first becomes visible and is allowed to descend with contractions.
- As the delivery of the shoulder proceeds, the baby's body is allowed to hang downwards to exert slight traction in the direction of the pelvic axis and suprapubic pressure may be applied to cause descend of head into the pelvis.

As soon as the head descends onto pelvic floor and nape of the neck can be seen below the pubic arch, the baby's legs are grasped, just above the ankles and by exerting slight traction, the baby's body is lifted upwards to the horizontal position. The face will then appear at the vulva and as the baby can now breathe; the head can be delivered slowly and carefully.

Complications

- **Delay in descent of breech:** If the breech had not entered the brim after 6–8 hours of labor, then disproportion may be present and cesarean section is the treatment of choice.
- **Extended arms:** Løvset's maneuver is the method of management. This is to assist the delivery of the posterior shoulder. Baby is held by the buttocks and pulled backwards and downwards, while rotating the body keeping the back anterior. This results in the posterior shoulder coming forward from the sacral hollow to appear under the pubic arch, thereby facilitating delivery.
- **Delay in descent of the head:** This may happen because of any of the following:
    - **Disproportion:** At this stage the baby will die, and perforation and crushing of the head will have to be performed.
    - **Extended head:** An attempt to flex and deliver the head is made by Mauriceau-Smellie-Viet maneuver.
    - **Incomplete dilatation of the cervix:** If the baby is alive, then anesthesia may be induced and the cervix is manually stretched or incised. If the baby is dead, wait for full dilatation.
    - **Rigid perineum:** This is easily overcome by an episiotomy and forceps. Forceps is applied to the after coming head, which

aids flexion, keeps traction off the cervical spine and allows a controlled delivery of the head.

BREECH EXTRACTION

Breech extraction carries a very high perinatal mortality and only has limited role in modern obstetrics. It may be indicated in the following conditions:
- Delivery of the second twin
- Acute fetal distress in second stage
- Cord prolapse.

Principles of Breech Extraction

- General anesthesia
- Full dilatation and adequate pelvis
- Generous episiotomy
- Traction should be downwards, backwards and continuous until umbilicus is born
- Keep the back uppermost
- Løvset's maneuver for the shoulders and arms
- Forceps to the after coming head.

HAZARDS OF BREECH DELIVERY

Maternal morbidity and perinatal mortality are considerably greater due to the following reasons:
- Labor tends to be prolonged, as breech is not an efficient dilator (except frank breech)
- Risk of cord prolapse is high
- Manipulative measures are frequently needed
- No time for molding of the head as it must pass through the pelvis in few minutes
- Delivery through an incompletely dilated cervix especially in footling and premature breeches
- Premature respiratory efforts and aspiration due to the stimulus of hypoxia or cold air and handling of the trunk
- Intracranial hemorrhage due to traumatic delivery of the after coming head

- Cord compression as the head enters the pelvic cavity
- Cord prolapse
- Delay in delivery of the head
- Prolonged anesthesia
- Asphyxia
- Intra-abdominal organ injuries due to rough handling during delivery, e.g. liver, spleen and adrenals.

MEASURES TO REDUCE PERINATAL MORTALITY

- Use of external cephalic version (ECV) wherever possible
- Careful pelvic assessment before attempting breech delivery
- Identify any associated or complicating factors early
- Delivery in a well-equipped hospital
- Delivery by a skilled obstetrician or under his supervision
- Local anesthesia in preference to general anesthesia
- Neonatologist to attend the delivery for expert resuscitation if it becomes necessary
- If there is arrest of labor and any doubt about adequacy of pelvis or size of baby, then cesarean delivery is best.

22. BROW PRESENTATION

Brow is the attitude adopted by the head between a face (complete extension) and a vertex (complete flexion). It is the most unfavorable of all cephalic presentations because its presenting diameter is the largest possible, mentovertical (13.5 cm). It therefore cannot pass through the pelvis unless it is unusually large or the fetus unusually small **(Fig. 22.1)**.

CAUSES

Maternal

- Multiparity with pendulous abdomen
- Lateral obliquity of the uterus
- Contracted pelvis
- Flat pelvis.

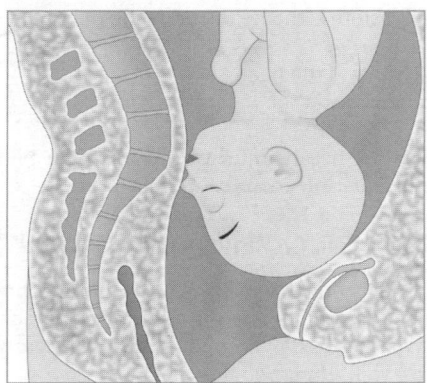

Fig. 22.1: Brow presentation.

Fetal

- Congenital malformations such as:
  - Congenital goiter
  - Dolichocephalic head with long anteroposterior diameter
  - Congenital bronchocele.
- Twist of the cord several times round the neck.

DIAGNOSIS AND MANAGEMENT

Brow presentation is not usually detected before the onset of labor.

On abdominal palpation: The head is high, appears unduly large and does not descend into pelvis despite good uterine contractions.

On vaginal examination: The presenting part is high and difficult to reach. The anterior fontanelle may be felt on one side of the pelvis and the orbital ridges and the root of the nose on the other side. There may be considerable molding and caput on the forehead.

Mechanism of Labor

In brow, the supraorbital ridges may be anterior or posterior. When the baby is average sized, the presenting diameter mentovertical is too large to pass through the normal pelvis and there is no mechanism of labor.

Management

The management depends on when the brow presentation is diagnosed:
- **In late pregnancy:** If the diagnosis has been made by radiograph or ultrasound during pregnancy, it is usual to await the onset of labor, because by then the fetus may have altered its attitude and present by the face or vertex.
- **In early first stage:** The diagnosis is usually made when a vaginal examination is done for lack of progress. In most cases, cesarean section is the safest treatment for mother and baby.
- **In late first stage:** If the baby is dead, an experienced obstetrician may consider performing craniotomy. In almost all cases of brow presentation, whatever the stage of labor, cesarean section is the safest method of delivery.

23. CESAREAN SECTION

Cesarean section is the delivery of a viable fetus, placenta and membranes through an incision in the abdominal wall and the uterine wall. The first cesarean section performed on a woman is known as primary cesarean section. An elective cesarean section is one which is performed before the onset of labor or before the occurrence of any complication, which calls for an emergency intervention.

INDICATIONS FOR CESAREAN SECTION

Maternal

General Indications

- Diabetes mellitus
- Chronic hypertension
- Coarctation of aorta
- Genital herpes.

Pregnancy Disorders

- Moderate to severe pregnancy-induced hypertension
- Placenta previa and abruption of placenta.

Past Obstetric History

- Elderly primigravida and prolonged previous infertility.
- Previous repair of genital prolapse or repair of vesicovaginal fistula (VVF)
- Previous difficult vaginal delivery and bad obstetric history
- Previous cesarean section, myomectomy, hysterotomy or uteroplasty
- Rh-incompatibility.

Labor Disorders

- Cephalopelvic disproportion (CPD), e.g. persistent brow presentation, mentoposterior position, breech presentation
- Umbilical cord prolapse
- Nonprogress of labor
- Soft tissue dystocia, e.g. cervical rigidity
- Disproportion due to uterine fibroids, impacted ovarian cysts
- Congenital anomalies of bony pelvis, e.g. Robert's pelvis, acquired deformities from fractures
- Failed forceps and threatened uterine rupture.

Fetal

- Previous unexplained fetal death
- Fetal distress in labor
- Intrauterine growth retardation (IUGR)
- Fetal macrosomia, e.g. maternal diabetes, post maturity
- Multiple pregnancies; triplets and over.

TYPES

- Lower segment cesarean section, the most commonly performed procedure
- Classical cesarean section, very rarely performed in present day obstetric practice.

PREPARATION OF THE PATIENT

- Psychological preparation of the mother/couple
- Physical preparation:
  - Shaving and cleaning of abdomen, back, private parts and upper parts of thighs
  - Bowel preparation in the evening before operation, if cesarean section is elective
  - Antacid therapy; molar sodium citrate 30 mL half an hour before surgery
  - Intravenous infusion started prior to surgery
  - Preliminary skin preparation with antiseptic solutions like savlon and betadine prior to induction of anesthesia
  - Indwelling catheter connected to sterile urosac.

COMPLICATIONS OF CESAREAN SECTION

Maternal

- Hemorrhage, shock and infection
- Extension of incision and hematoma formation
- Injury to bladder during opening of the parietal peritoneum
- Injury to ureters when attempts are made to suture the lateral portion of uterine incision
- Injury to bowel
- Paralytic ileus and peritonitis
- Formation of pelvis abscess, pelvic thrombophlebitis and later septic emboli
- Thromboembolism, disseminated intravascular coagulation (DIC) and pulmonary embolism
- Anesthetic complications, aspiration, hypotension, cardiac arrest.

Fetal

- Respiratory distress syndrome (RDS)
- Injury to the baby from surgical knife
- Birth asphyxia
- Fetal exsanguination, severe bleeding from placenta previa before extraction of baby
- Birth injuries during difficult extraction.

CESAREAN HYSTERECTOMY

Cesarean hysterectomy is an operation in which removal of the uterus is carried out after delivery of the fetus by cesarean section. The operation may be performed as a planned procedure, but more often it is an emergency operation to save maternal life in the following situations:
- Uncontrollable atonic postpartum hemorrhage
- Placenta accreta
- Multiple myomas where repair of incision is difficult
- Severely infected uterus
- Cancer cervix
- Rupture of the uterus.

NURSING PROCESS

Assessment

- Hypertension (escalating PIH)
- Nausea, vomiting, generalized edema (PIH)
- Fear of surgery
- Prolonged/dysfunctional contractile pattern (dystocia)
- Right upper quadrant/epigastria pain (PIH)
- Seizure activity (eclampsia)
- Hyperreflexia, clonus (PIH)
- Elevated temperature (infection/dehydration)
- Severe Rh-incompatibility
- Prolapsed cord
- Fetal distress
- Impending delivery for fetal distress
- Fetal macrosomia (estimated > 4000 g)
- Unsuccessful external cephalic version
- Membranes have ruptured for 24 hours or longer
- CPD; neoplasm/tumor obstructing the pelvis/birth canal
- Multiple pregnancy
- Placenta previa/abruptio placentae
- Previous cesarean delivery with classic incision; previous uterine or cervical surgery

- Presence of maternal complications/risk factors such as PIH, diabetes, cardiac disease, ascending infection, maternal age more than 35 years
- Failed induction.

Diagnostic Studies

- Complete blood count (CBC)
- Blood typing (ABO and cross match, Coomb's test)
- Urinalysis: Determines albumin/glucose levels
- Cultures: Identifies presence of herpes simplex type II
- X-ray pelvimetry: Determines CPD, presentation, position
- Amniocentesis: Assesses fetal maturity
- Ultrasonography: Locates placenta, determines fetal growth, lie and presentation as well as fetal anomalies/malformations, favoring cesarean delivery
- NST or CST: Assesses fetal responses to movements/stress of uterine contractions
- Continuous electronic monitoring: Validates fetal status/uterine activity.

Nursing Diagnoses

- Deficient knowledge regarding surgical procedure, expectations, postoperative regimen
- Anxiety
- Powerlessness
- Risk for acute pain
- Risk for infection
- Risk for impaired fetal gas exchange
- Risk for maternal injury.

Expected Outcomes

The client will:
- Verbalize understanding of indications for cesarean birth
- Appear appropriately relaxed and uses resources effectively
- Participate in decision making process whenever possible
- Verbalize reduced discomfort/pain

- Achieve timely wound healing without complications
- Manifest normal variability on monitor strip
- Remain free of injury.

Nursing Interventions

1. **Understanding the indications for cesarean birth:**
   - Assess learning needs
   - Note stress level and whether procedure is planned or unplanned
   - Provide accurate information in simple terms, clarify misconceptions
   - Encourage couple to ask questions and verbalise their understanding
   - Describe preoperative procedures in advance and provide rationale as appropriate
   - Provide preoperative teaching; including demonstration of leg exercises, coughing, deep breathing, splinting technique and abdominal tightening
   - Discuss anticipated sensations during delivery and recovery period.

2. **Reducing anxiety level:**
   - Assess psychologic responses to the event and availability of support
   - Ascertain whether procedure is planned or unplanned
   - Stay with client and remain calm, speak slowly and convey empathy
   - Reinforce positive aspects of maternal and fetal condition
   - Encourage client/couple to verbalise and/or express feelings
   - Support with expressed coping mechanisms
   - Discuss past childbirth experience/expectations as appropriate
   - Provide period of privacy if possible. Reduce environmental stimuli such as number of people present, as indicated by client's desires.

3. **Reducing feelings of powerlessness:**
   - Assess factors contributing to sense of powerlessness
   - Present options in care when possible (e.g. choice of anesthesia, IV placement)

- Identify client's expectations and desires regarding the delivery experience
- Provide personal space and time alone for the couple prior to surgery if possible. Remain with client if spouse is absent
- Provide information and discuss client's perceptions.

4. **Reducing discomfort/pain:**
   - Assess location, nature and duration of pain
   - Eliminate anxiety producing factors (e.g. loss of control), provide accurate information and encourage presence of partner if agency policy permits
   - Instruct in relaxation techniques: position for comfort as possible
   - Use therapeutic touch as appropriate
   - Collaborative intervention:
     - Administer sedative, narcotic or preoperative medication as needed.

5. **Reducing risk for infection:**
   - Review history of pre-existing conditions/risk factors. Note time of rupture of membranes
   - Assess for signs and symptoms of infection, e.g. abnormal odor of vaginal discharge, fetal tachycardia
   - Provide perineal care per protocol, especially once membranes have ruptured
   - Carry out preoperative skin preparation; scrub according to protocol
   - Obtain blood, vaginal and placental cultures as indicated
   - Note hemoglobin and hematocrit, and estimated blood loss during surgical procedure
   - Collaborative intervention:
     - Administer parenteral broad-spectrum antibiotic preoperatively.

6. **Reducing risk of fetal distress and achieving optimal FHR:**
   - Note presence of maternal factors that negatively affect placental circulation and fetal oxygenation
   - Continue monitoring FHR noting beat to beat changes or decelerations during and following contractions
   - Note presence of variable decelerations; change client's position from side to side

- Note color and amount of amniotic fluid when membranes rupture
- Auscultate FHR when membranes rupture
- Monitor fetal heart response to preoperative medications or regional anesthesia
- Collaborative intervention: As follows:
  - Provide supplemental oxygen to mother via mask
  - Administer IV fluid bolus prior to initiation of epidural/spinal anesthesia
  - Arrange for presence of pediatrician and neonatal intensive care nurse in delivery room for both scheduled and emergency cesarean births.

7. **Reducing risk of maternal injury:**
   - Remove prosthetic devices such as contact lenses, dentures/bridges and jewelry
   - Determine time and content of last meal. Report information to anesthesiologist
   - Restrict oral intake once decision for cesarean delivery is made
   - Review labor record noting, voiding frequency, output, appearance and time of last voiding
   - Monitor urine output and color following insertion of indwelling catheter. Note any blood-tinged urine
   - Assist with positioning for anesthesia; support legs during postoperative transfer to stretcher
   - Keep accurate instrument and sponge counts at critical times during closure, according to hospital protocol
   - Collaborative intervention:
     - Obtain urine specimen for routine analysis, protein and specific gravity. Ensure that laboratory results are available before surgery is started.
     - Insert indwelling catheter and connect to continuous gravity drainage system either just before surgical procedure or in the operating room.
     - Administer preprocedural medication, e.g. atropine.

24. CARCINOMA CERVIX

Carcinoma of the cervix is the most common cancer in women in most of the developing countries. It ranks first, the second being breast carcinoma.

VARIETIES OF CARCINOMA

- Squamous cell carcinoma (80-90%): These arise from the ectocervix
- Adenocarcinoma (10-15%): Develops from the endocervical canal either from the lining epithelium or from the glands.

MODE OF SPREAD

- By direct extension: The growth spreads directly to the adjacent structures, vagina and body of uterus
- By lymphatics: The commonly involved groups are parametrial nodes, internal iliac nodes, external iliac nodes and sacral nodes
- By bloodstream: Blood borne metastasis is late and usually by veins rather than arteries; lungs, liver and bones are generally involved
- By direct implantation.

STAGING OF CARCINOMA OF THE CERVIX

- Stage 0: Carcinoma in situ or intraepithelial carcinoma
- Stage I: Carcinoma strictly confined to the cervix
- Stage II: Carcinoma extends beyond the cervix, but has not extended to the pelvic wall. The carcinoma involves the vagina, but not the lower third
- Stage III: Carcinoma extends to the pelvic wall. The tumor involves the lower third of the vagina
- Stage IV: Carcinoma extends beyond the true pelvis or has clinically involved the mucosa of the bladder or rectum.

DIAGNOSIS

Early Carcinoma

- Maternal abnormalities such as bleeding on straining (during defecation) and intermenstrual bleeding

- Excessive white discharge, which may be offensive
- Erosion, nodular growth or ulcer on speculum examination
- Indurated, friable lesion that bleeds on touch on bimanual examination
- Confirmation by biopsy.

Advanced Carcinoma

- Irregular or continued vaginal bleeding
- Offensive vaginal discharge
- Pelvic pain of varying degree
- Bladder symptoms such as frequency of micturition, dysuria, hematuria or true incontinence due to fistula formation
- Rectal involvement evidenced by diarrhea, rectal pain, bleeding per rectum or rectovaginal fistula
- Ureteric colic due to pyelonephritis
- Patient cachectic, anemic with edema legs and uremia
- Ulcerative or fungating lesion, which bleeds on touch (on speculum examination)
- Induration of the bladder (on bimanual examination)
- Involvement of the rectum (on rectal examination)
- Confirmation of the diagnosis by biopsy.

COMPLICATIONS

- Frequent attacks of ureteric pain, pyelitis and pyelonephritis due to hydronephrosis
- Pyometra—especially with endocervical variety
- Vesicovaginal fistula
- Rectovaginal fistula.

Causes of Death

- Uremia: The patient may die of uremia due to ureteric obstruction following parametrial involvement with infection compromising kidney functions
- Hemorrhage: Vaginal bleeding from the growth may be brisk or continuous causing anemia and ill health
- Sepsis: Localized pelvic or generalized peritonitis may occur, which may be fatal

- Metastasis to distant organs especially to lungs may be fatal
- Cachexia: The cancerous tissues have a depressant action on general metabolism. Cumulative effect of complications leads to cachectic condition.

TREATMENT

Primary Prevention

Health education to identify and eliminate causative factors are:
- High-risk factors in women
- Early sexual intercourse
- Early age of first pregnancy
- Too many births or too frequent births
- Poor maintenance of local hygiene
- Sexually transmitted diseases
- Multiple sexual partners.

Secondary Prevention

Identifying and treating the disease earlier. Through regular screening, the disease can be identified in early stage.

Curative Treatment

- Primary surgery
- Primary radiotherapy
- Combination therapy
- Chemotherapy.

Surgery

The surgery involves removal of the uterus, tubes and ovaries of both sides and adjacent structures (radical hysterectomy).

Radiotherapy (Brachy Technique)

Small radioactive sources, mainly radium sulfate is mixed with some inert powder and packed in small needles or tubes are used for interstitial, intracavity or surface applications.

Combination Therapy

Either the surgery or the radiotherapy precedes or follows the other.

Chemotherapy

Chemotherapy is generally used as an adjuvant treatment. It is used along with surgery or radiotherapy in locally advanced metastatic or recurrent lesions in an attempt to improve the result. Chemotherapy can cause tumor regression. The drugs used are cisplatin, vinblastin and bleomycin (CVB).

25. CANCER UTERUS

Cancer of the uterus or endometrial carcinoma is higher amongst the white population of United States of America and lowest in India and Japan.

RELATED FACTORS

- **Estrogen:** Persistent stimulation of endometrium with estrogen
- **Age:** Seen in postmenopausal women, i.e. above 60 years
- **Parity:** Quite common in unmarried and married nulliparous women
- **Late menopause:** The chance of endometrial carcinoma increases, if menopause fails to occur beyond 52 years
- **Corpus cancer syndrome:** Obesity, hypertension and diabetes
- **Unopposed estrogen stimulation:** Conditions such as functioning ovarian tumors or polycystic ovarian syndrome is associated with increased risk of cancer. Estrogen therapy in postmenopausal women adds to the risk
- **Genetic inheritance:** Family history or personal history of cancer in colon, ovaries or breast increases the risk
- **Endometrial hyperplasia:** It precedes carcinoma in about one fourth of the cases.

SPREAD

- **Direct spread:** It may infiltrate the myometrium and spread to the parametrium or into the peritoneal cavity

- **Lymphatic spread:** A late development and can involve pelvic, paraaortic, inguinal and femoral lymph nodes
- **Blood borne spread:** It occurs late and the common sites of metastases are lungs, liver, bones and brain.

CLINICAL STAGING

- Stage I: Carcinoma confined to the corpus
- Stage II: Carcinoma has involved the corpus and cervix, but has not extended outside the uterus
- Stage III: Carcinoma has extended outside the uterus, but not outside the true pelvis.
- Stage IV: Carcinoma has extended outside the true pelvis or has involved the mucosa of the bladder and rectum.

CLINICAL FEATURES

- Postmenopausal bleeding, which may be irregular or continuous
- Irregular and excessive bleeding in premenopausal women
- Watery and offensive discharge in the presence of pyometra
- Colicky pain due to uterine contractions in an attempt to expel the polypoid growth
- Varying degrees of pallor
- On bimanual examination uterus may be atrophic, normal or enlarged.

DIAGNOSIS

- Postmenopausal bleeding
- Clinical findings and history listed above
- Endometrial biopsy
- Papanicolaou smear may be positive in about 50% of cases
- Ultrasound—transvaginal ultrasonography
- Hysteroscopy—direct visualization and biopsy
- Fractional curettage.

TREATMENT

Preventive

- Strict control of weight
- Restriction of estrogen usage after menopause

- Investigating any irregular bleeding per vagina
- Screening of high-risk women at least in menopausal period to detect premalignant or early carcinoma
- Cytological and histological examination of endometrial aspirate or curetted specimen
- Hysterectomy for premalignant lesions of the corpus.

Curative

Surgery

Hysterectomy is the treatment for Stage I carcinoma (endometrial carcinoma confined to the body). Surgery includes removal of the uterus, tubes and ovaries of both the sides and the cuff of vagina.

Radiotherapy

The primary treatment by radiotherapy is indicated in surgically risk patients and stage III and IV cancers. Whole abdomen is irradiated shielding the kidneys.

Combined Radiation Therapy

Hysterectomy followed by irradiation therapy 4–6 weeks after surgery is done to prevent tumor recurrence.

Intracavity radiation followed by extended hysterectomy 48 hours later is recommended in case of highly anaplastic tumor, deeply invasive cancer and growth extending to the cervix.

Chemotherapy

Chemotherapy is used in advanced and recurrent cases or in metastatic lesions. Drugs used are progestogens, tamoxifen, and cytotoxic durgs. The commonly used cytotoxic drugs are Adriamycin, cisplatin, carboplatin and cyclophosphamide.

FOLLOW-UP CARE

Following initial therapy, patient is examined every 4 months for the first 2 years, every 6 months for next 2 years and thereafter annually.

26. CARDIAC DISEASE IN PREGNANCY

Physiological changes during pregnancy place a considerable load on the heart and cardiovascular system. Most cases of heart disease with efficient and good management can go through pregnancy and labor successfully, but there is always an additional risk. The classification of cardiac diseases in pregnancy is given in **Box 26.1**.

PHYSIOLOGICAL CHANGES IN CARDIOVASCULAR SYSTEM DURING PREGNANCY

There are major cardiovascular changes in pregnancy:
- Increase in cardiac output from 4.5 L/min at 12th week to 6.8 L/min at 32 week
- Increase in blood volume, mainly plasma volume by nearly 30–40%
- Blood pressure (BP) drops in the first and second trimester and rises back to normal in the third trimester
- On examination, the apex of the heart is often displaced upwards and laterally
- Ejection systolic murmur may be heard over the precordium; continuous venous hums are often heard over the chest and neck.

Box 26.1: Classification of cardiac diseases.

- Rheumatic heart diseases:
  - Mitral stenosis
  - Mitral regurgitation
  - Aortic stenosis
  - Aortic regurgitation
- Congenital heart diseases:
  - Atrial septal defect
  - Ventricular septal defect
  - Patent ductus arteriosus
  - Tetralogy of Fallot
  - Eisenmenger's syndrome
  - Coarctation of aorta
- Cardiomyopathy

RHEUMATIC HEART DISEASE

Mitral Stenosis

In normal pregnancy the increased blood volume augments the venous return and the cardiac output. This increase in preload is transmitted to the left atrium where it encounters resistance from the stenosed mitral valve. The pressure in the left atrium increases and is transmitted backwards into the pulmonary circulation. The left ventricle, however, does not receive this augmented blood volume and so the cardiac output is low. The kidneys therefore retain fluid, further augmenting the hypervolaemia. Such patients are consequently at a very high-risk for pulmonary edema.

Clinical Presentation

Patients with mild disease have few if any symptoms, which includes:
- Dyspnea on exertion
- Palpitations
- Syncopal attacks or fatigue.

  As the disease becomes more severe, there is progressive increase of complications. Pulmonary edema with typical manifestations such as:
    - Orthopnea
    - Paroxysmal nocturnal dyspnea
    - Heart failure with peripheral edema
    - Tender hepatomegaly
    - Raised jugular venous pressure (JVP).

Classification

Classification of heart disease depending on the functional impairment that patient experiences according to New York Heart Association (NYHA).

Class 1: No limitation of physical activity, ordinary physical activity does not cause undue fatigue, dyspnea, palpitations or anginal pain.

Class 2: There is slight limitation of activity and patients are comfortable at rest. Ordinary physical activity results in fatigue, palpitations, dyspnea and anginal pain.

Class 3: There is marked limitation of physical activity. Patients are comfortable at rest. Less than ordinary physical activity results in fatigue, palpitations, dyspnea and anginal pain.

Class 4: Patient is unable to carry on physical activities without discomfort. Symptoms of cardiac insufficiency occur in the absence of physical activity.

Investigations

- Hemoglobin to ensure that patient does not develop anemia
- Urine examination (microscopic and culture)
- Electrocardiography (ECG) for diagnosis of arrhythmias
- Echocardiogram.

Management

- Patients of class 1 and 2 can be managed on an outpatient basis
- Patients in class 3 and 4 require immediate hospitalization
- The aim of antenatal care is to avoid situations that can result in tachycardia, stress, anemia, infection, arrhythmias and volume overload as in excessive salt and water ingestion
- Patient is advised, restriction of activity and restriction of emotional stress
- Sedative may be prescribed to overtly anxious patients to ensure greater compliance with bedrest
- Rest for a minimum of 2 hours in the afternoon and 8 hours at night
- Sodium restriction in diet to 2 g/day to limit edema and intravascular overload
- Excess weight gain or obesity to be discouraged
- Medications such as diuretics (Furosemide) digoxin and hematinics
- Infection prophylaxis
- Regular follow-up care in antenatal clinic
- Monitoring of vital parameters such as pulse rate, temperature, respiratory rate and BP.

Complications

- Pulmonary edema
- Cardiac arrhythmias
- Congestive heart failure (CHF).

Interventions/Preatment

Place of therapeutic MTP

The procedure is sometimes the safest line of therapy to be performed in the first trimester. It is indicated whenever there is:

- The CHF or pulmonary edema in the first trimester
- Active rheumatic fever or infective endocarditis in the first trimester
- Severe mitral stenosis with complications
- Coarctation of aorta
- Patient who decides on termination after counseling.

Intranatal care

During the intranatal period, as the uterine contraction squeezes blood into the circulation, cardiac output increases by 15–20%. This leads to a reflex bradycardia. Pain and apprehension further augment the basal cardiac output by almost 40%, putting additional strain on the heart. Careful management with adequate precautions is necessary during labor.

First stage of labor

- Bedrest in propped up position with oxygen and resuscitation cart to be available and handy
- Analgesia: A combination of narcotic with sedative is recommend as it ensures tranquil, cooperative patient and has minimal cardiovascular effects
- Intravenous fluids: Slow infusion rate is used in order to avoid fluid overload
- Fetal heart rate monitoring, ideally by a continuous electronic fetal monitor
- Clinical monitoring of progress of labor is documented on a partogram
- Invasive monitoring of pulmonary artery wedge pressure may be done in cases with pulmonary edema or severe mitral stenosis
- Antibiotic prophylaxis (endocarditis prevention).

Second stage of labor
In order to avoid additional strain on the heart by bearing down efforts the second stage may be shortened with the application of an outlet forceps. Furosemide 40 mg may be administered intravenously immediately after the birth of the baby. By augmenting renal blood flow, this diverts some of the excess blood volume that is added to the circulation by the contraction of the uterus after delivery.

Third stage of labor
Ergometrine intravenous or intramuscular is relatively contraindicated in these patients as the sudden and sustained uterine contractions can lead in addition of 500 mL of blood into maternal circulation increasing the left atria pressure, which can lead to pulmonary edema.

Puerperium

The patient must be observed closely for at least 24 hours. She needs to be given complete bedrest with monitoring of respiratory system, cardiovascular system and urinary output.

The postpartum hospital stay may be extended for 10–14 days till the pregnancy hypervolemia returns to normal. Ambulation is allowed earlier to prevent deep venous thrombosis. Temperature is monitored and antibiotics are continued.

Contraception

Tubal ligation or vasectomy for husband is recommended as an interval procedure (after correction of hypervolemia) for patients who have completed their family. For others, barrier contraception (condom) is the safest method. Intrauterine contraceptive device (IUCD) and oral contraceptive carry risks in these patients.

Mitral Regurgitation

This condition is common and usually rheumatic in origin and often occurs with others. It is usually well-tolerated and carries a low risk of heart failure. As they have a dilated left atrium, they are at risk for atrial fibrillation. Prophylactic dioxin is usually ordered. As there is risk of endocarditis, prophylaxis is recommended during labor.

Aortic Stenosis

This lesion is rheumatic is origin in 90% cases. In the rest it may be a congenital defect. The problem in patients with stenosis of aorta is maintaining adequate cardiac output without outflow obstruction. Inadequate cardiac output results in a state of reduced amount of blood ejected into the circulation at all times, so that in times of exertion, there is inadequate perfusion resulting in syncope, angina and even myocardial infarction.

Labor is particularly a dangerous period for these patients. Supine position and spinal anesthesia are avoided during labor as these can reduce venous return leading to inadequate cardiac output. Endocarditis prophylaxis is necessary.

CONGENITAL HEART DISEASES

Congenital heart disease complicating pregnancies are:
1. Atrial septal defect (ASD).
2. Ventricular septal defect (VSD).
3. Patent ductus arteriosus (PDA).
4. Tetralogy of fallot.
5. Eisenmenger's syndrome.
6. Coarctation of aorta.

Atrial Septal Defect

Atrial septal defect (ASD) is the most common lesion seen in adults. During pregnancy they may have increased pulmonary hypertension and supraventricular arrhythmias. Labor is usually uncomplicated. Patients with complications need to be delivered in a hospital with fully equipped cardiac care unit.

Ventricular Septal Defect

Patients with ventricular septal defect (VSD) in pregnancy usually have relatively small defects and are often asymptomatic. As in ASD, pulmonary hypertension may become aggravated in pregnancy. Management is similar to that of ASD.

Patent Ductus Arteriosus

Most patients with patent ductus arteriosus (PDA) are diagnosed and treated in childhood. Others with small defect tolerate pregnancy well. Hypervolemia of pregnancy leads to increased pulmonary blood flow, resulting complications such as pulmonary hypertension and supraventricular arrhythmias. In managing these patients, it is vital to avoid hypotension, e.g. due to epidural analgesia or hemorrhage as it could result in profound hypoxia and cyanosis. Bacterial endocarditis prophylaxis is needed.

Tetralogy of Fallot

In this anomaly, there is a right to left shunting of blood flow causing cyanosis. During pregnancy when the peripheral vascular resistance decreases, the right to left shunting of blood increases and cyanosis worsens.

Complications

- Congestive cardiac failure and vascular endocarditis
- Abortion, preterm labor and intrauterine growth restriction (IUGR)
- Cardiac arrhythmia.

Management

In the antenatal period, it is essential to diagnose and prevent the above mentioned complications. In labor, continuous oxygen and careful observation are mandatory. Systemic analgesics are preferred and general anesthesia is recommended if cesarean section becomes necessary. Patients with corrected lesions rarely experience any problem.

Eisenmenger's Syndrome

This condition is characterized by the occurrence of right to left or bidirectional shunting of blood at either the atrial or ventricular level, combined with an elevated pulmonary vascular resistance. The most common lesion with which it is associated is VSD, followed by ASD and PDA. The occurrence of this syndrome is an absolute indication for termination of pregnancy due to the high-risk for maternal and fetal mortality.

Coarctation of Aorta

This condition in pregnancy carries the risk of hypertension, which can lead to aortic rupture or rupture of associated cerebral vessel aneurysms or aortic dissection with rupture. Patients with severe disease are usually diagnosed and treated in childhood. With mild coarctation and no hypertension, pregnancy is usually uneventful. In patients with hypertension, antihypertensive therapy is given. However, care need to be taken to avoid hypotension and avert cardiovascular collapse. Cesarean section is usually favored for patients with severe aortic disease.

NURSING PROCESS

Assessment

- Tachycardia, palpitations and dysrhythmia
- History of congenital/organic heart disease and rheumatic fever
- The BP may be elevated or may be decreased with decreased vascular resistance
- Inability to carry on normal activities
- Nocturnal/Exertion related dyspnea or orthopnea
- Clubbing of toes and fingers may be present with systemic cyanosis in surgically untreated tetralogy of Fallot
- Urine output may be decreased
- May have edema of lower extremities
- May report chest pain with or without activity
- Cough; may or may not be productive
- Hemoptysis
- Respiratory rate may be increased
- Rales may be present on auscultation
- Repeated streptococcal infections
- Possible history of valve replacement, mitral valve prolapse, surgically treated/untreated tetralogy of Fallot.

Diagnostic Studies

- **White blood cell (WBC) count:** Leukocytosis is indicative of generalized infection, primarily streptococcal
- **Hemoglobin (Hb) and hematocrit:** Reveals actual or physiologic anemia
- **Maternal arterial blood gases (ABGs):** Provide secondary assessment of potential fetal compromise due to maternal respiratory involvement
- **Erythrocyte sedimentation rate (ESR):** Elevated in the presence of cardiac inflammation
- **Maternal electrocardiogram (ECG):** Demonstrates patterns associated with specific cardiac disorders
- Echocardiography
- **Serial ultrasonography:** Detects gestational age of fetus and possible IUGR.

Nursing Diagnoses

- Risk for cardiac output decompensation
- Risk for excess fluid volume
- Risk for impaired uteroplacental tissue perfusion
- Risk for maternal infection
- Risk for activity intolerance
- Knowledge deficit regarding condition, prognosis and treatment needs.

Expected Outcomes

The client will:
- Tolerate the stress of increasing blood volume as indicated by BP and pulse within normal/individually appropriate level
- Demonstrate adequate placental circulation and kidney function with fetal heart rate (FHR) and fetal movement within normal limits
- Demonstrate stable fluid balance with vital signs, appropriate weight gain and absence of edema
- Demonstrate adequate placental perfusion as indicated by reactive fetus with heart rate ranging from 120 to 160 bpm and size appropriate for gestational age

- Remain free of bacterial infection
- Adopt behaviors to maximize tolerance
- Verbalize understanding of individual condition, treatment needs and symptoms indicating need to notify physician.

Nursing Interventions

1. **Improving placental circulation:**
   - Determine/Monitor client's functional classification (as outlined by the NYHA)
   - Provide information about necessity of adequate rest (e.g. 8–10 hours at night and ½ hour after each meal)
   - Discuss use of left or right lateral position
   - Monitor vital signs
   - Auscultate client's breath sounds
   - Evaluate FHR, daily fetal movement count, and non-stress test (NST)
   - Assess for presence of venous stasis with resulting dependant edema of extremities or generalized edema. Instruct client to elevate legs when sitting down and periodically during the day
   - Instruct client to monitor fluid intake/output
   - Investigate report of chest pain and palpitations. Recommend limiting caffeine intake as appropriate
   - Collaboratiave interventions: As follows:
     - Participate in/coordinate multidisciplinary care as appropriate
     - Administer medications such as digitalis glycosides (digoxin or digitoxin) or propranolol (Inderal) as indicated. Monitor for early labor
     - Treat underlying infections as necessary and provide prophylaxis as required
     - Assess placental functioning using sequential serum/urine estriol levels and contraction stress test or NST
     - Obtain and review sequential ECGs
     - Monitor laboratory studies, such as clotting time and electrolyte levels
     - Encourage use of antithrombotic stockings

- Monitor hemodynamic pressures using arterial and central venous pressure lines or Swan-Ganz catheter to monitor pulmonary artery wedge pressure as indicated.

2. **Maintaining stable fluid balance:**
   - Obtain baseline weight. Instruct client to monitor her weight periodically as indicated
   - Review dietary intake, noting factors that may contribute to excessive fluid retention. Provide information as needed
   - Instruct client to monitor color and amount of urine. Measure specific gravity
   - Assess for and review with client signs of CHF such as dyspnea, distended neck veins, crackles, and haemoptysis
   - Collaboratiave interventions: As follows:
     - Investigate unexplained cough
     - Restrict fluids and sodium in presence of CHF
     - Administer diuretics, e.g. Chlorothiazide (Diuril), hydrochlorothiazide (HCTZ), furosemide (Lasix) as appropriate.

3. **Maintaining adequate uteroplacental tissue perfusion:**
   - Note individual risk factors and pregravid health history
   - Assess BP and pulse. Note behavior changes, cyanosis of mucous membranes and nail beds, activity intolerance, and signs of decompensation (i.e. excessive weight gain, unexplained cough, crackles/wheezes hemoptysis and increased pulse and respiratory rate
   - Provide information about use of modified upright position for sleeping and resting.
   - Collaboratiave interventions: As follows:
     - Monitor laboratory studies as indicated: Pulse oxymetry/ABGs/hematocrit (Hb)/Hct
     - The WBC, culture of upper respiratory secretions
     - Assess uterine/fetal blood flow using NST/contraction stress test (CST); check estriol levels and FHR.

4. **Avoiding bacterial infection:**
   - Assess for individual risk factors and history of rheumatic fever

- Provide information about risk of bacterial endocarditis during specific medical surgical procedures
- Review signs and symptoms suggestive of infectious processes requiring medical care (e.g. fever, malaise, cough, cloudy, odiferous urine)
- Assess urine periodically note pH and presence of bacteria
- Collaboratiave interventions: As follows:
  - Obtain cultures as indicated
  - Administer antibiotics when indicated.

5. **Adopting behaviors to maximise tolerance level:**
   - Assess for development of subjective and objective symptoms of activity intolerance (e.g. fatigue, cyanosis, inability to carry on normal daily activities, increasing dyspnea, change in pulse rate and development of respiratory symptoms)
   - Review signs and symptoms with the client and significant others
   - Assist client in setting priorities and restructuring daily routine to include needed rest and sleep periods
   - Identify energy conserving methods to accomplish necessary activites of daily living (ADLs)
   - Ascertain effectiveness of household assistance and available resources
   - Collaboratiave interventions:
     - Refer to appropriate allied health personnel such as occupational therapist and respiratory therapist.

6. **Enhancing understanding of individual condition and treatment needs:**
   - Assess understanding of pathology/complications regarding cardiac condition and pregnancy. Review history and incidence of complications
   - Discuss necessity for frequent monitoring/check-up, i.e. every 2 weeks during first 20 weeks, then every week until delivery
   - Provide information about symptoms indicative of cardiac involvement such as shortness of breath, cough, palpitations, unusual or rapid weight gain (i.e. 1–2 kg in 2 days period), edema or anorexia
   - Provide information regarding diet, rest/sleep, exercise and relaxation

- Review measures to avoid infection
- Review special considerations such as need to avoid foods high in vitamin K (raw, deep-green leafy vegetables) when on anticoagulants
- Review side effects of both prescription and over-the-counter drugs
- Provide appropriate information for protocol of care at home and hospital setting.

27. CEPHALOPELVIC DISPROPORTION

Cephalopelvic disproportion (CPD) exists when the maternal pelvis cannot accommodate the fetal head as it descends. It is the disparity in the relation between fetal head and maternal pelvis. Disproportion may be either due to an average size baby with a small pelvis or due to a big baby with normal size pelvis or due to a combination of both.

A contracted maternal pelvis and fetal macrosomia contribute to CPD (Bashore, 1992). A contracted pelvis refers to abnormalities in measurements that fall short of those required for a normal vaginal delivery. Congenital or acquired (from trauma) pelvic deviations may exist. Relative CPD is said to exist when the fetus is larger than the maternal pelvic inlet-outlet or when the fetal position places the head at an angle that is larger than the size, pelvis can facilitate.

DIAGNOSIS OF CEPHALOPELVIC DISPROPORTION

- Sonography
- X-ray pelvimetry
- Clinical methods:
  - Abdominal
  - Abdominoperineal.

Contributing Patterns

- Congenital non gynaecoid pelvic shape: Flattened, narrow or irregular
- Post-traumatic contractures as a result of crushed or fractured pelvis.

RISKS OF CPD

To Laboring Client/Mother

- Prolonged and painful labor
- Failure of the cervix to dilate
- Failure of fetal descend with resultant need for operative delivery
- Uterine rupture from prolonged thinning of lower uterine segment during non progressive, but active labor process.

To Fetus

- Extensive caput and molding from the prolonged labor
- Fetal intolerance with resultant hypoxia from prolonged labor
- Potential for birth injury related to difficult and traumatic delivery.

MANAGEMENT

Minor degrees of inlet contraction do not give rise to problems and have spontaneous vaginal delivery at term. The moderate and severe degrees are managed by one of the following methods:

Premature Induction of Labor

This is limited only to moderate degree of disproportion in selected multigravidae, 2–3 weeks prior to due date.

Elective Cesarean Section at Term

This is indicated in major degree of inlet contraction associated with outlet contraction or complicating factors such as elderly primigravida, malpresentation, postmaturity, toxemia, postcesarean delivery and medical disorders such as diabetes, heart disease, etc. If the expected date of delivery is known, the operation is planned and done in the last week of pregnancy. In cases where fetal maturity is not known, the operation is withheld till labor pains start or the membranes rupture, which ever occurs early.

Trial Labor

This is the preferred management method for a client with minor degree of cephalopelvic disproportion at the inlet (pelvic brim), particularly in a young primigravida with no other complications. The client is allowed to go in labor and then is carefully watched as the labor progresses.

Advantages

- Eliminates unnecessary cesarean section electively decided upon
- A successful outcome leading to a vaginal delivery secures the client's obstetric future.

Disadvantages

- Cesarean section may have to be performed for about half of the cases; because of fetal distress or abnormal uterine action
- Fetal morbidity and mortality may be higher than with elective cesarean section
- Maternal morbidity is higher
- When the trial fails and client has to face a surgical procedure, she is disappointed, dehydrated, frightened and in poor shape.

Contraindications

- Severe disproportion; true conjugate less than 9 cm
- If in a previous pregnancy, trial of labor had failed
- Maternal diseases such as diabetes, pregnancy-induced hypertension, cardiac condition
- Intrauterine growth restriction (IUGR)
- Cases of malpresentation, e.g. breech
- Previous cesarean section.

Conduct of Trail Labor

Trial labor should only be carried out in a well-staffed, well-equipped hospital with facilities for emergency cesarean section, which may be necessary at any time. Facilities to monitor fetal well-being must be present:

- Labor should be spontaneous and not induced
- As soon as the membranes rupture, vaginal examination must be performed to see the color of liquor and to exclude prolapse of cord
- Monitor carefully:
  - Maternal pulse, blood pressure and temperature
  - Fluid balance
  - Urine for acetone
  - Fetal heart rate
  - Uterine contractions and progress of labor
  - Cervical dilation, molding, position and station of head
- Graphic recording of progress of labor on partogram
- Adequate sedation, analgesics and reassurance
- Adequate hydration and nutrition (IV dextrose)
- Emergency cesarean section when indicated, e.g. fetal distress.

Favorable progress of cervical effacement and dilatation, descend of the head into the pelvis, and confirmation that the lower part of the pelvis is adequate are criteria for continuing the trial. Lack of progressive dilatation of the cervix and failure of the head to enter the inlet and descend to the ischial spines serve as evidence that the trial of labor has failed.

PROGNOSIS

- Rate of cesarean section is 40–50% depending on selection of cases
- Fetal wastage 2–3%.

28. CHROMOSOME ABNORMALITIES IN NEWBORNS

The normal human karyotype consists of 22 pairs of autosomes and 1 pair of sex chromosomes XX/XY. Chromosomal abnormalities may be numerical or structural. Both the autosomes and sex chromosomes can experience numerical and structural chromosomal abnormalities that have clinical consequences.

In numerical abnormality, chromosomes may be missing or present in excess of the normal pairs. Numerical alterations resulting in hyperploidy (3n, 4n and so on) produce a wide spectrum of malformations that render them incompatible with life. Small variations around the normal diploid number (46), such occur in trisomies (total chromosome number 47), are often found in clinical practice. The only monosomy compatible with life is a missing X-chromosome in persons with Turner's syndrome.

NUMERICAL ABNORMALITIES

Trisomy 21 (Down Syndrome)

Down syndrome is the most common aneuploidy compatible with development to full term with a reasonable quality of postnatal life. Physical and mental abnormalities vary enormously in affected individuals. Mean IQ is 50, with a range of 25–70. Physical anomalies includes:
- Craniofacial abnormalities such as flat occiput, low-set ears, oblique palpebral fissures, epicanthal folds, broad nasal bones and flattened profile and open mouth with protruding tongue
- Skeletal abnormalities such as broad, short fingers and clinodactyly of fifth finger
- Cardiac malformations, e.g. ventricular and atrial septal defects, patent ductus arteriosus
- Other abnormalities such as hypotonia, increased susceptibility to respiratory infections and acute leukemia; palmar simian crease and abnormal fingerprint pattern. Males with Down Syndrome are usually sterile.

Trisomy 18 (Edward's Syndrome)

This is a fairly common trisomy affecting mostly chromosome 18. In addition to severe mental retardation, children with this defect present with severe craniofacial abnormalities, e.g. dolichocephaly with a prominent occiput, low-set and malformed ears and micrognathia. Skeletal abnormalities seen are clenched fist with overlapping fingers, flexion deformities, adducted hips and 'rockerbottom' feet.

Cardiac anomalies includes ventricular and atrial septal defects and patent ductus arteriosus. Urogenital malformations may be 'horseshoe' kidneys, hydronephrosis, cryptorchidism and prominent genitals. Hypotonia is also common. Females are often affected and a few survive one year of age.

Trisomy 13 (Patau Syndrome)

Patau syndrome causes more severe malformations than the previous two trisomies which is consistent with the increased size of the extra chromosome and a greater gene imbalance. Craniofacial anomalies are much more pronounced: microcephaly, lowset and malformed ears, microphthalmia or anophthalmia and cleft lip and palate. Skeletal abnormalities include polydactyly and syndactyly, overlapping, flexed fingers and hypoplasia of pelvis. Systemic anomalies include cardiac defects and urogenital malformations. Mean life expectancy is 4 months.

Alterations in number may also involve the sex chromosomes. Some of the most common disorders are Klinefelter, Jacobs, Turner and triple X female syndromes.

47, XXY (Klinefelter Syndrome)

This syndrome is characterized by multiple X chromosomes and one Y chromosome. The greater the total chromosome number, the more severe the anomalies that result from increased gene imbalance. Physical abnormalities include elements of decreased masculinisation, such as gynecomastia, hypogonadism and increased pubis-to-sole length; reflecting elongated lower limbs. Mental development is normal in most cases. Mental retardation, if it occurs is in the range of 50–85. Delayed language skills, however, are common.

47, XYY (Jacob's Syndrome)

Individuals with an extra Y chromosome are of tall structure (more than 6 feet) and suffer skin disorders such as persistent adult acne. Mental retardation and aggressive tendency which were reported earlier (1960s) were not found significant.

45, XO (Turner Syndrome)

Clinical manifestations of this syndrome include low birth weight and short adult stature (4' 6"–4' 8"); low posterior hairline and webbing of the neck; shield-shaped chest with divergent nipples; short fourth metacarpals; cubitus valgus; coarctation of the aorta, urinary tract abnormalities, lymph edema of hands and feet in the newborn and hydrops. Intellectual development is normal, with verbal IQ exceeding performance IQ. Secondary sexual characteristics are decreased and growth is usually stunted.

47, XXX (Triple X)

This is a relatively common condition occurring in about 1:1,000 female live births. Triple X females display a normal phenotype, with perhaps a slight decrease in mental capacity, when compared to their euploid counterparts. Gynecologic complications include a delayed menarche and a premature menopause. The offsprings of XXX females are largely normal.

STRUCTURAL CHROMOSOMAL ABNORMALITIES

Structural abnormalities include a variety of chromosome defects (e.g. deletions and translocations) that do not alter the total chromosome number. The hallmark of these conditions is chromosomal breakage or rearrangement:

46, XX or XY, B5(P) (Cri du chat, or Cat's Cry Syndrome)

It is a rare (1 in 50,000 live births) chromosome deletion syndrome resulting from loss of the small arm of chromosome B(5). In early infancy, this syndrome presents with a typical, but non distinctive facial appearance, often a 'moon-shaped' face, with wide-spaced eyes. As the child grows this feature progressively diminishes and by age of 2 years, the child is undistinguishable from age matched children. Profound mental retardation persists throughout a short life. Most affected children die in infancy from multiple genetic imbalances. Typical of this disease is a crying pattern that is abnormal and cat-like. At times, it sounds like an angry cat; at others like a soft mewling sound. This is a result of laryngeal atrophy, which improves with age. By age of 3 years, the crying pattern acquires a normal pitch and looses its cat-like quality.

Fragile X-syndrome

The acquired name from the fact that in vitro conditions, the X chromosome frequently displays breaks and gaps in its terminal portions. This is an X-linked dominant condition with increased prevalence among males. Clinical features include mental retardation and a typical facial appearance, including an elongated face and long, elf-like ears.

Chromosome Instability Syndrome

This is a heterogeneous group of genetic disorders characterized by a high frequency of chromosome breakage that is observed in vitro. They include ataxia telangiectasia, Fanconi anemia and xeroderma pigmentosum. These syndromes are associated with decreased immune system and increased incidence of cancer, mostly lymphomas and leukemias.

PREVENTION AND MANAGEMENT

Because of the complexity and magnitude of genetic damage, treatment for these conditions is rarely successful. The primary weapon against increases in the prevalence of genetic and chromosomal conditions is an aggressive program of genetic screening and counseling.

Genetic Screening

Purposes

- To provide early recognition of diseases for which effective intervention and therapy exist, before symptoms occur, e.g. phenylketonuria
- To provide identification in carriers of genetic disease for the purpose of maximizing parenthood planning options, e.g. Tay-Sach's disease (an inherited disorder of lipid metabolism)

- To obtain population data on frequency, spectrum and natural history of genetic disorder, e.g. chromosomal disorders in newborns.

Scope

Screening for genetic disorders can occur at various times in a person's life:
- Screening of relatives of a known carrier or affected individuals within a family, for the purpose of reproductive decision making
- Preconception screening for carriers, e.g. screening of couples contemplating parenthood for specific condition such as Tay-Sachs disease
- Postconception (prenatal) testing for specific disorders, e.g. Tay-Sachs disease
- Newborn testing for conditions such as phenylketonuria (PKU) and congenital hypothyroidism
- Screening of selected population/group for heterogeneous carriers, e.g. screening for sickle cell disease.

Genetic Counseling

Genetic counseling consists of one or more encounters with the probands (affected) and their families with the objective of providing information about their genetic disease. Genetic counseling refers to a series of procedures that include processing the initial referral, assessing the needs, deciding on the appropriate tests, interpreting the results and finally communicating these findings to the proband, and family.

In the majority of families referred for genetic counseling, the precipitating event is the birth of an affected child. In the case of dominant diseases, usually one of the parents is affected, and there is some degree of preparation for the possibility of an affected child. In recessive disorders however, the parents are usually clinically normal, which prevents any warning of a potentially negative outcome. Maternal age is another reason for genetic counseling.

29. CONGENITAL UTERINE ANOMALIES/ABNORMALITIES

DEFINITION

Congenital anomalies of the uterus are defects of uterine development and shape that occur during intrauterine life.

DEVELOPMENT OF UTERINE ANOMALIES

Congenital anomalies, also called Mullerian duct anomalies are malformations that develop during embryonic life. During fetal development period, it actually starts as two small uteri which migrate down separately and ultimately fuses to form a single uterus. Normally the wall where the two uteri join, reabsorbs completely from the bottom to the top resulting in a triangular shape uterine cavity. Any alteration to this developmental process of cellular differentiation, migration, fusion and canalization leads to what is called congenital uterine anomaly.

Type of Uterine Anomalies

1. **Uterus didelphis (Fig. 29.1):** Didelphis uterus also called double uterus is a rare uterine abnormality in which the two halves of the uterus develop completely separate. There will be two separate uteri each one with a cervix. A uterus with double cervix is named a Bicollis and that with a single cervix is Unicollis. These may have double vagina or single vagina as seen in the figure. Women with this type of uterus often have successful pregnancies, however, they are at higher risk of preterm delivery or miscarriage. This is seen in 7.5% of women.
2. **Arcuate uterus (Fig. 29.2):** Here the uterus looks normal, but the internal surface of the single endometrial cavity shows a shallow groove of 1 cm or less which forms a short septum. This is seen in 7% of women.

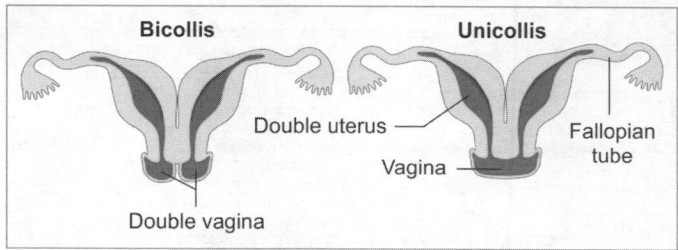

Fig. 29.1: Uterus didelphis.

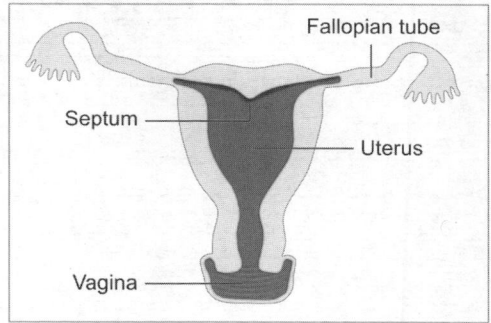

Fi. 29.2: Arcuate uterus.

3. **Unicornuate uterus (Fig. 29.3):** This abnormality of the uterus is also called single horned uterus and happens when the tissues that form the uterus do not develop properly. Only one half of the uterus develops from a single mullerian duct. The unicornuate uterus has only one fallopian tube. Seen in 15% of women.
4. **Bicornuate uterus (Fig. 29.4):** In this type, the uterus has an external indentation or groove marking its division internally into two endometrial cavities. The two halves of the uterus may appear almost completely separated except at the lower part.

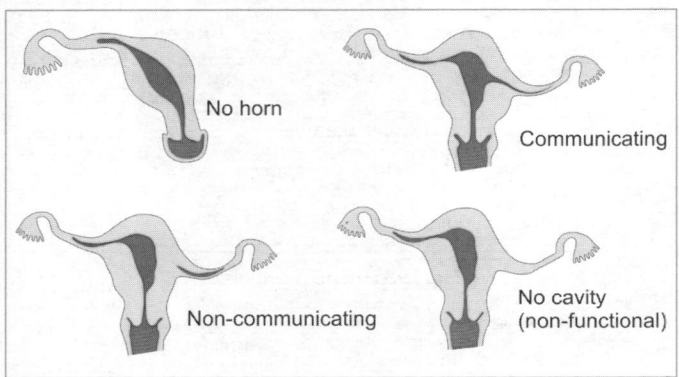

Fig. 29.3: Unicornuate uterus.

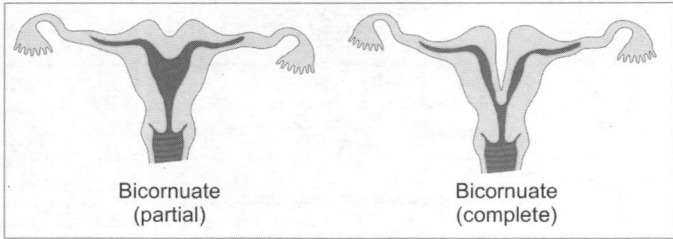

Fig. 29.4: Bicornuate uterus.

When pregnancy occurs, the baby has less space to grow in the uterine cavity. This makes up about 25% of such anomalies.

5. **Septate uterus (Fig. 29.5):** Here the uterus looks completely normal on the outside, but is separated on the inside into two different halves by a septum of varying size and thickness. Thus, there are two endometrial cavities. The septum may extend only partially into the uterus resulting in partial septate uterus or it may reach up to the cervix as complete septate uterus.

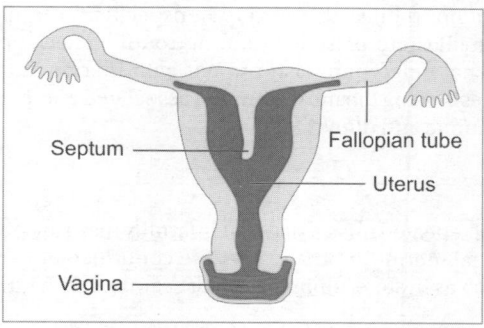

Fig. 29.5: Septate uterus.

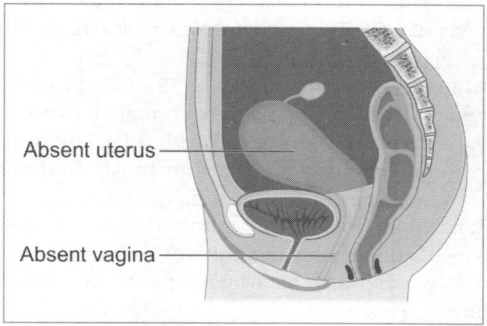

Fig. 29.6: Uterine agenesis.

6. **Uterine agenesis (Fig. 29.6):** The uterus fails to form at all in about 10% of women with uterine anomalies.

Clinical Features

Most women with uterine anomalies are not aware of any defect as their female physiology is typically unaffected. In most cases, fertility is unimpaired. In a few cases dysmenorrhea or painful periods may be a symptom, though this is very nonspecific. In fertile women, these anomalies are picked up during routine check-up. In some women, renal defects are also present with uterine anomaly with renal agenesis being the most common associated anomaly followed by renal ectopic and duplex kidney.

Diagnosis

A history of repeated miscarriages or infertility may cause a suspicion of congenital uterine anomaly. They are confirmed only by imaging studies such as hysterosalpingogram or scanning with ultrasound or MRI.

Management

Many women with congenital uterine abnormality do not require any treatment. If the anomaly causes a miscarriage, infertility or pain, a surgical correction is required.

Surgical repair or reconstruction is the only form of treatment for such women. If the defect is severe enough to cause obstruction of the reproductive tract, associated with infertility or miscarriage surgery is recommended. Septate uteri are most commonly repaired to improve the chances of having a baby, but the other types are generally left alone. The type of surgery recommended depends upon the type of abnormality and the woman's reproductive history and health. In women with bicornuate uterus, the dividing septum can be removed to open up the uterus. In case of unicornuate uterus, the obstructed hemi-uterus can be removed if the other part of the uterus is normal and functional.

Women who are at higher risk for preterm delivery or late pregnancy loss due to congenital uterine abnormality may need a stitch in the cervix (called cervical circlage). Most cases of anomalies can be corrected using a minimal invasive surgery like laparoscopy or hysteroscopy. In some cases, surgical correction may not result in improvement and hence, the women should be told what to expect beforehand.

Possible Complications Associated with Uterine Anomalies

- Dysmenorrhea
- Hematometra
- During pregnancy and labor:
  - Late miscarriage
  - Premature labor
  - Malpresentation
  - Obstructed labor
  - Uterine rupture
  - Retained placenta
  - Postpartum hemorrhage.

30. CONGENITAL ANOMALIES IN NEWBORNS

Congenital anomalies are abnormalities present at birth as a result of either genetic, prenatal or environmental factors or combination of these factors. Genetic anomalies are inherited defects that are transmitted from generation to generation. Major congenital defects are the leading cause of death in infants less than 1 year of age.

CENTRAL NERVOUS SYSTEM ANOMALIES

The most common anomalies of the central nervous system (CNS) occur during the primary neurulation period, which is during the first 3–4 weeks of gestation. These anomalies termed "neural tube defects" occur as a result of failure of the neural tube to close.

Encephalocele

A herniation of the brain and meninges through an opening in the skull. The defect is readily visible at birth (**Fig. 30.1**).

Manifestations

- Skin generally covers the encephalocele
- Skin may break open.

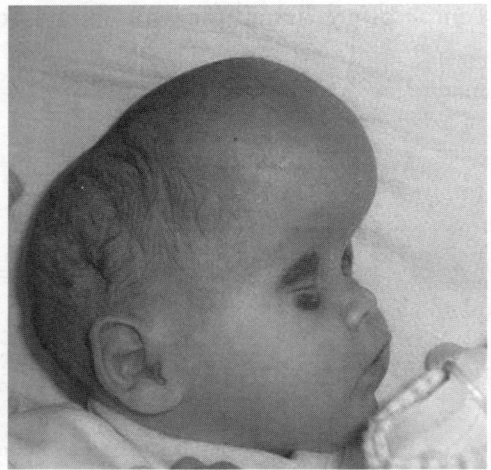

Fig. 30.1: Encephalocele.

Treatment

- Replacement of the brain contents and repair of the defect surgically
- If hydrocephalus is present, ventricular shunting 7–10 days after repair of the defect, from the ventricular system into the abdominal cavity.

Anencephaly

There is a complete or partial absence of cerebral hemisphere and skull **(Figs. 30.2A and B)**.

Features

Infants are usually stillborn or die within the first few hours of life.

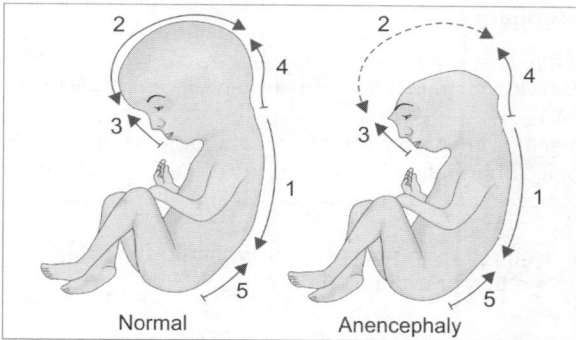

Fig. 30.2A: Normal head and anencephaly.

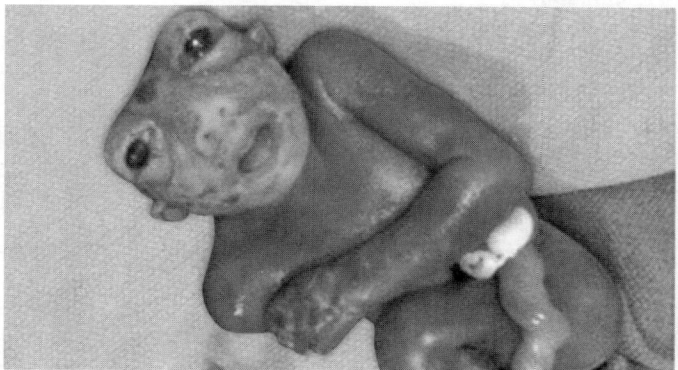

Fig. 30.2B: Baby born with anencephaly.

Management

- Nursing interventions for providing comfort until the infant dies from respiratory or cardiac failure
- Emotional and spiritual support to the parents.

Microcephaly

A condition in which there is small head, which contains an underdeveloped brain microcephaly may be congenital or acquired (**Fig. 30.3**):
- Congenital anencephaly may occur in conjunction with chromosomal abnormalities, intrauterine infections such as rubella, cytomegalovirus or toxoplasmosis and maternal exposure to X-rays.
- The acquired form may result from herpes infection (acquired from mother) or hypothyroidism.

Treatment

- No treatment and the condition generally results in mental retardation
- Supportive nursing care.

Hydrocephaly

A condition that results from an excess accumulation of cerebrospinal fluid (CSF) is the ventricles of the brain and subarachnoid space as a result of imbalance between CSF production and absorption (**Fig. 30.4**).

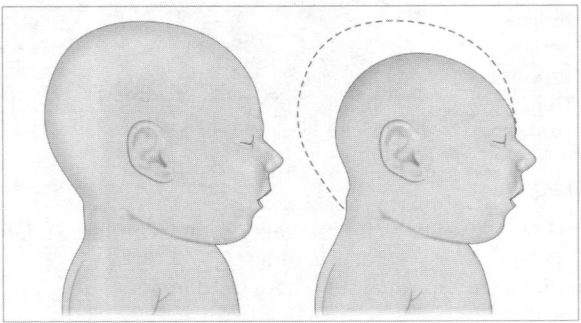

Fig. 30.3: Microcephaly.

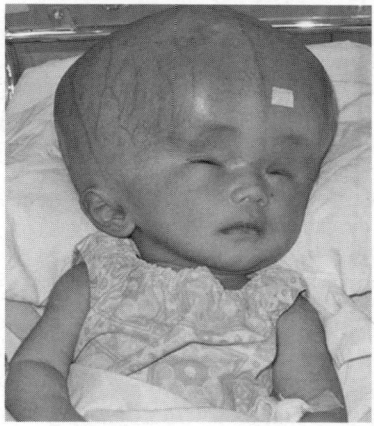

Fg. 30.4: Hydrocehalus.

Features

- Normal growth and development of the brain is altered due to CSF pressure
- Cesarean section is necessary to deliver the baby
- Infant is born with:
  - An enlarged head
  - Bulging fontaneles
  - Separated skull sutures
  - Prominent forehead
  - Depressed eyes that are rotated downward causing a 'setting sun' sign.

Nursing Care

- Observation and assessment of the neurological status
- Support to head while holding, turning, or positioning the infant
- Serial measurement of head circumference
- Observation to note any increase in intracranial pressure.

Treatment

- Surgical placement of a shunt from the ventricle in the brain to the abdominal cavity to allow drainage of excess CSF
- Postoperatively the infant to be placed in flat position to prevent rapid drainage of CSF and decompression.
- To educate parents about:
  - Care of infant with shunt such as positioning, and skin care
  - Signs of increased *intracranial pressure (ICP)*
  - Signs of shunt malfunction
  - Prevention of skin breakdown and infection.

Spina Bifida

A common CNS defect that results from failure of the spinal column to close. There are two categories **(Fig. 30.5)**.
- Spina bifida occulta
- Spina bifida cystica:
  - Spina bifida occulta is the failure of the spinal column to close when neither the cord nor the meninges herniate through the defect. There may be an overlying hairy patch over the defect
  - Spina bifida cystica includes meningocele and meningomyelocele.

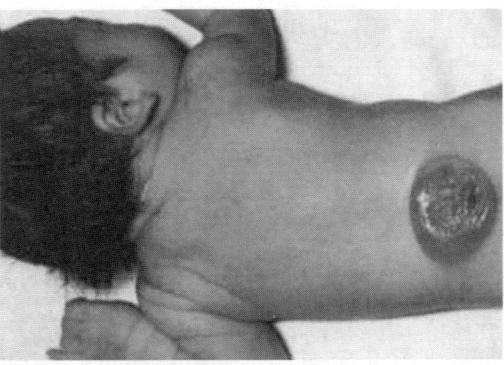

Fig. 30.5: Spina bifida.

- In a meningocele, there is an external sac that protrudes through the defect that contains meninges and CSF. However, the spinal cord and nerve roots are in their normal position.
- In meningomyelocele, the sac contains neural tissue in addition to meninges and CSF. It may be seen at any point in the vertebral column from C-1 to the coccyx, but is most common in the lumbar, lumbosacral and sacral segments.

Diagnosis

Diagnosis of neural tube defects can be made during pregnancy by:
- Testing amniotic fluid for presence of alphafetoprotein (AFP), which is from CSF that leaked into it
- Ultrasound examination to visualise the defect.

Management

- Closure of the defect within the 1st few hours of life
- Nurse the infant in prone or side lying position with a rolled towel to prevent pressure on the sac
- Infant's position to be changed every hour
- The sac should be covered with a moist, sterile gauze dressing
- The skin around the defect should be kept clean and dry to prevent skin breakdown
- Prescribed antibiotics to be administered
- Postoperative assessment include:
  - Signs and symptoms of infection
  - Signs of increased ICP
  - Bladder function.
- Manual emptying of bladder to stimulate urination
- Range of motion exercises.

RESPIRATORY SYSTEM ANOMALIES

Malformation of the respiratory system can be life-threatening and their recognition in the delivery room is imperative for proper treatment. The 1st few minutes of life are most crucial, so ensuring adequate oxygenation during this period is necessary to long-term positive outcome for the newborn.

Choanal Atresia

- A condition in which there is a bony or membranous separation between the nose and pharynx
- Unilateral atresia is more common than bilateral atresia and female newborns are affected more.

Manifestations

- Infants with choanal atresia usually have other anomalies such as:
    - Coloboma of eyes
    - Heart defects
    - Renal anomalies
    - Growth and mental retardation
    - Ear deficits
    - Gastrointestinal reflux
- Infants are nose breathers
- Respiratory distress especially in bilateral atresia
- Cyanosis at rest, but the color improves when the baby opens his/her mouth to cry.

Diagnosis

Checking patency by passing a catheter through each nostril.

Treatment

- Immediate surgical correction
- Prognosis is excellent if, there is no other concomitant-related medical conditions.

Diaphragmatic Hernia

Diaphragmatic hernia occurs during gestational life when diaphragm fails to close during the 7th or 8th week. Abdominal organs are displaced into the left side of the chest through an opening in the diaphragm.

Prenatal Diagnosis

- Ultrasound examination as early as 26 weeks gestation reveals abdominal contents in thoracic cavity and inadequate development of lung on affected side

- Respiratory distress at birth due to hypoplastic lung
- Breath sounds are diminished or absent on the affected side
- Bowel sounds are audible in the chest
- Large asymmetric chest and a flat, smaller abdomen.

Management

- Mechanical ventilation with 100% oxygen
- Positioning on the affected side with the head and chest elevated
- Gastric decompression with continuous low suction
- Surgical repair of the hernia after stabilizing the condition.

Prognosis depends on the degree of pulmonary development and success of closure.

CARDIOVASCULAR SYSTEM ANOMALIES

Development of the cardiovascular system is completed by 7th week of gestation. Congenital heart defects are anatomical abnormalities in the heart that are present at birth.

Patent Ductus Arteriosus

A vascular connection that during fetal life, short-circuits the pulmonary vascular bed and directs blood from the pulmonary artery to the aorta:
- Functional closure of the ductus normally occurs soon after birth
- If the ductus remains patent after birth, the direction of blood flow in the ductus reverses due to higher pressure in the aorta.

Ventricular Septal Defect

It is an abnormal opening between the right and left ventricles. VSDs vary in size and may occur in the membraneous or muscular portion of the septum.

Due to higher pressure in the left ventricle, a shunting of blood from right to left ventricle occurs during systole with resultant cyanosis.

Truncus Arteriosus

In this condition, there is a retention of the embryonic bulbar trunk. It is a failure of the normal septation and division of the trunk into an aorta and pulmonary artery. The single arterial trunk overrides the ventricles and receives blood from them through a VSD. The entire pulmonary and systemic circulation is supplied from this common arterial trunk.

Transposition of Great Vessels

This anomaly is an embryonic defect caused by a straight division of the bulbar trunk without the normal spiraling. The aorta originates from the right ventricle and the pulmonary artery from the left ventricle. An abnormal communication is present between the two circulations, which is necessary to sustain life.

Atrial Septal Defect

Atrial septal defect (ASD) is an abnormal opening between the right and left atria. Basically, three types of abnormalities result from incorrect development of the atrial septum:
- An incomplete foramen ovale
- An ostium secundum defect resulting from abnormal development of the septum secondum
- An ostium primum defect from improper development of ostium primum. Left to right shunting of blood occurs in all atrial septal defects.

Nursing Interventions

Continuous monitoring of the infants:
- Cardiac and respiratory status
- Thermoneutral environment
- Administering oxygen
- Administering medications as prescribed
- Offering comfort measures to minimise crying
- Gavage feeding
- Instructing parents about the defect, medication administration and how to observe for signs and symptoms.

GASTROINTESTINAL SYSTEM ANOMALIES

The primitive gut is formed during the 4th week of gestation. Many intricate steps are involved in the development of the complete gastrointestinal (GI) tract during which it is exposed to the possibility of various malformations, These malformations can occur anywhere in the GI tract and may be simple or complex.

Cleft lip and Palate

These are congenital anomalies that occur in the lip or palate or both, that results from failure of the maxillary and premaxillary processes to fuse during the 7th to 12th week of intrauterine life. These are seen in conjunction with other syndromes in relation to avitaminosis and viral infections of the mother during the first trimester **(Figs. 36A, B and C)**.

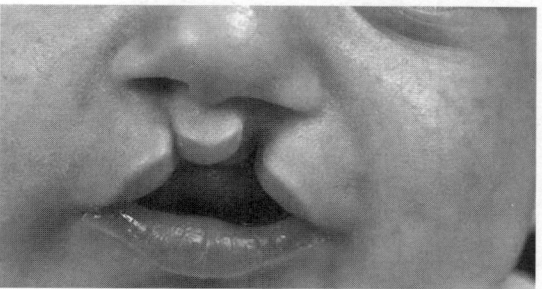

Fig. 30.6A: Cleft lip.

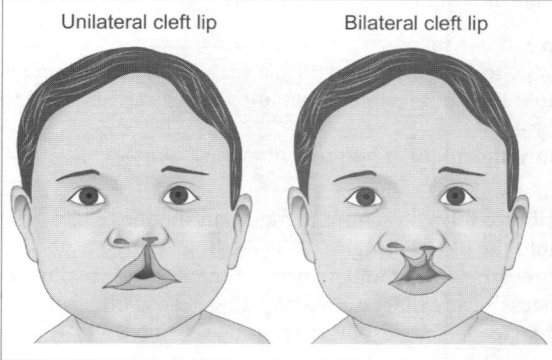

Fig. 30.6B: Unilateral cleft lip and bilateral cleft lip.

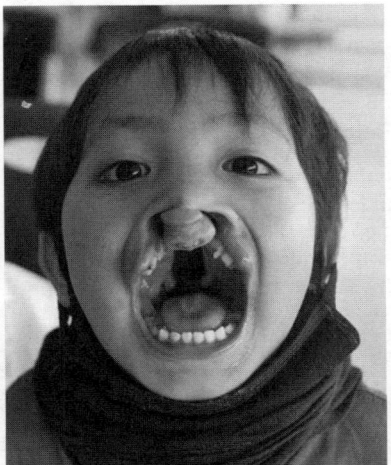

Fig. 30.6C: Cleft lip and cleft palate.

Diagnosis

- Physical appearance at birth
- Feeling for cleft palate with a gloved finger.

Difficulties and Measures to Help Feed

Cleft lip
- Inability to hold on to and form a seal around the nipple
- To hold the bottle while the infant's cheeks are grasped together to close the cleft
- To burp the infant at frequent intervals.

Cleft palate
- Inability to form a vacuum to maintain suction
- To hold the infant upright, while feeding
- To direct the flow of milk to one side of mouth to avoid choking
- With less severe defects breastfeeding is possible
- Syringe feeders are useful to feed successfully.

Management

- Education, counseling and emotional support to parents
- Surgical repair of cleft lip at 3 months of age
- Repair of cleft palate between 9 and 12 months of age
- Instruction to mothers on postoperative care and use of any appliances.

Esophageal Atresia and Tracheoesophageal Fistula

The esophageal atresia is a condition in which the esophagus ends in a blind pouch or narrows into a thin cord and is not connected to the stomach. The tracheoesophageal fistula occurs due to failure of separation of trachea and esophagus during 34th to 36th days of gestation. These defects may occur together or singly.

Manifestations

- With esophageal atresia (EA) and tracheoesophageal fistula (TEF), infants may appear well immediately after birth
- Copious secretions and inability to swallow oral feeds after the initial period
- Drooling, coughing and choking
- Regurgitation of feed
- Abdominal distention with a fistula at the distal end
- Cyanosis.

Diagnosis

- Inability to pass a nasogastric catheter any further, than 10 cm from the nares or into stomach
- X-ray, while inserting a radiopaque catheter.

Management

- Immediate surgical repair (if infant is medically unstable, surgery is delayed until infant's health status improves)
- Nothing to be given orally

- Continuous low suction to remove secretions and prevent aspiration
- Education of parents about the defect, management plan and care before- and after-surgery.

Omphalocele and Gastroschisis

An omphalocele is a defect covered by a peritoneal sac, located at the base of the umbilicus into which portions of the abdominal organs herniate (**Fig. 30.7**)

Manifestations

- The sac may contain both the small and large intestines, stomach, liver, spleen and bladder
- The peritoneal sac covering the defect may rupture during or after birth
- Omphalocele develops during the 10th to 12th weeks of gestation and is often seen in conjunction with other cardiac, genitourinary, neurologic or chromosomal anomalies

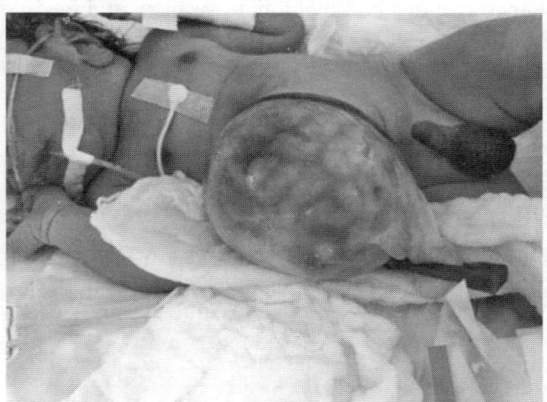

Fig. 30.7: Omphalocele.

- In gastroschisis, the bowel herniates through an abdominal wall defect to the right of the umbilicus and the contents lie openly on the abdomen (not contained in a sac). It is rarely associated with other anomalies.

Management

Immediate care
- Maintaining body heat and fluid and electrolyte balance
- Protecting the abdominal organs by covering with a warm, sterile, saline soaked gauze which in turn to be covered with a plastic wrap.

Surgical treatment
Replacement of the organs in the abdominal cavity in stages over 7–10 days. Parents need counseling to deal with the crisis and care of the baby.

Imperforate Anus

A group of congenital anomalies involving the rectum and anus, and result when the membrane separating the rectum from the anus fails to get absorbed during the 7th or 8th week.

Types of Imperforation

- If located low, there is stenosis of the anal opening or a thin, transparent membrane present over the normal opening
- If located high, the rectum ends in a blind pouch or there is no connection between the anus and rectum.

Treatment

- Surgical correction in stages with temporary colostomy in the interim
- For the low type, excision of the membrane followed by daily dilation.

GENITOURINARY ANOMALIES

Hypospadias

A congenital anomaly in which the urethral meatus is located on the ventral surface of the glans penis instead of at the tip. Surgical repair is generally completed during the 1st year of life **(Fig. 30.8)**.

Epispadias

In epispadias, the urethral meatus is located on the dorsal surface of the penis. This rare anomaly often occurs with extrophy of the bladder. Surgical repair is done, using the foreskin to close the defect **(Fig. 30.9)**.

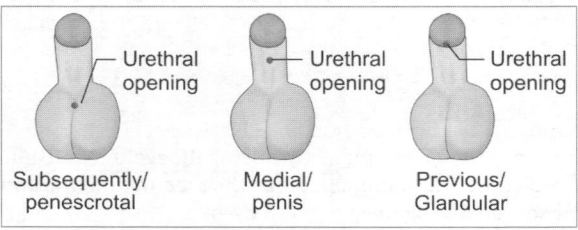

Fig. 30.8: Hypospadias.

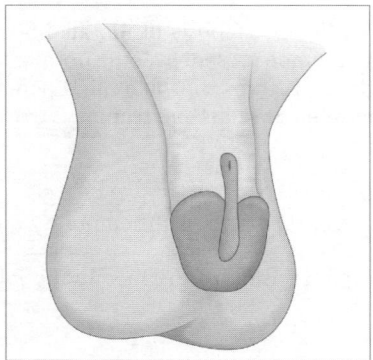

Fig. 30.9: Epispadias.

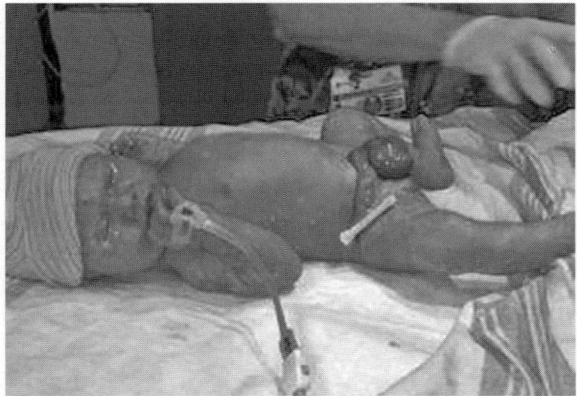

Fig. 30.10: Extrophy of bladder.

Exstrophy of Bladder

Bladder to lie open and exposed on the lower abdominal wall are absent, causing the bladder to lie open and exposed on the lower abdomen. Surgical reconstruction is often done in two stages. First stage within the first few hours of birth and second stage of creating a urethra before the child goes to school **(Fig. 30.10)**.

Ambiguous Genitalia

The gender of the newborn remains unclear at the time of birth. If reconstructive surgery is required, gender determination needs to be done within 3–6 months. In other cases, it should be done before the age of 2. Parents need great deal of support as they learn to live with the situation.

MUSCULOSKELETAL SYSTEM

Formation of the musculoskeletal system begins in the 4th week of gestation. Malformations are relatively minor and with treatment the outcome is usually favorable:

Developmental Dysplasia of the Hip

The condition includes malformation of hip involving various degrees of deformity that may be present at birth, ranging from subluxation to complete dislocation.

Treatment

- The hips must be maintained in a flexed and abducted position with triple diapering or Pavlik harness for 1–2 months
- Parents must be educated about the condition, management and care of the infant in a harness or cast.

Talipes Equinovarus (Club Foot)

A deformity in which portions of the foot and ankle are twisted out of the normal position. The foot is fixed in planter flexion (downward) and is deviated medically (inward) **(Fig. 30.11)**.

Treatment

- Gentle, repeated manipulations of the foot with serial castings done every few weeks, then every week or two until correction is satisfactorily completed
- Surgical correction.

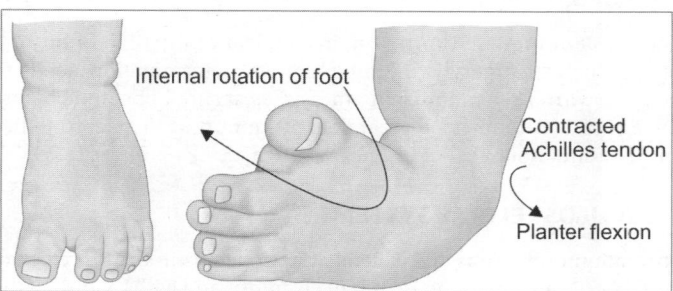

Fig. 30.11: Talipes eqinovarus (Club foot).

Talipes Calcaneovalgus

The foot is held in dorsiflexion and deviated laterally. Shortening of the soft tissues on the dorsum of foot limits the degree of planter flexion and inversion. It may result from an abnormal intrauterine position **(Fig. 30.12)**.

Treatment

- Passive stretching for mild deformity
- Exercise and application of plaster cast in some cases.

Polydactyly (Super Numerary Digits)

This anomaly occurs either on the hands or feet. Most frequently it occurs as an accessory and often as a hypoplastic appendage or a skin tag on the ulnar side of the little finger. At times, the thumb may be seen duplicated **(Fig. 30.13)**.

Treatment

- For simple skin tag, ligation and leaving it to slough
- Surgical correction.

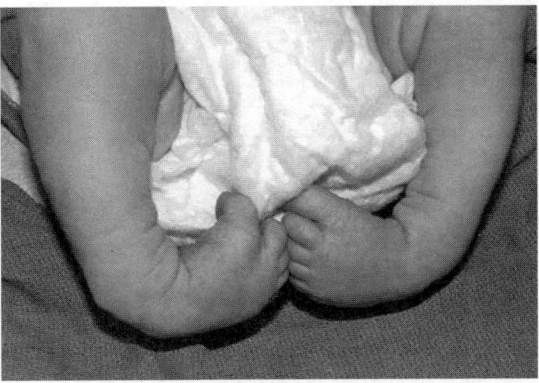

Fig. 30-12: Talipes calaneovalgus.

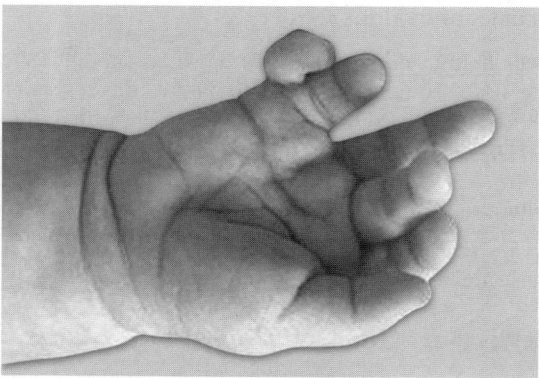

Fig. 30.13: Polydactyly.

Syndactyly

An abnormality of the upper extremity, which involves an abnormal fusion of the digits, either partial or complete. It may consist of interdigital webbing of the skin only, or bony structure or both. Often involves the third and fourth fingers or second and third fingers. It is often a hereditary abnormality **(Fig. 30.14)**.

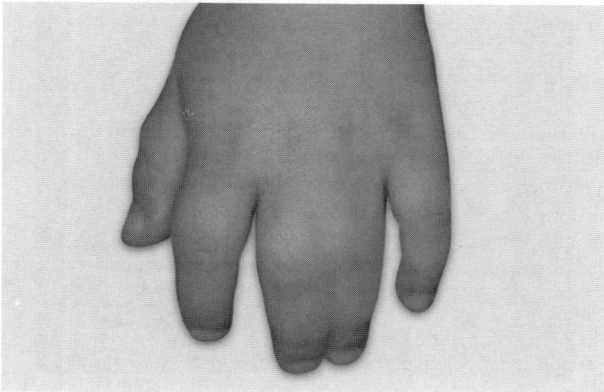

Fig. 3014: Syndactyly.

Treatment

Treatment is surgical correction.

Apert's Syndrome

A genetically inherited condition in which there is premature fusion of the sutures of vault of skull, cleft palate and complete syndactyly of both hands and feet.

Treatment

Surgical correction before the child enters school.

31. CONTRACTED PELVIS

A contracted pelvis may be defined as, one in which any of its essential diameters is so shortened as to alter the normal mechanism of labor. Any diameter of the inlet or outlet when shortened by more than 0.5 cm may produce obstruction in the passage of an average sized fetus. Such a pelvis may have a normal or an abnormal shape.

Cephalopelvic disproportion may be due to a relatively large baby or a contracted pelvis. Disproportion may be absolute or relative. It is absolute when under no circumstances can the baby pass through the birth passage. Relative disproportion is present when other factors contribute to the problem.

CLASSIFICATION

This classification is based on the etiological factors:
- Nutritional and environmental defects:
  - Minor variations
  - Major rachitic and osteomalacic.
- Diseases or injuries affecting the pelvis:
  - Pelvic: Tumors, fractures and tubercular arthritis
  - Spinal: Kyphosis, scoliosis, spondylolisthesis and coccygeal deformity
  - Lower limbs: Congenital dislocation of hip, poliomyelitis in childhood hip joint disease.

DIAGNOSIS

Past History

- Medical: Past history of rickets, osteomalacia, tuberculosis of pelvic joints or spine, poliomyelitis.
- Obstetrical: Prolonged and tedious labor followed by either spontaneous or difficult instrumental delivery. Difficult vaginal delivery ending in stillborn or early neonatal death or late neurological problems following difficult labor. Maternal injuries such as complete perineal tear, vesico-vaginal fistula or rectovaginal fistula.

Physical Examination

- Stature: Short stature of less than 5 feet
- Gait and bone deformities such as tilting pelvis, spine deformity and shortening of limb
- Dystocia dystrophia syndrome.

Abdominal Examination

- Pendulous abdomen in primigravidae
- Obstetrical: Non-engagement of the head beyond 37 weeks in primigravidae, malpresentation in primigravidae.

Assessment of the Pelvis

- **Clinical pelvimetry/bimanual examination:** The points to be noted in bimanual examination are:
  - Inlet: Diagonal conjugate and anterior arch of pelvis
  - Midpelvis: Sacrum, lateral pelvic wall, ischial spines and sacrosciatic notch
  - Outlet: Subpubic arch, intertuberous diameter.
- **Radiographic examination:** This method is more accurate, however, in current practice, it is seldom done.
- **CT pelvimetry:** The accuracy is greater and the procedure is easier than conventional X-ray pelvimetry.

MANAGEMENT

There are two methods to manage disproportion in cases of suspected contracted pelvis:
- Trial labor
- Cesarean section.

Trial labor is the preferred treatment in a patient with minor degree of contraction, particularly in a young primigravida with no other complications. The woman is allowed to go in to labor and then is carefully watched as labor progresses. In the presence of good contractions, the fetal head may undergo molding to overcome minor disproportion. If it fails because the labor does not progress or there is maternal or fetal distress, a cesarean section becomes necessary.

32. CONTRACTION STRESS TEST

A contraction stress test (CST) is performed to evaluate the response of the fetus to the stress of contractions. A CST stimulates uterine contractions for the purpose of assessing fetal response. It evaluates the presence or absence of fetal heart rate decelerations in the presence of uterine contractions. The presence of a late deceleration pattern of the fetal heart rate during a uterine contraction is indicative of uteroplacental insufficiency and altered fetal cardio-respiratory reserves.

PREPARATION

Timing and Indications

A CST usually is performed after a non-reactive finding on an non stress test (NST). The potential for preterm labor after a CST makes it contraindicated in clients with a predisposition to preterm labor or a gestation age at which the risk for preterm birth is greater.

Client Preparation

Because the CST is an invasive procedure, informed consent must be documented. A CST is potentially a dangerous procedure that can stimulate labor or titanic contractions. It must be performed in a hospital in the event that an emergency cesarean section becomes necessary.

PROCEDURE

To perform a CST, the client is placed in a semi-Fowler or left lateral recumbent position and baseline maternal vital signs and fetal heart tracings are obtained. Uterine contractions are induced by either nipple stimulation or administration of exogenous oxytocin. The results of a CST are documented as follows:
- **Negative:** No late decelerations with three adequate uterine contractions in a 10 minutes period, normal baseline fetal heart rate, and accelerations with fetal movement
- **Positive:** Late decelerations with more than half the uterine contractions
- **Suspicious:** Late decelerations with fewer than half the uterine contractions
- **Unsatisfactory:** Inadequate fetal heart rate recording or less than three uterine contractions in 10 minutes.

A CST is a lengthy procedure, averaging 90 minutes similar to the NST. The CST also has a high false positive rate of 50–70% (Paul and Miller, 1995). Therefore, external fetal monitoring as a surveillance technique identifies the healthy, well-oxygenated fetus, but is of limited use in identifying the at-risk or compromised fetus.

FOLLOW-UP

If the CST is negative, the oxytocin drip is discontinued. Intravenous fluids are continued until uterine activity has returned to preprocedure status. A negative CST is reassuring that the fetus is likely to survive labor, it should occur within 1 week if there are no other changes in either maternal or fetal condition. If the CST is positive, continue monitoring and assessment of fetal well-being are needed. A positive result may lead to a decision to end the pregnancy and care for the newborn in the nursery.

33. CONTRACEPTION

The term contraception includes all measures that are temporary and permanent **(Box 33.1)**, designed to avoid or postpone pregnancy.

TEMPORARY METHODS

Temporary methods are commonly used to postpone or space births.

Natural Methods

Rhythm Method

Couples using this method voluntarily avoid or interrupt sexual intercourse during the fertile phase of the woman's cycle. This method is appropriate for women who are unable to use other methods, those having regular menstrual cycles or those with religious beliefs that prevent them from using other contraceptive methods.

Cervical Mucus Method

The menstrual cycle is divided into three phases for the purpose of assessing the likelihood of conception. The three phases are detailed below.

Phase 1 (relatively infertile phase): Lasts from the start of the menses to the time just preceding ovulation.

Box 33.1: Contraceptive methods.

- Temporary/Reversible:
    - Natural methods
    - Barrier methods
    - Chemical contraceptives
    - Intrauterine contraceptive devices
    - Hormonal contraception
- Permanent/Irreverisble:
    - Female: Tubal ligation/tubectomy
    - Male: Vasectomy

Phase 2 (fertile phase): Lasts from a few days prior to ovulation until 48 hours after ovulation.

Phase 3 (infertile phase): Lasts from 48 hours after ovulation until onset of menstrual bleeding (18–28 days).

The phase of the cycle can be determined by testing the cervical mucus and/or checking basal body temperature. Testing the cervical mucus during the infertile phases 1 and 3 of the cycle shows that the mucus is scanty, thick and opaque and breaks easily on stretching. During the fertile phase 2 of the cycle, the mucus is copious, translucent, and thin and can be easily stretched between the testing fingers.

In the basal body temperature method, temperature is recorded in the morning on awakening. A sustained rise of temperature of 0.2–0.6°C is indicative of ovulation. The postovulatory infertile period begins from day 3 after the date of temperature rise until menses.

Calendar Method

The period of abstinence (fertile period) is calculated on the basis of record of previous twelve menstrual cycles. Subtracting 20 days from the shortest cycle gives the first unsafe day and deducting 10 days from the longest cycle gives the last unsafe day. Thus, if a woman had cycles ranging from 25 to 31 days, she would abstain from intercourse from the 5th day of her current menstrual cycle (25 – 20 = 5) until the 21st day of her current cycle 31 – 10 = 21)

Coitus Interruptus or Withdrawal Method

In this method, the sex act takes place as usual; however, the male partner withdraws the erect penis just prior to ejaculation so that the semen spills outside the female generative tract.

Lactational Amenorrhea

This method is appropriate for 6 months postpartum in women who are fully breastfeeding their infants. During lactation, ovulation is suppressed and the cervical mucus is thick.

Barrier Methods

Condoms

These are made of latex (plain or treated with spermicide) or vinyl. The spermicide immobilizes or kills the sperms, providing additional protection in case of breakage or leakage **(Fig. 33.1)**.

Directions for use

The condom should be donned on the erect penis prior to penetration. It should cover the entire length of the erect penis. Adequate lubrication should be used. The penis should be withdrawn before erection subsides. The rim of the condom should be firmly held at the time of withdrawal to avoid spillage. The condom should be suitably disposed off after use.

Advantages
- Best for prevention of sexually transmittted diseases (STDs)
- Prevents sperm allergy and formation of sperm antibodies
- Relatively inexpensive and easy to carry
- No systemic side effects
- Partner involvement not required
- Can be used along with other contraceptive methods to enhance protection.

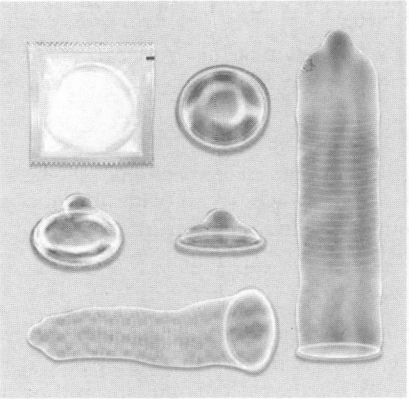

Fig. 33.1: Male condom.

Disadvantages
- Latex allergy
- Possible breakage of condom, slippage or leakage of semen
- Must be used with every act of intercourse
- Not reusable.

Diaphragm

A dome shaped-rubber cup attached to a flexible coiled spring in the rim. It prevents sperms from entering the upper genital tract. Diaphragms are appropriate for women who desire a user controlled method, are unsuitable for hormonal contraception, lactating mother or for couple having infrequent sex.

Fitting of the diaphragm

The diaphragm should be inserted deep into the cul-de-sac so that cervix is completely covered. The size of the diaphragm should be the largest that fits this space comfortably.

Instructions for use
- Apply spermicide prior to each use
- The diaphragm should be left in place for at least 8 hours following coitus.

Advantages
- Effective contraceptive if used properly and offers some protection against STDs
- There is some protection against cervical cancer as compared to women using no contraceptives.

Disadvantages
- Failure rate is 5–20%
- Increased risk of urinary tract infections
- Unsuitable for use by women with uterine prolapse, large cystocele and rectocele, and retroverted uterus.

Female Condom

The female condom is a polyurethane sheath 7.8 cm in diameter and 17 cm long. It has two polyurethane rings; one ring lies inside at the closed end of the sheath and other forms the external opening lying outside the vaginal orifice after insertion. It acts by providing a physical barrier by lining the vagina, occluding the cervix and partially covering the perineum.

Insertion technique
- Hold the pouch with open end hanging down
- Spread labia with fingers of one hand
- Using thumb and middle finger of the other hand squeeze the inner ring into the narrow oval for facilitating insertion. The inner ring and pouch are pushed deep into the vagina with the outer ring resting outside the vagina.

Removal
It is removed soon after intercourse by traction on the outer ring.

Advantages
- Impenetrable to the human immunodeficiency virus (HIV) virus
- Protective against STDs
- Available over the counter
- Easy to use and no hazards.

Disadvantages
- Relatively more expensive than male condom
- Anchoring ring visible outside the labia
- For every fresh act of coitus a new condom should be used
- Often makes disturbing and undesirable sound.

Chemical Contraceptives (Spermicides)

These are agents that immobilize and kill the spermatozoa. The usual agent is nonoxynol-9 and octoxynol. These are often used as an adjunct to barrier contraceptives. Spermicides offer protection against STDs. Efficacy is comparable to barrier methods and failure ranges from 0 to 50%.

Types

- **Foam:** Used along with condoms. It is effective immediately and its action lasts for about an hour.
- **Creams and gels:** May use along with/or in combination with diaphragm or cervical cap. Effective for about an hour when used singly, the duration of action is longer when used along with barrier contraceptive.

- **Suppositories:** May use alone or along with the condom. Action begins 10–15 minutes after insertion. Penile insertion prior to complete dissolution and dispersion may cause irritation to both partners. It remains effective for about an hour.
- **Sponge:** Needs to be moistened and squeezed just prior to use. Insert along the back wall of the vagina so that the cervix abuts against the dimple. Check placement to ensure that it has covered the cervix. It protects for about 24 hours. Repeated intercourse is possible, if sponge has not been disturbed. Removed by grasping the loop and giving traction.

Advantages

- Easy to use
- Offers some protection about STDs
- Protective against risks of cervical cancer.

Disadvantages

- Local irritation
- Allergy
- High failure rate of 10–25 per 100 women per year
- Interrupts spontaneity of love making
- Needs to be repeated at every act of coitus
- Considered to be messy.

Intrauterine Contraceptive Devices (IUCDs)

Intrauterine contraceptives have been in use for several decades. The closed devices such as Gräfenberg's ring and Birnberg bow are obsolete now. Open devices such as copper T, copper 7 and Lippes loop were in use in 1980s.

Types

Commonly used IUCDs in present day practice are: Cu T 200, Cu T 380 A, Multiload 250, Multiload 350, Progestasert, Levonorgesterel intrauterine device and others **(Fig. 33.2)**.

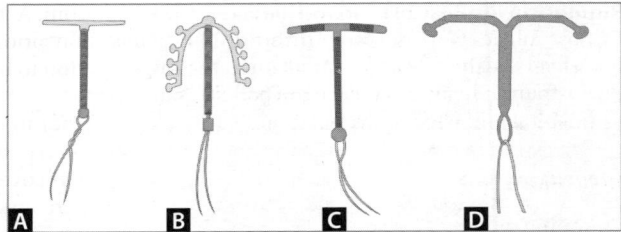

Figs. 33.2A to D: Commonly used intrauterine contraceptive devices (IUCDs). **A.** Cu T 200; **B.** Multiload 350; **C.** Cu T 380 A; **D.** Levonorgestrel containing IUD (LNG-IUS).

Mechanism of Action

Mechanism of antifertility effect of IUCDs is not yet clear.

Probable Factors

- It interferes with sperm transportation from the cervix to the fallopian tubes
- The IUCD inhibits sperm capacitation and survival (Speroff et al. 1999)
- It alters the biochemical or cellular composition of uterine fluid or both causing impairment of the viability of gametes
- The copper ions released from the device interferes with sperm motility and creates a reaction that results in a spermicidal endometrium (Nelson, 2000)
- Progestasert is thought to act through thickening the cervical mucus and rendering it impermeable to sperm.

Time of Insertion

- **Interval insertion:** Inserted 6 weeks after delivery or abortion. The timing should preferably be within 2–3 days of completion of menses. During the period of lactational amenorrhea it should be inserted after ensuring that the woman is not pregnant

- **Postabortal or Post-MTP insertion:**
  - Post placental insertion: Insertion immediately following delivery of the placenta. Expulsion rate is high
  - Postpartal: Insertion before the patient is discharged from the hospital following delivery.

Complications

- Cramping pain
- Syncope following a vasovagal attack
- Uterine perforation—partial or complete
- Pelvic infection—infertility
- Menorrhagia
- Intermenstrual bleeding
- Dysmenorrhea
- Unwanted pregnancy
- Spontaneous expulsion.

Advantages

- Provides excellent contraception
- May be used successfully in lactating women
- Indicated in women in whom oral contraceptives are contraindicated
- Can be used over long period of time
- Action easily reversible
- Progesterone IUCDs reduce dysmenorrhea and menorrhagia.

Disadvantages and Cautions

- IUCDs do not provide protection against STDs
- Cannot be used in patients with suspected pelvic infection
- Best avoided in women having multiple sex partners
- Menstrual disturbances such as menorrhagia
- Dysmenorrhea
- Women with valvular heart disease—risk of bacterial endocarditis
- Uterine anomalies
- Previous ectopic pregnancy
- Women with abnormal Pap smears.

Removal

This may be required because:
- The life span of the IUCD has been completed
- The patient does not tolerate the IUCD
- The patient has conceived with the IUCD in situ
- The IUCD has got displaced downwards
- The woman desires to conceive.

The median time from removal of IUCD to planned pregnancy is 3 months (Nelson, 2000).

Hormonal Contraception

Combined Oral Contraceptives or the Pill

The combined oral steroidal contraceptive is the most effective reversible method of contraception. Commonly used oral contraceptives are Mala N, Ovral L, Mala-D and Femilon. Combined oral contraceptives (COCs) contain third generation progestins and estrogens.

Mechanism of action

The oral pills act in various ways to ensure contraception:
- Inhibition of ovulation through the action on the anterior pituitary
- Altered cervical mucus—scanty, thick and not conducive to sperm transport
- Change in uterine environment—altered uterine secretions and altered endometrial bed.

Types of oral contraceptive pills

Oral contraceptive pills can be classified as monophasic, biphasic and triphasic depending on the variations in composition of active pills in the pack. Biphasic and triphasic pills are developed primarily with the objective of minimising midcycle spotting and to reduce the total estrogen dose per cycle. Market packs are available in two types:
- A 28 days pill pack containing 21 pills with pharmacologic activity and 7 iron or vitamin pills. The user takes one pill a day without fail
- A 21-day pill pack does not contain placebo pills, the user takes a 7 day break after completion of the 21 day pill course.

Efficacy

Failure rate is about 0.1% with perfect use and 2–3% with typical use.

Side Effects

Side effects are related to its hormonal constituents. Combination symptoms are as follows:
- Estrogen excess with progestin deficiency:
  - Bloating
  - Dizziness and syncope
  - Edema
  - Cyclic headaches
  - Irritability
  - Leg cramps
  - Nausea and vomiting
  - Visual disturbances
  - Cyclic weight gain.
- Estrogen and progestin excess:
  - Breast tenderness
  - Headaches
  - Hypertension
  - Myocardial infarction.

Advantages of oral contraceptives

- Highly effective
- Easily reversible
- Effective at all ages
- Regular menstruation
- Moderate blood flow
- Decrease in incidence of pelvic inflammatory disease
- Lowered incidence of ovarian neoplasms
- Decreased incidence of breast disease
- Lowered incidence of ectopic pregnancy
- Improvement in acne
- Not coitus dependant
- Decreased risk of osteoporosis
- Effective control of endometriosis.

Disadvantages and precautions
- The woman has to remember to take the pill daily
- There are many potential side effects—some resolve after few cycles and others persist
- The drug effect is diminished by certain drugs such as antituberculosis therapy and antiepileptics
- Not suitable for lactating mothers as it suppresses lactation
- Oral pills do not offer protection against STDs.

Contraindications
- Thrombophlebitis and history of thromboembolism
- Coronary artery disease
- Suspected breast cancer
- Estrogen dependant neoplasia
- Suspected pregnancy
- Hepatitis
- Presence of gallstones
- Undiagnosed vaginal bleeding (lower dose pills are safer for use)
- Hypertension
- Diabetes mellitus
- Migraine headaches
- Gallbladder disease
- Sickle cell disease.

Patient selection
Oral pills are best suited for the following classes of women:
- Young adolescent girls in unstable relationships
- Recently married women desirous of postponing their first pregnancy
- Women desirous of spacing their pregnancies
- Women with endometriosis
- Women who need reversible contraception
- Women suffering from acne
- Those suffering from menorrhagia, polymenorrhea, and dysmenorrhea
- Postpartum or postabortal contraception
- Women with polycystic ovarian disease—repeated anovulatory cycles
- Women with recurrent functional ovarian cysts.

Instructions to women who start taking pills

The following should be explained to women who are prescribed oral pills:

- Start the new pill pack on the first day of the menses
- The pill should be taken every day at the same time without fail like before going to bed; after brushing teeth, etc
- If using 28 pill pack, there should be no break between packs. Seven of the pills are dummies and contain either iron or vitamins
- A woman can start the pill up to day 5 of the bleeding. In that case she must use a condom additionally for next 7 days
- If following abortion, the pill should be started on the day after abortion
- Following childbirth, in non-lactating women it is to be started after 3 weeks and in lactating women, it is to be withheld for 6 weeks
- When a woman forgets to take a pill and it is within 12 hours, she should take it as soon as she remembers/take two pills at the usual time. It is safer to use backup contraception for 7 days for added protection
- If two pills have been missed, take two pills as soon as remembers, continue the pill pack as usual and observe additional backup contraception
- If three pills have been missed, start with a new pack, vaginal spotting and bleeding to be expected. Use additional backup contraception
- Women having nausea should take the pill soon after night meal. The symptom usually subsides after few cycles
- Women having smoking habit must stop smoking
- To report missed menses. Urine pregnancy test may be advised.

Duration of pill usage

Potential benefits of oral pills are greater, when compared to risks, in a well-selected individual. A woman, who does not smoke and has no risk factor for cardiovascular disease, may continue the pill (with careful monitoring) until the age of 50. For spacing of births, it can be used for 3–5 years safely.

Emergency Contraception

Amongst the various methods of emergency contraception, use of hormones constitutes an important contribution. The 'morning-after pill' reduces sperm transport and alters the endometrium, making fertilization less likely. It is appropriate for women who have had unprotected intercourse within the previous 72 hours, or in cases of victims of sexual assault or when the condom tears, slips or leakage occurs. The currently available product in India is the 'i pill'.

Indications
- Intercourse without contraception
- History of missed oral contraceptive pills with intercourse
- Broken or leaking condom
- Sexual assault
- IUCD expelled.

Advantages
The efficacy of the morning-after pill is 98% for prevention of pregnancy, provided that the pill is taken within 72 hours of coitus.

Disadvantages
Side effects include nausea and vomiting, spotting and irregular vaginal bleeding.

Caution
The morning-after pill should not be used by women in whom pregnancy is suspected or by women with history of thromboembolic episodes.

Injectable Contraceptives

Progestin given in the form of injection blocks the midcycle luteinizing hormone (LH) surge and causes suppression of ovulation, thickening of cervical mucus, atrophy of endometrial lining and altered tubal motility. The preparations available are:
- Depot medroxyprogesterone acetate (DMPA) or Depo-provera 150 mg IM once every 3 months
- Norethindrone [Noristerat, novethindrone enanthate (NET-EN)] 200 mg IM once every 2 months.

Advantages
- Effective in 24 hours and long acting
- Does not interfere with sexual intercourse
- Can be recommended to women over 35 years
- Safe for women with history of thromboembolism and smoking habit

- Offers protection against endometrial and ovarian cancers.
- Suitable for women having endometriosis
- Higher level of compliance of low rates of failure (0.3–0.9 per 100 women per year).

Disadvantages
- Return of fertility may be delayed for over 6 months
- Weight gain
- Irregular bleeding
- Amenorrhea on occasions
- Excessive bleeding
- Lack of protection from STDs.

Contraindications
- Known or suspected pregnancy
- Unexplained abnormal vaginal bleeding
- Known or suspected breast malignancy
- Allergy to DMPA
- Liver disease
- Suspected cervical cancer.

Side effects
- Irregular bleeding
- Weight gain
- Delayed return of fertility
- Headache, nausea, dizziness and breast tenderness
- Loss of libido, fatigue and nervousness
- Acne
- Loss of scalp hair.

It is important that the patient receive adequate counseling prior to accepting the method.

Hormonal Implants

The multiple capsule implants are called norplant. Norplant consist of six flexible closed capsules containing levonorgestrel or desogestrel that are inserted under the skin of the woman's arm. Each capsule is of 34 × 2.4 mm and conatins 36 mg levonorgestrel.

The single implant rod called implanon is 4 cm long and contains 60 mg of 3-keto-desogestrel. They (both types of implants) cause suppression of ovulation, thickening of the cervical mucus, thinning of the endometrium and altered tubal motility. Use of single rod makes implanon easier for insertion and removal **(Fig. 33.3)**.

Advantages
- Effective within 24 hours and provides long-term contraception (3–5 years)
- Fertility returns immediately on removal of the capsules
- No estrogen side effects
- Decreased incidence of anemia
- Low-risk of ectopic pregnancy
- No interference with breastfeeding
- Failure rate (pregnancy) 0.2–0.5 per 100 women per year.

Disadvantages
- Insertion and removal are minor surgical procedures
- No protection for STDs
- Diminished efficacy of epileptic treatment
- High cost.

Side effects
- Mastalgia
- Weight gain
- Irregular menses, amenorrhea

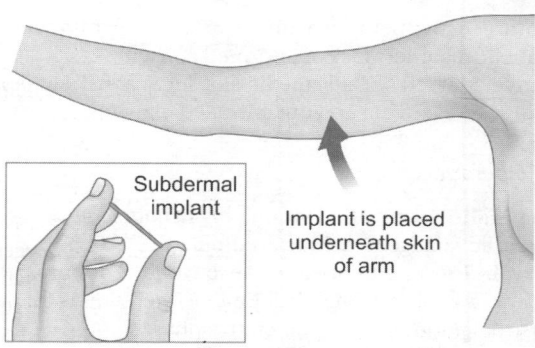

Fig. 33.3: Subdermal hormonal implant.

- Hirsutism and loss of scalp hair
- Altered libido.

Complications

- Inadvertent deep insertion of capsules
- Inadequate insertion
- Local infection and keloid formation.

PERMANENT METHODS OF CONTRACEPTION OR SURGICAL METHODS OF CONTRACEPTION

Female Sterilization

Female sterilization is an operation where resection of a segment of both fallopian tubes is done to achieve permanent sterilization.

Indications

- Couples who desire permanent sterilization
- Women with medical disorders in whom pregnancy carries risk of impairing health or being hazardous to life
- Women with severe inheritable genetic disorders in whom child bearing is not desirable.

Contraindications

- **Absolute:** Active peritoneal infection, severe cardiopulmonary or metabolic disorders lack of informed consent
- **Relative:** Marked obesity, medical or surgical risk factors present due to severe anemia and uncontrolled diabetes.

Time of Operation

- **Puerperal:** The operation is done 24–48 hours following delivery. Its chief advantage is technical simplicity
- **Interval:** The operation is done beyond 3 months following delivery or abortion. The ideal time of operation is following the menstrual period in the proliferative phase
- **Concurrent with Medical Termination of Pregnancy (MTP):** Sterilization is performed along with termination of pregnancy.

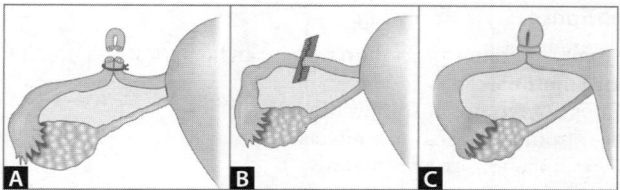

Figs. 33.4A to C: Female sterilization. **A.** Tubectomy (Tubal ligation); **B.** Filshie clip on fallopian tube; **C.** Falope ring on fallopian tube.

Methods of Surgery

- **Minilaparotomy:** The Pomeroy procedure is performed through a 3–4 cm suprapubic incision under local anesthesia or spinal anesthesia
- **Laparoscopic method:** Fallopian tubes are visualized at laparoscopy, and the tubes occluded by application of silastic rings (falope rings), clips or occluded and divided using the unipolar or bipolar cauterization **(Figs. 33.4A to C)**.

Advantages

- Method is highly effective
- Long-term sequelae are not significant
- Procedure can be performed in day care centers, in an outpatient or camp setting
- Very low failure rate 0.1–0.5 per 100 women per year.

Disadvantages

- The method is permanent and not easily reversible
- It does not offer protection against STDs
- There are small surgical risks involved.

Male Sterilization or Vasectomy

Male sterilization or vasectomy is a surgical procedure done in the male, where a segment of vas deference of both sides are resected and the cut ends are ligated.

Advantages

- Simple operative procedure which can be performed under local anesthesia
- Does not require hospitalization
- Free from long-term side effects
- Does not alter sexual functions
- Costs are lower
- Surgical reversal possible
- Failure rate is 3–4 per 1,000 procedures.

Disadvantages

- Procedure is permanent
- Does not protect against STDs
- Not effective immediately, requires about 20 ejaculations before becoming effective
- Not free from surgical risks
- Some men suffer from psychological ill effects.

34. CONVULSIONS IN NEWBORNS

Neonatal convulsion is usually a visible manifestation of some underlying pathology. The common causes of convulsion in the newborn are as detailed below.

Traumatic

- Hypoxic: Ischemic injury
- Intracranial injury.

Biochemical

- Hypo and hyperglycemia
- Kernicterus
- Hypocalcemia and hypercalcemia
- Inborn errors of metabolism
- Hyponatremia and hypernatremia
- Hypomagnesemia
- Pyridoxine dependence.

Infective

- High fever
- Meningitis
- TORCH infections [TORCH stands for 'toxoplasmosis, other (syphilis, varicella-zoster, parvovirus B19), rubella, cytomegalovirus (CMV) and herpes']
- Tetanus.

Iatrogenic

- Respiratory stimulants
- Analeptic drugs
- Drug toxicity and drug withdrawal.

Others

- Cerebral malformation
- Hyperthermia.

Diagnosis

- History of method of delivery
- Apgar score at birth
- Administration of analeptic or respiratory stimulant
- Type of feeding (breastfeeding or not).

Laboratory Studies

- Complete blood count (CBC)
- Blood, urine and cerebrospinal fluid (CSF) Cultures
- Serum immunoglobulin (IgM) and IgG: Specific TORCH titers
- Biochemical blood tests: Glucose, calcium, magnesium, bilirubin and electrolytes as needed
- Blood gas levels to detect acidosis and hypoxemia
- Ultrasonography and computed tomography (CT) scan of the head to detect intraventricular or subarachnoid hemorrhage
- Electroencephalogram.

Treatment

- Control of convulsions: Intravenous administration of phenobarbitone and phenytoin (Dilantin) in resistant cases
- Treatment of underlying cause:
  - Hypoglycemia: Glucose infusion to maintain blood glucose level at 40 mg/dL and above
  - Hypomagnesemia: Magnesium sulfate intravenous (IV) every 6 hours until magnesium level is normal
  - Infection: Appropriate antibiotic therapy following complete blood work up
  - Hypocalcemia: Calcium gluconate IV initially and followed by oral calcium
  - Pyridoxine deficiency: IV administration of pyridoxine.

Nursing Management

- Get assistance from physician while ensuring that the baby has a clear airway and adequate ventilation
- Turn the neonate to the semiprone position, with the head neither hyperflexed nor hyperextended
- Gentle oral and nasal suction to remove any milk or mucus
- Oxygen via mask if the baby is cyanosed
- Nurse baby in incubator without covering blankets for observation and maintenance of thermoneutral environment
- Accurate recording of convulsions observed, e.g. type of movement, the areas affected, the duration, any color change, any change in heart rate, respiratory rate or blood pressure
- Honest, clear explanation about the baby's condition to parents and follow-up discussions
- Supportive care to parents.

35. CORDOCENTESIS (PERCUTANEOUS UMBILICAL BLOOD SAMPLING)

Cordocentesis is a fetal evaluation procedure that provides direct access to the fetal circulation and involves direct aspiration of fetal blood. The most common site for needle placement is the umbilical cord, within 2 cm of the placental insertion site.

Timing and Indications

Cordocentesis can be performed anytime after 17 weeks gestation and is useful in diagnosing a variety of conditions including:
- Chromosomal alterations
- Intrauterine infections
- Coagulopathy
- Hemoglobinopathies and red blood cell (RBC) disorders
- Immunodeficiency states
- Platelet disorders
- Isoimmune diseases.
- In suspected IUGR, the test can be used to evaluate fetal hypoxia and determine fetal acid-base status. Percutaneous umbilical blood sampling (PUBS) can also be used for intrauterine transfusion and fetal drug therapy.

Client Preparation

Percutaneous umbilical blood sampling can be performed in either an outpatient or inpatient setting. The procedure takes about 10 minutes:
- An informed consent needs to be obtained, as it is an invasive procedure
- The client's needs to understand the reason, risks, benefits and nature of follow-up required
- Depending on the uterine size, a full bladder may be necessary
- The client needs to be informed that physical discomfort during procedure will be minimal
- Physical care of the woman includes documenting baseline vital signs and fetal cardiac activity
- When PUBs is performed after the fetus is viable (after 28 weeks), preparation for a cesarean birth in the event of fetal distress must be explained and considered by the client before procedure is implemented
- Preparation also involves ensuring that emergency equipment and personnel are available.

Procedure

Cordocentesis is performed under ultrasound guidance to identify the target sampling site.

- Antiseptic preparation of the maternal abdomen is done and a local anesthetic may be used
- A 20 or 22 gauge spinal needle is inserted through the abdominal and uterine walls and directed into the umbilical vessel, most commonly the umbilical vein
- A site approximately 1–2 cm from the insertion of the cord into the placenta is desirable.

This site minimizes the risk of cord injury and the chance of obtaining maternal blood from the placenta. If fetal movement interferes with the procedure, a sedative can be administered intravenously to the mother or intravenously or intramuscularly to the fetus.

After the blood specimen is obtained or the infusion is completed, the needle is removed, the site is inspected for bleeding and fetal cardiac activity is confirmed by ultrasonography.

Follow-up

Postprocedure care includes monitoring maternal vital signs, fetal heart rate and uterine activity. The fetal heart rate is evaluated for signs of reactivity and absence of distress. Because of the increased risk of infection, prophylactic antibiotics may be prescribed. The client should also be instructed to monitor her temperature twice a day to detect any temperature elevation.

36. CORD PRESENTATION

Definition

The umbilical cord lies alongside or in front of the presenting part with the fetal membranes intact **(Figs. 36.1A and B)**.

Predisposing Factors

Descend of the cord is more likely to occur when the presenting part imperfectly fits the pelvic brim leaving space for the cord to descend. Such situations are associated with:
- Malpresentations: Breech and shoulder presentations
- High parity: Presenting part may not be engaged when membranes rupture
- Prematurity: Smaller size of the fetus in relation to the pelvis

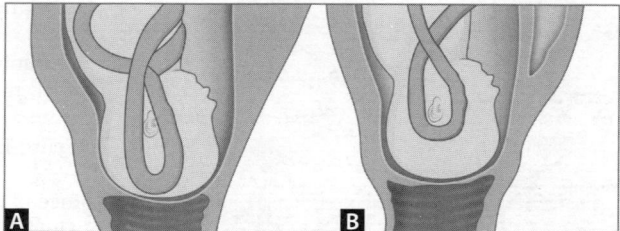

Figs. 36.1A and B: Cord presentations. **A.** Umbilical cord alongside fetal head upto the lower level of fetal head; **B.** Umbilical cord alongside fetal head upto ear level of the fetal head.

- Multiple pregnancies: Particularly of the second twin
- Polyhydramnios.

Diagnosis

- Cord presentation is rarely diagnosed before labor
- Vaginal examination is the only diagnostic method
- Signs of fetal distress in labor such as decelerations in fetal heart monitoring may lead to suspicion.

Management

When cord presentation is suspected or diagnosed:
- Avoid artificial rupture of membranes
- Discontinue vaginal examination in order to reduce the risk of rupturing the membranes
- Frequent or continuous fetal monitoring
- Cesarean section is the most likely outcome.

37. CORD PROLAPSE

Definition

The umbilical cord lies in front of the presenting part after the rupture of membranes. Occult cord prolapse is said to occur when the cord lies alongside, but not in front of the presenting part **(Figs. 37.1A and B)**.

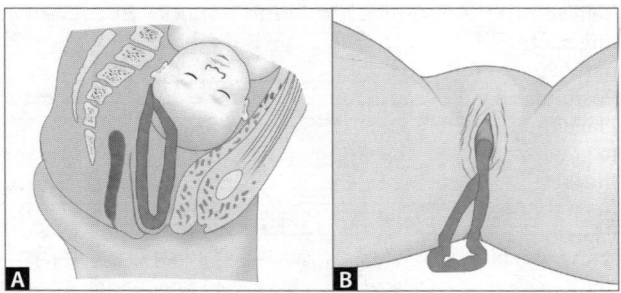

Figs. 37.1A and B: Cord prolapse. **A.** Cord in front of presenting part in vagina; **B.** Cord prolapsed outside vagina

Predisposing Factors

Predisposing factors are same as for cord presentation.

Diagnosis

- Cord is felt below or alongside the presenting part on vaginal examination
- An abnormal heart rate, particularly bradycardia following rupture of membranes
- A loop of cord may be visible at the vulva. The cord is more commonly felt in the vagina or in cases where the presenting part is very high, it may be felt in cervical os.

Immediate Care

- Call for immediate assistance
- Explain to mother and family the findings and measures that will be needed
- If an oxytocin infusion is in progress, it should be stopped
- Check if the cord is pulsating; if so, it should be handled as little as possible as spasm may occur through handling
- If cord is outside the vagina, it should be replaced gently to maintain temperature

- Relieve pressure on the cord during contractions by keeping a finger of the midwife in the vagina and holding the presenting part of the umbilical cord
- Position the mother with her pelvis and buttocks elevated
- Place the women in knee-chest position, which causes the fetus to gravitate towards the diaphragm relieving the compression on the cord
- Keep the foot of the bed raised until the delivery of the baby either vaginally or by cesarean section.

Management

- Assisted vaginal delivery: If the cervix is fully dilated or almost fully dilated, in a multipara, assisted vaginal delivery by forceps or vacuum extraction is indicated where the presentation is vertex
- Replacement of the umbilical cord and positioning: If the mother is not in a hospital or the cervix is only partially dilated, replacement of the cord and elevation of hips in lateral position must be carried out until she is transferred to a hospital.

Cesarean Section

Immediate cesarean section is the management of choice in those instances where the fetus is alive and delivery is not imminent or vaginal birth cannot be initiated.

Risks to the Fetus

- The risks to fetus are hypoxia and death as a result of cord compression; the average fetal mortality is 50%
- The risks are greater with prematurity and low birth weight
- The risk is less in multipara than in primigravida because of shorter labor in the former.

38. DIABETES IN PREGNANCY

Diabetes mellitus, a disease characterized by glucose intolerance occurs in about 1% of all pregnancies, making it the most common metabolic disorder complicating pregnancy.

Clinical Presentation

Diabetes is classified into three categories:
- Type 1: Diabetes mellitus or insulin-dependent diabetes
- Type 2: Diabetes mellitus or non-insulin-dependent diabetes
- Gestational diabetes or diabetes diagnosed during pregnancy.

Type 1, diabetes is an immune disorder in which the β-cells of the pancreas are destroyed, resulting in lack of insulin secretion. This type of diabetes is most often diagnosed before the age of 30 years and requires lifelong insulin therapy and dietary management.

Type 2, diabetes is characterized by abnormal insulin secretion and insulin resistance, and most often is found in persons over the age of 40 years and in overweight individuals. This type of diabetes may be managed by diet alone or with hypoglycemic agents, although oral hypoglycemic agents are contraindicated during pregnancy.

Gestational diabetes has the abnormal carbohydrate metabolism diagnosed during pregnancy.

Carbohydrate Metabolism During Pregnancy

Metabolic adaptations occur during pregnancy because the fetus depends on the mother for an uninterrupted supply of metabolic fuel, mainly glucose, in order to meet its growth demand.

Pregnancy is characterized by maternal hyperinsulinemia and insulin resistance, which become most marked in the third trimester. Beginning in early pregnancy, there are constantly elevated estrogen and progesterone levels, which stimulate the pancreatic cells, resulting in hyperplasia and hyperinsulinemia. This leads to decreased hepatic glucose production, increased peripheral glucose utilization and decreased maternal fasting glucose level, described as accelerated starvation.

As pregnancy advances, levels of human placental lactogen increase and along with cortisol, counter the effects of insulin, resulting in resistance. After meals, a state of facilitated anabolism ensues, with higher levels of triglycerides, prolonged hyperglycemia and enhanced lipolysis. Increased maternal use of fat for energy spares glucose for fetal consumption.

Effects of Pregnancy on Diabetes

- The diabetogenic effects of pregnancy on diabetes are:
  - Increased production of cortisol, estriol and progesterone
  - Insulin resistance
  - Increased lipolysis (mother uses fat for her caloric requirements and saves glucose for fetal needs)
  - Fetus uses alanine and other amino acids and deprives the mother of a major gluconeogenic source.
- Pregnancy unmasks diabetes: Gestational diabetes appears during pregnancy in women who were normal before pregnancy, but have potential to become diabetic later in life
- In patient with insulin-dependent diabetes mellitus (IDDM), a catabolic state ensues, which may lead to glycosuria, ketonuria and ketoacidosis requiring careful monitoring and increased dosage of insulin
- In patients with non-insulin-dependent diabetes mellitus (NIDDM), symptoms of clinical diabetes requiring insulin may get triggered off
- Ketoacidosis: Pregnant diabetics are more prone to develop ketoacidosis especially during periods of nausea and vomiting and with infections such as urinary tract infections
- Renal glycosuria: When glucose is detected in the second fasting urine specimen voided half-an-hour after the first, it becomes significant
- Insulin requirements: Immediately after delivery, insulin requirements fall requiring readjustment in dosage so as to prevent hypoglycemia.

Effects of Diabetes on Pregnancy

In prenatal period
- Spontaneous abortions in known diabetics with poor control
- Infections such as urinary tract infections and vaginal candidiasis are common
- Pregnancy-induced hypertension (PIH) is seen in 10–25% of patients, contributing to a worsened outcome
- Hydramnios occurs in 20% of patients and is seen associated with large placenta, macrosomia and malformations

- High incidence of chorioamnionitis and postpartum endometritis
- Higher incidence of postpartum hemorrhage caused by exaggerated uterine distension
- Higher incidence of cesarean section.

In labor
- Prolonged labor
- Shoulder dystocia due to macrosomia
- Operative deliveries with resultant genital tract injuries.

In puerperium
- Increased risk of sepsis
- Lactation failure.

Fetal Effects

- Congenital malformations: Commonly encountered fetal defects are anencephaly, spina bifida, meningomyelocele, ventricular septal defect, transposition of great vessels and coarctation of aorta
- Intrauterine fetal death: Occurs most commonly after 36 weeks in patients with poor glycemic control, vascular disease, hydramnios, macrosomia and preeclampsia. Chronic intrauterine hypoxia and fetal hypoglycaemia secondary to hyperinsulinaemia are likely complications
- Fetal macrosomia: These babies are large for gestational age with a birth weight greater than 3,500 or 4,000 grams. Infant of a diabetic mother, besides having a high birth weight, also has increased adiposity, with increased subcutaneous skin fold thickness, increased muscle mass and visceromegaly (e.g. liver). There is disproportionate increase in the size of the trunk and shoulders as compared to the head, often leading to shoulder dystocia and traumatic delivery
- Neonatal complications:
    - Hypoglycemia, due to fetal hyperinsulinemia
    - Respiratory distress syndrome (RDS)
    - Hyperbilirubinemia
    - Hypocalcemia
    - Birth injuries due to fetal macrosomia, operative delivery and shoulder dystocia
    - Perinatal mortality is increased twofold to threefold.

Diagnosis

History
- Family history of diabetes (genetic predisposition)
- History of having delivered large babies (> 4 kg), unexplained stillbirth or neonatal death, offspring with congenital anomalies, PIH, traumatic delivery with neurologically impaired child, recurrent spontaneous abortions and diabetes in a previous pregnancy
- Recurrent infection, i.e. urinary tract infection and moniliasis
- Chronic hypertension
- Maternal age over 30 years.

Clinical Examination

- Obesity: Weight over 91 kg (200 lbs) or more than 15% of non-pregnancy weight
- Hypertension
- Repeated urinary tract and monilial infection
- Polyhydramnios
- Evidence of vasculopathy
- Glycosuria.

Screening Test

- Random blood glucose: If blood glucose is more than 130 mg%, the test is considered positive and a glucose tolerance test is indicated
- Fasting and postprandial blood glucose: Fasting blood glucose of less than 100 mg/dL or post lunch blood glucose < 140 mg/dL, fall within normal range and the woman does not have diabetes. The

Table 38.1: Blood glucose values in non-pregnant and pregnant women.

	Non-pregnant (mg/dL)	Pregnant (mg/dL)
FBS	100.0	90
1 hour	160.0	165
2 hours	120.0	145
3 hours	110.0	125

test may be repeated at 32 weeks in high-risk cases. If any one value is abnormal, a glucose tolerance test (GTT) is recommended. When both tests are abnormal, the client is diagnosed to have diabetes
- Glucose tolerance test: After an overnight fast, fasting blood sugar (FBS) value is obtained. The patient is then asked to drink 100 grams of glucose in 200–400 mL of water over a period of 5 minutes. Blood glucose values are obtained at 1, 2 and 3 hour intervals. The results are interpreted according to O'Sullivan's criteria.

Interpretation

- When two or more values are abnormal, the GTT is abnormal and the woman suffers from diabetes
- If only one value is abnormal, the test is considered normal
- If all values are border line, the test should be repeated.

Investigations to Estimate the Severity of the Disease and the Prognosis

- Urine culture at initial visit and at 4–6 weeks intervals to rule out asymptomatic bacteriuria
- Ophthalmologic examination (fundoscopy) at initial visit and then serially in those that develop retinopathy
- Renal function, a baseline serum creatinine at initial visit and if the value is more than 0.8 mg/dL, a full 24 hours creatinine clearance is done
- Electrocardiogram (ECG): This is mandatory in patients where ischemic heart disease is either suspected or obtained from history
- Glycosylated hemoglobin (HbA1c): This test reveals the average glucose levels during the previous 4–6 weeks (the average red blood cell lifespan) when elevated above 10%, it is indicative of poor glycemic control in previous 6 weeks.

Management of Diabetes in Pregnancy

Objectives of antenatal care of diabetic pregnant client are:
- To achieve a metabolic control similar to that in normal pregnant clients

- To attain optimal fetal outcome (to avoid occurrence of fetal immaturity and sudden intrauterine death)
- To eliminate any maternal complication
- To educate patient about the nature of her disease and the steps necessary to achieve satisfactory outcome.

Diet

Dietary management is the first line of management. Recommended caloric consumption according to the American College of Obstetricians and Gynecologists is 2,000–4,000 kcal/day or 38 kcal/kg body weight and 300 kcal/day above basal requirements. Constituents of the diet may be:
- 50–60% carbohydrates
- 12–20% proteins (30 g additional per day)
- Less than 10% saturated fat, up to 10% unsaturated fat and the remainder as monounsaturated fat)
- Restrict cholesterol
- Avoid sugar
- Routine hematinic and calcium supplements.

Exercise

Light exercise after ensuring that they do not suffer from any of the vasculopathies and have intact autonomic symptoms.

Exercise must be avoided at peak time of insulin action and biscuits may be kept near at hand, should hypoglycemia occur.

Insulin

Ideal glucose levels are considered to be as follows:
- 2–6 AM: > 60 mg/dL
- Before breakfast: 60–90 mg/dL
- Before meals: 60–105 mg/dL
- 2 hours after meals: </120 mg/dL.

Indications for Use of Insulin

- The IDDM patients
- Gestational diabetics with:

- FBS ≥ = 100 mg/dL on two consecutive tests
- 1 h post-prandial blood sugar (PPBS) ≥ = 140 mg/dL.
- History of receiving insulin in a previous pregnancy
- History of previous fetal demise
- The NIDDM patients with poor glycemic control
- Patients on oral hypoglycemic therapy prior to pregnancy.

Management of Pregnancy in the Diabetic

- Counseling at the time of first antenatal visit
- Initial hospitalization to determine the blood glucose profile and to adjust the insulin dose
- The HbA1c level at 10–12 weeks to evaluate the risk of malformations aided with ultrasonography and maternal serum test for alphafetoprotein (AFP)
- Stable IDDM and gestational diabetic patients to be seen fortnightly until 28 weeks and thereafter weekly
- Admission of those patients with history of previous intrauterine fetal death at critical times
- Checks at each prenatal visit to include weight gain, uterine growth, fetal condition, pregnancy complications such as PIH and hydramnios
- Evaluation of the home blood sugar chart, fasting and post-lunch blood glucose and HbA1c every month.

Fetal Surveillance

Intensive fetal surveillance is required in the third trimester, after 32 weeks, when the risk of fetal death is increased. Modalities for surveillance are:
- Ultrasonography (USG):biophysical profile
- Fetal kick count
- Non-stress test
- Amniocentesis to determine AFP levels.

Intranatal Management

- Hospitalization of patient when she is near term in a well-equipped hospital with neonatal intensive care unit (NICU)

- Time of delivery is determined at 38 weeks considering the fetal risks and maternal complications
- Vaginal delivery is recommended if:
  - The expected fetal weight is less than 4 kg
  - The pelvis is adequate clinically
  - Intrapartum monitoring is available
  - The baby is in vertex presentation
  - There is no fetal distress.
- Lower segment cesarean section (LSCS) is indicated in cases of:
  - Elderly primigravida
  - Fetal malpresentation
  - Macrosomia
  - Unstable diabetes
  - Fetal compromise.
- Induction may be undertaken with amniotomy and oxytocin infusion when the cervix is ripe (either spontaneous or with use of prostaglandin)
- Accurate glycemic control using intravenous (IV) glucose and insulin to prevent maternal hypoglycemia and fetal hyperinsulinemia.

Management of Puerperium

- Insulin requirement declines immediately after delivery
- Determination of blood glucose levels and insulin requirement must be done to revert back to pre-pregnancy dose
- Prophylactic antibiotics to minimize infection
- Barrier method of contraceptives for those who desire spacing and permanent method for those who have completed their families may be advised.

Care of the Newborn

- A neonatologist must be present at the time of delivery
- The baby should be in neonatal intensive care unit (ICU) for 48 hours to detect and treat any likely complication:
  - Asphyxia
  - Congenital malformations
  - Hypoglycaemia.

- Early breastfeeding within ½ to 1 hour is advocated and to be repeated 3–4 hourly thereafter to minimize hypoglycemia
- If the baby is premature or lethargic and breastfeeding is inadequate 10% glucose may be given orally.

NURSING PROCESS

Assessment Database

- Pedal pulse and capillary refill of extremities may be diminished or slowed (with diabetes of long duration)
- Edema, elevated blood pressure (BP) (presence of associated PIH)
- Rapid pulse, pallor and diaphoresis (hypoglycemia)
- History of recurrent urinary tract infection, vaginal infection
- Polydipsia, polyphagia
- Nausea, vomiting
- Obesity; excessive weight gain
- May report episodes of hypoglycemia, glycosuria
- Fundal height may be higher or lower than normal for gestational age (hydramnios, inappropriate fetal growth)
- History of large for gestational age (LGA) neonate, congenital anomalies or unexplained stillbirth
- Family history of diabetes, gestational diabetes mellitus (GDM), PIH, infertility, LGA infant, neonatal death, stillbirth and congenital anomalies.

Diagnostic Studies

- Glucose tolerance test: Blood glucose level elevated above 140 mg/dL at 24–28 weeks gestation
- Glycosylated hemoglobin (Hb A1c): Elevated
- Random serum glucose level elevated
- Ultrasonography and pelvimetry: Evaluates fetal macrosomia and shoulder dystocia
- Amniocentesis for lecithin sphingomyelin (L/S) ratio and saturated phosphotidylcholine to determine fetal lung maturity.

Nursing Diagnoses

1. Risk for imbalanced nutrition: Less than body requirements.
2. Risk for fetal injury.
3. Deficient knowledge regarding diabetes, prognosis, treatment and selfcare needs.
4. Risk for impaired fetal gas exchange.
5. Risk for maternal injury.
6. Anxiety.

Expected Outcomes

1. Client will maintain normal serum glucose levels and be free of symptoms of ketoacidosis.
2. Fetus will be full-term with size appropriate for gestational age.
3. Client will verbalize understanding of procedures, tests and activities involved in controlling diabetes.
4. Neonate will display normal levels of serum glucose and be free of signs of hypoglycemia.
5. Client will be free of injury and complications.
6. Client will display appropriate coping strategies.

Nursing Interventions

1. Client will maintain normal serum glucose levels and remain free of symptoms of ketoacidosis:
   - Weigh client at each prenatal visit
   - Encourage client to periodically monitor weight at home between visits
   - Assess caloric intake and dietary pattern using 24 hour recall
   - Review/Provide information regarding any required changes in diabetic management (e.g. switch from oral agents to insulin, use humulin insulin, self-monitoring of glucose at least four times a day)
   - Review importance of regularity of meals and snacks (e.g. three meals and three or four snacks when taking insulin)
   - Note presence of nausea and vomiting, especially in first trimester

- Assess understanding of the effects of stress on diabetes; provide information about stress management and relaxation
- Teach client finger-stick method for self-monitoring of glucose; have client demonstrate procedure
- Recommend monitoring urine for ketones on awakening and when a planned meal or snack is delayed
- Review/Discuss signs and symptoms of hypoglycemia and hyperglycemia
- Instruct client to treat symptomatic hypoglycemia if it occurs, with an 8 oz glass of milk and to repeat in 15 minutes if serum glucose level remains below 70 mg/dL
- Adjust diet and insulin regimen to meet individual needs
- Monitor serum glucose levels on initial visit (FBS, 1 and 2 hour postprandial) and then as indicated by client's condition
- Ascertain results of HbA1c every 4 weeks.

2. Fetus will be full-term with size appropriate for gestational age:
   - Determine the classification of diabetes in which client is included, explain the significance to client and family
   - Obtain history of client's diabetic control before conception
   - Assess fetal movement and fetal heart rate (FHR) each visit as indicated
   - Encourage client periodically to count and record fetal movements daily from 34 weeks of gestation
   - Monitor fundal height at each visit
   - Provide information and reinforce procedure for home blood glucose monitoring and diabetic management
   - Monitor for signs of PIH
   - Provide information about possible effects of diabetes on fetal growth and development
   - Review procedure and rationale for periodic non-stress tests (NSTs)
   - Discuss procedure and rationale for carrying out periodic Oxytocin Challenge Test (OCT)/Contraction Stress Test (CST) beginning at 30–32 weeks gestation depending on diagnosis of IDDM or GDM
   - Review procedure and rationale for amniocentesis if required
   - Assess HbA1c every 4 weeks, as indicated

- Prepare for ultrasonoraphy at different stages as indicated
- Perform NST and OCT/CST as appropriate
- Assist as necessary with biophysical profile (BPP) assessment
- Assess with preparation for delivery of fetus vaginally or surgically if test results indicate placental aging and insufficiency.

3. Enhancing client's understanding of procedures, tests and activities for controlling diabetes:
   - Assess client's/couple's knowledge of disease process and treatment including relationships among diet, exercise, illness, stress and insulin requirements
   - Discuss importance of home serum glucose monitoring using reflectance meter and need for frequent readings as indicated
   - Review reasons why insulin to be used in pregnancy even though client used oral hypoglycemic agents prior to pregnancy
   - Provide information about action and adverse effects of insulin; assist client to learn administration of insulin if appropriate
   - Explain normal weight gain during pregnancy
   - Provide information about need for regular, daily mild exercise program (20 minutes after meals)
   - Provide information regarding the impact of pregnancy on the diabetic condition and future expectations
   - Discuss how client can recognize signs of infection
   - Review hemoglobin (Hb)/hematocrit (Hct) levels
   - Provide dietary information and sources of iron and the need for iron supplements.

4. Neonate will display normal levels of serum glucose and be free of signs of hypoglycemia (during labor):
   - Review prenatal course and maternal diabetic control
   - Check maternal urine at each voiding for glucose/ketones, and albumin
   - Monitor blood pressure
   - Monitor temperature as indicated; note character of vaginal discharge
   - Encourage lateral recumbent position for client during labor
   - Perform or assist with vaginal examination to determine progress of labor

- Review results of prenatal tests such as BPP, NST, CST, and estimation of fetal size
- Obtain or review results from amniocentesis and ultrasonography.
- Monitor maternal serum glucose level per protocol
- Monitor FHR with continuous fetal monitoring device, preferably with an internal electrode
- Initiate IV infusion of 5% dextrose solution as indicated
- Prepare for induction of labor using oxytocin (Pitocin) or for cesarean birth, if medically indicated as a result of complication
- Arrange for pediatrician, neonatologist or NICU nurse to be present in delivery room as indicated.

5. Client will be free of injury and complications (during labor):
   - Note time/content of last meal; amount/type/time of last dose of insulin
   - Ascertain recent serum glucose levels and any fluctuations
   - Observe for signs and symptoms of hypoglycemia
   - Check urine at each voiding for glucose, ketones and protein
   - Assess quality, duration and frequency of contractions
   - Evaluate skin turgor, pulse and temperature, and condition of mucous membranes
   - Note presence, quality and consistency of bloody show; if excess bleeding is present, notify physician
   - Have glucagons available at bedside
   - Review results of ultrasonography and pelvimetry
   - Monitor serum glucose level every hour until stable and then every 2–4 hours
   - Maintain glucose level between 60 and 100 mg/dL:
     - Initiate IV infusion of 5% dextrose solution as indicated
     - Administer regular insulin as appropriate.
   - Prepare for induction of labor by administration of oxytocin or cesarean section if indicated
   - Obtain complete blood count (CBC), blood type and crossmatch, if surgical procedure is planned.

6. Client will display appropriate coping strategies (during labor):
   - Arrange for continued presence of support person or primary nurse

- Position call light for easy access if the nurse goes out of the room and inform that calls will be answered promptly
- Ascertain response to labor and to medical management; assess effectiveness of support systems
- Involve couple in activities as much as possible
- Encourage use of relaxation and breathing techniques
- Explain all procedures; reinforce information from other healthcare providers
- Encourage questions and verbalization of concerns
- Keep client/couple informed of progress of labor; be positive in providing information
- Keep couple informed of fetal status.

39. DIAGNOSIS OF PREGNANCY

The average duration of pregnancy based on menstrual history has been calculated by clinicians to last for 10 lunar months or 9 calendar month and 7 days. This corresponds to 280 days or 40 weeks from the 1st day of last menstrual period (LMP). The duration of pregnancy is expressed as gestational weeks.

Diagnosis of Pregnancy in the First Trimester (First 12 Weeks)

The diagnosis of pregnancy is based on:
- Presumptive/Subjective symptoms
- Clinical examination
- Special investigations.

Presumptive/Subjective Symptoms

1. Cessation of menstruation: In normal menstruating women, the abrupt cessation of cyclic and regular periods is strongly suggestive of pregnancy.
2. Breast changes: Women experience heaviness, tingling, discomfort or tenderness in the breasts. As pregnancy advances, the breasts enlarge, feel nodular, the areola and nipples enlarge and become more deeply pigmented.

A clear or thin milk-like secretion can be expressed from the breasts. Tiny protuberances called 'Montgomery's tubercles' appear around the nipples.
3. **Nausea (with or without vomiting):** Most women (about 70%) experience some degree of nausea, usually in the early hours of the day. It may be accompanied by vomiting. This symptom generally passes away towards the end of first trimester.
4. **Frequency of micturition:** The enlarging gravid uterus exerts pressure on the bladder base causing frequency of micturition. This symptom is relieved when the growing uterus becomes an abdominal organ and returns towards full term when the fetal head engages in the pelvis.
5. **Fatigue:** Tiredness is an early symptom. Sleepiness and disinclination for work are experienced by some women and these symptoms often persist until mid-pregnancy.
6. **Feeling of warmth and sweating:** Some women complain of feeling feverish and experience excessive sweating due to altered circulation in the skin.

Clinical Examination

On examination, the clinician can elicit signs that strongly endorse the suspicion of pregnancy. These are due to early changes in the uterus and cervix and are objective signs:
- Goodell's sign: The cervix feels softened like the lips of the mouth
- Hegar's sign: The cervix and the bulky uterus feel separated because of the variation in consistency (lower part of the uterus (body) is empty and extremely soft and the cervix is comparatively firm). On bimanual examination the abdominal and vaginal fingers seem to appose below the body of the uterus
- Palmer's sign: On bimanual examination in early pregnancy, the uterus is felt to undergo regular, painless and rhythmic contractions
- Piskacek's sign: Asymmetrical enlargement of the uterus if there is lateral implantation where one half is felt more firm than the other
- Osiander's sign: Increased pulsation felt through the lateral fornices of vagina at 8th week of pregnancy
- Jacquemier's or Chadwick's sign: The discolorations due to local vascular congestion (bluish hue) of the vestibule and anterior vaginal wall can be seen at about 8th week of pregnancy.

Special Investigations

Immunological tests

Immunological tests for early detection of pregnancy are based on the detection of β subunit of human chorionic gonadotropin (hCG) in maternal serum or urine:

1. Direct agglutination test: Latex particles coated with anti-hCG monoclonal antibodies are mixed with urine. An agglutination reaction indicates a positive result when the urine sample contains hCG. Absence of agglutination (urine without hCG) indicates negative test.
2. The Gravindex test: This test is based on the latex agglutination inhibition technique. Absence of agglutination indicates presence of pregnancy.
3. Early icon II test: This is based on beta hCG monoclonal antibody detection by enzyme-linked immunosorbent assay (ELISA) technique. It is highly sensitive and can detect pregnancy on the 1st day of the missed period (28th day).
4. Pregcolor test kit and pregcolor card test: This is often used as a home kit for detection of pregnancy. It is based on color change. The card test is simpler and two lines confirm the pregnancy. This is positive by 5 days after the missed period (**Figs. 39.1A to D**).
5. Several pregnancy test kits for home use are presently available through drug stores. Some of the commonly used self-use kits are 'velocit eazy', 'i-can one step test device, 'instant pregnancy test' and 'first response test device'. Women can use these eazy-to-use kits to confirm the conception, when they realize that they have missed a menstrual period. Home pregnancy test kits.
6. Radioimmunoassay: This is a sensitive and specific test for early pregnancy. It can be used to detect the presence of hCG in the serum as early as 8–9 days after ovulation, probably on the day of blastocyst implantation.
7. Ultrasonography: This is the most reliable test. As early as the 5th week of intrauterine life, the gestational sac can be identified. The fetal node can be observed after the 6th week and fetal cardiac pulsation after the 7th week by transvaginal sonography.

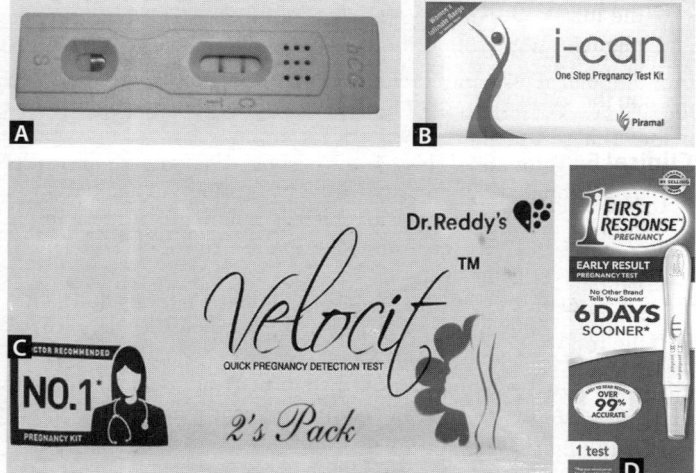

Figs. 39.1A to D: Home pregnancy test kits: **A.** Instant pregnancy test kit; **B.** i-can pregnancy test kit; **C.** Velocit eazy pregnancy test kit; **D.** First response pregnancy test kit.

Diagnosis of Pregnancy in the Second Trimester

Symptoms

1. Amenorrhea continues; nausea, vomiting and the complaint of frequent urination begin to subside. The breast changes continue.
2. Quickening between 16th and 20th weeks, women are able to appreciate the feelings of fetal movements, describing it as a flutter or feeling of bubbles inside. This is called quickening.
3. Enlargement of the abdomen: The enlarging pregnant uterus grows out of the pelvis and becomes palpable abdominally in the suprapubic region by about 12 weeks. It reaches the umbilicus at about 24 weeks.
4. Skin changes: Darkening of the skin occurs generally, but is particularly noticeable in the region of armpits, midline of

the lower abdomen (linea nigra) and breasts. A butterfly-like pigmentation around the cheeks called chloasma is observed around 24 weeks. Stretch marks called striae gravidarum appear on the lower abdomen, the flanks, breasts and hips.

Clinical Examination

1. Abdominal examination: Inspection reveals fullness in the lower abdomen, stretch marks or striae and linea nigra. On palpation, the uterus appears like a soft swelling arising out of the pelvis. Painless, periodic contractions (Braxton Hicks contractions) are felt. Fetal parts can be felt by 20th week. Around 20 weeks, the rocking of uterus between the palpating hands reveals the feeling of ballottement. This sign is called external ballottement. The examining hands can appreciate active fetal movements after 20 weeks.
2. Vaginal examination: Inspection with a speculum reveals the cervix and vaginal mucosa to appear congested and bluish, and the vaginal discharge creamy white.

    On bimanual examination after the 16th week, tapping the cervix reveals the presence of a body, which moves away from the examining finger and later returns with a thud. This sign is described as internal ballottement.
3. Auscultation: The fetal heart sounds are audible with a stethoscope or a fetoscope after 18th–20th weeks of gestation. The Doppler machine (sonic aid) can detect fetal heart tones as early as 12th week of gestation.

Investigations

ltrasonography: This can detect fetal skeleton and fetal organs, the location of placenta, amount of amniotic fluid and the state of internal os. It is used to detect normality of pregnancy. Whenever the LMP is in doubt, the scan helps to date the pregnancy accurately. Real-time ultrasound scan can detect multiple gestation and fetal abnormalities. It can reveal low-lying placenta, incompetent os and fibroids or cysts.

Diagnosis of Pregnancy in the Third Trimester

1. Symptoms: Amenorrhea continues and the enlargement of the abdomen progresses. Late in pregnancy, it may cause palpitation, breathlessness, pedal edema and difficulty in walking.

   About term when the presenting part engages in the pelvis, the woman experiences relief of pressure symptoms called lightening. Active fetal movements become more pronounced and sometimes cause discomfort. Frequency of micturition is experienced when the fetal head engages in the pelvis toward term.

2. Clinical examination.
   - Cutaneous pigmentation changes and striae gravidarum are more prominent
   - The uterine shape becomes more globular and the umbilicus becomes everted
   - The fundal height continues to grow
   - Braxton Hicks contractions are more evident
   - Fetal movements are easily appreciated and fetal parts can be palpated
   - Auscultation reveals a regular fetal heart rhythm.
3. Investigations
   - Sonography: This confirms pregnancy and determines the fetal lie, presentation and cardiac pulsations. Location of the placenta, amount of amniotic fluid and state of the internal os are determined. Gestational maturity is estimated and any abnormality is noted.

Differential Diagnosis of Pregnancy

1. Uterine Fibroids: This may enlarge symmetrically with intramural fibroids and they are sometimes soft enough to simulate the consistency of pregnant uterus. In later pregnancy, a fibroid in the pelvis may easily be mistaken for the fetal head on vaginal examination. Pregnancy tests and ultrasound examination will be of value to make correct diagnosis.
2. Ovarian Cysts: Generally on bimanual examination, the uterus can be felt separately from the ovarian cyst. Pregnancy test will be

negative and ultrasound examination will show an empty uterus and absence of fetal parts.

In pregnancy associated with an ovarian cyst, two swellings are usually evident. The combined swelling will then be larger than expected for the duration of pregnancy. Ultrasound scan will reveal the fetus within the uterus with the cyst as a separate entity.

3. Pseudocyesis: It is a psychological disorder in which the woman has a false but fixed idea that she is pregnant. Pregnancy fantasies may occur with other delusions in psychosis, but most women with pseudocyesis do not have serious mental illness. It is frequently, but not always seen near the menopause. It is more often seen in women without children. There may be amenorrhea and the woman may claim that she has morning sickness and breast tenderness, and that she can feel fetal movements. The abdomen may look distended due to voluntary aerophagy. The shape of the swelling is different from that of the pregnant uterus, fetal parts cannot be felt and the fetal heart cannot be heard. If the woman is fat, a pregnancy test and ultrasound scan may be required. The difficulty will be to convince the woman that she is not pregnant.

40. DIAGNOSTIC PROCEDURES IN GYNECOLOGY AND OBSTETRICS

I. PAPANICOLAOU TEST/PAP SMEAR/CERVICAL SMEAR

Definition

Papanicolaou test also known as Pap Smear or cervical smear is a screening test in which a sample of cells taken from the endocervical canal is smeared and screened under the microscope to detect potentially cancerous or precancerous cells.

Principles

- Follow aseptic technique.
- Screening should be done after 10 to 20 days of the first day of menstruation.

Purpose

To evaluate the condition of the internal female structures and to obtain specimens for cytological screening.

Indications

- As part of routine health check-up after the age of 21 years.
- To screen for cancer.
- To detect abnormal cells or precancerous cells.
- To diagnose inflammation and infection.

Articles (Figs. 40.1A to C)

A tray containing:
1. A drape sheet to expose the particular or needed area.
2. A bowl for antimicrobial solution.
3. A sponge holding forceps.
4. A Cusco's speculum to retract posterior vaginal wall.
5. A vulsellum to catch hold of the anterior lip of the cervix.
6. A pair of sterile gloves.
7. Cotton swabs for cleaning excess discharge.
8. An Ayer spatula to swab around the cervix.

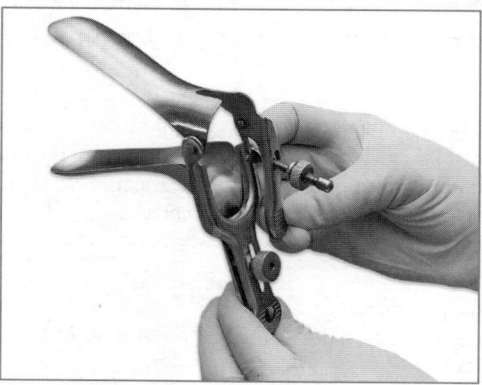

Fig. 40.1A: Vaginal speculum.

Diagnostic Procedures in Gynecology and Obstetrics

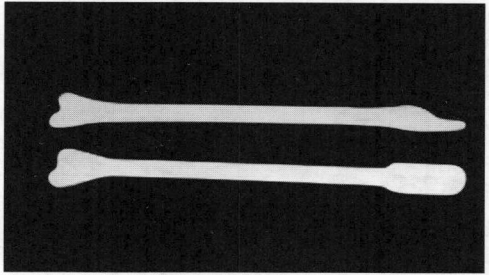

Fig. 40.1B: Ayer spatula (Pap smear sampling device).

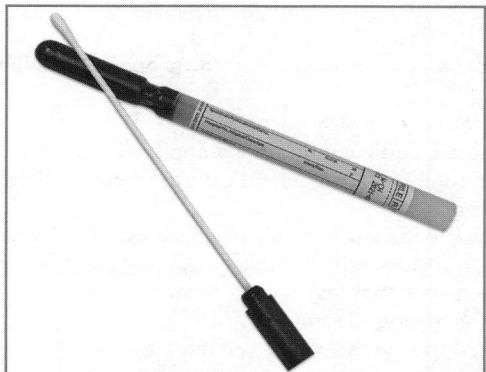

Fig. 40.1C: Cotton tipped applicator and tube for collecting specimen.

9. Cotton tipped applicators to swab the endocervix by rotating it 180°.
10. Glass slides to prepare the smear.
11. Spray fixative/Methanol spray
12. Ether/95% alcohol solution (1:1)
13. A graphite pencil.

Preparation of the Patient

- Explain the Pap cytology test to the patient.
- Reassure and provide psychological support.

- Ask the mother to empty her bladder and bowel to avoid discomfort during the procedure.
- Explain to patient not to use vaginal medications or vaginal contraceptive for 48 hours before the test. Intercourse should be avoided the night before the test.

Procedure

1. Ask the patient to undress from waist down.
2. Position her in supine position with knees flexed and legs abducted and drape the area with sterile sheet.
3. Wash hands and wear the sterile gloves.
4. Spread the labia and clean the vulva with antiseptic solution.
5. Insert the speculum gently into the vagina. Blades should be closed until inserted fully and slowly open the blades and lock them.
6. a. For endocervical smear:
      Insert a sterile cotton tipped applicator into the cervical os and rotate it 360 degrees. Leave the swab in place for 10 -20 seconds.
      Remove the swab gently and smear on to a glass slide and apply fixative (Fixative must be applied immediately, before the specimen dries).
   b. For ectocervical scraping:
      Insert the Ayre's spatula into the cervical os, rotate or scrape the squamocolumnar junction. Remove the spatula and smear on to a glass slide and fix it immediately.
   c. For cervical scraping:
      Insert the pointed edge of a wooden Ayre's spatula into the cervical os and rotate the spatula by 360°. Spread the cervical scrapings on a glass slide, fix it with an ether/95% ethyl alcohol solution, and dry the slide. A cervix-brush sampling device may be used, and it is recommended to rotate it a full 180° degrees to improve the sampling for abnormal cervical cells. Remove the speculum gently.
7. Give the patient a perineal pad after the procedure, to absorb any bleeding or drainage.

8. Watch for any bleeding for 15 minutes.
9. Make the mother comfortable and tell her to rest for 10-15 minutes.
10. Document the date, time smear obtained and any needed details about the procedure.

After Care

1. Replace all the articles.
2. Send the microscopic slide and cotton applicator for cytology.
3. Inform the mother that she may have some mild bleeding or discomfort which is normal.
4. Check the vital signs and general condition of the mother for the periods she is asked to rest.

Special Considerations

1. Smears that dry before fixative is applied cannot be properly interpreted.
2. Do not lubricate the speculum as it may distort the cells.
3. A smear taken any time other than the mid-menstrual cycle can result in abnormal findings.
4. Tetracycline or digitalis preparations can affect the appearance of squamous epithelium.
5. Blood, mucus or pus on the slide makes interpretation difficult.

2. VAGINAL SMEAR /VAGINAL WET MOUNT

Description

A vaginal smear or vaginal wet mount is a gynecological test wherein a sample of vaginal discharge is observed by wet mount microscopy by placing the specimen on a glass slide and mixing it with salt solution (saline). It is used to find vaginal thrush, bacterial vaginosis and trichomonas vaginalis.

Purpose of the test is to find the cause of vaginitis or vulvitis

Principles

- Follow aseptic precautions.
- Avoid contamination of swab in the lower perineum.
- Should not be done during menstruation

Indications

- Vaginitis
- Yeast infection
- Trichomonas infection
- Bacterial vaginosis
- Infections such as chlamydia, genital warts, syphilis, herpes simplex and gonorrhea
- It may also be done as rape investigation to detect the presence of semen.

Contraindications

- Acute human papilloma virus (HPV)/ herpes
- Abnormal Pap smear
- Active vaginal infection
- Undiagnosed vaginal bleeding
- Uncontrolled diabetes
- Rectal or vaginal injury
- Any active bleeding including menses.

Articles Needed (Figs. 40.2A to C)

A tray containing:
1. A vaginal speculum to visualize the vagina.
2. Sterile gloves to maintain asepsis.
3. Lubricant to avoid friction
4. A smear brush/vaginal smear kit/cotton tipped applicator for collecting sample.
5. A sterile drape
6. Methanol spray for fixation
7. An apron to avoid contamination/sepsis
8. Fixative.

Diagnostic Procedures in Gynecology and Obstetrics

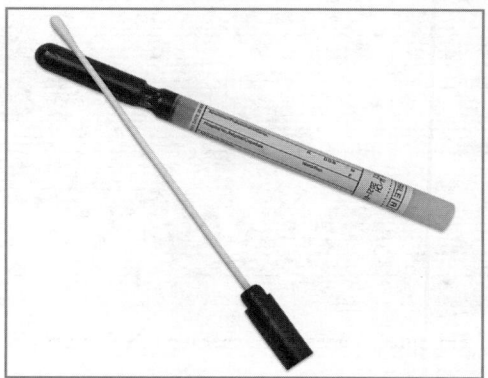

Fig. 40.2A: Cotton tipped applicator for collecting specimen.

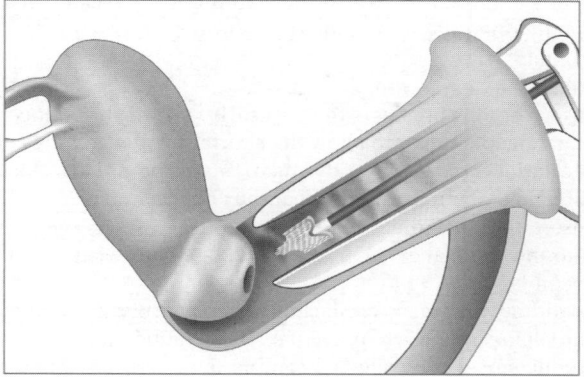

Fig. 40.2B: Cervical brush (Smear brush) in place.

Procedure

1. Place the woman on the examination table in lithotomy position for clear visualization.
2. Drape the area and expose only the needed part.

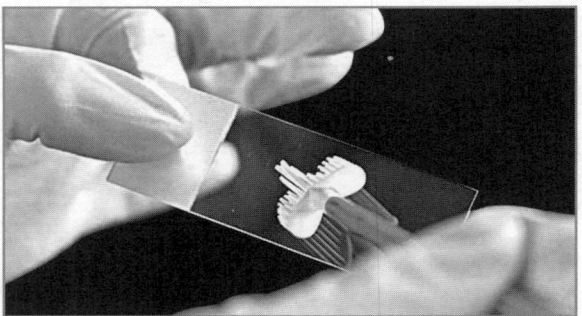

Fig. 40.2C: Smearing the specimen on glass slide.

3. Wash hands and put on gloves to prevent cross contamination.
4. Apply lubricant jelly on the speculum for easy insertion.
5. Separate the labia and insert the speculum in sideways direction gently and rotate it so that the clamp is at 12O' clock position. Gently open the speculum and view the inside to inspect the vagina.
6. Clean the vagina with plain gauze.
7. Insert the long bristles of the cervical brush into the endocervical canal deep enough to allow the shorter bristles to fully contact the endocervix. Push gently and rotate the broom in a clockwise direction, about 5 times to clear the cervical mucus.
8. Insert the specimen collection applicator or cervical brush into the cervical canal and gently rotate clockwise for 10 to 30 seconds.
9. Withdraw the brush/applicator carefully avoiding contact with the vaginal mucosa to prevent contamination.
10. Gently smear the collected sample on a glass slide and apply fixative.
11. Remove the speculum gently, watch for any bleeding.
12. Remove gloves, label the specimen and send it to the laboratory.
13. Reposition the mother, making her comfortable and ask her to take rest for 10 minutes.
14. Document the time of swab collection and needed details and any complications if identified.

Aftercare

1. Replace articles
2. Clean or soak the speculum immediately to dislodge secretions
3. Wash hands
4. Explain to the woman about follow up care.

3. ENDOMETRIAL BIOPSY

Definition

The endometrial biopsy is a gynecological procedure that involves taking a tissue sample from the inner lining of the uterus.

Purposes

- To determine the cause of abnormal uterine bleeding
- To evaluate infertility
- To test for uterine infection
- To monitor the response of endometrium with hormonal therapy.

Principles

- Strict aseptic technique to be followed
- The test should be done with the help of ultrasonography.

Indications

- Abnormal uterine bleeding
- Postmenstrual bleeding
- Screening for endometrial cancer after finding atypical cells
- Testing the response to hormonal therapy
- Abnormal Pap smear.

Contraindications

Absolute contraindications
- Pregnancy
- Acute pelvic inflammatory disease (PID)

- Clotting disorder or coagulopathy
- Acute cervical infection
- Acute vaginal infection
- Cervical cancer.

Relative contraindications
- Morbid obesity
- Uterine dehiscence
- Severe cervical stenosis.

Articles

A sterile tray containing:
1. Sponge holding forceps **(Fig. 40.3A-i)**
2. Bowl with povidone iodine solution
3. Draping sheet
4. Vaginal speculum to visualize vagina and cervix **(Fig. 40.3A-ii)**
5. Uterine sound to measure the length of uterine cavity **(Fig. 40.3A-iv)**
6. Endometrial suction catheter to aspirate the sample tissue
7. Cervical dilators to dilate the cervix **(Fig. 40.3A-iii)**
8. Scissors to cut the tip of catheter

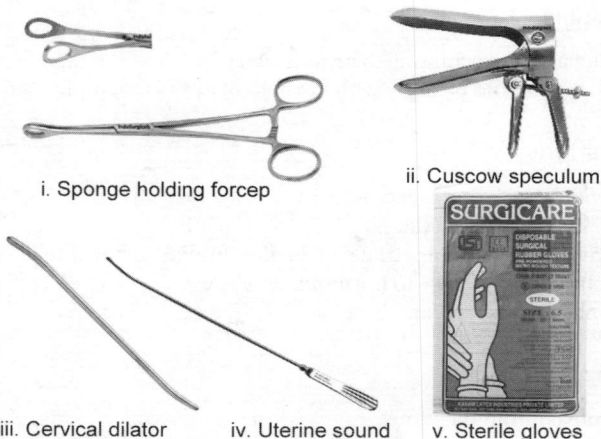

Fig. 40.3A: Instruments for endometrial biopsy (vaginal speculum, cervical dilator, uterine sound and sponge holding forceps).

A clean tray containing:
1. Sterile gloves **(Fig. 40.3A-v)**
2. Sterile sample container with formalin solution
3. Anesthetic gel or spray to use as local anesthetic agent.

Preparation of the Patient

- Get informed consent from the patient
- Check whether she is taking any medications
- Check whether she is allergic to any medication
- Advise the patient to empty her bladder
- Give analgesics 30-60 minutes before the procedure is scheduled.
    1. Explain the procedure to mother.
    2. Place the mother in lithotomy position with her feet on stirrups.
    3. Infiltrate with lignocaine if needed.
    4. Lubricate the speculum with antiseptic cream and insert the speculum into the vagina.
    5. Cleanse the cervix with antiseptic solution.
    6. Hold the cervix with Vulsellum.
    7. Insert the uterine sound till you feel resistance which indicates fundus.
    8. Insert the sampling catheter just beyond the internal cervical os.
    9. Holding the catheter sheath between the thumb and index finger of one of the hands, use the other hand to draw the internal piston out of the tube in one continuous motion.
    10. Hold the catheter sheath between the thumb and index finger and insert the tube up as far into the fundus as possible until resistance is felt (without perforating the uterine wall **(Fig. 40.3B)**.
    11. Slowly withdraw the tube using both hands in a spiral or swirling movement from the fundus toward the cervix while simultaneously moving the catheter back and forth within the uterine cavity between the fundus and internal os. Have the lumen of the sampling tube fill up with endometrial tissue.
    12. Place the removed tissue in formalin solution for preservation.
    13. Send the tissue to the laboratory.

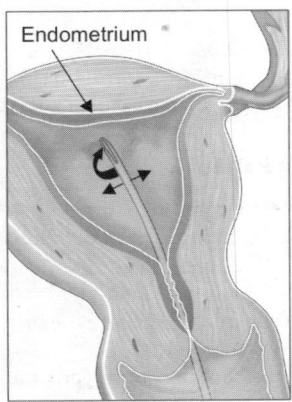

Fig. 40.3B: Site of endometrial biopsy showing biopsy catheter in place.

14. Remove the vulsellum and speculum and reposition the woman in supine or lateral position. Allow her to rest for some time.
15. Document in patient's chart the date and time of the procedure, type of anesthesia used and biopsy done.

4. HYSTEROSCOPY

Definition

Hysteroscopy is a Gynecological procedure that allows the doctor to look inside the uterus in order to diagnose and treat abnormal bleeding. Hysteroscopy is done using a hysteroscope, a thin lighted tube that is inserted into the vagina to examine the cervix and inside of the uterus **(Fig. 40.4)**.

Purposes

- To find the cause of abnormal bleeding.
- To find out the cause of infertility.
- To obtain a tissue sample/biopsy.
- To remove polyps or small fibroids.
- To remove adhesions caused by earlier infections or past surgery.

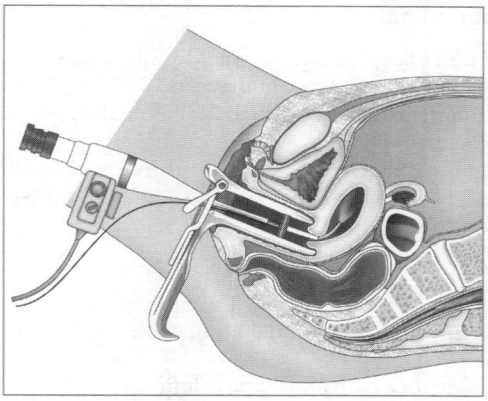

Fig. 40.4: Hysteroscope in place inside the uterus.

- To detect the cause of repeated miscarriages.
- To locate and remove an intrauterine device.
- To perform tubal ligation.
- To stop bleeding using electric current, freezing, heat or chemicals.

Indications

- Asherman's syndrome/intrauterine adhesions.
- Endometrial polyp.
- Endometrial ablation/ removal of layer of tissue (endometrium).
- Evaluation of retained products of conception.
- Removal of embedded IUCDs.
- Congenital uterine malformations.
- Postmenopausal bleeding.
- Abnormal Pap test results.

Contraindications

- During menstruation.
- Pelvic inflammatory disease
- Cervical cancer.
- Vaginal or cervical infection.

Preparation of patient

- Explain the procedure and obtain informed consent.
- Keep the patient on 'nil per oral' status.
- Advice mother to empty her bladder before the procedure.
- Perform skin preparation.
- Advice not to douche, use tampons or vaginal medications 24 hours prior to hysteroscopy.
- An IV line may be placed.

Procedure

- Position the patient on operating table supine with feet in stirrups.
- Vagina is cleaned with antiseptic solution.
- Cervix is then dilated and hysteroscope is inserted through the cervix into the uterus.
- The uterus is then expanded by injecting liquid or gas through the hysteroscope.
- The uterine cavity is then examined and required procedure is performed.

Aftercare

- Observe the mother for 2-4 hours
- Tell the patient that she may have cramping or mild sore throat due to anesthesia. This will get relieved after few days and salt water gargles help relieve throat symptoms
- Inform her that it is normal to have small amount of bleeding for a day
- Advise mother to avoid sexual intercourse and using tampons for a day after hysteroscopy
- Analgesics may be given to relieve pain
- Advise the mother to report to the hospital if she develops:
  - Heavy bleeding or discharge
  - Fever
  - Severe abdominal or pelvic pain.

5. HYSTEROSALPINGOGRAPHY (HSG)

Description

Hysterosalpingography, also known as uterosalpingography, is a radiologic procedure to investigate the shape of the uterine cavity and the shape and patency of the fallopian tubes. This is a special X-ray using a dye to look at the uterus and fallopian tubes. The type of X-ray used is called a fluoroscopy, which creates a video image rather than a still picture **(Fig. 40.5(1))**.

The radiologist can watch the dye as it moves through the reproductive system. H will then be able to see if there is any blockage in the fallopian tubes or other structural abnormalities in the uterus.

Indications

- Infertility.
- Suspected structural abnormalities in the uterus which may be congenital or required.
- Blockage of the fallopian tubes.
- Scar tissue in the uterus.

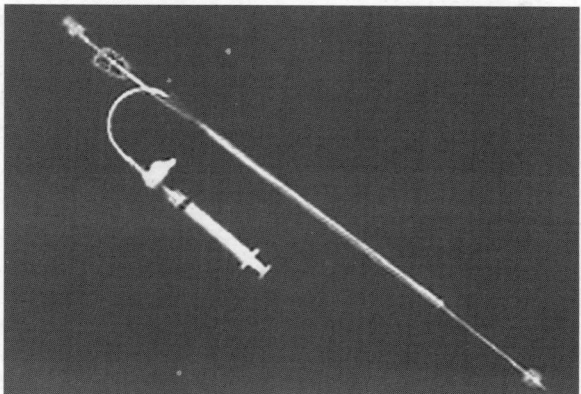

Fig. 40.5 (1): Syringe and catheter for injecting dye.

- Uterine polyps, tumors or fibroids.
- Post tubal pregnancy.

Patient Preparation

- Pain medication is given about an hour before the scheduled test.
- A sedative may be prescribed to help the patient relax, if she is nervous.
- The test will take few minute only and patient can go home after 2-3 hours.
- An antibiotic may be prescribed to take before or after the test to help prevent infection.
- The test will be scheduled a few days to a week after menstrual period.
- The patient will be asked to remove any metal from her body, such as jewelry and the metal can interfere with the X-ray machine.
- Explain to patient that a contrast dye will be used as instillation into the uterus to help highlight the uterine cavity and fallopian tubes. The dye will either dissolve or leave the body through urine. It is important to let your doctor know if you have had an allergic reaction to barium or contrast dye.

During the Test

The patient will need to put on a hospital gown and lie on her back with knees bent and feet spread, as would for a pelvic examination.

- The radiologist or doctor will then insert a speculum into the vagina. This is done to visualize the cervix, which is located at the back of the vagina.
- The cervix will then be cleaned and a local anesthetic injected to reduce discomfort.
- Next, a cannula will be inserted into the cervix and the speculum will be removed. The dye will be instilled through the cannula which will flow into the uterus and fallopian tubes.
- The patient will then be placed under the X-ray machine and X-rays will be taken. The patient will feel some cramping and pain as the dye will move through the fallopian tubes **(Fig. 40.5(2))**.
- After the X-rays are taken, the cannula will be removed.
- Medications for pain and to prevent infection are usually prescribed.

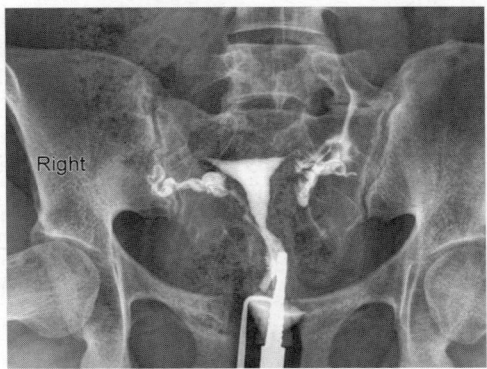

Fig. 40.5 (2): X-ray image of uterus and fallopian tubes.

Complications

Complications from a Hysterosalpingography is rare. Possible risks include:
- Allergic reaction to contrast dye.
- Endometrial or fallopian tube infection.
- Injury to the uterus, such as perforation.
- Vaginal bleeding.

Aftercare

- Tell the patient that small amount of spotting may be present following the procedure which is normal
- There may also be leakage of the contrast dye
- Wearing a sanitary pad for the rest of the day and for few days will protect her clothing.

6. ULTRASONOGRAPHY

Introduction

- Gynecologic ultrasonography refers to the application of medical ultrasonography to the female pelvic organs, especially the uterus, ovaries, fallopian tubes as well as bladder, the adnexa and the rectouterine pouch. The test is often referred to simply as an ultrasound or as a sonogram.

How is Ultrasonography Performed?

Sonography uses a device called a transducer to send out ultrasound waves at a frequency too high to be heard. The transducer is placed on the skin and the ultrasound waves move through the body to the organs and structures within. The organs like an echo return the waves to the transducer. The sound waves bounce through the organs like an echo and return to the transducer. The transducer processes the reflected waves, which are then converted by a computer into an image of the organs or tissues being examined.

An ultrasound gel is placed on the transducer and on the skin to allow for smooth movement of the transducer over the skin and to eliminate air between the skin and the transducer for the best sound conduction.

Types of Ultrasound Application

1. **Transvaginal/Pelvic ultrasound (through the vagina):** A long transducer is covered with a plastic or latex sheath and lubricated with conducting gel is inserted in the vagina. The transducer will be gently turned and angled to bring to focus the areas for study **(Fig. 40.6A)**.
2. **Transabdominal (through the abdomen) ultrasound:** The transducer is placed on the abdomen using the conductive gel **(Fig. 40.6B)**.
3. **Doppler ultrasound:** This is used on the abdomen to show the speed and direction of blood flow in certain pelvic organs. Unlike a standard ultrasound, some sound waves during the Doppler exam are audible. This is used in obstetrics to assess placental blood flow and fetal heart sounds.

The type of ultrasound procedure performed depends on the reason for the test. Only one method may be used or both methods may be needed to provide information needed for the diagnosis or treatment.

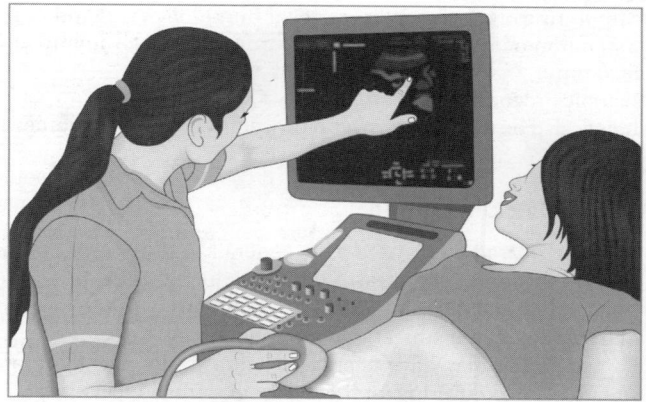

Fig. 40.6A: Pelvic ultrasound examination.

PELVIC ULTRASOUND/TRANSVAGINAL ULTRASOUND EXAMINATION (FIG. 40.6A)

Reasons for Pelvic Ultrasound

Pelvic ultrasound may be used for measurement and evaluation of female pelvic organs and include:
- Size, shape and position of the uterus and ovaries.
- Thickness, echogenicity (darkness or lightness of the image related to the density of the tissue) and presence of fluid or masses in the endometrium, myometrium, fallopian tubes or in or near the bladder.
- Length and thickness of the cervix.
- Changes in bladder shape.
- Blood flow through pelvic organs.
- Abnormalities in the anatomic structure of the uterus.
- Fibroid tumors, masses, cysts and other types of tumors within the pelvis.
- Presence and position of an intrauterine contraceptive device (IUCD).
- Pelvic inflammatory disease (PID).
- Postmenopausal bleeding.

- Monitoring of ovarian follicle size for infertility evaluation.
- Aspiration of follicle fluid and eggs from ovaries for invitro fertilization.
- Ectopic pregnancy.
- It may also be used to assist with procedures such as endometrial biopsy.

Risks of Pelvic Ultrasound

- There is no radiation used and generally no discomfort from the application of ultrasound transducer to skin during transabdominal ultrasound. Slight discomfort with the insertion of transvaginal transducer into the vagina.
- Some women may have allergic reaction to the plastic or latex sheath used as covering for the ultrasound transducer.
- During a transabdominal ultrasound some women experience discomfort from having a full bladder or lying on the examination table.
- Severe obesity.
- Barium within the intestines from a recent barium procedure.
- Intestinal gas.

Abdominal Ultrasound Examination (Fig. 40.6B)

Preparation of patient

Generally no fasting or sedation is required for abdominal ultrasound.

- Drink a minimum of 750 mL of clear fluid at least one hour before procedure. Do not empty the bladder until after the examination is completed.
- For vaginal ultrasound, bladder to be emptied before the procedure.

Explain to the patient:

- To remove any clothing, jewelry or other objects that may interfere with the scan and wear a hospital gown.
- To lie on her back on an examination table.

The physician will:

- Apply ultrasound gel on abdomen.
- Press the transducer against the skin and moved around over the area to be studied.

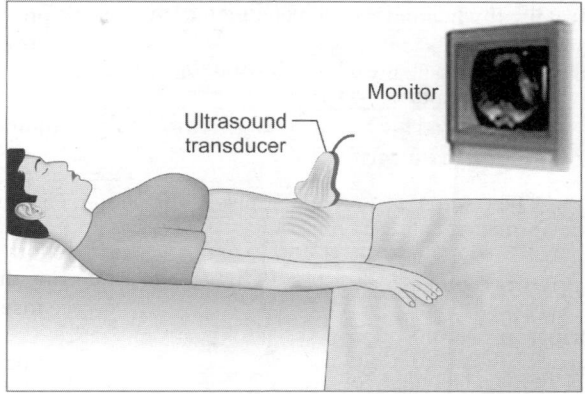

Fig. 40.6B: Abdominal ultrasound examination.

- If blood flow is being assessed, a 'whoosh' sound will be heard.
- Images will be displayed on the computer screen and recorded on various media for health record.
- Once the procedure is completed, the gel on abdomen will be removed.
  Patient will be asked to empty her bladder.

Procedure of Pelvic (Vaginal) Ultrasound

- For vaginal ultrasound examination, bladder needs to be emptied before the procedure.
- Instruct patient to remove any clothing or jewelry or other objects that may interfere with the scan and wear a hospital gown.
- Help patient to lie on the examination table with feet and legs positioned as for pelvic examination (lithotomy position).
- The physician will introduce the transvaginal transducer covered with a plastic or latex sheath and lubricated.
- The transducer will be gently turned and angled to bring to focus the areas of study.
- Images of organs and structures will be displayed on the computer screen. Images may be recorded on various media for health care record.

- Once the procedure has been completed, the transducer will be removed.
- Assist patient to get down from the examination table and instruct to change her clothes.

After Care of the Patient

No special type care is required after pelvic ultrasound. Patient may resume normal diet and activities.

7. CULDOSCOPY

Description

Culdoscopy is a technique of endoscopic visualization and/or minor operative procedure performed on the female pelvic organs in which the instrument is introduced through a puncture in the wall of the pouch of Douglas, an extension of peritoneal cavity, between the rectum and back wall (posterior wall) of the uterus. The word Culdoscopy is derived from the term cul-de-sac and refers to the recto-uterine pouch. Purpose of the procedure is to examine the recto-uterine pouch and pelvic viscera. Diagnostic value of the procedure is to diagnose pathologic conditions of the female pelvis and pelvic organs **(Fig. 40.7)**.

Indications

- Ectopic pregnancy
- Salpingitis
- Tubal ligation
- Tubal adhesions
- Assessment of diethylstilbestrol exposure in uterus.

Contraindications

- Chronic pelvic inflammatory disease (PID).
- Vaginitis and acute cervicitis.
- Vaginal atresia.
- Acute pelvic inflammation.

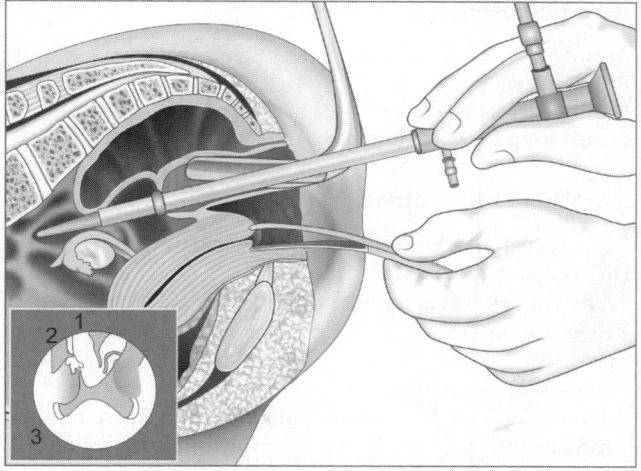

Fig. 40.7: Culdoscope in rectouterine pouch.

- Ruptured ectopic pregnancy.
- Inability to assume knee-chest position due to cardiac or respiratory disease.

Articles

A sterile tray containing:
1. A bowl with antiseptic solution and cotton swabs
2. A vulsellum to hold the cervix
3. A perineal retractor to hold the targeted tissue
4. A 10 mL syringe and sterile container to aspirate the fluid and collect the specimen
5. A draping sheet to expose the procedural site
6. A vaginal speculum to visualize the vagina and cervix
7. Catgut to suture the vaginal wound
8. Sterile trocar and culdoscope with lens to visualize the pelvic organs.

Preparation of the Environment

- Arrange all the articles
- Provide privacy.
- Ensure adequate lighting
- Ensure aseptic environment.

Preparation of the Patient

- Explain the procedure and get informed consent
- Do a pregnancy test prior to the test
- Administer enema for emptying the bowel
- Patient should be kept in 'nil per oral' status for 8 hours prior to the test
- Catheterize the bladder
- Administer premedication half hour before the procedure
- Perineum and vagina to be cleaned with antiseptic solution.

Procedure

1. Culdoscopy is performed with the patient in knee-chest position under local or general anesthesia.
2. Retract the perineum using a retractor.
3. Grasp the posterior lip of the cervix with a vulsellum.
4. Insert the sterile trocar of the culdoscope into the posterior fornix and then into the pelvis between two uterosacral ligaments.
5. Withdraw the trocar from the sheath, insert the sterile culdoscope through the sheath without touching the vaginal mucous membrane and view the uterus, tubes, broad ligaments, uterosacral ligaments, rectal wall, sigmoid and small intestine by manipulating the scope.
6. Remove the culdoscope after the examination and leave the sheath in position.
7. Suture the varginal wound and then remove the sheath, suture the wound and clean the perineum.
8. Document the indication for the procedure, date, time and any difficulties encountered.

Aftercare

1. Monitor the vital signs for about 1 to 2 hours.
2. Send the patient home after 4 to 6 hours if the procedure was done as out-patient.
3. Instruct the patient not to have sexual intercourse for 6 weeks, but can start normal activities as soon as she feels comfortable and fit.
4. Observe for any possible complications such as injuries, hydrosalpinx or bleeding.

8. DIAGNOSTIC LAPAROSCOPY

Definition

Laparoscopy is a surgical procedure in which a fiberoptic instrument is inserted through a small incision (about 0.5 to 1.5 cm) on the abdominal wall to visualize the abdominal or pelvic organs.

Purposes

- To reduce hemorrhage.
- To allow access to the inside of abdomen and pelvis without having to make a large incision in the skin.
- To keep the procedure as a key-hole surgery or minimally invasive surgery.
- To shorten the hospital stay allowing faster recovery and return to day-to-day activities.
- To reduce the exposure of internal organs to possible external contaminants reducing the risk of acquiring infections.

Indications

To rule out the cause of the following:
- Infertility: Site of tubal block, hydrosalpinx, pyosalpinx, tubo-ovarian mass, tubal kinks and peritubal adhesions, genital tuberculosis, polycystic ovarian disease and pelvic endometritis.
- Amenorrhea: Mullerian agenesis, genital tuberculosis.

- Acute pelvic pain:
  Ectopic pregnancy.
  Acute salpingo-oophoritis.
  Corpus luteum hematoma.
  Twisted ovarian cyst.
  Acute appendicitis.
- Chronic pelvic pain:
  Chronic PID
  Endometriosis
  Pelvic congestion syndrome
- Small pelvic masses:
  Ovarian cyst.
  Tuboovarian mass
  Broad ligament cyst or tumor.

Contraindications

- Severe cardiorespiratory disease.
- Generalized peritonitis.
- Bowel obstruction, ileus.
- Diaphragmatic or abdominal hernia.
- Second or third trimester pregnancy.
- Tuberculosis peritonitis with adhesions.
- Large pelvic mass.

Articles

A sterile tray containing:
1. Toothed thumb forceps to hold the tissues
2. Needle holder to hold the suturing needle
3. Dissection hook to dissect the tissues
4. Curved dissector
5. Scissors for cutting the tissues and suturing material
6. Trocar and cannula **(Fig. 40.8C)**
7. Suction catheter to suck out the blood and body fluids
8. Clip applicators with suitable clips to hold the surgical towels.

Other instruments:
9. A telescope usually 10 mm diameter and 25 cm long rod lens to visualize the abdominal/pelvic organs **(Fig. 40.8B)**

10. Inflation cannula (Rubin's cannula) **(Fig. 40.8A)**
11. Telescope for viewing
12. Laparoscope
13. A laparoscopic camera to use as a guide for procedure
14. Halogen or xenon light source

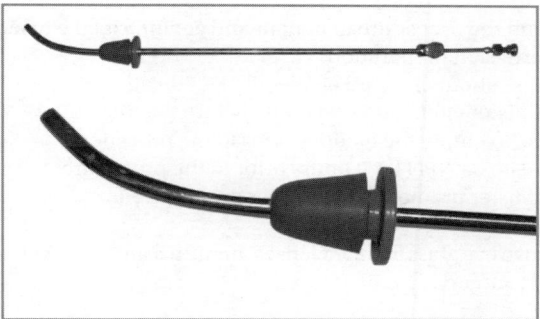

Fig. 40.8A: Rubin's cannula/Insufflation cannula.

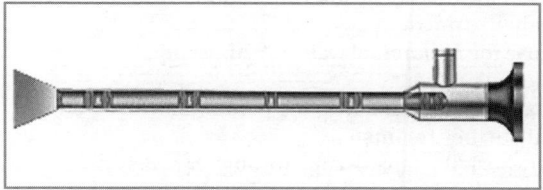

Fig. 40.8B: Telescope for viewing.

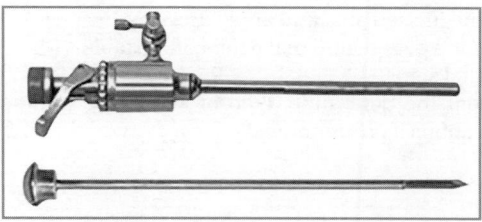

Fig. 40.8C: Trocar and cannula.

15. TV or video monitor to monitor the procedure
16. Suction- irrigation apparatus to collect the body fluids
17. Cautery machine with cables and foot control to cauterize the bleeding sites.

Preparation of the Patient

- Explain the procedure to patient and get informed consent
- Perform skin preparation
- Enquire about any kind of allergy to medication
- Administer enema several hours before the procedure
- Advise to empty the bladder prior to the procedure
- Advise to be NPO for 8 hours prior to the procedure
- Administer premedication as per prescription
- Remove jewelry
- Remove eye glass/contact lenses, dentures and removable bridge before surgery.

Procedure

- Position the mother in supine position.
- Anesthetize the mother.
- Cleanse the abdominal wall with antiseptic.
- Drape the mother.
- A small incision is made in the paraumbilical region.
- Insufflate the abdomen using CO_2 gas.
- Gently push the laparoscope through the incision.
- Visualize the internal organs in the TV monitor connected to the laparoscope **(Fig. 40.8D)**.
- Remove the laparoscope.
- Suture the incised area and apply dressing.
- Position the patient and make her comfortable.
- Check vital signs.
- Document the date, time, type of anesthesia and surgery and complications if any is noticed.

Aftercare

- Monitor vital signs for 2-3 hours
- Check the dressing for any oozing of blood.

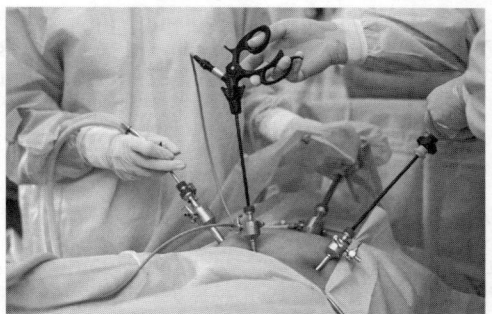

Fig. 40.8D: Laparoscopy procedure.

- Administer analgesics and antibiotics as prescribed.
- Tell the mother that she may experience sore throat which is due to the tube in throat applied during anesthesia.

9. LASER PROCEDURES/SURGERIES FOR GYNECOLOGICAL CONDITIONS

Important terms

- Conization: A cone shaped piece of abnormal tissue is removed from the cervix.
- Laser vaporization: Use of laser heat to destroy cells usually of the cervix, vagina and vulva that have dysplastic (premalignant) cells in them.
- Ablation: Laser ablation or photo ablation is the process of removing material from a solid surface (an organ) by irradiating it with laser beam. The material or tissue is heated by the absorbed laser energy and evaporated or sublimated.

Introduction

Laser surgery is the use of a type of energy that uses special light beams instead of instruments for surgical procedures. Laser stands for "Light Amplification by Stimulated Emission of Radiation". Lasers were first developed in 1960. In gynecological surgeries CO_2 (carbon dioxide) and iridium lasers are used for the treatment of many female genital tract diseases with applications in colposcopy, laparoscopy and hysteroscopy, obtaining many advantages against more traditional techniques or open surgeries. CO_2 laser coupled with colposcope has become an indispensable tool for ablation and excision of numerous lesions of the lower genital tract especially when it is necessary to minimize tissue removal.

Indications for Laser Surgery

In gynecology, laser surgery is recommended for the treatment of:
- Condylomata accuminata (warts) in the anogenital region.
- Dysplasia (abnormal cells within the tissue or organ) of the vulva, vagina and cervix which were treated with colposcopy.
- Intrauterine and endometrial pathologies which were treated with hysteroscopy or laparoscopy depending on the location of the lesion.

Contraindications

- Active vaginal or vulvar lesions such as herpes, candida, STDs
- Pregnancy or within three months postpartum.
- History of radiation to vaginal or colorectal tissue.
- History of reconstructive pelvic surgery.
- History of impaired wound healing and keloid formation.
- Known anticoagulant therapy or thromboembolic condition.
- Vaginal prolapse of uterus beyond the hymen.

Specific Laser Equipment and Instruments are used with Colposcopy, Laparoscopy or Hysteroscopy Laser Machine (Figs. 40.9A and B)

- Laser wave guides
- Hand pieces
- Couplers.

Gynecological Conditions for which Laser Surgery is Used

- Cervical intraepithelial neoplasia (CIN) and vulvar-vaginal intraepithelial neoplasia (VIN).

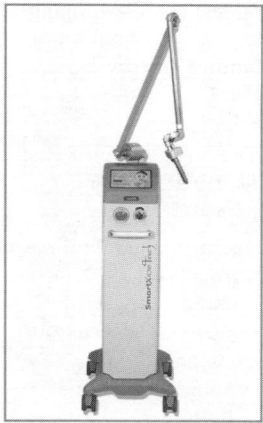

Fig. 40.9A: CO_2 laser machine.

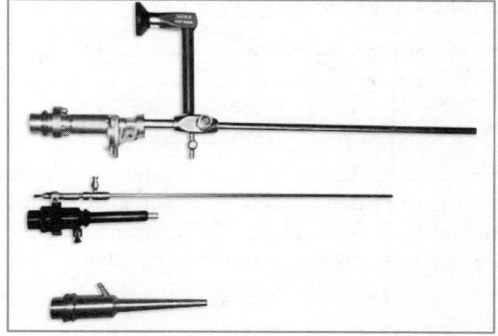

Fig. 40.9B: Laser instruments: Head piece and coupler, laser wave guides.

- Condyloma of cervical, vulvar or perineal tissue.
- Leukoplakia (vulvar dystrophies).
- Incision and drainage of Bartholin's and Nabothian (mucus filled) cysts located on the surface of the cervix or cervical canal).
- Urethral caruncle.
- Cervical dysplasia.

- Benign or malignant lesions of external genitalia.
- Erythroplasia.
- Uterine tumors (Myomas) and cysts.
- Endometriosis.
- Adhesions.

Advantages of Laser Surgery

- High degree of clinical efficacy.
- Bloodless field by sealing small blood vessels.
- Microscopic precision.
- Sparing of normal tissue.
- Rapid healing with normal scar formation.
- Significant reduction of pain.
- Small number of complications.
- Accurate removal of tumors.
- Low perioperative and postoperative morbidity.

Disadvantages of Laser Surgery

- Absence of histologic sample when vaporization is performed.
- Expense of laser machine.

Patient Preparation and Procedure

Preparation and procedure will be in accordance with the condition for which surgery is determined. As laser instruments are used in combination with those required for the endoscopic surgeries (colposcopy, laparoscopy or hysteroscopy), patient preparation and procedure are same as for those procedures described earlier in the same chapter.

Possible Discomforts of Patients During and After Laser Vaporization of Cervical, Vulvar or Vaginal Lesions

- Initial impact of the beam on cervix is experienced as a pinch similar to that experienced with applying a Tenaculum or taking a punch biopsy.

- As vaporization progresses, many women complain of uncomfortable warmth. Stopping the treatment for a moment usually gives relief.
- Menstrual like cramping due to liberation of prostaglandin like substances. This can be relieved by administration of prostaglandin synthetase inhibitor (Motrin) 30 minutes prior to laser vaporization.

Possible Complications

Complication rates are very low
- Cervical stenosis occurs in 1.3% of cases.
- Cervical incompetence in 0% cases.
- Major bleeding in less than 1% of all patients.

10. MAGNETIC RESONANCE IMAGING (MRI)

Definition

Magnetic resonance imaging is a non-invasive imaging technique that uses a magnetic field and computer-generated radio wave to create detailed images of the organs and tissues inside of the body. It produces three dimensional detailed anatomical images. An MRI scanner is a large tube that contains powerful magnets. The patient lies inside the tube/drum during the scan **(Fig. 40.10)**.

Purposes

MRI scan is used to:
- Detect tumors, cysts and other anomalies in various parts of the body.
- Screen for breast cancer.
- Evaluate pelvic pain related to fibroids and endometriosis.
- Detect uterine anomalies in women undergoing evaluation for infertility.
- Detect congenital abnormalities of the fetus, mainly central nervous system anomalies.

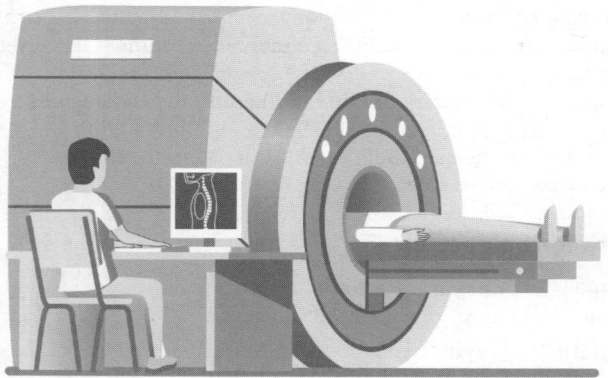

Fig. 40.10: MRI scanner.

Preparation of Patient

No special preparation is required. Patient may be asked to:
- Change into a hospital gown.
- Ensure that no metal jewelry or accessories are present on or inside the body such as cochlear implants.
- Individuals who are anxious or nervous about being in closed spaces should inform the doctor, who may be given medication prior to the MRI, to help make the procedure more comfortable.
- Patients will sometimes receive an injection of intravenous (IV) contrast liquid to improve the visibility of a particular tissue that is relevant to the scan.
- Once the patient has entered the scanning room, the radiologist will help her on to the scanner table to lie down. Staff will ensure that they are as comfortable as possible by providing blankets or cushions.
- Earplugs or headphones will be provided to block out the loud noises of the scanner, especially for children to calm them off any anxiety during the procedure.
- Allow the patient to lie on a padded stretcher face down and breasts placed through a depression in the table that slides into a chamber.

- If contrast medium is needed, inject gadolinium intravenously (after kidney function is verified.
- Series of images are then taken.

During an MRI Scan

Once inside the scanner, the MRI technician will communicate with the patient via the intercom to make sure that they are comfortable. They may not start the scan until the patient is ready. During the scan, it is vital to stay still. Any movement will disrupt the images much like a camera trying to take a picture of a moving object.

- Inform the patient that loud and changing noises will come from the scanner and this is perfectly normal.
- If the patient feels uncomfortable, during the procedure, they can speak to the technician via the intercom and request that the scan be stopped or press the buzzer to inform the technician, whichever facility is provided.
- After the can, the radiologist will examine the images to check whether any more are required. If the radiologist is satisfied, the patient can go home.

Side Effects

It is extremely rare that a patient will experience side effects from an MRI scan. However, the contrast dye if used, can cause nausea, headache and pain or burning at the point of injection in some people. Allergy to contrast material is also seldom seen but possible and can cause hives or itchy eyes. Notify the technician if any adverse reactions occur. People who experience claustrophobia or feel uncomfortable in enclosed spaces, sometimes express difficulties with undergoing an MRI scan.

41. DIARRHEA IN NEWBORNS

The frequent passage of stool in the newborn is common. Often times it is related to feeding and occasionally due to infection.

A. Feeding-Related Diarrhea

- Overfeeding: Increased amount and/or frequent feeds lead to undue irritation of the gut and intestinal hurry causing frequent stools
- Underfeeding: Inadequate feeding results in frequent passage of small green stools. This is called hunger diarrhea
- Excessive carbohydrate: Increased intake of carbohydrate produces flatulence, frequent frothy stools with excoriation of the buttocks. The reaction of the stool is acidic
- Excessive fat: More fat in feed may lead to vomiting and diarrhea with pale stool
- Protein excess: This is associated with colic and screaming, vomiting and frequent bloody stools.

B. Infective Diarrhea (Gastroenteritis)

Infective diarrhea in newborn is caused by organisms such as *Escherichia coli (E.coli), Staphylococcus* or virus.

Clinical Features

- Frequent watery stools, generally green in color due to unchanged bile
- Presence of mucus and blood in stool
- Colic and screaming
- Dry, inelastic skin due to dehydration
- Sunken eyes, depressed fontanelle
- Loss of weight
- Circulatory collapse.

Treatment of Infective Diarrhea

- Isolating the baby
- Culture and sensitivity test of the stool
- Milk feeding to be stopped
- Oral rehydration solution (ORS) to be started and continued at 2–3 hourly intervals
- Parenteral fluids if the baby refuses to take adequate ORS

- Antibiotics
- After diarrhoea is controlled, breastfeeding to be resumed.

42. DISSEMINATED INTRAVASCULAR COAGULATION

Definition

A coagulation disorder with bleeding tendency due to consumption of clotting factors and platelets due to thrombin generation in blood stream.

Physiological Changes During Pregnancy Affecting Coagulation

During pregnancy, there is increase in concentration of clotting factors II, V, VII, VIII, IX, X and XII. Plasma fibrinogen level is significantly increased. There is a small decrease in platelet count, due to low-grade intravascular coagulation. Plasma fibrinolytic activity is suppressed during pregnancy and labor. It returns to normal within 1 hour of delivery of placenta.

Conditions of Coagulopathy in Pregnancy

- Abruptio placentae
- Amniotic fluid embolism
- Severe preeclampsia, eclampsia and 'HELLP' syndrome (HELLP stands for 'hemolysis, elevated liver enzymes and low platelets')
- Instillation of intra-amniotic hypertonic saline
- Dextran infusion
- Hydatidiform mole
- Endotoxemia: Septic abortion, chorioamnionitis
- Prolonged retention of dead fetus in uterus
- Cesarean section.

All these clinical conditions may trigger the delicate hemostatic mechanism either by endothelial injury or by release of thromboplastin and phospholipids. It is always a secondary phenomenon. Because of the hypercoagulable state in pregnancy, presence of any provocative factor can easily upset the normal balance culminating into disseminated intravascular coagulation (DIC). The blood fibrinogen level of 100 mg/100 mL is arbitrarily considered to be the critical level.

Clinical Manifestations

Manifestations of blood coagulation disorder are evidenced by hemorrhage from various sites.

Before Delivery

- Signs of bruising
- Prolonged bleeding at injection sites (venipuncture or intramuscular)
- Gum bleeding
- Hemorrhage from gastrointestinal tract.

After Delivery

In addition to the manifestations already described:
- Postpartum hemorrhage in spite of a hard, well-contracted uterus (traumatic bleeding excluded), occurring about 1–2 hours following delivery
- Bleeding from the suture sites of episiotomy or hematoma formation in the abdominal wound following cesarean section
- Vulval hematoma following vaginal delivery.

Investigations

- Bleeding time
- Coagulation time
- Clot observation test
- Peripheral smear
- Circulatory fibrinolysis test
- Tests to detect defects in the coagulation mechanism:
  - Platelet count
  - Partial thromboplastin time
  - Prothrombin time
  - Thrombin time

- Fibrinogen estimation
- Fibrin degradation products (FDP)
- Euglobulin clotlysis time.

Treatment

1. Preventive:
   - Management of abruptio placentae with adequate blood transfusion, delivery by low rupture of membranes supplemented by oxytocin drip or early cesarean section
   - Emptying uterus within 2 weeks in case of intrauterine death
   - Effective antenatal care and judicious and timely termination of pregnancy in preeclampsia, eclampsia and 'HELLP' syndrome.
2. Precautions:
   - Avoiding bloody tap while instilling hypertonic saline for induction of abortion
   - Infusion of polymolecular gelatin (hemacel or gelofusine) as plasma expander in preference to dextran.
3. Curative:
   - Whole blood transfusion for volume replacement and to restore hemostatic competence
   - Administration of fibrinogen as replacement therapy
   - Administration of fibrinolytic inhibitors and heparin to correct appropriate disorders
   - Immediate volume replacement with hemacel, till properly crossmatched whole-blood is available to maintain perfusion
   - Massive whole blood transfusion to replenish the fibrinogen and clotting factors
   - Fresh frozen plasma to replace fibrinogen and certain clotting factors.
   - Cryoprecipitate, platelet concentrates and commercially available fibrinogen are used as required
   - Heparin is used in acute conditions such as amniotic fluid embolism and intrauterine fetal death to arrest the process of coagulation
   - Prompt replacement of blood volume and coagulation factors is an important step in the management of coagulation disorders in obstetrics.

43. DRUGS IN OBSTETRICS

Drugs are prescribed very cautiously to pregnant and lactating women because of the risks involved to fetus and newborn. Drugs taken by a mother during pregnancy can be potentially harmful or even teratogenic to the fetus. When absolutely indicated, drugs of proven safety are used for minimal effective period.

OXYTOCICS

Oxytocics are drugs of varying chemical nature that have power to excite contractions of uterine muscles. Important drugs in this group are:
- Oxytocin
- Ergot derivatives
- Prostaglandins.

OXYTOCIN

Endogenous oxytocin is a hormone synthesized in the hypothalamus and stored in the posterior pituitary. It stimulates contractions of the uterine smooth muscle during gestation and causes milk ejection after childbirth. Synthetic preparations of oxytocin are used in clinical practice.

Preparations Used

1. Syntocinon (Sandoz)-Ampoules of 5 IU/mL;
   Pitocin (Parke-Davis) 10 IU/mL.
2. Syntometrine (Sandoz); Syntocinon 5 units and Ergometrine 0.5 units.
3. Desamino oxytocin, buccal tablets containing 50 IU.
4. Oxytocin nasal solution 40 units/mL.

Effectiveness of Oxytocin

- First-trimester: No effect on uterine muscle
- Second-trimester: Supplements abortifacient agents in induction of labor

Drugs in Obstetrics

- In later months of pregnancy and labor, the uterus is highly sensitive to oxytocin.

Indications

Therapeutic

In pregnancy:
- To accelerate abortion
- To expel hydatidiform mole
- To stop bleeding following evacuation of uterus.

In labor:
- For initiation of labor
- For augmentation of labor
- For active management of labor (Pitocin 5 units is given when the anterior shoulder is delivered)
- Following expulsion of placenta.

Diagnostic:
- Oxytocin challenge test (OCT)
- Oxytocin sensitivity test (OST).

Methods of Administration

- Controlled intravenous infusion
- Intramuscular injection.

Dosage and Administration for Induction of Labor

Oxytocin is diluted and administered as controlled intravenous infusion in dose of 0.5–2 milliunits/min. The rate of infusion may be slowly increased at 1–2 milliunits/min increments at 15–60 minutes intervals until the required contraction pattern is established. The rate of infusion is then decreased slowly at 15–60 minutes intervals and continued till labor has progressed to 5–6 cm dilatation of cervix.

Nursing Management of Patient on Oxytocin Infusion

- Prior to infusion, assess client to exclude any fetopelvic disproportion
- Ensure that the infusion begins with the correct dose and increased at correct intervals

- Do not leave the mother unattended when the infusion is running
- Check the uterine response every 15–30 minutes
- Check the fetal heart tones every 15–30 minutes
- Check the mother's blood pressure at regular intervals
- Note the urinary output is > 20 mL/min
- Check the progress of labor and descend of fetal head periodically
- Note any untoward symptom.

Indications to Stop to Infusion

- Abnormal uterine contractions, i.e.; frequency every 2 minutes or less, lasting more than 60 seconds
- Increased tone between contractions
- Any evidence of fetal distress
- Evidence of maternal exhaustion.

Contraindications

- Grand multipara
- Contracted pelvis
- Previous cesarean section or hysterotomy
- Malpresentation
- Obstructed labor
- Incoordinate uterine action
- Hypovolaemic state
- Cardiac disease.

ERGOT DERIVATES

Ergometrine and methergine are the two commonly used ergot derivatives. Ergometrine (ergonovine) is an alkaloid isolated from ergot, a fungus that develops commonly in cereals. Methergine (methylergonovine) is a semi-synthetic product derived from lysergic acid. The preparations are available in different forms and strengths **(Table 43.1)**.

Mode of Action

Ergometrine causes sustained uterine contractions with hypertonicity (tonic uterine contractions).

Table 43.1: Composition of different preparations.

Preparation	Form and strength
Ergometrine	Ampoules 0. 25 mg/mL Tablets 0.125 mg
Methergine	Ampoules 0. 2 mg Tablets 0.125 mg

Effectiveness

Highly effective in hemostasis, i.e. stops bleeding from uterine sinuses following delivery or abortion.

Indications

- To stop atonic uterine bleeding
- As prophylactic against postpartum hemorrhage (PPH), it is given after delivery of anterior shoulder or following delivery of placenta.
  Ergot preparations can be used parenterally or orally.

Contraindications

- Suspected pleural pregnancy
- Organic cardiac disease
- Severe preeclampsia and eclampsia
- Rh negative mother.

Nursing Considerations

- Assess client for nausea, vomiting, weakness, muscular pain or paresthesia of extremities
- Monitor blood pressure and pulse for changes that may indicate hemorrhage
- Note fundal tone and check for relaxation
- If intramuscular (IM) injection, give deep in large muscle.

TOCOLYTIC AGENTS

Tocolytic agents are drugs used to arrest preterm labor, avert fetal distress and as a prophylaxis against preterm labor. Action, dosage and side effects of tocolytic drugs are outlined in **Table 43.2**.

Table 43.2: Tocolytic drugs.

Preparation	Action	Dosage	Side effects
Isoxsuprine (Duadilan)	Stimulation of adrenergic receptors	10 mg intravenous (IV) 6-hourly for 24 hours –10 mg PO, 6–8 hourly –0.2–0.8 μg per min IV	Hypertension, dizziness, palpitation, nausea, vomiting, abdominal distress, rash
Terbutaline (Brycanyl)	β adrenenergic receptor agonist, sympathomimetic	2.5–5.0 mg PO Q 4–6 hour 0.25–0.5 mg SC Q 3–4 hours	Hypertension, hypoglycemia, hypocalcemia, cardiac insufficiency
Ritodrine (Yutopar)	Same as Terbutaline	0.05–0.35 mg/min IV in 5% dextrose for 12 h 10–20 mg PO before termination of IV	Tachycardia, arrhythmia, palpitation, headache, nausea, vomiting, pulmonary edema, anaphylaxis
Magnesium Sulfate	Intracellular calcium antagonism	4–6 gm IV over 10 min, followed by 2 g/h and then 1 g/h in 5% dextrose using infusion pump	Hypotension, muscle weakness, flushing, sweating, confusion, depressed knee reflexes, flaccid paralysis, respiratory depression, cardiac arrhythmia

Note: Tocolytics are continued for 2 h after the contractions cease.

Contraindications of Tocolytics

Maternal:
- Unstable maternal conditions such as preeclampsia, trauma or hemorrhage
- Renal and pulmonary disease.

Fetal:
- Fetal death
- Intrauterine infection
- Severe intrauterine growth restriction
- Anomalies incompatible with life.

Nursing Considerations

- Monitor intake-output and check for decrease in urine output
- Monitor fetal status by checking fetal heart tones
- Monitor uterine contractions
- Monitor pulse rate and blood pressure
- Tocolytics are not administered for more than 48 hours.

ANTIHYPERTENSIVE DRUGS USED IN PREGNANCY

Antihypertensive drugs are used in hypertensive disorders of pregnancy such as preeclampsia, eclampsia and chronic hypertension. The commonly used antihypertensive drugs and their dosages are outlined in **Table 43.3**.

Table 43.3: Antihypertensives used in pregnancy.

Preparation	Dose	Dosages
Methyldopa (Aldomet)	250–500 mg	Four to six time/day
Propranolol (Inderal)	30–40 mg	Four time/day
Hydralazine (Apresoline)	20–40 mg	Four time/day
Labetalol	100 mg	Two to three time/day
Nifedipine	25 mg	Thrice daily

Mechanism of Action and Side Effects

1. Methyldopa (Aldomet):
    - This is the most widely used drug in women with mild to moderate pregnancy-induced hypertension, as it is effective and safe for both mother and fetus
    - It has central and peripheral antiadrenergic action
    - Side effects are postural hypotension hemolytic anemia, sodium retention and exessive sedation for the mother and intestinal ileus for the fetus.
2. Propranolol (Inderal):
    - This is a beta-adrenergic receptor blocker
    - It decreases the force of contraction, rate and conduction of myocardium
    - It also decreases cardiac output, which leads to reduction of blood pressure
    - Side effects include severe hypotension, sodium retention, bradycardia and bronchospasm for mother; for fetus, bradycardia and impaired response to hypoxia are possible.
3. Hydralazine (Apresoline):
    - It acts by causing peripheral vasodilation probably by inhibiting the movement of calcium into the smooth muscles.
    - It increases the cardiac output and renal blood flow
    - Side effects are maternal hypotension, dizziness, postural hypotension and edema
    - The drug is reasonably safe for fetus.
4. Labetalol:
    - Labitalol is a beta-blocker
    - Side effects include postural hypotension, sodium retention and sedation.
5. Nifedipine:
    - This drug acts as a calcium-channel blocker
    - It causes arteriolar vasodilation by inhibition of calcium ion influx in vascular smooth muscle
    - Side effects are flushing, hypotension, headache, tachycardia and inhibition of labor.

Nursing Considerations

Teach patients on antihypertensive medications:
- Not to discontinue medication abruptly
- To have blood pressure checked biweekly
- To report bradycardia, dizziness, confusion, shortness of breath and edema
- To avoid alcohol and smoking.

PROSTAGLANDINS

Prostaglandins are derivatives of prostanoic acid. Chemically prostaglandins are 20-carbon carboxylic acid with a cyclopropane ring formed from polyunsaturated fatty acids. Prostaglandins act as 'local hormones'.

Varieties used in Obstetrics

- PGE_2 (Dinoprostone)
- PGF_{2a}.

Available forms include vaginal tablet, vaginal suppository, vaginal pessary and gel for placement into cervical canal. Injectable forms include Prostin E2 and F2a. Oral preparation is misoprostol (PGE1).

Mode of Action

- Prostaglandins have direct effect on uterine muscle like oxytocin; particularly PGF_{2a}, which is used for induction of labor in cases of intrauterine death, shorter period of gestation or in elderly primigravida
- They have a cervical ripening effect by lysis of rigid collagen fibers (PGE_2), when used intravaginally or intracervically.

Indications

- Induction of abortion: MTP and missed abortion
- Termination of molar pregnancy
- Induction of labor

- Augmentation or acceleration of labor
- To stop bleeding in refractory cases of PPH.

Contraindications

Absolute:
- Hypersensitivity
- Asthma
- Acute pelvic inflammatory disease.

Relative:
- Hypertension
- Cardiovascular disease
- Peptic ulcer
- Hepatitis
- Uterine scar.

Nursing Considerations

- For cervical or vaginal application, make sure that the patient is in dorsal position
- Teach patient to remain supine for 10–15 minutes after insertion of suppository, 2 hours following insert and 15–20 minutes following gel
- Apply prostaglandins after warming to room temperature
- Instruct patient to report excessive cramping, bleeding, chills or fever
- Monitor cervical dilatation, uterine contractions and fetal status.

ANTICONVULSANT DRUGS

The commonly used anticonvulsants in obstetrics are:
- Magnesium sulfate
- Diazepam
- Phenobarbitone
- Phenytoin.

Magnesium Sulfate

Mode of action:
- Increases cerebral blood flow
- Reduces cerebral ischemia

- Reduces neuromuscular irritability
- Decreases intracranial edema and helps in diuresis
- Improves uterine blood supply.

Indications

Control of convulsion in eclampsia.

Dose for Different Regimens

1. Pritchard regimen:
   - 4 g $MgSO_4$ (20 mL of 20% solution) IV given slowly over 3–4 min
   - Followed immediately by 10 g (in 10 mL) given as deep IM in buttocks
   - Followed with 5 g, IM in alternate buttocks 4 hourly till 24 hours postpartum.
2. Zuspan regimen:
   4 g IV over 5–10 minutes followed by 1–2 g/hour IV, diluted in 5% dextrose using IV pump
   - Therapeutic level of serum magnesium is 4–7 mEq/L
   - Infusion continued only if:
     - Knee jerks are present
     - Urine output exceeds 30 mL/h
     - Respiration rate is more than 12/min.
   - For recurrence of fits, further 2 g IV bolus is given over 5 minutes
   - Antidote for toxicity is calcium gluconate 10% 10 mL IV (evidenced as diminished knee jerks respiratory failure and reduced renal function).

Diazepam

Acts as central muscle relaxant and anticonvulsant.

Dose

20–40 mg IV initially, followed by an infusion of 40 mg in 500 mL of IV dextrose at 30 drops/minute.

Side Effects

- Mother: Hypotension
- Fetus: Respiratory depression
- Newborn: Respiratory depression, hypotonia and thermoregulatory problems.

Phenobarbitone

Acts by inhibiting reticular activating system.

Dose

About 120–240 mg IV in divided doses.

Side effects

- Mother: Sedation
- Fetus: Withdrawal syndrome and bleeding seen after birth.

Phenytoin (Dilantin)

Phenytoin inhibits spread of seizure activity in motor cortex by altering ion transport.

Dose

About 10 mg/kg IV followed by 5 mg/kg after 2 hours.

Side Effects

Drowsiness, dizziness, paresthesia, confusion and peripheral neuropathy.

Nursing Considerations When Patient is on $MgSO_4$

- Position client in left lateral position and maintain fetal monitoring
- Monitor BP, respiratory rate and deep tendon reflexes (absence of deep tendon reflexes and/or respiratory rate less than 12/min indicates toxicity)

- Monitor intake and output to assess renal function; urine output to be > 30 mL/h
- Monitor serum magnesium levels periodically
- Keep 10% calcium gluconate ready for emergency use
- Institute measures to prevent fall and injury
- Ensure that her air passage is kept clear
- When other anticonvulsants are used, watch for development of any side effect
- Watch for signs of onset of labor
- Monitor fetal status.

ANALGESIA IN NORMAL DELIVERY

Analgesic drugs are used for pain relief in labor. When medications are used, care should be taken as most/all of them have depressing effect on the respirations of the fetus and uterine activity.

Methods of Pain Relief

- Sedatives and analgesics
- Inhalation agents
- Regional analgesia
- Patient controlled analgesia
- Transcutaneous electronic nerve stimulation
- Psychoprophylaxis.

Sedatives and Analgesics

- Opioid analgesics:
  - Pethidine (Demerol)
  - Pentozocin (Fortwin).
- Tranquillizers:
  - Diazepam
  - Midazolam (versed).

Pethidine

Used as analgesic in labor; it has strong sedative effect; dose is 75–100 mg IM (1.5 mg/kg).

Side effects
Mother: Nausea, vomiting and delayed gastric emptying.
Fetus: Depresses respiration as it crosses placenta and accumulates in fetal tissue.

Pontazocin

Dose is 30–40 mg IM.

Side effects: Nausea, vomiting, anorexia and dry mouth.

Diazepam

Dose 5–10 mg IV.

Side effects: Dizziness, drowsiness, headache, insomnia.

Midazolam

Midazolam is a sedative, hypnotic and antianxiety drug.

Dose: 0.07–0.08 mg/kg.

Side effects: Nausea, vomiting, hiccups, increased salivation, pruritus and rash.

Regional Analgesia

1. Epidural block:
   a. Medication: Dilute solution of a local anesthetic and an opioid are used.
   b. Route of administration: Administered into the epidural space through a small catheter that is left in place.
   c. Advantages:
      - Provides excellent analgesia
      - Titratable when administered as a continuous infusion.
   d. Disadvantages:
      - Client is confined to bed
      - Frequent vital signs check is needed as hypotension is a possible side effect
      - May interfere with maternal pushing effort
      - Possible headache as the dura is punctured.

2. Paracervical block:
   a. Medication; local anesthetic.
   b. Route of administration: Medication is injected into the vaginal wall near the cervix at 3 and 9 O'clock positions.
   c. Advantage: Good pain relief for the first-stage of labor.
   d. Disadvantages.
      - Short acting and may need to be repeated
      - Associated with fetal bradycardia.
3. Perineal infiltration: Infiltration with a local anesthetic produces loss of sensation in a small area. This is done prior to episiotomy and instrumental delivery.

MATERNAL DRUG INTAKE AND BREASTFEEDING (TABLE 43.4)

Drugs taken by breastfeeding mothers may have adverse effect on lactation and also on the baby as it may be present in her breast milk.

Table 43.4: Maternal Medications with Established Teratogenic Properties and their effects on fetus.

Medication	Effect on fetus	Use in therapy
Alcohol	Growth retardation, congenital defects	Avoided
Amphetamines	Congenital heart defects	Avoided
Antimetabolites	Eye abnormalities	Avoided
Anesthetics	Depressed fetal vital centers	Avoided
Antithyroid drugs	Causes goiter	Avoided
Anticonvulsants	Cleft lips/palate, congenital heart defects, abnormalities of fingers and toes	Avoided
Chloroquine	Affects ears (hearing)	Avoided
Chlorpromide	Intrauterine death	Avoided
Chloramphenicol	Neonatal grey baby	Avoided

Contd...

Contd...

Medication	Effect on fetus	Use in therapy
Chlorthiazide	Decreased blood count	Avoided
Caffeine	Abortion, growth retardation, stillbirth	Avoided
Carbamazepine	Neural tube defects	Avoided
Cocaine	Growth retardation, uterine rupture and placental insufficiency	Avoided
Glucocorticoids	Intrauterine growth retardation	Avoided
Lithium	Heart defects	Avoided
LSD	Chromosome abnormalities	Avoided
Metronidazole	Embriotoxic	Avoided
Estrogen	Vaginal carcinoma	Avoided
Progestogens	Masculinization of female fetus.	Avoided
Phenobarbitone	Fetal bleeding is a rare complication	Used with vitamin K
Prednisolone	Cleft palate, fetal death	Used with care
Phenytoin	Fetal congenital anomalies	Avoided
Streptomycin	Fetal congenital anomalies	Avoided
Sulphonilamide	Neonatal jaundice	Avoided at term
Steroids	Congenital deformities	Used with care
Tetracycline	Effects on bones and teeth	Avoided
Trimethoprim	Antifolate action	Avoided
Thalidomide	Limb deformities	Avoided
Tolbutamide	Multiple deformities	Avoided
Valporic acid	Neural tube defects	Avoided
Warfarin	Skeletal and limb defects, low birth weight	Avoided

The concentration of the medication in breast milk is usually low compared to blood levels in mother.

Some drugs taken by the mother may cause toxicity to the infant as the milk concentration of the drug may increase. Drugs in breast milk may cause hypersensitivity in the infant even when used in therapeutic doses.

44. DYSMENORRHEA

Definition

Painful menses or cramping during menstruation. Typically dysmenorrhea begins up to 48 hours before onset of menses and resolves within 2–4 days of onset or by the end of menstrual period.

Dysmenorrhea can be classified as primary or secondary.

Primary Dysmenorrhea

Primary dysmenorrhea is painful menses with a uterine cause, but without pelvic pathology and usually occurs within 1–3 years of menarche (Ugarriza, Klinger and O'Brien, 1998).

Cause

Painful uterine contractions stimulated by prostaglandin produced by endometrium during menses are most often identified as the cause for primary dysmenorrhea.

Symptoms

- Sharp, intermittent suprapubic pain radiating to the back or thighs
- Headache, fatigue, backache, flushing, dizziness and syncope
- Adolescents typically experience the problem only after menstrual cycles become ovulatory
- Women often experience reduction in dysmenorrhea after pregnancy.

Therapeutic Interventions

- Nonsteroidal anti-inflammatory drugs (NSAIDs) started 1–3 days prior to the onset of menstrual flow (to decrease prostaglandin production)

- Oral contraceptives, to decrease endometrial proliferation and therefore production of prostaglandin.

Secondary Dysmenorrhea

Secondary dysmenorrhea is painful menses resulting from a pathologic process, such as pressure from outside the uterus, tissue ischemia, cervical stenosis, congenital abnormality (imperforate hymen), endometriosis, ovarian cysts, pelvic inflammatory disease (PID) or uterine fibroid tumors.

Symptoms may begin earlier in the cycle and last longer than the symptoms of primary dysmenorrhea with specific symptoms other than pain. Those symptoms include breast tenderness and a change in bowel habits.

Therapeutic intervention usually involves correction of the cause.

45. DYSPAREUNIA

Dyspareunia is occurrence of pain during sexual intercourse. It is the most common sexual dysfunction.

Male Causes

- Impotence
- Premature ejaculation
- Congenital anatomic defect of the penis
- Improper technique of coital act.

Female Causes

1. Superficial or entrance dyspareunia:
   - Narrow introitus
   - Tough hymen
   - Bartholin gland cysts
   - Tender perineal scar
   - Vulval infection
   - Urethral pathology
   - Vulvar vestibulitis syndrome.

2. Vaginal causes.
   - Pain along the barrel of vagina either during or following intercourse
   - Vaginitis
   - Vaginal septum
   - Tender scar following gynecologic operation or delivery
   - Secondary vaginal atresia
   - Tumor
   - Vaginal atrophy following menopause.
3. Deep dyspareunia.
   - Patient experiences pain while the penis penetrates deep into the vagina
   - Endometriosis especially on retrovaginal septum
   - Chronic cervicitis
   - Chronic PID
   - Retroverted uterus (retroverted and fixed)
   - Prolapsed ovary in the pouch of Douglas.

Treatment

Treatment depends upon the cause:
- Sex education of both partners
- Treatment for any infection if present
- Excision of scar if present
- Surgical correction of retroverted uterus or prolapsed ovary
- Treatment for any organic lesion if present.

46. ECLAMPSIA

Occurrence of convulsions in a patient with preeclampsia with no coincidental neurologic disease is called eclampsia.

Eclampsia may be antepartum (50%), intrapartum (25%), postpartum (25%) or rarely intercurrent, wherein the patient seems to recover after her convulsion and the pregnancy continues. In the concurrent type, there always remains the risk of a future fulminant eclampsia. Eclampsia is more common in primigravidae (75%), five times more common in twins than in singleton pregnancies and occurs between the 36th week and term in more than 50%.

The typical eclamptic seizure is described in four phases:
1. *Initial or prodromal phase:* There may be an aura, followed by convulsive movements that begin around the mouth. There is twitching of the muscles of the face, tongue and limbs. Eyeballs roll or are turned to one side and become fixed. This stage lasts for about 30 seconds.
2. *Tonic phase:* The entire body becomes rigid, the trunk opisthotonos, limbs are flexed and hands clenched. Respiration ceases and the tongue protrudes between the teeth. Cyanosis appears and eyeballs become fixed. This stage lasts for 20–30 seconds.
3. *Clonic phase:* Jerky movements then appear starting form the facial muscles to involve the entire body. There is frothing of sputum at the mouth. Biting of the tongue may occur. Cyanosis is often present. Duration of this phase is about 1 minute.
4. *Recovery phase/coma:* Following the seizure, the patient passes on to the stage of coma. It may last for a brief period or in some patients deep coma persists till another convulsion. On occasion, the patient appears to be in a confused state following the seizure and fails to remember the happenings.

The convulsions are usually multiple, recurring at varying intervals. When it occurs in quick succession it is called status eclampticus. Eclampsia can have disastrous consequences such as pulmonary edema due to cardiac failure or aspiration and sudden death, coma, or hemiplegia due to cerebral hemorrhage. Besides these, the patient is at a risk for injuries such as tongue bite and falling out of bed.

Management

- Assess for signs of impending eclampsia:
  - Hyperactivity of deep tendon reflexes (3 + to 4+)
  - Ankle clonus
  - Decreased pulse and respirations
  - Epigastric pain
  - Oliguria (< 50 mL/hour).

- Institute measures to reduce likelihood of seizures:
  - Keep room quiet and dimly lit
  - Limit visitors
  - Plan and coordinate care activities and promote rest.
- Implement seizure precautions per protocol:
  - Prop up the side rails of bed to prevent injury and fall out of bed
  - Keep a padded tongue depressor at bed side
  - Keep oxygen supply, suction articles and crash cart ready.

  In the event of seizure:
  - Turn patient on her side to reduce the risk of aspiration
  - Insert a padded airway if mouth is relaxed to prevent tongue from occluding the airway and biting of tongue
  - Remove restrictive clothing
  - Administer oxygen
  - Document motor involvement, duration of seizure and postseizure behavior.
- Start a large-bore intravenous line to administer fluids and medication
- Monitor signs and symptoms of labor such as uterine contractions
- Assess fetal well-being, noting FHR
- Emergency laboratory investigations include:
  - Complete blood count, platelet count, liver and renal function tests, arterial blood gases, serum electrolytes bleeding time and clotting time, prothrombin time (PT), partial thromboplastin time (PTT), blood type and cross match.
- Maintain oxygenation as dictated by the patient's condition and arterial blood gases
- Introduce a self-retaining catheter, test urine for protein; maintain continuous drainage and hourly measurement of output
- Anticonvulsant therapy:
  - Magnesium sulfate ($MgSO_4$) is the drug of choice; administer $MgSO_4$ per protocol
  - Pritchard regimen: 4 g IV as loading dose, followed by 4 g IM hourly in alternate buttock
  - Suspan regimen: 4 g IV as loading dose, followed by 1–2 g/h IV infusion.

- Nurse the patient in lateral position to facilitate drainage of secretions and to prevent aspiration; oral suctioning to be done frequently as required
- Antihypertensive medications and diuretics are administered if blood pressure remains more than 160/100 mm Hg
- Precise recordings of vital signs, intake-output and occurance of convulsions to be done
- Monitor for signs of labor such as periodic restlessness
- Monitor fetal heart sounds periodically
- Delivery should be accomplished speedily and with as little trauma as possible.

Complications of Eclampsia

Eclampsia patients are at risk for several complications and as such preventive measures and careful monitoring are essential:
- Cardiovascular: Vasospasm, pulmonary edema
- Renal: Ischemia, oliguria and renal failure
- Hematological: Hypovolemia, thrombocytopenia, hemorrhage and disseminated intravascular coagulation
- Neurological: Cerebral edema, cerebral hemorrhage
- Hepatic: Hepatocellular damage, hepatic rupture
- Fetal: Placental abruption, fetal distress and intrauterine death.

Nursing Process: Refer Chapter 86 (PIH).

47. ECTOPIC PREGNANCY

Any pregnancy where the fertilized ovum gets implanted in a site other than in the normal uterine cavity is said to be an ectopic gestation. The incidence is approximately 1:300 normal pregnancies worldwide.

Sites of Ectopic Pregnancy

- Fallopian tube: 95–99%, most frequently in the ampullary portion
- Ovarian: About 0.5%
- Abdominal: About 0.1%.

Etiology

- Any factor that causes delayed transport of the fertilized ovum through the fallopian tube:
  - Congenital flaws such as tubal hypoplasia, tortuosity, congenital diverticuli, accessory ostia and partial stenosis
  - Acquired factors such as inflammation of the tubal mucosa, e.g. salpingitis secondary to pelvic inflammatory disease (PID)
  - Surgical procedures on the fallopian tubes or in the pelvis causing intraluminal or extraluminal adhesions
  - Neoplastic conditions such as broad ligament myomas and ovarian tumors, which can elongate the overlying fallopian tube.
- Intrauterine contraceptive devices
- Endometriosis
- Assisted reproductive procedures such as in vitro fertilization (IVF) and gamete intrafallopian transfer (GIFT)
- Prior induced abortion
- Previous ectopic pregnancy
- Tubal spasm and impaired tubal mobility related to use of hormones such as progestin only pill or postcoital estrogen pill.

Mode of Termination

Once implanted, the pregnancy could proceed along one of several pathways leading to various presentations of such patients **(Figs. 47.1A to C)**.

Tubal Abortion

Tubal abortion is the common mode of termination, if implantation occurs in the ampulla or infundibulum. Choriodecidual hemorrhage occurs around the ovum, which gets detached and is expelled into the tubal lumen. This may get expelled through the abdominal ostium resulting in a complete abortion. If the abortion is incomplete, part of the products of gestation remain attached to the endosalpinx and bleeding continues. The blood may collect in the pouch of Douglas to form a pelvic hematocele. Rarely the dead ovum remains in the tubal lumen surrounded by layers of clotted blood. The outcome is

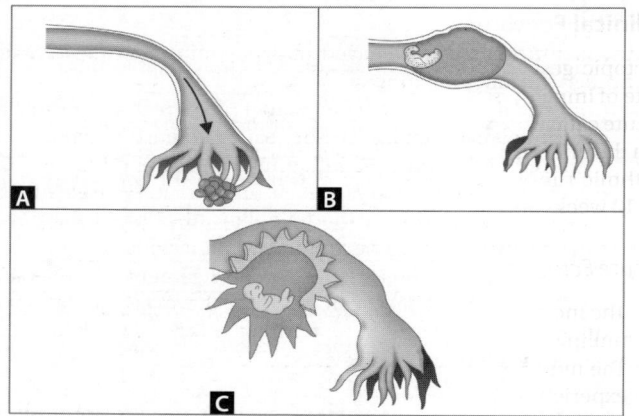

Figs. 47.1A to C: Possible outcomes of tubal pregnancy. **A.** Tubal abortion; **B.** Tubal mole; **C.** Tubal rupture.

similar to a missed abortion and the product is termed as carneous mole.

Tubal Rupture

When the fertilized ovum implants in the isthmic or interstitial portion of the tube, then tubal rupture is more common. Due to distension and erosion of large arterioles, rupture of the tube produces heavy and continuous bleeding. The patient may present in shock. Intraperitoneal hemorrhage and pelvic hematocele are common. With isthmic implantation, extraperitoneal rupture occurs, which is rare compared to implantation in the interstitial portion.

Tubal Mole

The formation of tubal mole is similar to that formed in uterine pregnancy. Repeated small hemorrhages occur in the choriocapsularis space separating the villi from their attachments. The mole then ends up as complete absorption or expulsion through the abdominal ostium as tubal abortion. The expelled mole may become a pelvic hematocele due to internal hemorrhage.

Clinical Features

Ectopic gestations have varied presentations depending upon the site of implantation. Tubal ectopic gestation can either present as an acute catastrophic event or as a subacute or chronic form depending on the underlying pathophysiology and the location of implantation. Isthmic rupture usually occurs at 6–8 weeks, the ampullary one at 8–12 weeks and the interstitial one at about 4 months.

Acute Ectopic Rupture

- The incidence is maximum between the age of 20 and 30 years, in nulliparous women following a period of infertility
- The mode of onset is acute, however, about one third of patients experience unilateral uneasiness before the appearance of symptoms. The classic triad of symptoms is amenorrhea followed by abdominal pain and lastly appearance of vaginal bleeding
- Short period of amenorrhea of 6–8 weeks, or a delayed period or spotting on the expected date
- Acute, agonising and colicky pain, which is initially experienced in the lower abdomen and later spreads all over the abdomen
- Vaginal bleeding may be slight, sanguineous or dark colored and usually continuous
- Feeling of nausea, vomiting and fainting attacks
- On examination: Patient is often in shock with pallor, restlessness, tachycardia, hypotension and cold, clammy extremities
- Abdominal examination:
  - Often reveals distension, extreme tenderness, guarding and rigidity
  - Signs of free fluid such as shifting dullness and fluid thrill in patients where hemorrhage has been severe.
- Speculum examination would reveal a pale vaginal mucosa and possibly a bluish cervix that has tenderness on movement. Vaginal mucosa blanched white
- Vaginal examination would reveal normal-sized uterus, soft cervix and tenderness on movement. The fornices are tender and rarely an adnexal mass may be palpable. The pouch of Douglas is often felt as soft, with fluctuant fullness and is tender due to the pelvic hematocele.

Investigations

- Complete blood count with hemoglobin
- Blood group and cross-match (at least 2–3 units of blood to be reserved)
- Ultrasonography: The findings of an empty uterine cavity with an adnexal mass and fluid in the pouch of Douglas are most suggestive of ectopic gestation. The findings of a gestational sac, fetal pole and fetal heart within the adnexal mass is an added confirmation
- Culdocentesis: Aspiration of fresh, non-clotting blood is suggestive of intraperitoneal bleeding
- Laparoscopy: Done in cases of confusion in diagnosis and if the patient's condition is stable.

Management

- Resuscitation of the patient with intravenous fluids, blood, oxygen and medications
- Once the patient's condition becomes relatively stable and the diagnosis is confirmed, an immediate exploratory laparotomy is indicated
- When the diagnosis is in doubt, laparotomy is the investigation of choice.

Surgical Treatment

- Linear salpingostomy for pregnancy in the ampullary part of the tube
- Segmental excision for isthmic pregnancies
- Salpingectomy if there is repeat ectopic pregnancy on the same side, the tube is severely damaged or there is uncontrolled hemorrhage from salpingostomy site
- Milking of the tube in cases of ampullary pregnancy where the products can be easily dislodged.

Medical Treatment

The mode of treatment depends upon clinical presentation, investigations and patient's further desire for fertility. Medical treatment is offered to those patients whose hCG level is less than 2000 IU and size of the mass is less than 3 cm. The patient must be clinically stable and reliable for follow-up.

Methotrexate (Mx), prostaglandins and potassium chloride (KCl) can be used in cases of ectopic pregnancy. Intralesional administration under USG guide is preferred over administration via other routes. Single dose of methotrexate given intramuscularly is done in selected patients.

Prevention of Recurrence of Tubal Pregnancy

Precautions taken during surgery for prevention of recurrence includes:
- Removal of blood clots
- Squeezing out of blood from the contralateral tube
- Removal of the ipsilateral ovary
- Bilateral salpingectomy in ectopic pregnancy following tubal ligation.

Nursing Diagnoses

Numbers 55, 59, 78, 81, 99 and 156 in Appendix.

48. ENDOMETRIOSIS

The presence of functioning endometrium (glands and stroma) in sites other than uterine mucosa is termed as endometriosis. The ectopic occurrence of endometrial tissue frequently forms cysts containing altered blood. Such tissues when found in the endometrium are called endometriosis interna or adenomyosis. When endometrial tissues are seen present in tissues other than uterus, it is referred to as endometriosis externa or endometriosis.

GENERAL INFORMATION

Causes

- Delayed marriage and conception
- Postponement of first conception
- Small family norm.

Prevalence

- Fertile women 10%
- Infertile women 30–40%.

Sites of Occurrence (Fig. 48.1)

- **Abdominal:** Confined to the abdominal structures below the level of umbilicus such as ovary, pouch of Douglas, uterosacral ligament, broad ligament, retrovaginal septum and pelvic lymph nodes. Rare sites are intestines, appendix, ureter and urinary bladder.
- **Extra-abdominal:** Common sites are abdominal scar of hysterectomy, cesarean section, tubal ligation and scars in vagina and cervix.
- **Remote sites:** Pleura, lungs and deep tissues of arms and legs.

PATHOLOGY

The endometrium in the ectopic sites has the potential to undergo changes under the action of ovarian hormones. Cyclic growth and shedding will continue till menopause. As the blood is an irritant, there is dense tissue reaction surrounding the lesion with fibrosis. The cysts enlarge with cyclic bleeding. The serum gets absorbed in between the periods and the content inside becomes chocolate colored. The appearance may vary at different sites. In the uterosacral

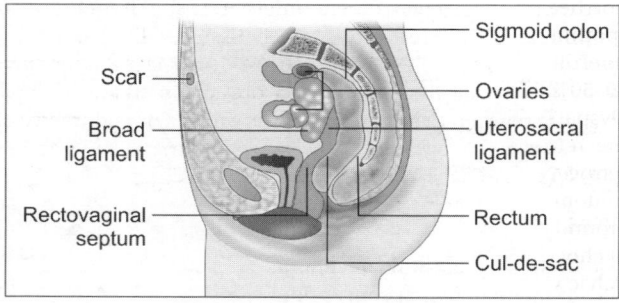

Fig. 48.1: Common sites of endometriosis.

ligaments and pouch of Douglas they appear as small, black dots. Lesions in other sites vary in appearance such as red flame-shaped areas, red polypoid areas, yellow-brown patches, or white peritoneal patches.

Patient Profile

- Age 30–45 years
- Infertility or voluntary postponement of first conception until late age
- Nulliparous or have had one or two children several years prior to appearance of symptoms
- Family history of endometriosis.

SYMPTOMS

About 25% have no symptoms and are discovered during laparoscopy or laparotomy and symptoms are not related to the extent of lesions. Pain occurs with lesions that:
- Penetrate more than 5 mm
- Are non pigmented and respond to prostaglandin F (PGF)
- Are situated in the midline.

  The degree of pain is not related to the spread or severity of endometriosis.
- Dysmenorrhea: Starts few days prior to menstruation, gets worsened during menstruation and subsides gradually after cessation of menstruation. Increased PGF_2 is the cause of pain
- Abnormal menstruation: Menorrhagia, polymenorrhea, epimenorrhea (prolonged and profuse menstruation) and premenstrual spotting
- Infertility: Endometriosis is found in 20–40% of infertile women. 40–50% of patients with endometriosis suffer from infertility
- Dyspareunia: Mostly found in patients with endometriosis of the retrovaginal septum or pouch of Douglas and with fixed retroverted uterus
- Abdominal pain: Variable degrees of abdominal pain occur around periods. Sometimes the pain may be acute due to rupture of chocolate cyst
- Pelvic pain: The pain varies from pelvic discomfort, lower abdominal pain or backache

- Other symptoms: These are related to the organs involved and cycle associated:
  - Bladder—frequency, dysuria, and hematuria
  - Sigmoid colon and rectum—painful defecation (dyschezia), diarrhea, rectal bleeding and melena
  - Chronic fatigue.

DIAGNOSIS

- **Clinical diagnosis:** Classic symptoms of progressively increasing dysmenorrhoea, dyspareunia and infertility. Pelvic findings of nodules in the pouch of Douglas, nodular feel of uterosacral ligaments, fixed retroverted uterus and unilateral or bilateral adnexal mass
- **Serum marker cancer antigen 125 (CA-125):** Moderate elevation of CA 125 is noticed in patients with severe endometriosis (CA 125 is a glycoprotein and values over 35 u/mL is suggestive of epithelial ovarian cancer)
- **Ultrasonography:** Transvaginal ultrasonography can detect ovarian, endorectal and rectosigmoid endometriosis
- **Laparoscopy:** On double puncture laparoscopy 'powder burns' or matchstick spots can be seen on the peritoneum of the pouch of Douglas.

TREATMENT

Preventive

- Encourage women with family history of endometriosis not to postpone first conception and to complete the family
- Avoid forcible pelvic examination during or shortly after menstruation
- Avoid tubal patency test immediately after curettage or around the time of menstruation.

Curative

- Encourage to have conception. Pregnancy usually cures the condition

Hormonal Treatment

- Combined oral pills to produce pseudo-pregnancy
- Progestogens to produce pseudo menopause
- Gonadotropin-releasing hormone (GnRH) analogues to cause medical oophorectomy
- Levonorgestrel: Releasing IUCD to reduce dysmenorrhea.

Surgical

- Ablation and adhesiolysis for endometriosis with severe symptoms, deeply infiltrating type and endometriomas of more than 1 cm
- Laparoscopic ovarian cystectomy and adhesiolysis
- Hysterectomy with bilateral salpingo-oophorectomy for women in whom other methods of treatment have failed and who have completed their family.

Treatment for endometriosis at special sites:

- Abdominal scar—excision
- Umbilicus—excision
- Bladder—local excision of bladder wall and repair.
- Gut—hormone therapy, resection and anastomosis or oophorectomy in patients above 40 years, depending on the location and response to therapy years
- Cervix and vagina—surgical excision.

COMPLICATIONS OF ENDOMETRIOSIS

- Endocrinopathy (disorder of endocrine glands)
- Rupture of chocolate cyst
- Infection of chocolate cyst
- Obstructive features:
  - Intestinal obstruction
  - Ureteral obstruction leading to hydroureter, hydronephrosis or renal infection.
- Adenocarcinoma—a very rare complication.

49. ENDOSCOPIC SURGERY IN GYNECOLOGICAL PATIENTS

Surgical procedures performed in gynecology patients with the use of either a laparoscope or a hysteroscope are designated as endoscopic surgeries. The procedures are:
- Laparoscopic surgery
- Laparoscopic assisted vaginal hysterectomy (LAVH)
- Hysteroscopy
- Hysteroscopic myomectomy.

LAPAROSCOPIC SURGERY

Laparoscopy refers to examination of the contents of abdominopelvic cavity with a laparoscope passed through the abdominal wall. When a surgical procedure is performed with the aid of a laparoscope, it is called laparoscopic surgery.

Indications

Minor Procedures

- Tubal ligation
- Adhesiolysis
- Aspiration of simple ovarian cysts
- Ovarian biopsy.

Moderate Procedures

- Ectopic pregnancy:
  - Salpingostomy
  - Segmental resection
  - Salpingectomy
  - Salpingo-oophorectomy
- Endometriosis:
  - Ablation by diathermy or laser.
- Ovary:
  - Diathermy for polycystic ovary syndrome (PCOS)

- Drainage of endometriomas
- Ovarian cystectomy
- Salpingo-ovariolysis.
- Uterus:
  - Myomectomy
  - LAVH
  - Adhesiolysis.

Contraindications

- Severe cardiopulmonary disease
- Patient hemodynamically unstable
- Generalized peritonitis
- Hemoperitoneum
- Intestinal obstruction
- Extensive peritoneal adhesion
- Large pelvic tumor
- Pregnancy above 16 weeks
- Previous periumbilical surgery
- Extreme obesity.

LAPAROSCOPIC ASSISTED VAGINAL HYSTERECTOMY

Laparoscopic procedure is done to visualize the structures, dissect surrounding structures and free the entire uterus from its attachments. An umbilical incision of 10 mm for the laparoscope connected to a video camera and three incisions of 5 mm [medially (1) and laterally (2)] above the symphysis pubis are generally used for the laparoscopic surgery. Uterus is removed through a vaginal incision as in a vaginal hysterectomy.

Complications of Laparoscopy

- Surgical emphysema from extraperitoneal insufflations
- Omental emphysema
- Cardiac arrhythmia
- Injury to pelvic or abdominal vessels/injury to organs such as bowel, bladder or ureter

- Thermal injury such as electrode burns
- Gas embolism (carbon dioxide) resulting in hypotension and cardiac arrhythmia
- Anesthesia complications.

HYSTEROSCOPY

Hysteroscopy is a procedure that allows direct visualization inside the uterus. It can be used for diagnostic as well as therapeutic purposes.

Indications

For Diagnostic Procedure

- Abnormal uterine bleeding:
  - Menorrhagia
  - Postmenopausal bleeding:
- Infertility
- Mullerian anomalies such as arcuate, subseptate or bicornuate uterus
- Recurrent miscarriage due to intrauterine pathology such as fibroids and polyps
- Misplaced intrauterine contraceptive device (IUCD)
- Chronic pelvic pain.

For Operative Hysteroscopy

- Polypectomy and myomectomy
- Lysis of intrauterine adhesions
- Endometrial ablation for dysfunctional uterine bleeding (DUB)
- Endometrial resection for DUB
- Metroplasty (resection of uterine septum)
- Removal of foreign body or IUCD when the thread is missing
- Biopsy of endometrium
- Tubal cannulation under hysteroscopic guidance
- Sterilization by blocking the interstitial portion of the tube. Essure, a 4 cm long microcoil (spring-like device) made of nickel-titanium alloy within which lie dacron fibers is inserted into each

50. EPISIOTOMY

An episiotomy is the surgical incision made to enlarge the vaginal opening for delivery of the baby's head. An episiotomy involves incision of fourchette, the superficial muscles and skin of the perineum and posterior vaginal wall.

INCISION

Types

1. Median or midline episiotomy is the incision made in the midline downward.
2. Mediolateral episiotomy is the incision that begins in midline and is directed laterally and downward away from rectum **(Fig. 50.1)**.

Timing of the Incision

The episiotomy incision is made at the time of crowning when the largest diameter of the fetal head, first becomes visible and the perineum is stretched extremely thin. Local anesthetic (lignocaine 1%) is injected prior to episiotomy.

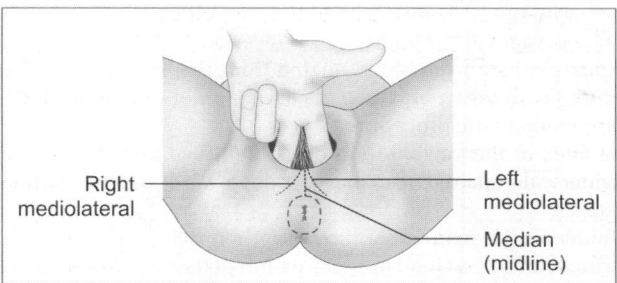

Fig. 50.1: Types of episiotomy.

MAKING THE INCISION/EPISIOTOMY

The incision is best made during a contraction, when the tissues are stretched, so that there is a clear view of the area and bleeding is likely to be less severe. Two fingers are inserted into the vagina and open blades of a straight bladed blunt ended scissors is positioned before the beginning of a contraction and at the height of the following contraction, a single, deliberate cut of 4–5 cm long is made at the correctangle.

Delivery of the head should follow immediately and its advance must be controled in order to avoid extension of the episiotomy. If there is delay before the head emerges, pressure should be applied to the episiotomy site between contractions in order to minimize bleeding.

REPAIR OF EPISIOTOMY

The episiotomy is best repaired as soon as possible after delivery in order to secure hemostasis, while the tissues are still anesthetized and before edema sets in:

- The trolley with appropriate instruments, antiseptic solution, and suture materials should be ready
- The midwife scrubs her hands and puts on sterile gown and gloves
- Prior to commencement, the mother is made as warm and comfortable as possible
- The mother is placed in lithotomy position
- The perineum is cleaned with antiseptic solution
- A taped vaginal tampon may be inserted into the vault of the vagina to absorb the blood oozing from the vagina. The tape is secured with a pair of forceps as a remainder to remove it at the completion of the procedure
- The apex of the vaginal incision is identified and the posterior vaginal wall repaired from the apex downwards using continuous suturing
- The deeper interrupted sutures are then inserted to repair the perineal muscles. Good approximation of tissues is important for subsequent strength of the pelvic floor

- Skin closure is done next with interrupted transcutaneous suturing or continuous subcuticular sutures
- The sutured areas should be inspected in order to confirm hemostasis before removing the vaginal pack
- A vaginal examination is made to ensure that the introitus has not been narrowed
- Upon completion, a rectal examination is done in order to ensure that no sutures have penetrated the rectal mucosa. Any such sutures must be removed to prevent fistula formation
- The area is cleaned and a sterile vaginal pad positioned over the vulva and perineum
- The mother's legs are then gently and simultaneously removed from lithotomy support and she is made comfortable.

CARE OF THE VULVA AND PERINEUM WITH AN EPISIOTOMY WOUND

- Care of the vulva after delivery includes applying ice packs to the perineum for the first 24 hours to help decrease edema and pain. Ice packs also assist in constricting blood vessels minimizing the risk of hematoma formation, muscle irritability and spasm. Ice packs should not be applied directly to the skin; they should be wrapped with an absorbent, disposable type of covering
- From the 1st postpartum day, assess the episiotomy and perineum every shift. For assessment, have the client lie on her side, flexing her upper leg toward her hip. The nurse can then lift the buttocks to expose the perineum. Using a good light source visualize the repaired area. The REEDA (redness, edema, echymosis, discharge and approximation) scoring scale can be used when assessing the episiotomy.
- After the first 24 hours of delivery, a sitz bath with warm water may be used to reduce the local discomfort. Sitz bath may be given until the episiotomy heals.
- A squeeze-bottle filled with warm tap water may be used to clean the perineum. Daily washing with warm water and mild soap to be encouraged.
- Mother should be taught to wipe the perineum from front to back to avoid contamination from the anal region.

- Explain/Encourage practices such as changing the perineal pad after each voiding and bowel movement or at least four times a day, removing the pad from front to back and hand washing to decrease the risk of infection and promote wound healing of episiotomy or repaired lacerations.
- Use of a heat lamp such as infra-red light, two–three times a day also will assist in the healing process.
- The vagina returns to its prepregnant state by 6–8 weeks postpartum. Vaginal rugae returns by 4 weeks.

51. EXTERNAL CEPHALIC VERSION

External cephalic version (ECV) is the use of external manipulation on the mother's abdomen to convert a breech to a cephalic presentation.

PREPARATION

- The procedure is offered at term by a skilled obstetrician
- The ECV is planned to be performed after 37 completed weeks' of gestation
- A tocolytic agent such as Terbutaline or isoxsuprine IV is started 15–30 minutes before hand
- A contraction stress test is performed to ensure that the fetus is not stressed
- The woman is given adequate explanation about the reasons and procedure and an informed consent obtained
- An ultrasound scan is performed to localize the placenta and to confirm the position and presentation of the fetus
- Maternal blood pressure and pulse are recorded prior to starting
- The woman is asked to empty her bladder. She is then assisted into a comfortable supine position
- The foot of the bed may be elevated to help free the breech from the pelvic brim
- The abdomen is dusted with talcum powder to prevent pinching of the mother's skin during the procedure.

PROCEDURE

- The breech is displaced using both hands from the pelvic brim towards an iliac fossa towards, which the back of the fetus lies
- The podalic pole is grasped by the right hand in a manner like that of Pawlik's grip, while the head is grasped by the left hand
- Simultaneous force is then used to make the fetus perform a forward somersault. Flexion of the head and back is maintained throughout
- Pressure is exerted on the head and breech simultaneously until the head is lying at the pelvic brim
- If the fetus does not turn easily, then the procedure is abandoned and may be tried again after few days
- The fetal heart should be auscultated soon after the procedure or an non-stress test (NST) performed. If fetal bradycardia persists beyond 10 minutes, cord entanglement should be suspected and in such cases, reversion may have to be considered
- The patient is to be observed for 10 minutes in order to allow the (FHR) to settle down and to note for any vaginal bleeding or evidence of premature rupture of membranes
- If the woman is Rh-negative, an injection of anti-D immuno-globulin is given as prophylaxis against isoimmunization caused by any placental separation
- The woman is checked on the following day for the position of the fetus.

POSSIBLE COMPLICATIONS

- **Knotting of the umbilical cord:** This should be suspected if bradycardia occurs and persists. The fetus is immediately turned back to breech presentation and the woman is admitted for observation, and if necessary prepare for cesarean delivery
- **Separation of the placenta:** Pain or vaginal bleeding during and after the procedure is indicative of this
- **Rupture of the membranes:** If this occurs, the cord may prolapse because neither the head nor the breech is engaged.

CONTRAINDICATIONS

- Preeclampsia or hypertension because of the increased risk of placental abruption
- Multiple pregnancy
- Oligohydramnios
- Ruptured membranes
- A hydrocephalic fetus
- Any condition, which would require delivery by cesarean section.

52. FACE PRESENTATION

Face presentation occurs when the attitude of the head is one of complete extension, the occiput of the fetus is in contact with its spine and the face will present. The attitude of the fetus shows complete flexion of the limbs with extension of the spine. Incidence is 1:500 deliveries.

TYPES OF FACE PRESENTATION

- **Primary face presentation:** Face presents during pregnancy
- **Secondary face presentation:** The presentation develops after the onset of labor. It occurs more often in multiparae.

ETIOLOGY

The cause of extreme extension of the head is not clear in all the cases. The following are the factors, which are often associated.

Maternal

- Multiparity with pendulous abdomen
- Lateral obliquity of the uterus, especially if it is directed to the side towards, which the occiput lies
- Contracted pelvis; flat pelvis favors face presentation.

Fetal

- Congenital malformations such as anencephaly, congenital goiter, dolicocephalic head and congenital branchiocele swelling or growth arising from pharynx

- Twist of the cord several times round the neck
- Increased tone of the extensor group of neck muscles
- Intrauterine death of fetus (toneless fetus).

POSITIONS

- Left mentoanterior
- Left mentoposterior
- Right mentoanterior
- Right mentoposterior.

DIAGNOSIS

Antenatal diagnosis is rarely made. Diagnosis is made only during labor and in about 50% the detection is made at the time of delivery **(Figs. 52.1A to F)**.

Abdominal Findings

- **On inspection:** There is no bulging of the flanks because of the 'S' shaped spine.
- **On palpation:** In mentum anterior, the occiput feels prominent, with a groove between head and back, but it may be mistaken for the sinciput. The limbs may be palpated on the side opposite to the occiput and the fetal heart is best heard through the fetal chest on the same side as the limbs. In a mentoposterior position, the fetal heart is difficult to hear because the fetal chest is in contact with the maternal spine.

On Vaginal Examination

The presenting part is high, soft and irregular when the cervix is fully dilated, orbital ridges, eyes nose and mouth may be felt. Confusion between mouth and anus could arise. The mouth may be open, and the hard gums are diagnostic. The fetus may suck the examining finger. As labor progresses, the face becomes edematous, making it more difficult to distinguish from a breech presentation.

Sonography

This should be done to confirm the diagnosis, to exclude bony congenital malformation of the fetus and to note the size of the baby.

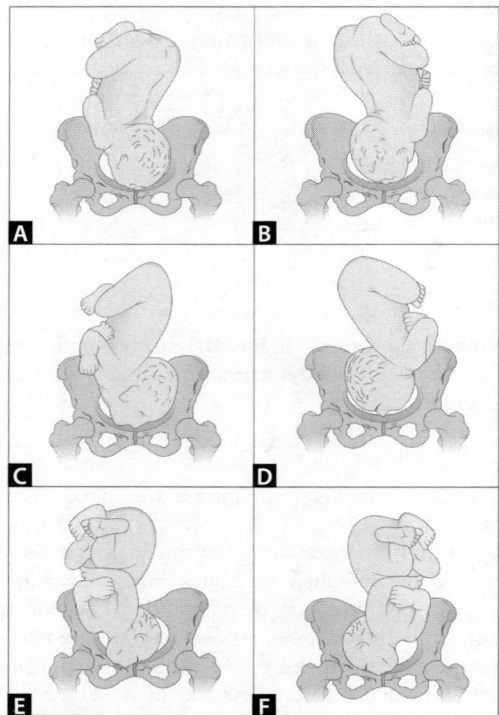

Figs. 52.1A to F: Six positions of face presentation. **A.** Right mentoposterior; **B.** Left mentoposterior; **C.** Right mentolateral; **D.** Left mentolateral; **E.** Right mentoanterior; **F.** Left mentoanterior.

MECHANISM OF LEFT MENTOANTERIOR POSITION

- The lie is longitudinal
- The attitude is one of extension of head and back
- The presentation is face
- The position is left mentoanterior
- The denominator is mentum
- The presenting part is the left malar bone.

Extension

Descend takes place with increasing extension. The mentum becomes the leading part.

Internal Rotation of the Head

This occurs when the chin reaches the pelvic floor and rotates forwards 1/8th of a circle. The chin escapes under the symphysis pubis.

Flexion

Flexion takes place and the sinciput, vertex and occiput sweep the perineum, the head is born by flexion followed by extension to deliver the face.

Restitution

This occurs when the chin turns 1/8th of a circle to the woman's left.

Internal Rotation of the Shoulders

The shoulders enter the pelvis in the left oblique diameter and the anterior shoulder reaches the pelvic floor first and rotates forwards 1/8th of a circle along the right side of the pelvis.

External Rotation of the Head

This occurs simultaneously. The chin moves a further 1/8th of a circle to the left.

Lateral Flexion

The anterior shoulder escapes under the symphysis pubis, the posterior shoulder sweeps the perineum and the body is born by a movement of lateral flexion.

POSSIBLE COURSE AND OUTCOMES OF LABOR

- **Prolonged labor:** Labor is often prolonged because the face is an illfitting presenting part and does not therefore stimulate effective contractions. In addition, the facial bones do not mold and for the mentum to reach the pelvic floor and rotate forwards the shoulders must enter the pelvic cavity at the same time as the head.

- **Spontaneous delivery in mentoanterior positions:** With good uterine contractions, descent and rotation of the head occurs and labor progresses to a spontaneous delivery.
- **Conversion to mentoanterior position:** After the mentum reaches the pelvic floor, if the contractions are effective, the mentum will rotate forward and the position becomes anterior.
- **Persistent mentoposterior position:** In this case, the head is incompletely extended and the sinciput reaches the pelvic floor first and rotates 1/8th of a circle, which brings the chin into the hollow of sacrum. There is no further mechanism. The face becomes impacted.
- **Reversal of face presentation:** A face presentation from a persistent mentoposterior position may, in some cases be manipulated to an occiput anterior position with bimanual pressure.

POSSIBLE COMPLICATIONS

- **Obstructed labor:** The face does not mold, a minor degree of pelvic contraction may result in obstructed labor. In a persistent mentoposterior position, the face becomes impacted and cesarean delivery is necessary.
- **Cord prolapse:** A prolapsed cord is more common when the membranes rupture, because the face is an ill-fitting presenting part.
- **Facial bruising:** The baby's face is always bruised and swollen at birth with edematous eyelids and lips.
- **Cerebral hemorrhage:** The lack of molding of the facial bones can lead to intracranial hemorrhage by excessive compression of the fetal skull.
- **Neonatal infection:** This is due to bacterial contamination within the vagina.
- **Maternal trauma:** Excessive perineal laceration due to the large submentovertical and biparietal diameters distending the vagina

and perineum. Due to the increased incidence of operative delivery such as forceps delivery or cesarean section, maternal morbidity is increased.
- **Postpartum hemorrhage:** This is due to atonic uterus and trauma following operative delivery.

53. FETAL CIRCULATION

The growing human embryo at about 20 days of intrauterine life establishes a communication between the vascular circulation in the chorionic villi and the vessels in the umbilical stalk, so that placental circulation is established for circulatory exchanges between mother and fetus. Fetal circulation differs from adult circulation in several ways and is designed to ensure supply of well-oxygenated blood to the brain and myocardium.

CHARACTERISTICS OF FETAL CIRCULATION

- Placenta is the source of oxygen
- Fetal lungs receive less than 1% of blood volume and lungs do not exchange gas
- Right atrium of the fetal heart is the chamber with the highest oxygen concentration.

STRUCTURES THAT PLAY MAJOR ROLES

Fetal circulation contains five unique structures:
- **Umbilical vein:** Carries oxygenated blood laden with nutrients to the fetus.
- **Ductus venosus:** Shunts blood from the umbilical vein to the inferior vena cava.
- **Foramen ovale:** The oval opening between the atria shunts oxygenated blood from the right atrium to the left atrium bypassing the lungs.
- **Ductus arteriosus:** Shunts blood from the pulmonary artery to the aorta.
- **Umbilical arteries:** Two umbilical arteries carry deoxygenated blood and waste products from the fetus.

- **Hypogastric arteries:** Blood from descending aorta returns to the placenta though hypogastric arteries which becomes umbilical arteries when they enter the umblilical cord.

PATTERN OF ALTERED BLOOD FLOW (FIG. 53.1)

- The blood from the placenta flows through the umbilical vein, which penetrates the abdominal wall of the fetus at the site of the umbilicus
- If divides into two branches, one of which circulates a small amount of blood through the fetal liver and empties into the inferior vena cava through the hepatic vein

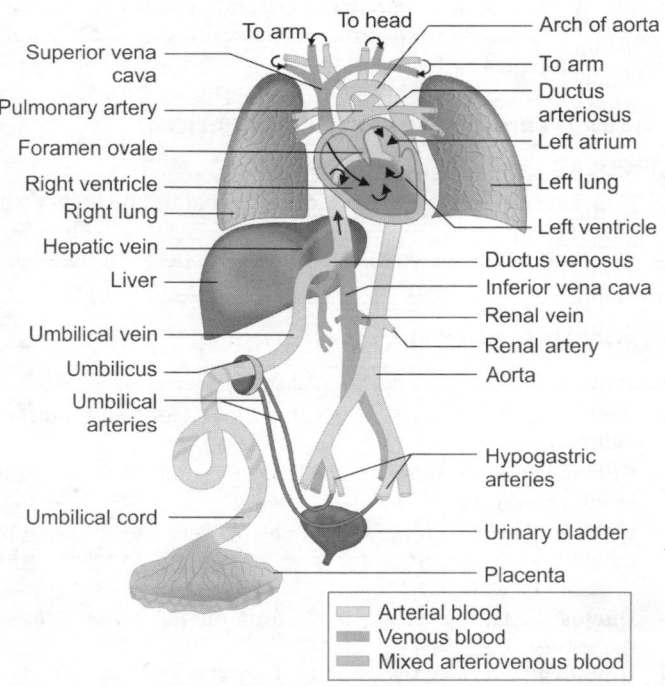

Fig. 53.1: Fetal circulation.

- The second and larger branch, called the ductus venosus, empties directly into the inferior vena cava
- The blood then enters the right atrium, passes through the foramen ovale into the left atrium and pours into the left ventricle, which pumps it into the aorta for distribution through carotid arties to cerebral circulation
- Some blood returning from the head and upper extremities by way of superior vena cava is emptied into the right atrium and passes through the tricuspid valve into the right ventricle. This blood is pumped into the pulmonary artery, and a small amount passes to the lungs and provides nourishment only
- The larger portion of blood passes from the pulmonary artery through the ductus arteriosus and into the descending aorta, below the exit of carotid arteries. The mixed blood is distributed to the viscera and lower extremities
- Finally blood returns to the placenta through the two umbilical arteries and the process is repeated.

CIRCULATORY CHANGES AT BIRTH

When the umbilical cord is clamped or severed, the blood supply from the placenta is cut off and oxygenation must then take place in the newborn's lungs. As the lungs expand with air, the pulmonary artery pressure decreases and circulation to lungs increases. This leads to the following structural changes to occur in the vascular system.
- Obliteration of umbilical vein, which becomes ligamentum teres of the liver
- Obliteration of ductus venosus, which becomes ligamentum venosum
- Closure of foramen ovale
- Closure of ductus arteriosus
- Obliteration of the umbilical arteries.

54. FETAL DISTRESS

Fetal distress is a term used to express intrauterine fetal jeopardy as the fetus suffers oxygen deprivation and becomes hypoxic. Severe hypoxia may result in the baby being stillborn or may be asphyxiated at birth and suffer brain damage.

SIGNS

- Fetal tachycardia, which is an early sign
- Fetal bradycardia or fetal heart rate decelerations related to uterine contractions
- Passage of meconium stained amniotic fluid.

MANAGEMENT

- When signs of distress occur, the nurse must call the physician if he is not already present
- Place the mother in left lateral position to improve placental circulation
- Stop oxytocin drip, if it is being infused
- Administer oxygen in case of maternal oxygen lack such as eclampsia or shock due to antepartum hemorrhage
- Terbutaline is given SC or IV if the uterus is hypertonic
- Infusion of crystalloid (Ringer's solution) to correct maternal hypotension if present
- Expedite delivery if fetal distress is more than transient. In the first stage, cesarean section is indicated. In the second stage, episiotomy and forceps delivery
- Avail pediatrician's help during delivery.

55. FETAL HEART RATE MONITORING CARDIOTOCOGRAPHY (CTG)

Fetal heart rate monitoring is a procedure used to evaluate the well-being of the fetus by assessing the rate and rhythm of the fetal heart beat. Monitoring of fetal heart rate and other functions is done during late pregnancy and labor. The average fetal heart rate is between 120 and 160 beats per minute, and can vary about 5–25 beats per minute. The fetal heart rate may change as the fetus responds to conditions in the uterus. An abnormal fetal heart rate or pattern may indicate that the fetus is not getting enough oxygen or that there are other problems.

METHODS OF MONITORING

There are two methods of fetal heart rate monitoring, i.e. external and internal.

External Fetal Heart Rate Monitoring

A fetoscope is the most basic type of external monitor. Another type of monitor is a hand-held electronic Doppler ultrasound device. These methods are often used during prenatal visits to count the fetal heart rate. They may also be used to check the fetal heart rate at regular intervals during labor. For continuous fetal heart monitoring, during labor and birth, an electronic fetal monitor is used (**Fig. 55.1**).

An ultrasound transducer placed on the mother's abdomen conducts the sounds of the fetal heart to a computer. The rate and pattern of the fetal heart are displayed on computer screen and printed on to special graph paper (monitor strip).

Internal Fetal Heart Rate Monitoring

Internal fetal heart rate monitoring uses an electronic transducer connected directly to the fetal skin. A wire electrode is attached to the fetal scalp through the cervical opening and is connected to the monitor. This type of electrode is called 'spiral or scalp electrode'.

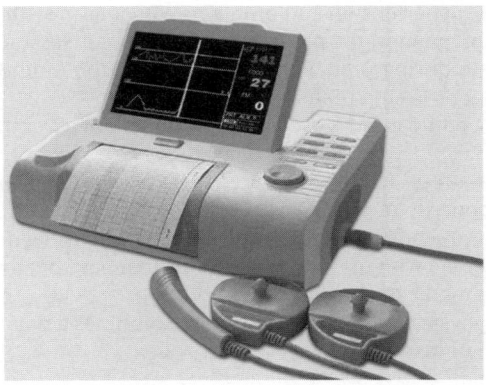

Fig. 55.1: Fetal heart rate monitor.

For the electrode to be placed on he fetal scalp, amniotic sac (membranes) must be ruptured. Internal monitoring provides more accurate and consistent transmission of the fetal heart rate than external monitoring, because factors such as movement does not affect it. Internal monitoring is used when external monitoring of the fetal heart rate is inadequate or closer surveillance is needed.

During labor, uterine contractions are usually monitored along with the fetal heart rate. A pressure-sensitive device called tocodynamometer is placed on the mother's abdomen over the area of strongest contractions to measure the length, frequency and strength of uterine contractions. Because the fetal heart rate and uterine contractions are recorded at the same time, these results can be examined together and compared.

Internal uterine pressure monitoring is sometimes used along with internal fetal heart monitoring. A fluid-filled catheter is placed through the cervical opening into the uterus beside the fetus, which transmits uterine pressure readings to the monitor.

REASONS FOR FETAL HEART RATE MONITORING

- Fetal heart rate monitoring is used in nearly every pregnancy to assess fetal well-being and identify any changes that might be associated with problems during pregnancy or labor. Monitoring is especially helpful in high-risk pregnancy conditions such as diabetes, hypertension and problems with fetal growth
- During pregnancy, the procedure is useful for assessment of fetal heart rate during prenatal visits and when the mother is given medications to stop preterm labor
- This procedure may be used as a component of other procedures such as:
  - Non-stress test (procedure that measures heart rae in response to movement)
  - A contraction stress test (procedure in which fetal heart rate is observed with uterine contractions that have been simulated with medication or other methods)
  - Biophysical profile (BPP) test that combines a non-stress test with ultrasound).

- During labor monitoring is indicated in the presence of conditions that can affect the fetal heart rate such as:
  - Variations of uterine contractions
  - Pain medications and/or anesthetic agents given to the mother during labor
  - Procedures performed during labor
  - Pushing during second stage of labor.

PROCEDURE

For External Monitoring (Fig. 55.2)

- The woman will be asked to undress from waist down or wear a hospital gown and lie on her back on the bed or examination table
- A clear gel, which will as a conductor will be applied on the abdomen
- A transducer will be placed on the abdomen, where fetal heart is heard best
- For continuous monitoring, the transducer will be connected to the monitor with a cable and a wide elastic belt will be placed around the abdomen to secure the transducer in place

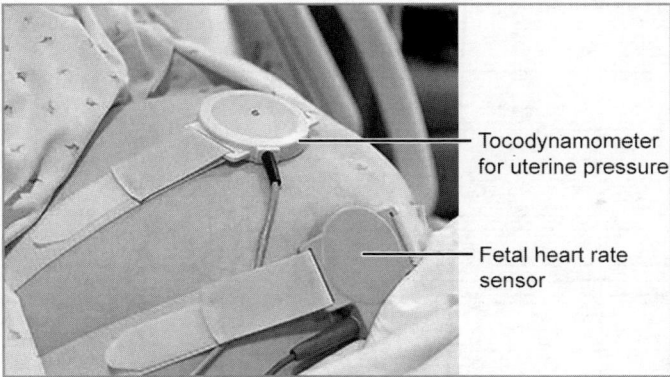

Fig. 55.2: External fetal monitoring.

- The fetal rate will be printed on to a graph paper on the monitor
- The patient will have to stay in bed till the procedure is completed and the gel is wiped off.

For Internal Monitoring (Fig. 55.3)

- The patient will be asked wear a hospital gown and lie on a labor bed
- The amniotic sac if intact and the cervix is dilated up to about 3 cm, the physician may perform an artificial rupture
- A long plastic electrode guide will be inserted into the cervix and small spiral wire at the end of the electrode will be placed against fetal head and gently rotated into the scalp skin. The guide will be removed and the electrode left in place on the fetal scalp
- The electrode wire will be connected to the monitor cable and secured with a band around the mother's thigh
- Once the baby is born, the electrode will be removed.

Internal fetal monitoring is contraindicated in women with active herpes lesions on the cervix or vagina; because of the risk in infection to the fetus. During labor, uterine contractions are usually monitored along with fetal heart rate. A pressure-sensitive device called tocodynamometer, is placed on the mother's abdomen over the area of strongest contractions to measure the length, frequency

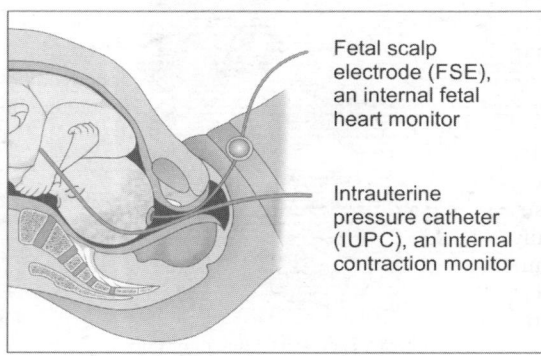

Fig. 55.3: Internal fetal monitoring.

and strength of uterine contractions. Because the fetal heart rate and uterine contractions are recorded at the same time recordings can be examined together and compared. Internal uterine pressure monitoring is sometimes used along with fetal heat monitoring.

56. FETAL IMAGING

The primary means of fetal imaging include ultrasonography, Doppler studies and magnetic resonance imaging (MRI).

ULTRASONOGRAPHY

Ultrasonography is the use of high frequency (> 20,000 Hz) sound waves to detect differences in tissue density and visualize outlines of structures within the body. It provides physical measures of tissue density, size and location. The translation of these measures lead to estimates of gestational age or fetal weight. Real-time ultrasonography is most commonly used in obstetrical practice, because of its capability to display motion picture like- two-dimensional sectional images.

Timing and Use of Ultrasound Examination

Ultrasound examinations may be one of the following three forms or levels:
- Level I or basic
- Level II or comprehensive
- Level III or targeted.

Level I or Basic Ultrasonography

It is used to:
- Detect the gestational sac as early as 5 weeks after the last menstrual period
- Identify the number of fetuses
- Document fetal life
- Detect gross fetal structural abnormalities
- Determine fetal position
- Locate the placenta
- Estimate amniotic fluid volume.

The basic level examination takes about 20 minutes and is a component of standard prenatal care.

Level II or Comprehensive, Ultrasound Examination

It is done when there is suspicion that the fetus has anatomical or physiological abnormality. Indications for this type of ultrasonography include abnormal findings on clinical examination, history of an abnormal fetus and validation of information obtained in the level one examination. The focus of comprehensive examination is to survey fetal anatomy for specific malformation. It is used to:
- Evaluate gestational age
- Measure fetal growth
- Perform specific examinations of the brain, kidney and cord insertion
- Quantify amniotic fluid volume
- Determine placental location.

The examination is performed after 18 weeks of gestation.

Level III Examination

It is limited or targeted is performed when specific information is needed. This type of examination is performed during amniocentesis, percutaneous umbilical blood sampling (PUBS) or biophysical profile to confirm fetal cardiac activity as a result of decreased fetal movement and identify fetal presentation or locate the placenta after the onset of spontaneous bleeding or labor.

Client Preparation

The client needs to be informed about the purpose of the examination, content and limitations. Before tansabdominal examination, the client will need to fill her bladder by drinking 1–2 liters of water 1 hour before the procedure. During transabdominal ultrasonography, a lubricating gel is applied on the abdomen and the probe is moved over the abdominal surface. The lubrication reduces friction and enhances transmission of the sound waves by the probe.

If transvaginal ultrasonography is planned (usually in the first trimester), a hand held probe is inserted into the vagina, allowing detailed examination of the pelvic anatomy and earlier diagnosis of intrauterine pregnancy.

Follow-up

Ultrasonography being a non-invasive procedure follow-up is primarily education, counseling and support as referral for additional testing or treatment based on ultrasound findings may be implemented.

DOPPLER STUDIES

Doppler study or Doppler ultrasonogaphy is the measurement of blood flow velocity, and direction in major fetal and uterine structures.

Timings and Indications

Velocity waveforms can be detected as early as 15 weeks gestation:
- Intrauterine growth restriction (IUGR)
- Pregnancy-induced hypertension (PIH)
- Postdated pregnancy, when it exceeds 42 weeks
- Exposure to nicotine from maternal smoking.

Decreased umbilical vessel flow and/or decreased blood flow velocity are seen in such cases.

Client Preparation

Physical preparation is similar to the preparation for imaging ultrasonography. Additional education and counseling needed are specific to the indications.

Procedure

The technique of transabdominal ultrasound is used to obtain blood flow velocity measurements. Color-enhanced flow imaging is used as an extension of Doppler velocimetry.

Follow-up

Follow-up care includes providing information and support to the client, and her family; explaining the management plan and making referrals as needed.

57. FETAL SKULL

The fetal skull is oval shaped and larger in proportion to the fetal body at term. Bones of the face are completely ossified at birth, and are fused together. Bones of the vault are much flatter and pliable. Ossification of the bones is incomplete at birth and the gaps between bones form the sutures and fontanels. The ossification center on each bone appears as a protuberance.

LANDMARKS OF THE SKULL (PARTS OF THE SKULL) (Fig. 57.1)

The skull is considered as divided into three parts, vault, face and base:
- The vault is the large, dome-shaped part above an imaginary line drawn between the orbital ridges and the nape of the neck. The bones are thin and pliable, which allow the skull to alter slightly in shape during birth.
- The face is firm and non-compressible and forms 1/3rd of the cranium.
- The base is composed of bones, which are firmly united to protect the vital centers in the medulla.

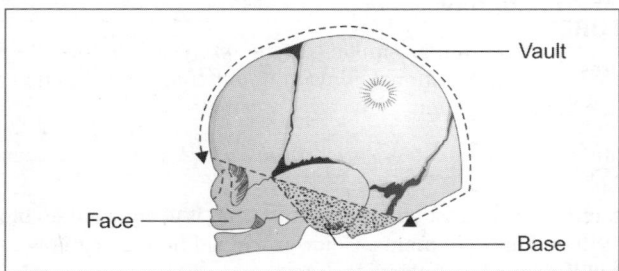

Fig. 57.1: Regions of the skull showing the vault, face and base.

Bones of the Vault

There are five main bones in the vault of the skull:
- **Two frontal bones:** These bones form the forehead or sinciput. At the center of each is a frontal eminence. The frontal bones fuse to form a single bone by 8 years of age.
- **Two parietal bones:** The two parietal bones lie on either side of the skull. The ossification center of each is called the parietal eminence.
- **Occipital bone:** The occipital bone lies at the back of the head and forms the region of the occiput. Part of it contributes to the base of the skull as it contains foramen magnum, which protects the spinal cord as it leaves the skull. At the center is the occipital protuberance.

REGIONS OF THE FETAL SKULL

- **Vertex:** It is bounded by the anterior fontane, the two parietal eminences and the posterior fontane.
- **Sinciput or brow:** It extends from the anterior fontanelle and the coronal suture to the orbital ridges.
- **Face:** It extends from the orbital ridges and roof of the nose to junction of chin and neck. The point between the eyebrows is known as glabella. The chin is called mentum.
- **Occiput:** It lies between the foramen magnum and the posterior fontanelle. The part below the occipital protuberance is known as the suboccipital region **(Fig. 57.1)**.

SUTURES OF THE FETAL SKULL

Sutures are cranial joints are formed where two bones adjoin. They are composed of fibrous tissue and allow mobility between the cranial bones. They permit molding of the skull during labor. Identification of suture lines helps to determine the position of the fetal presenting part during vaginal examination in labor:
- **Frontal suture:** It lies between the two frontal bones extending from bregma to the glabella.
- **Sagittal suture:** It lies centrally between the two parietal bones running anteroposteriorly between the two fontanels

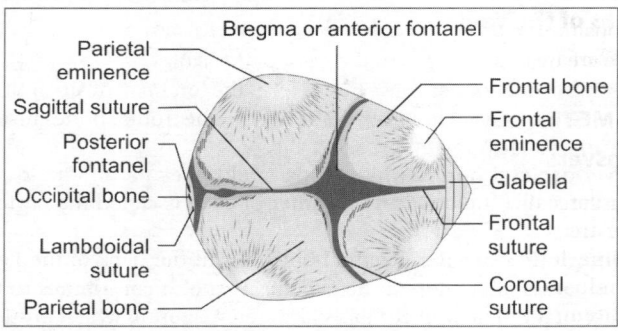

Fig. 57.2: Landmarks head at term showing fontanelles and sutures.

- **Coronal suture:** There are two coronal sutures. It extends transversely outwards from the anterior fontanel, running between the parietal and frontal bones
- **Lambdoidal suture:** There are two lambdoidal sutures. It extends transversely outwards from the posterior fontanel between the parietal bones and the occipital bone **(Fig. 57.2)**.

FONTANELS (FIG. 57.2)

These are membrane filled spaces at the intersections of the suture lines. The two fontanels of obstetric significance are anterior fontanelle and posterior fontanel. Recognition of the fontanel helps to diagnose the position of the fetal head in the pelvis during labor.

Anterior Fontanelle or Bregma

It is located at the junction of the sagittal, coronal and frontal sutures. It is broad, diamond-shaped and recognizable vaginally. It measures 3–4 cm long and 1.5–2 cm wide and normally closes by the age of 18 months. Pulsations of cerebral vessels can be felt through it. It facilitates molding during labor.

Posterior Fontanel or Lambda

It is located at the junction of the sagittal and lambdoidal sutures. It is small, triangular and shaped-like an inverted 'Y'. It helps determine the position of the fetal head during labor. This fontanel closes by 6 weeks of age.

DIAMETERS OF THE FETAL SKULL (Fig. 57.3)

Transverse Diameters

Transverse diameters, which are concerned with the mechanism of labor are:
- **Biparietal diameter 9.5 cm:** It extends between the two parietal eminences.
- **Bitemporal diameter 8.5 cm:** It is the distance between the furthest points of coronal suture at temples.

Anteroposterior or Longitudinal Diameters

- **Suboccipitobregmatic diameter 9.5 cm:** Measures from below the occipital protuberance to the center of the anterior fontanel or bregma.
- **Suboccipitofrontal diameter 10 cm:** From below the occipital protuberance to the center of the frontal suture.
- **Occipitofrontal diameter 11.5 cm:** From the occipital protuberance to the glabella.

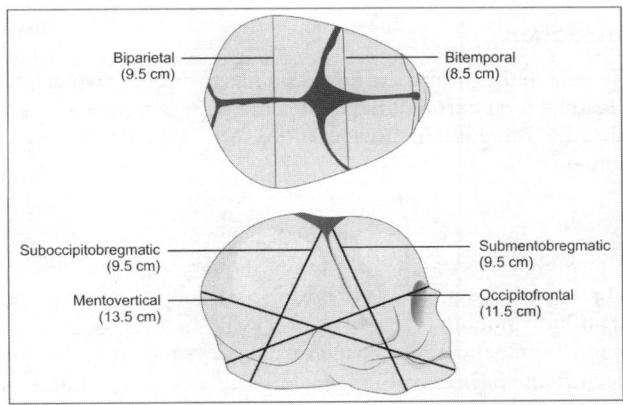

Fig. 57.3: Diameters of the fetal skull.

- **Mentovertical diameter 13.5 cm:** From the midpoint of chin to highest point on the vertex.
- **Submentovertical diameter 11.5 cm:** From the point where the chin joins neck to the highest point on vertex.
- **Submentobregmatic diameter 9.5 cm:** From the point where chin joins the neck to center of bregma.

FETOPELVIC RELATIONSHIPS

The terms used to describe the relationship between the fetus in utero and the mother are defined here:

Lie

This denotes the relationship between the long axis of the fetus to the long axis of the maternal spine. The lie of the fetus may be:
- Longitudinal: When the long axis of the fetus corresponds to the long axis of the maternal spine, e.g. in vertex presentation and breech presentation
- Transverse: When the long axis of the fetus is perpendicular to the long axis of the mother
- Oblique: When the fetal long axis crosses the maternal long axis obliquely at an angle other than right angle.

Presentation

This refers to the part of the fetus that lies over the pelvic inlet. It is the leading fetal part that negotiates the maternal passages during labor. The three main presentations are cephalic, breech and shoulder.

Attitude

This term refers to the relationship of the fetal parts to each other. The basic attitudes are those of flexion and extension. The common fetal attitude in utero is that of flexion, with the head bent forwards the chin approaching the chest, arms and legs folded in front to the body, with the back curved.

Denominator

It is the name of the part of presentation, which is used when referring to the fetal position, which refers to the different quadrants of the maternal pelvis. In vertex presentation, denominator is the occiput. In breech presentation, it is the sacrum. In face presentation, it is the mentum and in shoulder presentation, acromion process. In the brow presentation, no denominator is used.

Position

This term refers to the relationship between the denominator of the presentation and six points on the pelvic brim (front, back and sides of the maternal pelvis). Positions in vertex presentation are **(Fig. 57.4)**:
- Left occipitoanterior (LOA)
- Right occipitoanterior (ROA)
- Left occipitolateral (LOL)
- Right occipitolateral (ROL)
- Left occipitoposterior (LOP)
- Right occipitoposterior (ROP).

Presenting Diameters

The diameters of the fetal head present at right angles to the curve of Carus. There are two diameters—an anteroposterior and a transverse diameter. Diameters presenting in different head positions are as follows:
- Vertex presentation: When the head is well flexed, the occipitobregmatic 9.5 cm and the biparietal diameter 9.5 cm present
- Brow presentation: When the head is partially extended, the mentovertical diameter 13.5 cm and the bitemporal 8.5 cm present
- Face presentation: When the head is completely extended, the presenting diameters are the submentobregmatic 9.5 cm and the bitemporal 8.5 cm present.

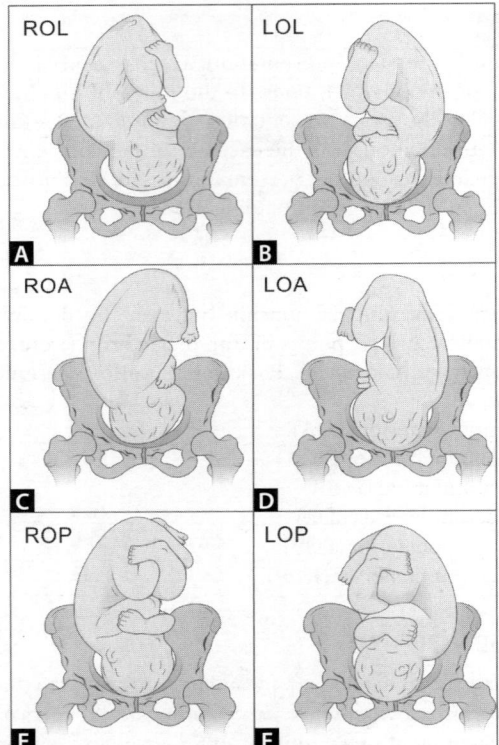

Figs. 57.4A to F: Diagrammatic presentation of six positions of the vertex. **A.** Right occipitolateral; **B.** Left occipitolateral; **C.** Right occipitoanterior; **D.** Left occipitoanterior; **E.** Right occipitoposterior; **F.** Left occipitoposterior.

Molding

This is the term applied to the change in shape of the fetal head that takes place during its passage through the birth canal. The suture lines permit the skull bones to slide over each other. Molding helps to reduce the presenting diameters.

58. FIBROID TUMORS IN UTERUS

These are benign tumors arising in the myometrium that can protrude into the uterine cavity, bulge through the outer layer or grow within the myometrium.

Incidence

These are more common in nulliparous women and those having one child. The prevalence is highest between 35–45 years. About 20% of women develop fibroid by the age of 30 and most remain asymptomatic.

Growth of Tumors

Fibroids are estrogen-dependant tumors and show following characteristics such as:
- Growth is limited during childbearing period
- Increased growth occurs during pregnancy
- Tumors do not occur before menarche
- Cessation of growth is seen; following menopause
- It contains more estrogen receptors than the adjacent myometrium
- Frequent association of anovulation.

Types of fibroids
- **Corporeal or body fibroids:** These are fibroids located in the body of the uterus. They are usually multiple and cause marked distortion in the shape of the uterus.
- **Interstitial or intramural fibroids:** Some get pushed outwards or inwards and in about 70% remain in that position.
- **Subperitoneal or subserous:** The intramural fibroids that get pushed outwards towards the peritoneal cavity and get covered partially or completely by peritoneum. The fibroid that develops pedicle is called pedunculated subserous fibroid. Fibroids that develop omental or mesenteric adhesions are called wandering or parasitic fibroid.
- **Submucous fibroids:** When the fibroid bulges towards the uterine cavity and lies underneath the endometrium, it is called

364 Manual of Midwifery and Gynecological Nursing

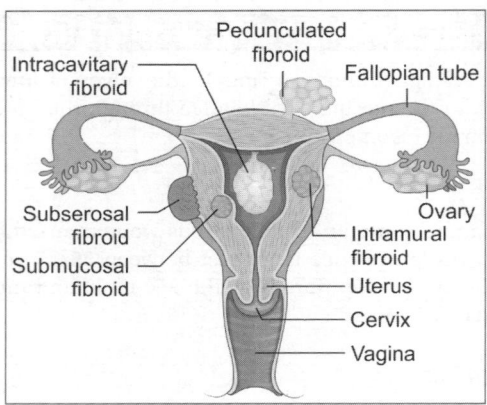

Fig. 58.1: Uterine fibroids.

submucous fibroid. Submucous fibroid can make the uterine cavity irregular and distorted. Pedunculated submucous fibroid may come out through the cervix (**Fig. 58.1**).

Clinical Features and Patient Profile

Primary or secondary infertility with peak incidence is between 35 and 45 years. Majority of fibroids remain asymptomatic (75%) and are discovered during physical examination, laparotomy or laparoscopy. Clinical features and patient profile are as detailed below:

1. Menstrual abnormalities:
    - Menorrhagia: Menstrual loss progressively increases with successive cycles
    - Metrorrhagia or irregular bleeding
    - Dysmenorrhea due to associated pelvic congestion or endometriosis
    - Infertility due to distortion or elongation of uterine cavity causing sperm ascent difficult
    - Dyspareunia.
2. Pregnancy-related problems:
    - Abortion, preterm labor and intrauterine growth restriction

- Pain in lower abdomen
- Abdominal swelling and pressure symptoms

3. Abdominal examination findings:
   - If the tumor is enlarged to 14 weeks size or more it can be felt per abdomen.
4. Pelvic examination findings:
   - Bimanual examination reveals the uterus, irregularly enlarged
   - Cervix moves with the movement of the tumor felt per abdomen.

Investigations

- Ultrasound examination confirms the diagnosis
- Laparoscopy in cases where uterine size is less than 12 weeks and associated pelvic pain and infertility
- Hysteroscopy in suspected submucous fibroid and unexplained infertility
- Uterine curettage in the presence of irregular bleeding to detect any coexisting pathology and to study endometrial pattern.

Management

1. Medical management:
   The objectives of medical treatment are:
   - To improve menorrhagia and to correct anemia before surgery
   - To minimize the size and vascularity of the tumor in order to facilitate surgery
   - As an alternative to surgery in perimenopausal women or women with high-risk factors for surgery
   - Where postponement of surgery is planned temporarily.
2. Drugs used to minimize blood loss:
   - Progestogens
   - Antifibrinolytics
   - Prostaglandin synthetase inhibitors
   - Danazol
   - Gonadotropin-releasing hormone (GnRH) analogues.

Surgery

Myomectomy

Myomectomy is the enucleation of myomata from the uterus leaving behind a potentially functioning organ capable of future reproduction.

Factors to be Considered Prior to Myomectomy

- It should be done mainly to preserve the reproductive function
- Myomectomy is a more risky operation when the fibroid is too big and too many
- There is a chance of recurrence in 5-10%
- There is chance of persistence of menorrhagia in 1-5%
- Pregnancy rate is about 40-60%
- Pregnancy following myomectomy should have a mandatory hospital delivery.

Pre-requisites Prior to Myomectomy

- Examination of the husband from fertility point of view including semen analysis
- Hysteroscopy or hysterosalpingography to detect a fibroid encroaching the uterine cavity or a polyp or tubal block
- Diagnostic D and C in cases of irregular cycles, to exclude endometrial carcinoma.

Contraindications

- Husband proved infertile
- Associated bilateral infective tubo-ovarian mass
- Infected fibroid
- Big broad ligament fibroid
- Too many fibroids.

Vaginal Myomectomy

Submucous pedunculated myoma can be removed vaginally. Morcellation (removal by piecemeal) is needed if the tumor is large.

A moderate size fibroid is removed by twisting after grasping it with a sponge holding forceps.

Hysterectomy

Hysterectomy is the surgical removal of the uterus, either through an incision in the abdominal wall (abdominal hysterectomy) or through the vagina (vaginal hysterectomy). Hysterectomy is the operation of choice in symptomatic fibroid.

Indications for Hysterectomy

- Absence of indications for myomectomy
- Patients over the age of 40 years
- Clients not desirous of having a child.
- Total hysterectomy (removal of the whole uterus) is done in women with fibroids over 12 week's size.
- Subtotal hysterectomy (removal of the body of uterus leaving the cervix in place) is done in situations where the patient's condition deteriorates during surgery or with associated endometriosis.

Advantages of Hysterectomy

- There is no chance of recurrence
- Adnexal pathology and unhealthy cervix are also removed.

Vaginal Hysterectomy

Fibroids with size of 10–12 weeks of pregnancy associated with uterine prolapse are generally removed by the vaginal route. Vaginal hysterectomy with repair of pelvic floor is the operation of choice.

Indications of Emergency Surgery in Fibroid

- Torsions of subserous pedunculated fibroid
- Massive intraperitoneal hemorrhage following rupture of veins over subserous fibroid
- Uncontrolled infected fibroid
- Uncontrolled bleeding fibroid.

Cervical Fibroid

Cervical fibroids cause symptoms due to pressure on the surrounding structures. Symptoms vary depending on the location of fibroid are:
- Anterior cervical fibroids: Cause bladder symptoms such as frequency or retention of urine
- Posterior cervical fibroids lead to rectal symptom in the form of constipation
- Lateral cervical fibroids may lead to hemorrhoids and edema of legs the ureter is pushed laterally below the tumor
- Central cervical fibroids produce predominantly bladder symptoms. The cervix is expanded on all sides. The uterus sits on the expanded cervix.

In pregnancy cervical fibroids remain asymptomatic, but produce obstruction during labor. Fibroids arising from the vaginal part of the cervix may remain asymptomatic during non-pregnant state, but produces obstruction during labor. If pedunculated, there may be a sensation of something coming down or if infected, there may be a foul smelling discharge.

Treatment

- Myomectomy, if the patient is young and desirous of having a baby
- Enucleation followed by hysterectomy.

Fibroid Polyp

The fibroid polyp may arise from the body of the uterus or from the cervix. Almost always this is due to extrusion of a submucous fibroid into the uterine cavity. During this process it attains a pedicle, which is often broad and usually attached to the posterior wall. The uterus contracts to expel the polyp out and as a result, the polyp may be pushed out through the cervix to lie even in the vagina. The polyp is usually single of varying sizes. There may be evidence of necrosis, infection and hemorrhage especially at the tip. The pedicle may be broad and there may be associated other fibroids in the uterus.

Cervical fibroid polyp usually arises from the ectocervix and from its posterior lip. It may be small, large and at times big enough to distend the vagina or even comes out of the introitus confusing the diagnosis of uterine inversion.

Signs and Symptoms

- Intermenstrual bleeding, often continuous specially in fibroid polyp arising from the body
- Colicky pain in the lower abdomen due to uterine contraction in an effort to expel the polyp out of the uterine cavity
- Excess vaginal discharge
- Sensation of something coming down when the polyp becomes big distending the vagina
- Varying degrees of anemia
- Uterus bulky
- Cervix patulous and polyp felt distinctly outside the external os.

Treatment

- Hysterectomy with the polyp inside
- For fibroid/fibroid polyp associated with uterine inversion, enucleation of the fibroid followed by hysterectomy at a later date
- If infection is present, antibiotics are administered.

NURSING PROCESS

Assessment

- Dysfunctional uterine bleeding
- Colicky pain in abdomen
- Signs of pelvic infection: Foul-smelling discharge
- Anemia
- Enlargement of uterus
- Prolapse
- Dyspareunia
- Infertility.

Diagnostic Studies

- Pap smear
- Pelvic ultrasound or computed tomography
- Hysteroscopy (fiberoptic viewing of endometrial cavity)
- Laparoscopy
- Endometrial sampling (D and C with biopsy)
- Schiller's test (staining of cervix with iodine to identify abnormal cells)
- Complete blood count.

Nursing Diagnoses

- Situational low self-esteem.
- Impaired urinary elimination, retention.
- Risk for constipation/diarrhea.
- Risk for ineffective tissue perfusion.
- Risk for sexual dysfunction.
- Risk for dysfunctional grieving.
- Deficient knowledge regarding condition, prognosis, treatment and self-care.

Expected Outcomes

Client will:
- Verbalize acceptance of self and adaptation to change in body/self.
- Empty bladder regularly and completely.
- Maintain usual/normal pattern of elimination.
- Demonstrate adequate perfusion, as evidenced by stable vital signs, palpable pulses, good capillary refill and adequate urinary output.
- Identify satisfactory/acceptable sexual practice.
- Verbalize reality of perceived loss and sense of acceptance and hope for future.
- Verbalize understanding of therapeutic needs.

Nursing Interventions

1. Accepting self and adapting to change:
   - Provide time to listen to concerns and fears of client
   - Discuss client's perceptions of self, related to anticipated changes and her specific lifestyle
   - Provide accurate information, reinforcing information previously given
   - Ascertain individual strengths and identify previous coping behaviors
   - Provide open environment for client to discuss concerns about sexuality.
     *Refer to psychiatric or other counseling as necessary.
     *Denotes collaborative intervention.
2. Improving urinary elimination:
   - Note voiding pattern and monitor urinary output once urinary catheter is removed
   - Palpate bladder, investigate reports of discomfort, fullness and inability to void
   - Provide routine voiding measures, e.g. privacy, normal position, running water in sink and pouring warm water over perineum
   - Provide/Encourage good perineal cleansing and catheter care (when present)
   - Assess urine characteristics, noting color, clarity and odor
   - Catheterize when indicated/per protocol if client is unable to void or is uncomfortable
   - Maintain patency of indwelling catheter; keep drainage tubing free of kinks
   - Check residual urine volume after voiding is completed.
3. Improving bowel elimination:
   - Auscultate bowel sounds
   - Note abdominal distention, presence of nausea/vomiting
   - Assist client with sitting on edge of bed and walking
   - Encourage adequate fluid intake, including fruit juices when oral intake is started

- Provide sitz bath
- Restrict oral intake as indicated
- Maintain nasogastric tube if present
- Provide clear/full fluids and advance to solid food as tolerated.
  *Administer medications such as stool softeners, mineral oil and laxatives as prescribed.
  *Denotes collaborative intervention.
4. Maintaining adequate tissue perfusion:
   - Monitor vital signs, palpate peripheral pulses, assess urinary output, and evaluate changes in mentation
   - Inspect dressing and perineal pads, noting color, amount and odor of drainage
   - Weigh client and compare with dry pads if client is bleeding heavily
   - Turn client and encourage frequent coughing and deep breathing exercises
   - Avoid high Fowler's position and pressure under the knees or crossing legs
   - Assist with/instruct in foot and leg exercises and ambulate as early as possible
   - Note erythema, swelling of extremity or reports of sudden chest pain with dyspnea.
     *Administer intravenous (IV) fluids and/or blood products as indicated and prescribed.
     *Denotes collaborative intervention.
5. Improving acceptance of future sexual practice:
   - Assist patient to be aware of/deal with the stage of grieving
   - Encourage client to share thoughts/concerns with spouse
   - Assist patient to identify solutions to potential problems, e.g. postponing sexual intercourse when fatigued, substituting alternative means of expression, using vaginal lubricants
   - Discuss expected physical sensations/discomforts and changes in response to surgical trauma and altered hormone levels.
     *Refer to counselor as required/ordered.
     *Denotes collaborative intervention.

6. Improving the sense of acceptance and hope for future related to dysfunctional grieving:
   - Provide an open environment in which the client feels free to realistically discuss feelings and concerns
   - Determine client's perception and meaning of current and past loss
   - Assist spouse/significant others to cope with the patient's responses
   - Note withdrawn behavior, negative self-talk, over concern with actual or perceived changes
   - Discuss healthy ways of dealing with difficult situations.
   *Refer to other resources, e.g. counseling, spiritual care, and psychotherapy as indicated and ordered.
   *Denotes collaborative intervention.
7. Improving understanding of condition and potential complications:
   - Review effects of surgical procedure and future expectations, e.g. client needs to know that she will no longer menstruate or bear children
   - Discuss complexity of problems anticipated during recovery, e.g. emotional liability, feeling of sadness/depression, excessive fatigue, sleep disturbances
   - Discuss resumption of activity; encourage light activities initially with frequent rest periods and increasing activities/exercises as tolerated
   - Identify individual restrictions, e.g. avoiding heavy lifting and strenuous activities such as vacuuming, staining at stool and prolonged sitting/driving
   - Discuss dietary modifications, medical bulk agents, stimulation by suppository, etc. to manage constipation
   - Identify dietary needs, e.g. high-quality protein, complex carbohydrates, addition of iron, include information about foods to include and avoid in managing menopausal symptoms.
   *Review hormone replacement therapy (HRT) when used.
   *Discuss potential side effects of hormone replacement therapy, e.g. skin pigmentation or acne, breast tenderness, headaches and photosensitivity.

*Review incisional care when appropriate.
*Stress importance of follow-up care.
*Denotes collaborative intervention.

59. FORCEPS DELIVERY

Obstetrical forceps are metal instruments designed to assist and expedite delivery of the baby's head.

Design of Forceps

The obstetric forceps consist of two matched metallic halves that articulate with each other at the lock. Each half consists of a blade, shank, lock and handle. Each blade has two curves; the cephalic curve, which permits an accurate and safe grip of the fetal head and the pelvic curve that conforms to the axis of the birth canal **(Fig. 59.1)**.

The blades are referred to as the right blade and left blade corresponding to the side of the maternal pelvis they occupy after application. The left blade is applied first, until it is in place closely apposed to the fetal head; and the right blade is applied thereafter. In this way the shaft of the right blade comes atop the shank of the left blade and locks in position as the handles are approximated **(Figs. 59.2A to C)**.

Varieties of Obstetric Forceps

Conventional traction forceps:

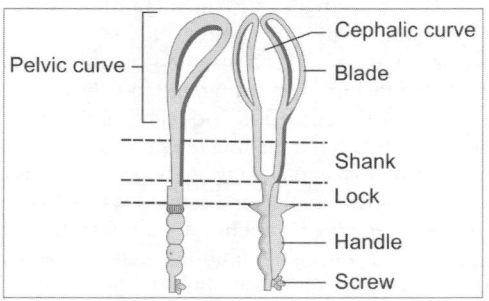

Fig. 59.1: Different parts of a long-curved obstetric forceps.

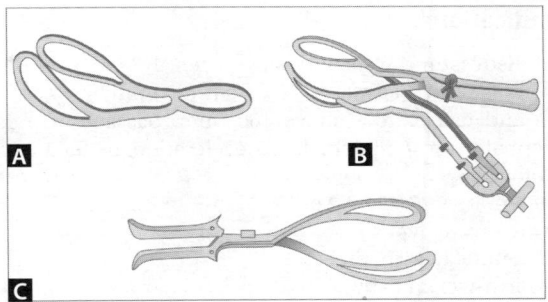

Figs. 59.2A to C: Different types of obstetric forceps. **A.** Short forceps; **B.** Axis traction forceps; **C.** Long forceps.

Short forceps	Wrigley's forceps Short Simpson's forceps
Long forceps	Das's forceps Simpson's forceps
Long forceps with axis traction	Milne Murray's forceps Haig Ferguson's forceps Neville Barnes forceps
Rotation forceps	Kielland's forceps Barton's forceps
Forceps for special use	Piper's forceps for after coming head in breech

Classification of Forceps Application According to Station of the Head

- Outlet forceps:
  - When head is crowning/scalp is visible at the introitus
  - Sagittal suture in the anteroposterior diameter.
- Low forceps: When head is at + 2 station or lower, but not yet crowning
- Mid forceps: When head is above + 2 station, but engaged.

Indications for the Use of Forceps

The obstetric forceps is used to cut short labor in both maternal and fetal interests.

Fetal Indications

- Fetal distress in the second stage when the prospect of vaginal delivery is safe (bradycardia less than 100 bpm between contractions and tachycardia above 160 bpm, passage of meconium in cephalic presentation, late deceleration of fetal heart rate monitoring)
- Acute emergencies, e.g. cord prolapse or cord around the neck causing severe hypoxia
- After coming head of breech
- Low-birth-weight baby
- Postmature baby.

Maternal Indications

- Maternal exhaustion following prolonged labor
- Prolonged second stage of labor
- Maternal distress as shown by maternal tachycardia, dehydration, presence of acetone in urine or mild pyrexia
- Maternal medical disorders such as cardiac disease, severe anemia, tuberculosis, pregnancy-induced hypertension, eclampsia or debilitating illness, in order to shorten the second stage of labor
- Failure of descend or internal rotation for 2 hours in a primigravida and 1 hour in a multipara in the second stage of labor.

Situations Predispose to Arrest of Progress of Labor

- Poor uterine contractions
- Malpositions such as right or left occipitoposterior positions
- Deflexed head
- Prominent spines in lower pelvic strait
- Heavy sedation, epidural analgesia.

Contraindications for the Use of Forceps

The use of forceps is contraindicated in the following situations:
- Absence of full dilatation of cervix
- In case of cephalopelvic disproportion
- High station of fetal head
- Cessation of uterine contractions.

Prerequisites for Forceps Application

Certain conditions must be satisfied prior to forceps application:
- Fetal head must be engaged, flexed and preferably well-rotated
- There should be no obvious cephalopelvic disproportion
- Cervix must be fully dilated, effaced and with absent membranes
- Uterus must be contracting and relaxing
- The bladder must be empty.

Prophylactic Forceps/Elective Forceps

The method refers to forceps delivery, only to shorten the second stage of labor when maternal and/or fetal complications are anticipated. The indications are:
- Eclampsia
- Heart disease
- Previous cesarean section
- Post maturity
- Low-birth-weight baby and patients under epidural analgesia.

It prevents possible fetal cerebral injury due to pressure on the perineum and spares the mother from the strain of few bearing down efforts.

Trial Forceps

This method is a tentative attempt of forceps delivery in a case of suspected midpelvic contraction with a preamble declaration of abandoning it in favor of cesarean section, if moderate traction fails to overcome resistance. The procedure is performed in an operating room set up, with full preparation for cesarean section.

If the blades apply easily and descent occurs with gentle traction, the delivery is accomplished vaginally with the forceps.

Failed Forceps

When a deliberate attempt at a vaginal delivery with forceps has failed to expedite the process, it is called failed forceps. The cases of failed forceps include:
- Incompletely dilated cervix
- Unrotated occipitoposterior position

- Unrecognized cephalopelvic disproportion
- Undiagnozed brow or hydrocephalus, or fetal ascitis
- Constriction ring
- Large baby with the shoulders impacted at the brim.

In such cases, there is a high incidence of maternal and perinatal morbidity and mortality resulting from trauma due to ill-conceived intervention.

60. GENE DISORDERS, GENETIC SCREENING AND GENETIC COUNSELING

The majority of traits in the human body are controlled by several genes working together to produce the final effect or polygenic traits; for example, the distribution of height or the distribution of various shapes of individuals.

Several pathologic conditions are polygenic and multifactorial. There is genetic disposition to conditions such as diabetes mellitus, hypertension, obesity and common psychiatric illnesses such as bipolar disorder and schizophrenia along with environmental factors such as lifestyle, dietary habits and stressful events.

Gene disorders are inherited through the genes in the ovum or sperm. Genetically determined disorders are classified as:

1. Chromosomal disorders:
   a. Structural abnormalities:
      - 46XX or 46XYB (5) P/cri-du-chat syndrome
      - Fragile X syndrome
      - Chromosome instability syndrome.
   b. Numerical abnormalities of autosomes:
      - Trisomy 21/Down syndrome
      - Trisomy 18/Edwards syndrome
      - Trisomy 13/Patau syndrome.
   c. Numerical abnormalities of sex chromosomes:
      - 47XXY/Klinefelter syndrome
      - 47XYY/Jacob's syndrome
      - 45XO/Turner syndrome
      - 47XXX/Triple X syndrome.

2. Single gene disorders:
   a. Atuosomal dominant gene disorders:
      - Achondroplasia
      - Familial hypercholesterolemia
      - Marfan syndrome
      - Neurofibromatosis
      - Osteogenesis imperfecta
      - Polycystic kidney disease
      - Ehlers-Danlos syndrome.
   b. Autosomal recessive gene disordes:
      - Cystic fibrosis
      - Mucopolysacharidoses
      - Phenylketonuria
      - Sickle cell disease
      - Tay-Sachs disease.
   c. X-linked disorders:
      - Duchennes muscular dystrophy
      - Glucose-6-phosphate dehydrogenase deficieny (G6PD)
      - Hemophilia
      - Lesch-Nyhan syndrom.
3. Plygenic and multifactorial disorders:
   a. Coronary heart disease, diabetes mellitus, hypertension, obesity and psychiatric illnesses.

Chromosomal Disorders

Chromosomal abnormalities may result from alteration in individual chromosomes (structural abnormalities) or from alterations in the total number of chromosomes (numerical abnormalities). Either situation may cause significant and observable characteristics and pathogenic conditions. Structural abnormalities include a variety of chromosome defects such as deletions and translocations.

Structural Abnormalities

1. 46XX or XYB (5) P (Cri-du-chat or Cat's cry syndrome).
   This is a rare chromosome deletion syndrome resulting from loss of the small arm of chromosome B (5). In early infancy this

syndrome presents with a typical, but non-distinctive facial appearance, often non-distinctive facial appearance, often moon shaped face with wide-spaced eyes. As the child grows, this feature diminishes and by age 2, the child is undistinguishable from age-matched children. Profound mental retardation persists throughout a short life. Most affected children die in infancy. Typical of this disease is a crying pattern that is abnormal and cat-like. At times it sounds like an angry cat's cry and other times like a soft mewling sound. This is a result of laryngeal atrophy, which improves with age.

2. Fragile X syndrome.

   This syndrome acquired its name from the fact that in *in vitro* conditions, the X-chromosome frequently displays breaks and gaps in its terminal portions. This is an X-linked dominant disorder with increased prevalence among males. Clinical features are mental retardation and typical facial appearance, including an elongated face and long elf-like ears.

3. Chromosome instability syndrome.

   This is a heterogeneous group of genetic disorders characterized by high frequency of chromosomal breakage that is observed in vitro (outside body). These include 'ataxia-telangiectasia (Louis-bar syndrome), Fanconi anemia and xeroderma pigmentosum. These syndromes are associated with decreased immune function and an increased incidence of cancer, mostly lymphomas and leukemias.

Numerical Abnormalities of Autosomes

Numerical alterations of the autosome include some of the most common trisomies such as trisomy 21, 18 and trisomy 13.

1. Trisomy 21 (dowm syndrome): Down syndrome is the most common condition having abnormal number of chromosomes compatible with development to full term, with a reasonable quality of postnatal life. Physical and mental abnormalities vary and the IQ ranges from 26–75. Physical abnormalities include flat occiput, fissure on eye lids (palpebral fissures), epicanthal folds, broad nasal bones and open mouth with protruding tongue. Skeletal abnormalities seen are broad and short fingers. Several

cardiac malformations and increased susceptibility to infections is seen. Palmar simian crease and abnormal finger print are also common. Males with down syndrome are usually sterile.

2. **Trisomy 18 (Edward's syndrome):** Edward's syndrome is a fairly common trisomy affecting mostly chromosome 18. Children with this disorder have severe mental retardation and craniofocal abnormalities (dolichocephaly, prominent occiput, low set and malformed ears, and micrognathia). Skeletal abnormalities seen are overlapping fingers, flexion deformities and aducted hips. Cardiac anomalies, urogenital malformations and hypotonia are common. Females are more affected. Most children die in infancy itself.

3. **Trisomy 13 (Patau syndrome):** Patau syndrome causes more severe malformations than the previous two trisomies discussed. Craniofacial anomalies are much more pronounced; microcephaly, low set and malformed ears, microphthalmia or anophthalmia, polydactyly and syndactyly, and overlapping flexed fingers are seen. Systemic anomalies include cardiac defects and urogenital malformations. Mean life expectancy is 4 months.

Numerical Abnormalities of Sex Chromosomes

1. **47XXY (Klinefelter syndrome):** Klinefelter syndrome is characterized by multiple X chromosomes and one Y chromosome. Physical abnormalities include elements of decreased masculinization and increased pubis-to-sole length, reflecting elongated lower limbs. Mental development is normal in most cases. Mental retardation occurs in some children with reduced or delayed language skills.

2. **47XYY (Jacob's syndrome):** Individuals with an extra Y cromosome are tall statured and develop skin disorders such as adult acne. Mental retardation and aggressive tendency were seen in some cases. A majority of children produced by XYY fathers have normal chromosomal constitution.

3. **XO (Turner syndrome):** Clinical manifestations of this condition include low birth weight and short adult stature, low posterior hair line, webbing of neck, shield-shaped chest with

divergent nipples. limb deformities, cardiac anomalies, urinary tract abnormalities cystic hygromas and hydrops are seen in newborns. Intellectual development is normal.
4. 47XXX: Triple X females display a normal phenotype with their euploid sisters with a slight decrease in mental capacity. Gynecologic complications include delayed menarche and premature menopause. Offsprings of XXX females are largely normal.

Single Gene Disorders

Autosomal Dominant Gene Disorders

1. Achondroplasia.
   This is the most common form of dwarfism (adult stature is 120–125 cm (48–50 inches), that is characterized by shortened limbs and a normal length torso. Common features include lordosis, prominent forehead with flattened nasal bridge and short hands with stubby fingers. Life span and IQ are within normal limits among heterozygotes. Gynecologic problems include premature menarche, enlarged breasts and premature menopause, increased paternal age is seen as a factor in producing achondroplasia.
2. Familial Hypercholesterolemia hyperlipoproteinemia): This is one of the most common single gene disorders in which the manifestations are sensitive to dietary variations. Individuals who are homozygous for this gene, (possessing two identical alleles at a given locus that are descended from a single source as may occur in consanguineous mating) tend to develop severe and life-threatening atherosclerotic disease that affects the coronary artery, and cerebral and peripheral circulation.
3. Marfan syndrome: It is a disorder of connective tissue involving a triad ocular, skeletal and cardiovascular alterations. The most common ocular deformity is a partial dislocation of the lens. Common skeletal findings include tall stature, arachnodactylic (spider-like) hands and feet and scoliosis. The major life-threatening risk, however, is the frequent occurrence of aortic fusiform or dissecting aneurysms. 50% of aortic aneurysms in

affected women under age 40 occur during pregnancy, with rupture most likely to occur in the third trimester. Aortic valve abnormalities found in Marfan syndrome also contribute to an increased mortality rate during pregnancy. Average life span with the syndrome is 40–50 years.

4. Neurofibromatosis: This condition also referred to as von Recklinghausen disease, is the development of multiple soft tumors of peripheral nerves or neurofibromas and abnormal skin pigmentation. In the early childhood, the disease presents with multiple brown spots, usually on the torso and then progresses from adolescence onwards, in the form of neurofibromas. About 75% of individuals go through life without developing complications of the disease. Others develop some of the complications such as scoliosis, moderate-to-severe mental retardation, learning difficulties, hypertension, seizures, spinal cord compression, optic gliomas, pheochromocytoma and malignant changes in the neurofibromas.

5. Osteogenesis imperfecta type 1: It is characterized by blue sclera, conductive deafness and discolored teeth resulting from dentinogenesis defects. Type 2 results in perinatal lethality with multiple fractures during gestation and birth. Life span of type 1 is usually normal in spite of multiple fracrtures throughout life. Certain forms of osteogenesis imperfecta involve osteoporosis and recurrent fractures of long bones with minimal trauma.

6. Polycystic kidney disease: This is a fairly common disorder that causes cysts in the kidneys, liver, pancreas and spleen. Renal cysts may remain asymptomatic until third or fourth decade of life, when the onset of renal failure or hypertension prompts a diagnosis of polycystic disease.

    Occasionally an enlarged kidney is detected on X-ray studies before the onset of other symptoms such as hematuria and proteinuria. Polycystic renal disease accounts for approximately 10% of all adult cases of chronic renal failure.

7. Ehlers-Danlos syndrome:
   This genetic disease includes a group of disorders of connective tissue that result in hyperplasticity of skin, hyperflexible joints, vascular fragility and poor wound healing. Common complications include a tendency for bruising, hernias and varicose veins,

all of which increases during pregnancy. Poor wound healing and predisposition to hemorrhage are risk factors during and after delivery (e.g. episiotomy wound healing may be delayed or complicated by these factors). The lifespan may be limited by vascular events such as aneurisms or rupture of large vessels.

Autosomal Recessive Gene Disorders

The most common autosomal recessive gene disorders include cystic fibrosis, mucopolysacharidoses, phenylketonuria, sickle cell disease and Tay-Sachs disease.

1. Cystic fibrosis: It is a lethal genetic disease more common in Caucasians (white race). Clinical manifestations include abnormal exocrine gland function with pancreatic insufficiency and malabsorption, chronic pulmonary disease and excessive salt in sweat. The pancreatic insufficiency results in pancreatic juice that lacks trypsin, an enzyme that must be endogenously supplied throughout life. Chronic lung disease occur secondary to recurrnet infections resulting from the inability of ciliated epithelium to secrete adequate mucus. Pulmonary function progressively deteriorates and a large number of affected children die before the age of 10.

2. Mucopolysaccharidosis: These are a group of lysosomal storage diseases that have in common a disorder in metabolism of mucopolysaccharidosis as evidenced by excretion of various mucopolysaccharidosis is in urine and infiltration of these substances into connective tissue resulting in various defects of bone, cartilage, connective tissue and other organs. The primary types are: Type 1—Hurler syndrome, type 2—Hunter syndrome, type 3—Sanflippo's syndrome and type 4—Morquio syndrome.

3. Phenylketonuria (PKU): It results from an enzyme (phenylalanine hydroxylase) deficiency and consequent accumulation of he amino acid, phenylalanine and its byproducts, which cause mental retardation and other manifestations. Management of PKU consists of removing phenylalanine from the infant's diet and maintaining a low-phenylalanine intake throughout life. If a low phenylalanine diet is initiated within the first days of life, normal development and life span can be expected. However, the offspring of women rescued or treated are at risk

for mental retardation, microcephaly, congenital heart disease and intrauterine growth retardation. The condition develops as a result of intrauterine exposure to high levels of maternal phenylalanine and its metabolities.

4. Sickle cell disease: It is a serious, chronic, hemolytic anemia that results from homozygosity for a mutant allele (one of two or more alternative forms of gene, only one of which can be present in a chromosome) hemoglobin S (HbS) gene. As a result of his genetic imbalance, HbS, an abnormal hemoglobin replaces the normal adult hemoglobin A. HbS has decreased oxygen carrying capacity and red blood cells acquire a sickle-shaped appearance, a morphologic change that greatly contributes to obstruction of small vessels and further ischemia. Infarctions in the lungs, kidneys, spleen and bones are common. The result is a life-long series of sickle cell crises with recurrent pneumococcal infections, painful ulcers, osteomelitis, priapism and other symptoms. Renal failure is a common and serious complication. The life span is seriously shortened even with aggressive management.

5. Tay-Sachs diseases: It is a lipid shortage disorder, with accumulation of GM_2 ganglioside in cells of the nervous sysem, resulting in a progressive neurologic disorder. The genetic defect results in decreased production of the enzyme β-hexosaminidase A (HexA). During their short life, children with TSD experience a progressive and steady deterioration in a series of mental and motor deficits, which begin at approximately 6 months of age. Symptoms at various ages include loss of developmental milestones acquired before the onset of the disease, along with deafness, blindness, seizure activity and death by age 3–5.

X-Linked Disorders

Genetic disorders whose causative gene is located on the X-chromosome include Duchenne's muscular dystrophy, glucoce-6-phosphate dehydrogenase deficiency (G_6PD) and Lesch-Nyhan syndrome.

1. Duchenne's muscular dystrophy: It is a progressive, muscular weakening atrophy and contractures beginning in early childhood. In the majority of cases, the age of onset is 5

years and the disease is characterized by delayed walking. A pseudohypertrophy of the calf (in which the muscle is replaced by adipose tissue) may mask the disease. Affected children are usually unable to run and 95% of affected children are using a wheelchair by age 12. Mild mental retardation occurs in about one of four cases. Death is often from respiratory insufficiency that occurs in the second decade.

2. Glucose-6-phosphate dehydrogenase deficiency: The common self-limiting hemolytic anemia is a disorder due to deficiency of G6PD and is usually asymptomatic until the affected male is exposed to one of many environmental triggers such as certain drugs (antimalarial agents, aspirin, and sulfonamides) or certain foods. The hemolytic episodes may also be precipitated by infections. Carrier females remain asymptomatic even when exposed to a trigger agent. Pregnant women with deficiency suffer several complications. Hemolytic episodes are more frequent; urinary infections which are common in pregnancy cannot be treated with sulpha based drugs; and exposure of fetus with G6PD deficiency suffer several complications. Hemolytic episodes are more frequent; urinary infections, which are common in pregnancy cannot be treated with sulfa-based drugs; and exposure of fetus with G6PD deficiency to maternally ingested trigger substances may result in fetal hemolysis, hydrops fetalis and death. The incidence of anemia, hperbilirubinemia and kernicterus is also increased among newborns with G6PD deficiency.

3. Hemophilia A: Type A or classic hemophilia is a fairly common X-linked recessive disorder of coagulation resulting from deficiency of clotting factor VIII C. In 10% of clients, the factor VIII C level is normal, but activity is reduced. Variable degrees of deficiencies are probably caused by genetic heterogeneity (different mutations). In the presence of severe factor VIII C deficiency, massive hemorrhage occurs following trauma and surgical procedures (including dental procedures). Spontaneous bleeding frequently occurs in areas subject to trauma such as joints, resulting in hemarthroses. Petechiae and ecchymoses are usually absent. Prenatal diagnosis by measurement of factor VIII is possible.

4. **Lesch-Nyhan syndrome:** This syndrome is a rare X-linked recessive disorder caused by an enzyme deficiency resulting in an overproduction of uric acid. Affected boys are mentally retarded and suffer from spasticity and gouty arthritis. They also have a compulsion for self-mutilation. Prenatal diagnosis is made by determination of hypoxanthine-guanine phosphoribosyl transferase (HGPRT).

Polygenic and Multifactorial Disorders

The majority of traits in human body are controlled by several genes working together to produce the final effect; these are polygenic traits. When environmental factors also contgribute to the expression of the phenotype (the observable characteristic of an individual), these are multifactorial traits, e.g. distribution of height or body shape.

The pathologic conditions that are polygenic and multifactorial in nature are coronary artery disease, diabetes mellitus, hypertension, obesity and common psychiatric illnesses such as schizophrenia and bipolar disorder. Even through an undeniable genetic predisposition exists for these conditions, they are heavily influenced by environmental factors, such as lifestyle, dietary habits and stressful events. Risk determination of these conditions is made on the basis of empirical observation of a large number of cases, followed by specific statistical analysis of each trait.

Genetic Screening

Genetic screening is the process by which individuals or populations can be assessed for various genetic disorders to detect the presence of a gene before it expresses a genetic disease or to identify the carrier of a recessive state. Treatment for genetic disorders is rarely successful because of the complexity and magnitude of genetic damage. The primary weapon against increase in the prevalence of genetic disease is an aggressive program of genetic screening and counseling. The requirement of any such intervention must include voluntary participation, equal access to all and confidentiality (both in conducting the tests and in handling records and results). In addition, education and counseling about tests and procedures must be an integral part of any screening program.

Purposes of Genetic Screening

- To provide early recognition of a disease for which effective intervention and therapy exist before symptoms occur, e.g. phenylketonuria.
- To provide identification of carriers of genetic disease for the purpose of maximizing parenthood planning options, e.g. Tay-Sachs disease.
- To obtain population data on frequency, spectrum and natural history of genetic disease, e.g. chromosomal abnormalities in newborns.

Timings of Genetic Screening

Screening of genetic disorders can be performed during various times in a person's life:
- Screening of selected populations for heterogeneous carriers, e.g. sickle cell disease
- Preconception screening for carrier or affected individuals within a family, for the purpose of reproductive decision-making
- Preconception screening for carriers, e.g. screening for Tay-Sachs disease among couples contemplating parenthood
- Post-conception (prenatal) testing, e.g. screening for Tay-Sachs disease in the product of conception by two heterozygous carriers
- Newborn testing, e.g. testing for PKU in all newborns as mandated by law in some countries.

Among prenatal benefits of screening for carrier is the removal/reduction of anxiety and restoration of self-esteem when the results do not reveal carrier status. It also facilitates genetic counseling and reproductive planning. Testing newborns for genetic defects provide for early detection and treatment initiation, maximizing quality of life.

Risks incurred in genetic screening include the potential stigmatization of those identified as carriers of affected individuals and for the development of feelings of inadequacy and guilt often seen in conjunction with genetic disease. A positive test result for one family member may result in the disclosure of genetic risks to other family members who did not seek or want to know the outcome of the tests.

Candidates for Genetic Screening

- Women over 35 years
- Family history of neural tube defects
- Previous baby born with neural tube defect
- One or both parents, carriers of sex-linked autosomal traits
- A mentally retarded child with or without congenital anomaly
- History of recurrent abortion.

Detection Tests

Improved prenatal screening and diagnostic techniques are now available for detection of abnormalities in early pregnancy, which include:
- Maternal serum alpha-fetoprotein (MSAFP)
- Triple test: MSAFP, unconjugated estriol (E3) and human chorionic gnadotropin (hCG)
- Amniocentesis
- Chorion villus biopsy
- High resolution ultrasonography
- Fetoscopy
- Embryo biopsy.

Termination of pregnancy is considered following early detection of certain genetic disorders, chromosomal abnormalities and structural abnormalities.

Management of at Risk Couples

Preconceptional counseling is an important step in the management, so that the couple has adequate information before hand. Option of termination of pregnancy is offered if the fetus is affected with serious genetic, chromosomal or structural abnormality.

Genetic Counseling

Genetic counseling consists of one or more encounters with the probands and their families with the objective of providing information about their genetic disease. A proband is a clinically identified individual who displays the characteristics or features of the disease in question. The information includes risk figures and options, and provides a framework for a course of action to be taken by the individual or family.

It also includes an assessment of psychosocial family dynamics, which are an integral part of a genetic disease and exploration of feelings and perceptions often elicited by the newly obtained knowledge. Genetic counseling in its broader definition refers to a series of procedures that include processing the initial referral, assessing the needs, deciding on the appropriate tests, interpreting the results, and finally communicating these findings to the proband and family counseling. However, two factors make genetic counseling a unique process:

1. Counselors must work with the grief and anticipatory grief issues. Even with the knowledge of a potentially negative outcome, a certain amount of hope and denial usually prevails, until the birth of the affected child brings the family back to the reality.
2. The parent's knowledge that they are biologically responsible for their child's condition is a burden often too heavy to carry without emotional damage. The physical contact with the individual, sometimes for a lifetime is a constant reminder of what may be perceived as reproductive failure. Emotional support can be provided by family members, counselors, social workers or even through question-answer column in newspaper, television and internet.

Many genetic disorders are not treatable with conventional techniques. In many instances, the prevention of a genetic disease is only possible though genetic counseling of persons at risk.

Stages of Counseling Interview

1. In the first interview, the counselor gathers pertinent information from family members. Once a detailed pedigree chart is generated, the counselor identifies the mode of inheritance and confirms the initial diagnosis. Testing of other family members if recommended is initiated at this time. The family members are made to feel at ease and ample time is allotted for answering all questions.

2. In the second interview, with all the previous information processed, the counselor discusses with the family all the implications of the findings, presents options and clarifies possible outcomes. For example, possibility of therapeutic abortion or sterilization. It is of topmost importance that genetic counseling remains a nondirective process, with the counselor remaining supportive, but neutral about decisions that must be made. It must be remembered that the family members are the ones who will have to live with their decision, and therefore their decision, once made must be respected and supported by all health team members.

Prenatal Diagnosis for Genetic Counseling

One of the tools for genetic counseling is prenatal diagnosis of genetic disorder. These include a trisomy profile test, an ultrasound assisted nuchal translucence test, a mid-trimester amniocentesis and chorionic villi sampling:

1. Trisomy profile test.
   This involves testing of maternal serum for MSAFP, hCG levels and unconjugted estrogen (uE_3). The MSAFP levels are found lower in pregnancies affected by down syndrome. Serum levels of hCG are found twice as high in down syndrome pregnancy. This test presently includes maternal age, MSAFP, hCG and uE_3 has high rate of identification of common chromosome disorders.

2. Nuchal Translucency on intravaginal ultrasonography.
   This high resolution ultrsonography is used to detect increased nuchal (backside of neck) translucency as an indicator of Down syndrome. An increased nuchal translucency or presence of cystic hygromas (septated fluid-fluid sacs in the nuchal region) is a common feature of several aneuploidy conditions including the common trisomies; 13,18 and 21. The procedure can be performed earlier in pregnancy than serum screening and it may decrease the need for future chorionic villi sampling (CVS) or amniocentesis.

3. Midtrimester amniocentesis.
   This procedure is commonly performed between 14th and 16th weeks of gestation, under ultrasound guidance, and

consists transabdominally withdrawing approximately 20 mL of amniotic fluid for analysis of cells sloughed off by the developing embryo. Chromosomal analysis and biochemical analysis of the fluid are also done to detect the defects.

4. Chorionic Villi Sampling.

This test can be performed at an earlier time than amniocentesis, i.e. 9th–12th week and yields results sooner. The test is accurate in about 99% of cases, provided true chorionic villi material is obtained. One major disadvantage of CVS is that alpha-fetoprotein determination for detection of neural tube defects cannot be obtained and must be attempted at a later date, when the concentration of this substance increases.

Nursing Implications

One of the most important advances in biomedical science is the mapping of the human genome. This has the potential to make dramatic changes in all health care and certainly will affect the care of women and infants.

The nurse is likely to interact with client and their families in a number of ways related to genetics. The involvement can vary depending on the setting and level of education. The nurse should have a general knowledge of genetic terminology to answer client questions and direct them to resources.

There are major implications in supporting couples in reproductive decision-making and in coping with potential genetic risks. Nurses may also be in the position to provide education and support for risk management for clients who have their own risk factors.

61. GYNECOLOGICAL DISORDERS IN PREGNANCY

1. FIBROID UTERUS

Description

Fibroid uterus is the common benign tumor of the uterus during pregnancy. These are benign smooth muscle tumors that occur within the uterus and are the most common tumors of the female genital tract **(Fig. 61.1)**.

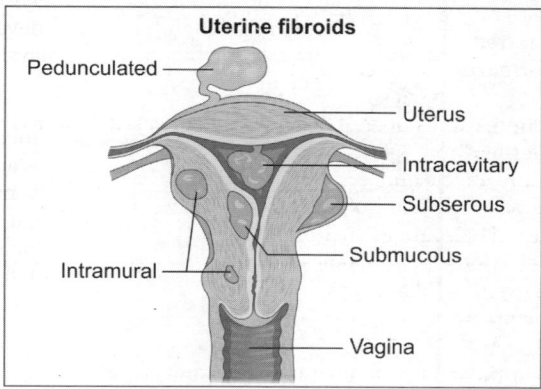

Fig. 61.1: Location of uterine fibroids.

Incidence

The incidence of fibroid in pregnancy is about 1 in 1000.

Causes

- The exact cause is unknown.
- Women who smoke tend to be relatively estrogen deficient and have been found to have a lower incidence of fibroid uterus.

Risk Factors

- Age 35 – 45 years.
- Nulliparous or low parity.
- Obesity.
- Early menarche.
- Family history of diabetes, hypertension.

Signs and Symptoms

- More than 50% are asymptomatic.
- Acute onset of pain over the tumor.

- Malaise or even rise of temperature.
- Dry, tarred tongue.
- Abnormal uterine bleeding.
- Pelvic pain or backache, acute pain occurs in case of torsion, infection, expulsion, red degeneration or vascular complications.
- Tenderness and rigidity over the tumor.
- Pressure effects on:
  Bladder – Frequency of urine, retention with overflow.
  Ureter – Hydroureter, hydronephrosis.
  Bowel – Constipation, tenesmus.
  Pelvic veins – Edema legs.
- Pelvic pressure with large fibroids.
- Leukocytosis.
- Sometimes fetal parts are not easily palpated or fetal heart sounds (FHS) are not auscultated properly.
- Size of the uterus may be more than the weeks of gestation.

Diagnosis

Confirmed diagnosis usually by an ultrasound examination.

Effects of Fibroid on Pregnancy, Labor and Puerperium

a. **Pregnancy**
   In majority of cases, fibroids cause no problems in pregnancy. Problems occur occasionally in few women as listed below.
   - **Abortion**
     Submucous fibroid can lead to recurrent abortions. With subserous and intramural fibroids, incidence of abortion is very low. Abortion occurs due to distortion of the uterine cavity, and interference with growth of fetus. Abortion may be incomplete type.
   - **Pressure symptoms**
     Growing fibroid during pregnancy affects functions of surrounding organs like bladder, ureters and rectum.
   - Malpresentation.
   - Retro displacement of uterus.
   - Non engagement of the presenting part.

b. **Labor**

Malpresentation—due to distortion of the cavity.
- Uterine inertia—due to interference with uterine contractions, particularly with multiple fibroids.
- Premature labor—due to overstretching and irritation of the uterus
- Dystocia—when fibroid is situated in isthmic or cervical region or in broad ligament, it causes obstruction for the descent of the presenting part.
- Postpartum hemorrhage—usually occurs with submucous fibroid. There is an increased chance of retained products. If placenta is implanted on fibroid, proper contraction and retraction cannot occur.
- Manual removal of placenta becomes necessary if placenta is adherent on fibroid.

c. **Puerperium**
- Subinvolution
- Secondary postpartum hemorrhage.
- Puerperal sepsis.
- Inversion of uterus with fundal submucous fibroid.

Effects of Pregnancy and Labor on Fibroid Size, Shape, Consistency

- As fibroid is an estrogen dependent tumor, during pregnancy there is increased secretion of estrogen which leads to increased size of fibroid.
- Microscopically, there is increased edema; hypertrophy and hyperplasia of muscle as well as increased vascularity. These changes make the fibroid soft.
- Shape of fibroid is also changed sometimes making it flat and difficult to palpate.
- Upward displacement of fibroid can occur if situated above isthmic level.

Torsion

In pedunculated subserous fibroid, torsion can occur and give rise to symptoms of acute abdomen.

Degeneration

Red degeneration:
- Rate of growth of fibroid is more; blood supply cannot cope up so that the surface area becomes necrosed. This usually occurs in second trimester of pregnancy.
- Obstruction to the venous outflow from the tumor is considered possible. Microscopically there is vascular thrombosis and necrosis.
- Severe constitutional symptoms like pain, malaise, fever and vomiting can occur.

Cystic degeneration:
- Due to increase in size, necrosis and hyaline degeneration occur and ultimately fibroid becomes cystic.
- Impaction in pelvis.
- Infection: After delivery, submucous fibroid may get infected and can cause puerperal sepsis.
- Injury: During passage of fetus through birth canal, fibroid gets bruised and compressed between fetal head and pelvis and leads to PPH.
- Expulsion: With delivery of fetus and placenta, pedunculated submucous fibroid may be expelled out.
- Rupture of subserous veins of the fibroid causing intraperitoneal hemorrhage is rare.

Treatment

- In asymptomatic and uncomplicated patients, no treatment is required.
- Frequent antenatal visits and counseling of patient about possible complications.
- In complicated and symptomatic patients treatment is given according to the complication.
- In cases of impaction, manual removal of impaction is done.
- In retention of urine, self-retaining catheter may be placed.
- In red degeneration, treatment is always conservative. That is bed rest, higher antibiotics, analgesics and sedation.

- Torsion of subserous, pedunculated fibroid: It causes acute abdomen and laparotomy with myomectomy is indicated.

During Labor
- Labor should be managed according to the site and size of fibroid.
- Very vigilant observation during labor for any developing complication.
- Cesarean section is indicated in cases of malpresentation, dystocia, precious pregnancy and fibroid situated in cervical canal, isthmic region or broad ligament causing mechanical obstruction.
- During cesarean section, myomectomy is avoided as blood loss is more due to increased vascularity and increased size. Cesarean hysterectomy may be required for uncontrollable PPH.
- If patient has completed child bearing, cesarean hysterectomy may be performed.
- Pedunculated, subserous fibroid can be removed during cesarean section.

2. UTERINE PROLAPSE IN PREGNANCY

Description
Pregnancy with first degree uterine prolapse with mild cystorectocele is common; but pregnancy with third degree prolapse is rare. Uterine prolapse presents a severe uterine problem in which the uterus protrudes through the pelvic floor aperture. It is usually associated with a cystocele and/or rectocele.

Incidence
The incidence is about 1 in 200 to 1 in 300 pregnancies.

Causes
- Previous vaginal deliveries (multiparous women).
- Obesity.
- Chronic pulmonary disease.
- Uterine or ovarian tumor.

- Chronic cough.
- Chronic constipation.

Clinical Manifestations

- Patients with first degree prolapse may report sensation of heaviness or fullness and feeling that something is coming down in the vagina.
- In more severe prolapse, when cervix protrudes at the introitus, the patient may complain of feeling like she is sitting on a ball.
- With severe prolapse, the woman is clearly aware of the mass.
- Vaginal bleeding, discharge and infection may be present.
- Woman may have dyspareunia.
- A feeling of heaviness in the pelvis and backache.
- Bowel or bladder problems.
- Abortion.
- Premature labor.
- Premature rupture of membranes.
- Ascending infection.

Effects of Pregnancy on Prolapse

- Symptoms like lower abdominal pain and backache increases.
- Increased vaginal discharge and difficulty in micturition and defecation as well as symptoms of urinary infection.
- Abortion.
- Premature labor.
- Premature rupture of membranes.
- Ascending infection.
- Aggravation of changes associated with prolapse.
- Marked hypertrophy and edema of the cervix.
- Increase in uterine descend during pregnancy as well as after delivery.
- Cystocele and rectocele become pronounced.
- Uterus may become incarcerated, if it fails to rise above the pelvis by 16th week.

Effects of Prolapse on Pregnancy

- Symptoms like lower abdominal pain and backache increases.
- Increased vaginal discharge and difficulty in micturition and defecation as well as symptoms of urinary infection.
- Abortion.
- Premature labor.
- Premature rupture of membranes.
- Ascending infection.

Labor and Puerperium

- Early rupture.
- Prolonged labor due to delayed dilatation of cervix and sagging of cystorectocele.
- Puerperal sepsis.
- Subinvolution.

Management

During Pregnancy

- If the cervix is outside the introitus: The cervix is to be placed inside the vagina and is kept in position by a ring pessary.
- The pessary should be kept in place until 18th to 20th week of pregnancy when the body of the uterus will be sufficiently enlarged to sit on the brim of the pelvis.
- The patient is to lie in bed with the foot end raised by about 20 cm as the pelvic floor is too much lax.
- To relieve edema and congestion, the mass should be covered with gauze, soaked in glycerin and $MgSO_4$ solution.
- This treatment is continued till 18 to 20 weeks of pregnancy till prolapsed mass is reduced in size and replaced in vagina.
- If reposition is not possible and there is incarceration, termination of pregnancy is indicated.
- If the cervix remains outside the vaginal introitus even in the later months, it is preferable to admit the patient at 36th week.

During Labor

- The patient should be on bed rest, not only to prevent early rupture of membranes but also to facilitate replacement of the prolapsed cervix inside the vagina.
- Intravaginal plugging with gauze soaked with glycerin and acriflavine, not only helps in reduction of cervical edema, but also it facilitates dilatation of cervix.
- Prophylactic antibiotics, in case of premature rupture of membranes or when the cervix remains outside vagina, should be administered.
- Manual stretching of the cervix or pushing up the cystocele and rectocele during contraction facilitates progressive descend of the head.
- If the head is deeply engaged with the cervix remaining thin but undilated, delivery may be facilitated by Duhrssen's incision at 2 O' clock and 10 O' clock positions followed by Ventouse extraction or forceps application.
- If the head is higher up or cervix is thick, edematous and non-dilated, cesarean section is a safe procedure.

Puerperium

- The patient should lie flat in bed.
- If the mass remains outside, it should be covered with gauze soaked in glycerin and $MgSO_4$.
- If subinvolution is evident, a ring pessary may be put in, until involution is completed.
- Prophylactic antibiotic is administered.
- Surgery for prolapse is contraindicated in antepartum and post-partum period.
- Definitive surgery is done only after six months of delivery and preferably after the patient starts menstruating.

3. OVARIAN TUMORS IN PREGNANCY

Description

Benign tumors of the ovary are many and varied. The cause of most of them is unknown. The benign tumors develop from a variety of physiological imbalances.

Incidence

Ovarian tumor with pregnancy is about 1 in 2000.

Effects of Ovarian Tumor on Pregnancy and Labor

- Pressure symptoms.
- Increased chance for impaction leading to retention of urine.
- Mechanical distress in presence of large tumor.
- Malpresentation.
- Non-engagement of the fetal head at term.
- Obstructed labor.

Clinical Manifestations

- In about 50% of cases, it is asymptomatic.
- Symptomatic tumors present with vague abdominal discomforts.
- Retention of urine due to impaction of tumor.
- Mechanical distress due to large cyst.
- Acute abdomen due to complications of tumor.

Diagnosis

- Abdominal examination reveals the cystic swelling felt separated from the gravid uterus.
- Ultrasonography.

Treatment and Management

During Pregnancy

- For uncomplicated tumors, the best time of elective operation is between 14th and 18th week, as the chance for abortion is less and access to pedicle is easy.
- Beyond 36 weeks: The operation is better to be withheld till delivery and the tumor is removed as early in puerperium as possible.
- If the tumor causes non-engagement of head or obstructs labor, LSCS and cystectomy or ovariotomy is performed.

During Labor

- If the tumor is well above the presenting part, a watchful expectancy hoping for vaginal delivery is followed.

4. CANCER CERVIX WITH PREGANCY

Pre-invasive Cancer/Cervical Intraepithelial Neoplasia (CIN)

- Cytological examination can be done during pregnancy, considering that some features of dysplasia are seen as increased cells showing mitosis are normally present during pregnancy.
- If CIN I or CIN II is detected, follow up is done till one month after delivery and then conization or hysterectomy is done as indicated.

Invasive Cancer Cervix

This is a very rare cancer (1 in 10,000) as the mean age of cancer cervix is 45–50 years and associated infection prevents conception.

Effects of Invasive Carcinoma Cervix on Pregnancy and Labor

- Abortion and preterm labor due to hemorrhage, infection and affection of general health.
- Cervical dystocia, obstructed labor, cervical laceration and/or uterine rupture may occur.
- Puerperal sepsis.

Effects of Pregnancy on Invasive Carcinoma

- Rapid growth of tumor.
- Rapid spread if vaginal delivery is allowed.

Management

In Early Pregnancy

- Wertheim's operation or hysterectomy followed by radiation therapy.

In Late Pregnancy

- Upper segment cesarean section followed by either "Wertheim's operation or radical hysterectomy".

During Puerperium

- Tumor should be removed as early in puerperium as possible.

5. DISPLACEMENT OF PREGNANT/GRAVID UTERUS

Description

Minor variations in position of the uterus occur constantly with changes in posture with straining, with full bladder or loaded rectum. Only when the uterus rests habitually in a position beyond the limit of normal variation, it is called displacement.

Retroverted Gravid Uterus

Retroverted uterus, either congenital or acquired is considered as a normal variant of uterine position. Retroversion in pregnancy is either pre-existing or may be due to pregnancy.

Definition of Retroversion

Retroversion is the term used when the long axis of the corpus and cervix are in line and the whole organ turns backwards in relation to the long axis of the birth canal. Retroflexion signifies a bending backwards of the corpus on the cervix at the level of internal os; the two conditions are usually present together and are loosely called retroversion or retrodisplacement.

Incidence

The incidence is about 10% during first trimester of pregnancy.

Degrees

Conventionally, three degrees are described.
1. First degree: The fundus is vertical and pointing towards the sacral promontory.

2. **Second degree:** The fundus lies in the sacral hollow, but not below the internal os.
3. **Third degree:** The fundus lies below the level of the internal os.

Causes

Developmental

Retrodisplacement is quite common in fetuses and young children. Due to developmental defect, there is lack of tone of the uterine muscles. The infantile position is retained. This is often associated with short vagina with shallow anterior vaginal fornix.

Acquired

Puerperal
The stretched ligaments caused by childbirth fail to keep the uterus in its normal position. A subinvoluted, bulky uterus aggravates this condition.

Prolapse
Retroversion is usually implicated in the pathophysiology of prolapse which is mechanically caused by traction following cystocele.

Tumor
Fibroid, either in the anterior or posterior wall produces heaviness of the uterus and hence, it falls behind.

Pelvic Adhesions
Adhesions either inflammatory, operative or due to pelvic endometriosis pull the uterus posteriorly.

Anatomic Changes

Favorable
In the majority, spontaneous rectification occurs. As the uterus grows, the fundus rises spontaneously from the pelvis beyond 12 weeks. Thereafter, the pregnancy continues uneventfully.

Unfavorable
In the majority, spontaneous rectification fails to occur between 12 to 16 weeks. The developing uterus gradually fills up the pelvic cavity and becomes incarcerated.

Changes following incarceration and resulting complications:
- **Changes in the uterus:** The cervix is pointed upwards and forwards and is placed even on the upper border of the symphysis pubis. Rarely, the uterus continues to grow at the expense of the anterior wall called anterior sacculation while the thick posterior wall lies in the sacral hollow.
- **Changes in the urethra and bladder:** The major brunt falls on the lower urinary tract, predominantly on the bladder. Urethral changes include marked elongation due to stretching of the anterior vaginal wall by the cervix. This causes retention of urine.
- **Bladder changes:** As a result of retention of urine, the bladder gets distended and becomes an abdominal organ reaching even up to the umbilicus. If retention is not relieved, the following may happen:
  - The bladder walls become thickened due to edema.
  - Severe cystitis or pyelonephritis leading to uremia.
  - Intraperitoneal rupture resulting in peritonitis in neglected cases.

  Swelling due to full bladder disappears after catheterization.

Effects on Pregnancy

- **Abortion**

  If pregnancy continues with anterior sacculation, there is increased chance of malpresentation, non-engagement of fetal head, preterm delivery and rupture of uterus during labor.
- **Management**

  a. Before incarceration
  - Periodic checkup up to 12 weeks until the uterus becomes an abdominal organ. The woman is advised to empty her bladder frequently and to lie in prone position as far as possible.

  b. After incarceration
  - To empty the bladder slowly by continuous drainage with a Foley's catheter.
  - To put the patient in bed and advice to lie on her face or in Sim's position as far as practicable.

- Culture and sensitivity test of urine and administration of antibiotics. With this regimen, the uterus is expected to be corrected spontaneously within 48 hours.
- **If spontaneous correction fails**
  - Manual correction by pushing the uterus digitally through the posterior fornix under anesthesia. After correction, a Hodge-Smith pessary is to be inserted and to be kept up to 18th – 20th week.
  - In obstinate cases, when the above method fails due to adhesions, laparotomy may have to be done. Adhesiolysis may be attempted, failing which, termination of pregnancy may be indicated.
  - In diagnosed cases of anterior sacculation of the uterus, delivery by cesarean section is the method of choice.
- **Preventive measures**
  The following guidelines are helpful during the weeks after abortion or childbirth.
  - To empty the bladder at regular intervals.
  - To increase the tone of pelvic muscles by regular exercise.
  - To encourage lying in prone position for half to one hour once or twice daily for 4 to 6 weeks postpartum.

62. HYALINE MEMBRANE DISEASE/RESPIRATORY DISTRESS SYNDROME

Respiratory distress syndrome (RDS) is the most common cause of respiratory disease in preterm neonates. The disease manifests as surfactant deficiency characterized by collapsed alveoli and low lung volume. Hyaline membrane is made up of protein that is extended into the alveoli and airways of a baby with premature lungs. It is caused by deficiency of surfactant in the baby's lungs. Surfactant is made by cells in the alveolar walls. Its production slowly increases from 20 weeks gestation with a surge at 30–34 weeks and at term with the onset of labor.

Causes of Surfactant Deficiency

- Prematurity
- Perinatal asphyxia

- Maternal diabetes
- Delivery by cesarean section
- Breech delivery
- Hypothermic and hypovolemic baby.

Clinical Features

The clinical manifestations usually appear abruptly, 4–6 hours after birth:
- Respiratory rate more than 60 per minute
- Rib retraction
- Expiratory grunt
- Cyanosis.

Prevention

- Administration of betamethasone to mothers anticipating preterm delivery specially before 36 weeks
- Assessment of lung maturity before premature induction of labor and to delay induction as much as possible without any risk to the fetus
- Prevent fetal hypoxia in diabetic mothers.

Treatment

- The baby to be nursed in a warm incubator with high humidity; air passage is cleaned periodically through endotracheal suction
- Warmed, humidified oxygen therapy in concentration of 35–45% under positive pressure to be administered through endotracheal intubation to relieve hypoxia and acidosis
- Prevention and treatment of infection
- Correction of hypovolemia with albumin or other colloid solutions
- Correction of anemia and electrolyte imbalance, if any.
- Frequent monitoring of partial pressure of oxygen (pO_2), partial pressure of carbon dioxide (pCO_2), pH and base excess to detect metabolic and respiratory acidosis
- Surfactant therapy
- Intragastric feeding if possible
- Intravenous administration of 10% glucose if there is chance of vomiting and aspiration.

Complications

Important complications of hyaline membrane disease are:
- Intraventricular hemorrhage
- Bronchopulmonary dysplasia
- Pulmonary hemorrhage
- Pneumothorax
- Retrolental fibroplasia
- Neurological abnormalities.

Prognosis

About one third of the babies die with it. Babies with mild affection may survive, if acidosis and biochemical abnormalities are corrected effectively. Infants who survive usually have no untoward effect in the long run.

63. HYDATIDIFORM MOLE/VESICULAR MOLE

Hydatidiform mole is an abnormal conceptus in which the chorionic villi will show hydropic degeneration of the connective tissue stroma and hyperplastic changes of the trophoblastic epithelium. The resulting conceptus appears like an amorphous conglomeration of grape-like semitranslucent cystic vesicles of varying sizes. It is regarded as a benign neoplasm of the chorion with a high malignant potential.

Clinical Features

Hydatidiform mole is prevalent amongst teenaged and elderly patients with high parity. The patient gives history of amenorrhea of 8–12 weeks with initial features suggestive of pregnancy, but subsequently presents with the following manifestations:
- Vaginal bleeding: It may be preceded by a brownish or watery discharge. The blood may be mixed with fluid from ruptured cysts giving the appearance of 'white currant in red currant juice'
- Lower abdominal pain: This is due to overdistension of the uterus, concealed hemorrhage, infection, perforation or uterine contraction to expel out the contents

- Constitutional symptoms: It is like excessive vomiting, breathlessness, thyrotoxic features of tremors or tachycardia and feeling sick without any apparent reason
- Expulsion of grape-like vesicles per vagina
- Features of early pregnancy
- Pallor out of proportion to the visible blood loss
- Features of preeclampsia (hypertension, edema and/or proteinuria)
- The size of the uterus is more than that expected for the period of amenorrhea
- The feel of the uterus is firm elastic (doughy) due to the absence of amniotic fluid
- Fetal parts are not felt or any fetal movements
- Absence of fetal heart sounds.

On Vaginal Examination

- Internal ballottement cannot be elicited
- Unilateral or bilateral enlargement of ovaries
- Findings of vesicles in the vaginal discharge.

Investigations

- Complete blood count, ABO and Rh grouping
- Hepatic, renal and thyroid function tests
- Sonography: 'snow storm' appearance
- Estimation of chorionic gonadotropin (hCG titer) positive in urine diluted up to 1 (in 200) to 1 (in 500) beyond 100 days is very much suggestive
- X-ray abdomen. If the uterine size is more than 16 weeks, a negative fetal shadow is suggestive.

Management

Evacuation of the hydatidiform mole is to be achieved as soon as the diagnosis is made. Any of the following methods of termination may be followed:
- Suction evacuation supplemented by oxytocin drip
- Slow dilatation of the cervix with PGE_2 (dinoprostone) followed by oxytocin drip and evacuation

- Hysterotomy is indicated when the vaginal bleeding is profuse, cervix unfavorable and general condition is poor
- Hysterectomy is indicated in patients with age over 35 years and in those who completed their families.

Follow-up Protocol

- A curettage is usually done 5–7 days following evacuation, when uterine wall gets thicker and firmer and cavity becomes smaller
- Prophylactic chemotherapy is administered if the hCG titers fail to become negative in 4–6 weeks or the level of excretion exceeds 40,000 IU. Drugs commonly used are methotrexate and actinomycin D
- Follow-up is mandatory to all cases for at least one year. The objective is to diagnose persistent trophoblastic proliferation that is considered malignant. The occurnce of choriocarcinoma is mostly confined to this period
- Initially the check-up should be at intervals of one week till the hCG titers in urine becomes negative by immunological test. Once negative, the patient is followed-up at 1 month interval for 1 year
- Follow-up protocols include history and physical examination, hCG assay and chest X-ray
- Contraceptive advice: The patient is advised not to become pregnant for at least 2 years. Barrier method of contraception can be used safely.

Other Entities of Hydatidiform Mole

Partial Hydatidiform Mole

Partial hydatidiform mole is an abnormal conceptus with an embryo/fetus that tends to die early. Part of the placenta may reveal molar changes, and the rest would remain as the functional organ. There is focal villous swelling and focal trophoblastic hyperplasia, usually involving the syncytiotrophoblast only.

The clinical picture does not differ markedly from complete mole and may be confused with threatened or missed abortion. Once the diagnosis is made and the fetus is not alive, termination of pregnancy is to be done. Even if the fetus is alive, the patient should be warned about the risks to the baby if the pregnancy is continued.

Post-termination follow-up protocol should be the same as outlined in complete mole. As the chance of malignancy is much less, follow-up care is advised for 3–6 months and till the hCG level returns to normal.

Persistent Trophoblastic Disease

Persistence of active molar tissue with continued elevation of serum or urine hCG levels 8 weeks after evacuation of hydatidiform mole.

Diagnosis

This state is diagnosed during post-evacuation follow-up period. The diagnostic features are:
- Continued vaginal bleeding
- Persistent theca lutein cysts
- Persistent soft and enlarged uterus
- The hCG titers in urine and blood fail to become negative by 8 weeks postmolar evacuation
- Diagnostic curettage when performed, exhibits either hydatidiform mole or choriocarcinoma.

Treatment

- Hysterectomy for those nearing 40 years or completed her family
- Chemotherapy is indicated in young patients where the uterus is to be preserved. Methotrexate and Actinomycin D are used either singly or in combination. Regular follow-up is essential following hysterectomy or during chemotherapy.

64. HYDRAMNIOS/POLYHYDRAMNIOS

Polyhydramnios (hydramnios) is a pathologic condition characterized by an excessive amount of amniotic fluid. It is arbitrarily defined as the presence of more than 2,000 mL of liquor amni, because it becomes clinically evident beyond this:
- Incidence: Hydramnios is detectable in 0.5–1.5% of pregnancies. Polyhydramnios sufficient to cause clinical symptoms (over 3–4 L) occurs in 1 in 1,000 pregnancies

- Etiology: In many cases it is idiopathic and no cause can be found.
  Maternal causes:
  - Diabetes mellitus
  - Cardiac or renal disease.
- Fetal causes
  - Fetal malformations such as anencephaly, spina bifida, hydrocephaly and meningomyelocele
  - Multiple pregnancy
  - Hydrops fetalis in Rh incompatibility
  - Esophageal or duodenal atresia
  - Facial clefts and neck masses.
- Clinical features: Acute polyhydramnios occurs earlier in pregnancy and rapidly in rare cases. This variety generally occurs in the second trimester of pregnancy before the fetus is viable. Preterm labor before 28 weeks is frequent in such cases. Chronic polyhydramnios occurs usually between 32 and 40 weeks. Manifestations are:
  - Dyspnea especially in the lying down position
  - Palpitation
  - Edema of legs, varicosities in legs or vulva and hemorrhoids
  - Evidence of preeclampsia (edema, hypertension and proteinuria).
- Inspection of abdomen:
  - Abdomen is markedly enlarged, appearing globular with fullness at the flanks
  - The skin is tense, shiny with large striae.
- Palpation:
  - Height is of the fundus is more than the period of amenorrhea
  - Girth of the abdomen is more than normal
  - Fluid thrill can be elicited in all directions over the uterus
  - Fetal parts, presentation and position cannot be made out easily; external ballottement can be elicited more easily.
- Auscultation:
  - Fetal heart sounds are not heard distinctly, although they can be picked up by Doppler.
- Ultrasonography:
  - Detects large, echo-free space between the fetus and the uterine wall
  - Fetal abnormalities can be detected if present.

- Differential diagnosis:
  - Multiple pregnancy
  - Pregnancy with huge ovarian cyst
  - Maternal or fetal ascitis.
- Management:
  - Supportive therapy includes bedrest, if needed with a back rest, analgesics and sedatives when required, and treatment of associated conditions such as pregnancy-induced hypertension (PIH), and diabetes
  - If patient is responsive to therapy, pregnancy is to be continued awaiting spontaneous delivery at term
  - In unresponsive cases with maternal distress, slow decompression with amniocentesis is done
  - About 500–1,000 mL of fluid is drained to provide relief to the patient; the procedure may be repeated as re-accumulation occurs; a beta mimetic drug (isoxsuprine and ritodrine) may be given to reduce the risk of premature labor
  - Termination of pregnancy is done in the presence of fetal abnormality irrespective of the period of gestation.
- Complications of polyhydramnios:
  - Fetal malpresentations.
  - Premature rupture of membranes and associated problems such as preterm labor, abruption of placenta or prolapse of umbilical cord.
  - Inefficient uterine contractions and prolonged labor.
  - Postpartum atony and postpartum hemorrhage (PPH).
  - Amniotic fluid embolism may follow oxytocin induction without amniotomy.

Nursing Considerations for Client in Late Pregnancy and Labor

Nursing considerations depend also on the contributing causes and maternal symptoms. When the client is admitted in preterm labor, nursing care focuses on tocolysis, fetal and maternal monitoring and prevention of side effects of therapy. In addition, maternal comfort is usually challenging because of dyspnea due to uterine distention some of the nursing considerations are:

- Elevation of head of bed, pulse oxymetry and oxygen supplementation by nasal cannula are beneficial during labor
- Once delivery is inevitable, the neonatal team should be notified of the premature labor and anticipated fetal anomalies
- Diligent education, emotional support and encouragement are nursing interventions, which may support the client to cope with her situation.

ACUTE POLYHYDRAMNIOS

Acute polyhydramnios is an extremely rare condition. The onset is acute and the fluid accumulates within a few days. It usually occurs before 20 weeks of pregnancy. It is usually associated with uniovular twins or chorioangioma of the placenta:

- Clinical manifestations:
  - Features of acute abdomen such as abdominal pain, nausea and vomiting
  - Edema of the legs or presence of features of preeclampsia
  - Enlarged abdomen, more than the period of amenorrhea
  - Presence of fluid thrill
  - Fetal parts not felt
  - Patient appears ill
  - Sonography reveals multiple features or fetal abnormalities.
- Treatment:
  - Decompression through amniocentesis in an attempt to prolong the pregnancy, if no fetal abnormalities
  - If fetal abnormalities are detected, pregnancy is terminated by low rupture of membranes, with care to allow slow escape of fluid.

OLIGOHYDRAMNIOS

Oligohydramnios refers to the condition where the amount of amniotic fluid is less than expected for pregnancy. The volume is 500 mL or less between 32 and 36 weeks of pregnancy.

Etiology

The cause is not known, but oligohydramnios is seen associated with the following conditions:

- Renal agenesis in the fetus (Potter's syndrome) or an obstruction to the fetal urinary tract
- Intrauterine growth retardation associated with placental insufficiency
- Pregnancies that are prolonged several weeks beyond term.

Diagnosis of Oligohydramnios

- Uterine size much smaller than the period of amenorrhea
- Less fetal movements
- The uterus is 'full of fetus' as the liquor is scanty
- Malpresentations such as breech
- Evidence of intrauterine growth retardation
- If membranes are artificially ruptured, there is scanty escape of liquor, which is often meconium stained.

Complications

Fetal

- Deformities due to intra-amniotic adhesions or due to compression, e.g. alteration in shape of skull, amputation of fetal limbs
- Pressure deformities such as club foot
- Pulmonary hypoplasia
- Dry, lethargy and wrinkled skin
- Increased fetal mortality due to hypoxia.

Maternal

- Prolonged labor due to inertia
- Increased operative intervention due to malpresentation.

Treatment

Premature rupture of membranes for early termination of pregnancy.

Nursing Considerations for Client in Labor

- Thorough maternal-fetal assessment with fetal monitoring
- Monitoring for signs of infection in the event of the membranes ruptured early or leaking
- Anticipatory grief support if the fetus has significant anomalies

- Ongoing fetal monitoring if amnioinfusion is done during labor to relieve cord and fetal compression
- Supplemental oxygenation by face mask to improve fetal status
- Intravenous (IV) hydration to avoid perfusion complications that increases fetal stress
- Neonatal resuscitation equipment and team should be ready
- Acknowledge the parents' loss and accept their grief in the event of perinatal loss
- Support with the grieving process according to protocol.

65. HYPEREMESIS GRAVIDARUM

Hyperemesis gravidarum is a severe type of vomiting of pregnancy, which has adverse effects on the health of the mother and incapacitates her in her day-to-day activities.

Predisposing Factors

- Psychological and emotional stress
- Primigravid status
- Women with multiple pregnancies
- Molar pregnancies
- Familial tendency
- Unplanned pregnancies.

Clinical Manifestations

- Vomiting independent of food, spread throughout the day (Vomitus consists of bile-stained fluid, pogresses to coffee ground or blood stained)
- Oliguria
- Constipation and at times diarrhea
- Epigastric pain
- Progressive emaciation with loss of weight
- Loss of skin elasticity
- Weight loss
- Electrolyte imbalance and starvation-induced ketoacidosis
- Neurological damage
- Liver damage (jaundice)

- Kidney impairment (oliguria, anuria)
- Metabolic disturbances
- Anxious look and sunken eyes
- Tongue dry, thickly coated or red and raw
- Teeth covered with sordes
- Blood pressure low
- Temperature raised to 100°F or more
- Korsakoff's psychosis—loss of memory of recent events
- Eye complications—diplopia, dimness of vision or even blindness.

Investigations

- Urinalysis: Small quantity, dark color, high specific gravity with acid reaction. Presence of acetone and rarely bile pigments
- Serum electrolytes
- Ophthalmoscopic examination if patient is seriously ill. Retinal hemorrhage and retinal detachment are possible unfavorable signs
- Electrocardiogram (ECG) when there is abnormal potassium levels
- Pelvic ultrasound to exclude molar pregnancy.

Management

- Hospitalization for skillful management to eliminate neurogenic element
- Correction of fluid and electrolyte imbalance with IV fluids
- Oral feeding is withheld for at least 24 hours after the cessation of vomiting
- Medications including:
  - Antihistamine and antiemetic drugs, e.g. promethazine (Phenergan), prochlorperazine (Stemetil)
  - Sedatives, e.g. diazepam
  - Vitamins: Vitamin B_6, vitamin C and B complex
  - Hydrocortisone in case of hypotension.
- Therapeutic termination of pregnancy, if the woman's condition deteriorates in spite of therapy.

Complications

- Neurological complications: Wernicke's encephalopathy, peripheral neuropathy, Korsakoff's psychosis
- Stress ulcer in stomach
- Jaundice.

Nursing Considerations

- Sympathetic yet firm handling
- Regular oral hygiene
- Maintaining record of:
  - Fluid intake and output
  - Character of vomitus
  - Total peripheral resistance (TPR) and blood pressure (BP)
  - Urine tests for specific gravity, acetone, protein, bile and chloride
  - Serum electrolytes
  - Body weight on admission and again when out of bed
  - Electrocardiogram (ECG) to ascertain potassium status
  - Findings of ophthalmoscopic examination.
- Identify, record and report change in condition/improvement as manifested, e.g. feeling of hunger, better look, disappearance of acetone from urine, moist tongue, falling pulse rate and rising blood pressure and increase in urine output
- Start oral feeding before intravenous fluid is omitted
  - At first, dry carbohydrate foods such as biscuits, bread and toast are given
  - The diet needs to be normalized quickly as the stomach is more likely to retain solids than liquids
  - Meals at frequent intervals such as six times a day are tolerated better
- Psychological preparation and support to women who do not respond to treatment and for whom termination of pregnancy is decided as the preferred line of management
- Prepare client and assist for the termination procedures, which may be vaginal or through hysterotomy.

Nursing Diagnoses

Numbers 59, 67, 81, 91 and 94 in Appendix.

66. HYSTERECTOMY

Hysterectomy is the surgical removal of the uterus.

Types of Hysterectomy

- Total hysterectomy: Removal of the uterus and cervix
- Subtotal hysterectomy: Removal of the uterus with the cervix spared
- Pan hysterectomy: Removal of the uterus along with the tubes and ovaries on both sides
- Radical hysterectomy: Removal of the uterus, tubes and ovaries on both sides, upper one third of vagina, adjacent parametrium and the pelvic lymph nodes
- Extended hysterectomy: Pan hysterectomy with removal of cuff of vagina.

Routes of Surgery

- Abdominal:
  - Through abdominal incision
  - Through laparoscope.
- Vaginal:
  - Through vaginal incision
  - Laparoscopy assisted.

Indications

Benign lesions:
- Dysfunctional uterine bleeding
- Fibroid uterus
- Tubo-ovarian mass
- Endometriosis
- Cervical intraepithelial neoplasia
- Endometrial hyperplasia
- Benign ovarian tumor in perimenopausal age.

Malignancy:
- Carcinoma ovary, endometrium or cervix
- Uterine sarcoma
- Choriocarcinoma.

- Traumatic:
- Uterine perforation
- Cervical tear
- Rupture of uterus.

Obstetrical:
- Atonic PPH
- Morbid adherent placenta
- Hydatidiform mole > 35 years
- Septic abortion.

Preoperative management:
- History, physical examination and pelvic examination
- Physical preparation as for a laparotomy—local preparation of lower abdomen, pubic and perineal region
- Bowel to be emptied by giving an enema
- Bladder to be emptied prior to sending to operating room
- Antiseptic vaginal douche previous evening
- Preoperative instructions
- Psychological preparation
- Preoperative medications.

Postoperative Management

- General postoperative care as for abdominal surgery patient
- Particular attention to peripheral circulation to prevent thrombophlebitis and deep vein thrombosis (DVT), such as leg exercises and elastic compression stockings
- Attention to voiding problems following vaginal hysterectomy
- Education regarding outcome of surgery, possible feelings of loss and options for management of symptoms of menopause.

Nursing Diagnoses

- Anxiety related to diagnosis
- Fear of pain, possible perception of loss of feminity or childbearing potential
- Acute pain related to surgery and other adjuvant therapy
- Deficient knowledge of postoperative aspects of hysterectomy and postoperative self-care.

67. HYSTEROSALPINGOGRAPHY

An X-ray study of the uterus and the fallopian tubes after injection of a contrast agent.

Purpose

To evaluate infertility or tubal patency and to detect any abnormal condition in the uterine cavity.

Patient Preparation

- Hysterosalpingography (HSG) is done between day 6 and day 10 of the cycle
- Antibiotic prophylaxis is given
- Laxatives and enema may be administered to evacuate the intestinal tract to avoid any gas shadow in the X-ray findings
- Analgesics may be prescribed.

Procedure

- Patient to be in lithotomy position
- Cervix is exposed with a bivalve speculum
- A cannula is inserted into the cervix and the contrast agent injected into the uterine cavity and fallopian tubes
- X-rays are taken to show the path and distribution of the contrast agent.

Patient Management

- Some patients experience nausea, vomiting, cramps and faintness
- After the test, the patient has to be instructed to wear a perineal pad for several hours as the radio opaque contrast agent may stain the clothing.

Possible Complications

- Uterine perforation and hemorrhage
- Peritoneal irritation and pelvic pain

- Vasovagal attack
- Intravasation of dye within the venous or lymphatic channels
- Flaring up of pelvic infection.

Contraindications to HSG

- Pelvic infection
- Presence of hydrosalpinx
- Presence of adnexal mass (PID)
- Pelvic tenderness on bimanual examination.

68. IMMEDIATE CARE OF THE NEWBORN

INTRODUCTION

Immediate care of the newborn baby is an important first step in allowing term babies to transition safely between intrauterine and newborn life. The majority of babies will make this transition without requiring anything other than the basic care. Unfortunately some babies "will be born compromised" before or during the birth process. These are sometimes recognized through intrauterine monitoring, whilst others will be unexpected. Such babies require high quality resuscitation at birth.

Whether it is a term newborn or a premature newborn, knowledge of the physiology underlying the transition from intrauterine to extrauterine life is essential to support babies effectively.

PHYSIOLOGICAL CHANGES AT BIRTH

Amazing physiological changes occur with birth. When the baby is delivered the umbilical cord is clamped and cut close to or near the navel. This ends the baby's dependence on the placenta for oxygen and nutrition. As the baby takes its first breath, air moves into the lungs.

Before birth, the lungs are not used to exchange oxygen and carbondioxide, and need less blood supply away from the lungs through special connections in the heart and large blood vessels. When a baby starts to breathe air at birth, the change in pressure in the lungs helps close the fetal connections and redirect blood flow. Now blood is pumped to the lungs to help with the exchange of oxygen and carbon dioxide. Some babies have too much fluid in their lungs. Stimulating the baby to cry, by massaging and stroking the skin can help bring the fluid up where it can be suctioned from the nose and mouth.

Care of the Baby in the Delivery Room

- Providing warmth for the newborn.
  A newborn baby is wet from the amniotic fluid and can easily become cold. Drying the baby and removing wet linen is an important first step. Drying the baby and using warm blankets and heat lamps can help prevent heat loss. Often a knitted hat is placed on the baby's head in cold climate. Placing a baby skin to skin on mother's chest or abdomen also helps to keep the baby warm. This early skin to skin contact reduces crying, improves interactions with mother and breast feed successfully. Before transferring to mother's chest, most institutions carry out initial steps in a radiant warmer which provides warmth and convenience for providing care **(Fig. 68.1)**.

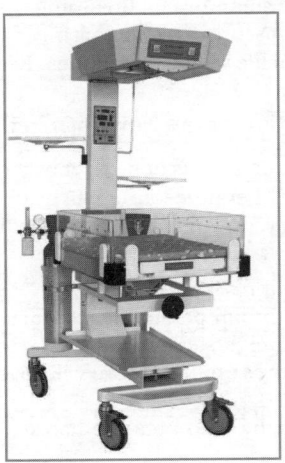

Fig. 68.1: Radiant warmer.

- Health assessment of the new baby must start right way. One of the first assessment is the Apgar scoring. This is to evaluate the condition of the newborn at one minute and five minutes after birth. The midwife or nurse will evaluate the signs and give a point value.

Apgar Scoring System

Indicator	0 - Point	1 - Point	2 - Points
A-Activity (Muscle tone)	Absent	Flaccid arms and legs	Active
P-Pulse	Absent	Below 100/bpm	Over 100/bpm
G-Grimace (Reflex irritability)	Floppy	Minimal response to stimulation	Prompt response to stimulation
A-Appearance (skin color)	Blue/Pale	Pink body, blue extremities	Pink
R-Respiration	Absent	Slow and irregular	Vigorous cry

A score of 7–10 is considered normal. A score of 4–6 may mean that the baby needs some rescue breathing measures, oxygen and careful monitoring. A score of 3 or below means that the baby needs rescue breathing and life saving techniques (Resuscitation).

Physical Examination of the Newborn in the Delivery Room

A brief physical examination is done to check for obvious signs that the baby is healthy. Other procedures will be done over the next few hours in the delivery room, in the nursery or in the room, depending on the hospital policy.

Some of these procedures include:
- Measurement of the temperature, heart rate and respiratory rate.
- Measurement of weight, length and head circumference.
- Cord care: The baby's umbilical cord will have a clamp. It needs to be kept clean and dry.
- Bath: Once the baby's temperature has stabilized the first bath can be given.

- Eye care: The baby will be given antibiotic or antiseptic eye drops or ointment either right after delivery or later to prevent eye infection that can occur from mother's birth canal.
- Footprints: These are often taken and recorded in the mother's medical record.

Before the baby leaves the delivery area, ID bracelets with matching numbers are placed on the baby and mother. Babies often have two ID bands, one on the wrist and another on the ankle. The first hour or two after birth, for babies of normal vaginal birth, it is the best time to start breast-feeding. Babies have an innate ability to start nursing right away after they are born. Most healthy babies are able to breastfeed in these first few hours.

Care of Newborns after Cesarean Section

Babies born by cesarean section may have trouble clearing some of the lung fluid and mucus, they often need extra suctioning of the nose, mouth and throat. In some cases they need deeper suctioning in the trachea and oxygen administration.

Babies born by C-sections are brought to mother to see and touch, after the baby is checked and wrapped warmly and then watched in the nursery for a short time till the mother recovers from anesthetic effects.

Babies who may have trouble at birth include those born prematurely, those born in a difficult delivery or those born with a birth defect. These babies need treatment and care in Neonatal Intensive Care Units (NICU).

69. IMMUNIZATION

Immunization is the process by which an individual's immune system becomes fortified against an infectious agent. A person becomes protected against a disease through vaccination or inoculation. WHO definition states that immunization is the process whereby a person is made immune or resistant to an infectious disease **(Table 69.1)**.

Table 69.1: National Immunization Schedule (NIS) for Infants, Children and Pregnant Women 2021.

Vaccine	When to give	Dose	Route	Site
For Pregnant Women				
TT-1	Early in pregnancy	0.5 mL	Intra-muscular	Upper arm
TT-2	4 weeks after TT-1	0.5 mL	Intra-muscular	Upper arm
TT- Booster	If received 2 TT doses in a pregnancy within the last 3 years	0.5 mL	Intra-muscular	Upper arm
For Infants				
BCG	At birth or as early as possible till one year of age	0.1 mL (0.05 mL until 1 month age)	Intra-dermal	Left upper arm
Hepatitis B - Birth dose	At birth or as early as possible within 24 hours	0.5 mL	Intra-muscular	Antero-lateral side of mid-thigh
OPV-0	At birth or as early as possible within the first 15 days	2 drops	Oral	Oral
OPV 1, 2 and 3	At 6 weeks, 10 weeks and 14 weeks (OPV can be given till 5 years of age)	2 drops	Oral	Oral
Pentavalent 1, 2 and 3	At 6 weeks, 10 weeks and 14 weeks (can be given till one year of age)	0.5 mL	Intra-muscular	Antero-lateral side of mid-thigh
Rotavirus	At 6 weeks, 10 weeks and 14 weeks (can be given till one year of age)	5 drops	Oral	Oral

Contd...

Contd...

Vaccine	When to give	Dose	Route	Site
IPV	Two fractional dose at 6 and 14 weeks of age	0.1 mL	Intra-dermal two fractional dose	Intra-dermal: Right upper arm
Measles /MR 1st dose	9 completed months–12 months (can be given till 5 years of age)	0.5 mL	Sub-cutaneous	Right upper arm
*JE - 1	9 completed months–12 months	0.5 mL	Sub-cutaneous	Left upper arm
Vitamin A (1st dose)	At 9 completed months with measles, rubella	1 mL (1 lakh IU)	Oral	Oral
For Children				
DPT booster-1	16–24 months	0.5 mL	Intra-muscular	Antero-lateral side of mid-thigh
**Measles/MR 2nd dose	16–24 months	0.5 mL	Sub-cutaneous	Right upper arm
OPV Booster	16–24 months	2 drops	Oral	Oral
*JE-2	16–24 months	0.5 mL	Sub-cutaneous	Left upper arm
Vitamin A (2nd to 9th dose)	16–18 months. Then one dose every 6 months up to the age of 5 years	2 mL (2 lakh IU)	Oral	Oral
DPT Booster-2	5–6 years	0.5 mL	Intra-muscular	Upper arm
TT	10 years and 16 years	0.5 mL	Intra-muscular	Upper arm

*JE Vaccine- Japanese Encephalitis Vaccine. Introduced in select endemic districts after the campaign.

**Phased introduction, at present in five states namely Karnataka, Tamil Nadu, Goa, Lakshadweep and Puducherry.

Source: www:/nhm.gov.in

Vaccination versus immunization
- Vaccination is the use of vaccines to stimulate a person's immune system to protect that individual against an infection or disease.
- Immunization is the process of making an individual immune or resistant to an infectious disease typically via vaccination. Immunity or resistance to a disease occurs due to vaccination, it is a process that happens in one's body. It can also happen from exposure to pathogens. Inoculation has come to mean the same as immunization

Immunization prevents several illnesses, and safeguards from vaccine-preventable diseases. Some of the vaccine preventable diseases include Hepatitis, Poliomyelitis, Pertussis, Diphtheria and Tetanus. Immunization is a key component of primary health care and an indisputable human right. It is also one of the best health investments. Childhood immunization not only protects children from deadly diseases, but they also keep other children from getting such illnesses. Vaccination or immunizing them strengthens their immune system and helps them stay free of preventable diseases.

Immunization is essential as it is important for prevention of childhood diseases and disabilities and is thus a basic need for all children. This starts in the early neonatal period itself where early protection is desirable. The following schedule has been recommended by the Indian Academy of Pediatrics in 2021 for children aged 0 – 18 years.

Nursing Responsibilities for Child Immunization

Nursing personnel are mostly responsible for administration of immunization and its related activities in collaboration with other health team members. The nursing personnel should shoulder the responsibility to organize the immunization sessions and to ensure the achievement of the benefit of universal immunization programme. Though administration of vaccine is the main assignment, other related activities are also vital for the success of the programme. The nursing responsibilities at various levels can be summarized as follows.

- Motivation of people about the importance of immunization and its benefits.
- Estimation of beneficiaries of the area and identification of nonparticipants and dropouts.
- Assessment of problems and reasons for non-acceptance and intervening to solve the problems.
- Providing information, health education and communication sessions regarding time, place, available vaccines and other health facilities related to immunization.
- Organization of immunization clinics at different institutions, immunization camps, out-reach and home-based services.
- Arrangements and maintenance of required amount of vaccines and other necessary articles for the particular immunization center or clinic. Maintenance of cold- chain system at the center and during transportation to the clinic with necessary precautions to preserve the efficiency and potency of vaccines.
- Administration of vaccines in accordance with the basic nursing skills and instructions related to the use specific vaccines.
- Observation of possible reactions after vaccination and providing necessary instructions about care of the child following immunization, to the parent and family.
- Providing information about the next date of visit to complete the immunization as per schedule and dangers of default.
- Maintenance of immunization card with required information and next date of visit.
- Reporting about immunization coverage and problems of particular area.
- Updating own knowledge regarding advancement of immunization practices and changing attitudes.

70. INDUCTION OF LABOR

Induction of labor is deliberate termination of pregnancy beyond 28 weeks of gestation by a method that aims to secure a normal vaginal delivery. The procedure, if possible is deferred until after the 36th week when the fetus attains reasonable maturity.

INDICATIONS FOR INDUCTION

Induction of labor is indicated in those conditions where continuation of pregnancy may adversely affect the maternal or fetal wellbeing.

Fetal

- Postmaturity
- History of unexplained intrauterine death
- Chronic placental insufficiency
- Rh-isoimmunization
- Unstable lie after correcting into longitudinal lie
- Intrauterine death of fetus.

Maternal

- Chronic polyhydramnios with maternal distress
- Congenital malformations of the fetus
- Uncontrolled chorea gravidarum.

Combined

- Preeclampsia and eclampsia
- Minor degree of placenta previa
- Abruptio placentae (early termination to save mother and baby from complications)
- Premature rupture of membranes
- Chronic hypertension
- Chronic renal disease.

Elective Induction

Deliberate termination of pregnancy at term for the convenience of the patient, obstetrician or hospital.

CONTRAINDICATIONS

- Contracted pelvis and cephalopelvic disproportion
- Persistent malpresentation
- Previous classical cesarean section (CS)
- Elderly primigravida with associated medical or obstetric complications
- Heart disease
- High-risk pregnancy with compromised fetus
- Pelvic tumor
- Pregnancy following repair of vesicovaginal fistula
- Presence of active herpetic genital lesions.

ASSESSMENT FOR INDUCTION

Prior to induction of labor the following factors have to be considered carefully:
- The period of gestation, the expected date of delivery (EDD) and ultrasound reports
- Pelvic capacity in relation to size of fetal head
- Fetal presentation
- The state of the cervix and the station of the presenting part.

SELECTION OF TIME

When the termination is done for maternal interest, induction is done ignoring the gestational period. When the induction is done for fetal interest, a fair idea about the maturity of the fetus has to be obtained prior to induction. Assessment of the fetal well-being has also to be ascertained.

SUCCESS OF INDUCTION

Success of induction depends on:
- Period of gestation—the uterus is more sensitive nearer to term or post-term
- Patient profile—the induction is more successful in parous women and in cases with premature rupture of membranes. In

Table 70.1: Bishop scoring system.

Factors	0	1	2	3
Cervix dilation	Closed	1–2 cm	3–4 cm	5–6 cm
Effacement	1–30%	40–50%	60–70%	80+%
Consistency	Firm	Medium	Soft	–
Position	Posterior	Midline	Anterior	–
Fetal head station	– 3	– 2	– 1	+ 1, + 2

Table 70.2: Predictive value of Bishop scores.

Scores	Rate (%)
0–4	Induction failure rate (40–50%)
5–9	Induction failure rate (10%)
10–13	Failure rate (0%)

elderly primigrvidae and intrauterine death of fetus, the uterus is likely to be less responsive
- Sensitivity of the uterus—the induction is likely to be successful if the uterus readily contracts on massaging and sensitive to oxytocin as seen on sensitivity test (the response occurs with 0.04 units or less of oxytocin)
- Preinduction scoring—a favorable score on Bishop scoring **(Table 70.1)** indicates better results.

Predictive value: It is mentioned in **Table 70.2**:
- Total score: 13
- Favorable score: 6–13
- Unfavorable score: 0–5.

METHODS OF INDUCTION

Medical Induction

Medical induction is done in cases of:
- Intrauterine death
- Premature rupture of membranes

Induction of Labor

- Failed surgical induction
- Along with surgical induction to shorten the induction-delivery interval.

Drugs used: Oxytocin and prostaglandins.

Oxytocin Induction

Oxytocin is an octapeptide (8 amino acids) containing a pentapeptide ring and a tripeptide side chain. Synthetic oxytocin preparations, syntocinon and pitocin are commonly used. Syntocinon is available in ampules containing 2 IU/mL and pitocin in 5 IU/mL. The drug is widely used as intravenous infusion. Its infusion may be started without rupture of membranes or in conjunction with artificial rupture of the forewaters.

Dose

Five units of oxytocin in 500 mL of dextrose give approximately 0.5 μ in one drop of infusion. The drip is started with 5 μ/min (10 drops), increasing at intervals of 15–30 min, according to the strength and frequency of uterine contractions, to a maximum of 30 μ/min.

Dangers of oxytocin

- In coordinate uterine action, especially uterine hyperstimulation
- Fetal hypoxia
- Uterine rupture in multipara
- Water intoxication, due to mild antidiuretic effect of oxytocin.

Nursing considerations

- Constant supervision is essential for the patient receiving intravenous oxytocin infusion
- Uterine contractions and fetal heart rate need to be observed constantly as sudden alterations in response may occur
- The progress of labor needs to be monitored carefully using a partogram.

Nursing alert

Oxytocin should always be administered through an infusion pump and inserted by piggyback through the main intravenous (IV) line as an accidental bolus can be life-threatening to both mother and fetus. In case of hyperstimulation of uterus, turn off the pitocin, change client's position to left lateral, administer oxygen and notify physician.

Prostaglandin Induction of labor

Prostaglandins are drugs that are like the actual hormones that trigger off labor and are used to "prime" the cervix. This process makes the cervix softer and shorter preparing it for induction of labor.

Forms of Medications

- Prostaglandin E_2, also known as Dinoprostone is a naturally occurring prostaglandin with oxytocic properties that is used as a medication. Dinoprostone is used in labor induction, in cases of bleeding after delivery, in termination of pregnancy, and in newborn babies to keep the ductus arteriosus open.
- Prostaglandin F_2a, is a different formulation of prostaglandin. Both E_2 and F_2a, are used as gels, tablets and pessaries.
- Misoprostol is a synthetic analogue of prostaglandin E_1. Misoprostol has uterotonic properties. By contracting the smooth muscle fibers in the myometrium and causing relaxation of cervix, it facilitates ripening of the cervix.

Use of Prostaglandins

- Prostaglandin E_2 and F_2 are used for induction of labor.
- Different formulations of prostaglandins- PGE_2 and PGF_2a, are used as gels, tablets and pessaries.
- Misoprostol is administered orally as 50 mcg tablets or vaginally as 25 mcg suppositories. Vaginal application is repeated every 4 hours if contractions do not appear or are not painful.

Advantages

- Effective method for use in cases of intrauterine death or in cases of unfavorable cervix.
- No antidiuretic effect.

Drawbacks

- More systemic side effects when used orally or intravenously, but vaginal administration has minimal side effects.
- The adverse uterine effect (hyperstimulation) if occurs, usually lasts for a longer period compared to oxytocin.
- Systemic side effects include pyrexia, diarrhea and vomiting.

Other Drugs used for Induction

Nitric oxide donors (Glyceryl trinitrate, isosorbide mononitrate)
- It has been suggested that nitric oxide compounds which stimulate cervical ripening without stimulating uterine contractions and may be used as an effective outpatient cervical ripening method.
- They have been found to be less effective than prostaglandins, but have fewer safety concerns and higher patient satisfaction.
  Used in combination with prostaglandins (inpatients), their use may be synergistic resulting in shorter induction to vaginal delivery time and reduced uterine tachysystole.

Surgical Induction

The initiation of labor is attempted by surgical method and is almost exclusively done by rupture of the membranes.

Amniotomy (Artificial Rupture of Membranes)

With the usual aseptic care, the index or middle finger is inserted through the cervical os. The membranes below the presenting part overlying the internal os are ruptured with a Kocher's forceps. Some amount of liquor drains out. After rupture of the membranes, color of the amniotic fluid, status of the cervix, station of the head, presence or absence of cord prolapse and quality of fetal heart rate (FHR) are to be noted.

Advantages

- A relatively easy procedure when the cervix is ripe
- Quite effective when combined with oxytocin infusion; in 80% of patients labor starts within 8 hours
- It is a safe method of delivery if completed within 24–48 hours.

Contraindications

Chronic hydramnios; sudden decompression may precipitate early separation of the placenta and accidental hemorrhage.

Hazards

- Cord prolapse
- Uncontrolled escape of amniotic fluid
- Injury to the cervix or the presenting part
- Rupture of vasa-previa leading to fetal blood loss
- Amnionitis.

Hindwater Rupture (High Rupture of Membranes)

This procedure is performed by introducing a specially designed metal instrument—Drew Smythe catheter above the presenting part. The membranes are then ruptured by pushing up a sharp stilette.

This procedure is rarely performed in modern obstetrics. The claimed advantages were that the forewaters were intact and infection is less likely and the risk of cord prolapse is not increased. But it is not as effective as rupture of the forewaters. There is also the possibility of trauma to the placenta, and accidental injury to the uterine wall.

Stripping the Membranes

Stripping of the membranes off the lower uterine segment with the examining finger is an effective procedure for induction if the cervical score is favorable. It is used as a preliminary step prior to rupture of membranes. It is also used to make the cervix ripe. Stretching of the cervix and liberation of endogenous prostaglandins either help in ripening the cervix or at times in initiation of labor.

Combined Method

The combined medical and surgical methods are commonly used to increase the efficacy of induction by reducing the induction-delivery interval.

The oxytocin infusion is started either prior to or following rupture of membranes depending upon the state of the cervix and head-brim relation. With the head nonengaged, it is preferable to induce with prostaglandin gel or to start oxytocin infusion followed by artificial rupture of membranes.

Advantages of combined method
- More effective than single procedure
- Shortens the induction—delivery interval and thereby minimises the risk of infection and lessens the period of observation.

71. INFECTIONS IN NEWBORNS

Neonates are more susceptible to infection because they lack in natural immunity and take some time for the acquired immunity to develop. There is also deficiency of leukocytic response to infection.

MODE OF INFECTION

Antenatal
- **Transplacental:** Maternal infections that can affect the fetus through transplacental route are mainly the viruses. They are rubella, cytomegalovirus, herpes virus, human immunodeficiency virus (HIV), chicken pox and hepatitis B virus. Bacterial infections include syphilis, toxoplasmosis and tuberculosis.
- **Amnionitis:** Amnionitis following premature rupture of membranes can affect the baby following aspiration or ingestion of infected amniotic fluid.

Intranatal
- Aspiration of infected liquor in prolonged labor following early rupture of membranes. This may lead to congenital or neonatal pneumonia
- Contamination, while passing through the vagina:
    - Ophthalmia neonatorum (gonococcal infection)
    - Oral thrush *[Candida albicans (C. albicans)]*.
    - Cord sepsis from improper asepsis, while cutting cord.

Postnatal
- Transmission from infected mother, relatives or hospital staff
- Cross infection from another infected baby
- Infected articles used for feeding, bathing, clothing or air-borne.

COMMON INFECTIONS

Umbilical Sepsis (Omphalitis)

Infection of the umbilical stump in the neonatal period:

Causative organisms: Staphylococcus aureus, Streptococcus, Escherichia coli (E. coli).

Manifestations: Serous or seropurulent umbilical discharge, which may be offensive, base of stump moist and red, swollen periumbilical skin, delay in falling off the cord. Pyrexia, features of toxemia and jaundice in severe infection.

Treatment: Cleaning with alcohol (spirit), topical antibiotic cream, systemic antibiotic after taking skin swab for culture and sensitivity.

Oral thrush (candidiasis): Infection of the buccal mucous membranes and the tongue by the fungus, C. albicans.

Source of infection: From genital tract during birth, feeding utensils, breasts.

Manifestations: Milky white, elevated patches resembling milk, curd, which cannot be wiped off:
- Lesions appear late in the 1st week or during 2nd week
- May spread to respiratory tract or gastrointestinal (GI) tract.

Treatment: Nystatin suspension dropped under tongue. Local application of 1% aqueous solution of gentian violet on mucous membrane.

Conjunctivitis (Ophthalmia Neonatorum)

Inflammation of the conjunctiva during the first 3 days of life:

Causative organisms: Chlamydia trachomatis, Staphylococcus, Pseudomonas, Pneumococcus, herpes virus, gonococcus.

Source of infection: Contamination from vaginal discharge—common in face and breech deliveries.

Clinical manifestations: As follows:
- Watery, mucopurulent or frank purulent discharge in one or both eyes
- Sticky, swollen eyelids.

Treatment: As follows:
- Gonococcal infection: Saline irrigation followed by gentamycin eyedrops, four times a day for 7 days. Penicillin or cefotime intravenously
- Chlamydia infection: Erythromycin suspension orally and erythromycin eyedrops
- Herpes simplex: Acyclovir intravenously for 2 weeks. Idoxuridine ointment topically.

Skin Infections

Causative organism: Staphylococcus aureus.

Source of infection: Unhygienic environment, cross infection or carriers.

Manifestations: As follows:
- Mild form—superficial pustules, single or scattered, on face, axilla or scalp
- Severe form—manifests as pemphygus neonatorum with superficial blisters on any part of the skin and pustules, which break and raw area becomes infected.

Treatment: As follows:
- Isolation of the baby
- Blisters pricked open with sterile needle
- Antibiotic ointment application on skin
- Erythromycin 25 mg/kg per day
- Cloxacillin 50 mg/kg per day in 3–4 divided doses. Pemphygus due to syphilis show blisters on palms, soles or trunk. Treatment is antisyphilitic therapy.

Systemic Infections

Life-threatening systemic infections are usually caused by bacteria from the maternal genital tract acquired during the process of birth. This presents early in the first 3 days or late after 7–10 days.

The commonly implicated organisms are group B β-hemolytic *Streptococcus, E. coli, Klebsiella, Pseudomonas, Haemophilus, Pneumococcus, Staphylococcus aureus* and in preterm infants, *Staphylococcus epidermis*.

MANIFESTATIONS

- Respiratory distress
- Lethargy
- Poor temperature regulation (hypothermia more common than fever)
- Poor feeding
- Vomiting
- Apnea
- Pallor
- Abdominal distension.

DIAGNOSIS

- Complete blood count and smears: Neutropenia (< 2,000/mL) or neutrophilia (> 8,000/mL), presence of band forms and toxic granules in neutrophils
- Blood culture
- Urine culture
- Lumbar puncture to exclude meningitis
- Chest radiography to detect signs of pneumonia.

TREATMENT

- Transfer newborn to a special care unit to allow close observation
- Provide neutral thermal environment
- Supportive measures such as oxygen, respiratory support and intravenous colloids
- Specific antibiotic based on culture results.

MEASURES TO PREVENT NEONATAL INFECTIONS

- Washing and cleansing mother's vulval area with soap and water
- Preparation with non-irritating detergent preparation such as dettol or hibitane solution
- Shaving or clipping perineal hair
- Bathing and wearing clean gown in labor room
- Antiseptic and aseptic precautions during vaginal examination

- Use of facial mask, while performing vaginal examination and conducting delivery
- Washing hands and forearms before vaginal examination and conducting/assisting with delivery
- Avoiding health personnel with respiratory tract infection.

NURSING MANAGEMENT OF INFANTS

- Monitoring vital signs hourly
- Temperature regulation
- Maintenance of respiratory and cardiovascular functions
- Management of fluid and electrolyte balance
- Maintenance of neutral thermal environment
- Administration of intravenous fluids as prescribed
- Measurement of intake and output, and daily weight
- Blood glucose monitoring
- Administration of medications including specific antibiotics
- Encouraging parent-infant bonding and parental involvement in the care of infant
- Health education to parents and assistance to families with special needs and problems.

72. INFECTIOUS CONDITIONS OF PELVIC ORGANS

VULVOVAGINITIS

Vulval and vaginal infection occurs when the defence is lost following constant irritation by vaginal discharge or urine (incontinence) or following menopause when there will be atrophic changes.

Causative Organisms and Clinical Manifestations

Bacterial Infections

These are caused by sexually transmitted organisms *(Chlamydia, Gonorrhea, Trichomonas)*. Patients present with symptoms of:
- Increased vaginal discharge
- Musty or fishy odor of discharge following sexual intercourse
- Homogenous, grey-white discharge.

Treatment is local antiseptics and systemic antibiotics.

Monilial Infection

Caused by *Candida albicans*. Symptoms include:
- Itching and burning
- Thick curd-like discharge
- Dyspareunia
- Vulvar or vaginal erythema
- Edematous cervix.

Treated with clotrimazole cream and Griseofulvin oral preparation.

Viral Infection

Caused by varicella zoster virus. Produces painful eruptions of groups of vesicles distributed over the skin. Vesicles may rupture or become dry with scab formation.

Treated with analgesics, antibiotics (to prevent secondary infection) and acyclovir.

Atrophic Vulvovaginitis

Manifestations: As follows:
- Vaginal dryness
- Irritation, burning and itching
- Vulvar and vaginal atrophy
- Pale, thin, friable vaginal mucosa
- Sparse pubic hair
- Dyspareunia.

Treatment: As follows:
- Intravaginal applications of estrogen cream
- Systemic estrogen if there is no contraindication
- Treatment of infection if present.

CERVICITIS

Cervicitis refers to infection of the endocervix including the glands and stroma. The infection may be acute or chronic. Usually occurs following childbirth, abortion or any operation on cervix.

Causative Organisms

Streptococcus, Staphylococcus, Escherichia coli (E. coli), gonococcus or *Chlamydia trachomatis.*

Clinical Features

- Spotting after sexual intercourse
- Yellowish white discharge
- Red, edematous, friable cervix
- Cervical motion tenderness.

Treatment

Antibiotics based on identified drug sensitivity.

ENDOMETRITIS

Endometritis is an inflammation of the lining of the uterus—the endometrium.

Causes

Endometritis can stem from several underlying causes the most prevalent of which are bacterial infections:
- Amniotic fluid can become infected from stool excreted by the fetus or from other sources of pathogenic bacteria during pregnancy
- Sexually transmitted disease (STD) such as gonorrhea and chlamydia are often the causes
- Pelvic inflammatory disease (PID) may also lead to endometritis
- Tuberculosis
- Normal vaginal bacteria can be a reason for endometritis
- Remnant tissues such as the placenta retained after a delivery or abortion is the most common cause of postpartum infection. Such infection may spread to the entire uterus, ovaries and pelvis.

Risk Factors

The risk of developing endometritis increases by number of factors:
- A cesarean section significantly heightens the chances of postpartum infection

- Extended labor or premature rupture of fetal membranes
- Anemia may be a pre-existing condition or it may result from heavy bleeding during labor
- Steroid medications—sometimes used to assist fetal lung development and functioning when premature birth is expected, are another risk factor
- The presence of an intrauterine device (IUD) can induce or exacerbate inflammation
- Use of special instruments and procedures such as hysteroscopy, and D and C can induce inflammation.

Signs and Symptoms

Postpartum endometritis develops in 49–72 hours:
- Abdominal distention or swelling
- Abnormal vaginal bleeding
- Abnormal vaginal discharge often with a foul odor
- Lower abdominal or pelvic pain
- Fever with chills (temparature 100–104°F)
- Discomfort with bowel movement (constipation may occur)
- Malaise and general discomfort.

Tests and Investigations

- Abdominal palpation to discover tenderness or soreness
- Pelvic examination
- Blood tests such as white blood cells (WBC), complete blood count (CBC), erythrocyte sedimentation rate (ESR)
- Cultures from cervix for organisms
- Pap smear to detect the presence of abnormal cells
- Laparoscopy/Hysteroscopy and endometrial biopsy
- Computed tomography (CT) scan to assess the uterus and other internal organs.

Treatment

Patients with serious symptoms and postpartum infection need to be hospitalized and treated. Treatment measures include:

- Administration of intravenous antibiotics for 2–7 days
- Administration of oral or intravenous fluids to prevent dehydration
- Aspiration to drain pus from uterus
- Evacuation of remnant tissue from the uterus (placenta, membranes)
- Adequate rest
- A postpartum hysterectomy to remove a hopelessly damaged or infected uterus
- Analgesics for pain and fever, and isolation to avoid cross-infection are often instituted. Mild cases may be treated on an outpatient basis.

Prognosis

Most cases of endometritis clear up with antibiotics. Untreated endometritis can lead to more serious infection and complications with pelvic organs, reproduction and general health.

Possible Complications

- Infertility
- Pelvic peritonitis
- Pelvic or uterine abscess formation
- Septicemia
- Septic shock.

Prevention

Endometritis caused by STI can be prevented by:
- Early diagnosis and complete treatment of sexually transmitted diseases
- Educating women on safe sex practices

The risk of endometritis will be reduced by following sterile techniques by healthcare workers, while delivering a baby or performing an abortion, intrauterine device (IUD) placement or other gynecological procedures.

73. INFECTIONS IN PREGNANCY

Pregnancy produces a degree of altered immunoresponsiveness, which helps to prevent fetal infection, but predisposes the woman to infection. The physiological changes of childbearing also predispose her to urinary and vaginal infections. Exposure to viral infections is increased if she has small children in the family.

VIRAL INFECTIONS IN PREGNANCY

Rubella or German Measles

The disease is transmitted by droplet exposure. Fetal affection is by transplacental route. Risk of major anomalies to fetus is present when infection occurs in the first 3 months of pregnancy. There is increased chance of abortion, stillbirth and congenital malformations due to the teratogenic effects of the virus.

Test for rubella-specific antibody should be done within 10 days of exposure to rubella virus to know if the woman is immune or not. Rubella-specific antibodies are present for life after natural infection or vaccination. If the mother is found not immune, therapeutic abortion is usually considered.

Active immunity can be conferred in non-immune subjects by giving rubella vaccine. When given during childbearing period, pregnancy should be prevented for 3 months by contraceptive measures.

Measles

Infection causes high fever, which can lead to abortion, stillbirth or premature delivery. Non-immunized women coming in contact with measles may be protected by intramuscular injection of immune serum globulin within 6 days of exposure. The infection does not interfere with normal embryogenesis.

Influenza

With Influenza the course of pregnancy remains unaffected, but if the infection is virulent, it may cause abortion or premature labor. There is no evidence of teratogenic effect even if it is contracted in the first trimester.

Chickenpox (Varicella Zoster)

Varicella virus does cross the placenta and may cause congenital or neonatal chicken pox. Varicella immune globulin should be given to exposed non-immune patients to reduce the morbidity. It should be given to exposed newborns, within 5 days of delivery. The fetal congenital malformations, include hypoplasia or limb deformity, cataracts, microcephaly and cutaneous scarring.

Cytomegalovirus Infection

Transmission may be sexual, respiratory droplet or transplacental. Virus is also excreted in urine and breast milk. The consequences of infection include abortion, stillbirth, intrauterine growth restriction (IUGR), microcephaly, intracranial calcification, hepatosplenomegaly, thrombocytopenia, choroidoretinitis, mental retardation and deafness.

Maternal mumps has no ill effects on the course of pregnancy or embryogenesis. Incidence is seen low in women who had childhood vaccination with measles-mumps-rubella (MMR) vaccine.

Herpes Simplex Virus

The virus is transmitted mostly by sexual contact. Primary infection may occur during pregnancy and recurrent infection with or without symptoms and viral shedding occurs later. Primary infection in the third trimester can cause premature labor or IUGR. The fetus can get affected by virus shed from the cervix or lower genital tract during vaginal delivery or in utero from contaminated liquor following rupture of membranes. Cesarean delivery is indicated in an active primary genital HSV infection where the membranes are intact or recently ruptured. When virus culture is positive, patient is treated with acyclovir 200 mg, five times daily for 5 days.

Acquired Immunodeficiency Syndrome

The acquired immunodeficiency syndrome (AIDS) is caused by human immunodeficiency virus (HIV), which is a group of retrovirus. The virus reduces CD4 cells leading to immunodeficiency. As a result, the individual becomes susceptible to infections by opportunistic organisms and specific tumors. Incubation period is from 2 months to 10 years.

Mode of Transmission

- Sexual contact (homosexual or heterosexual)
- Transplacental
- Exposure to infected blood or body fluids
- Through breast milk.

Clinical Presentation

- Initial presentation may include fever, malaise, headache, sore throat, and lymphadenopathy and maculopapular rash
- Primary illness may be followed by an asymptomatic period
- Progression of the disease manifests as opportunistic infections such as candidiasis, tuberculosis and pneumocystis
- Neoplasms such as cervical carcinoma, lymphoma and Kaposi's sarcoma
- Associated constitutional symptoms such as weight loss, lymphadenopathy and diarrhea.

Diagnosis

- Screening test for specific antibodies using enzyme-linked immunosorbent assay (ELISA)
- Western blot test to confirm positive ELISA
- Clinical progression monitored by evaluating the CD4 cell counts.

Decreasing CD4 counts indicates medical intervention (500/mL, no evidence of immunosuppression, 200–500/mL, greater likelihood of developing symptoms, less than 200/mL indicate that client is at increased risk of developing complicated diseases).

Management

Prenatal care
- Prenatal HIV counseling to all pregnant women
- Monitoring of immune status
- Prophylaxis of opportunistic infections
- Assessment for presence of other STDs
- Aerosolized pentamidine spray or trimethoprim-sulfamethoxazole prophylaxis for *Pneumocystis carinii* pneumonia

- Prevention of vertical transmission by preventing chorioamnionitis, shortening the duration of labor, delaying rupture of membranes and preventing vaginitis
- Prophylactic treatment with zidovudine to all HIV-infected women after appropriate counseling.

Intrapartum care
- Avoid procedures that might produce break in the skin and mucous membranes of newborns such as amniotomy, placement of scalp electrodes and scalp blood pH
- Limit vaginal examinations
- Use of masks, gowns, double gloves and goggles by health workers
- All linen to be collected in a vessel containing hypochlorite solution
- All cotton swabs, perineal pads, mops, etc. must be discarded in a container with hypochlorite solution
- All needles and sharp blades must be deposited in puncture proof containers
- Any spills on floors must be cleaned with antiseptic solution observing all precautions
- Fumigate labor room/operating room after delivery
- Autoclave all instruments after proper washing and cleaning
- Wash off any blood contamination on skin immediately.

Postpartum care
- Provide counseling and help mother make informed choice regarding breastfeeding
- Zidovudine oral syrup administered to all newborns for 6 weeks
- Barrier contraception recommended to the couple.

74. INFERTILITY

DEFINITION

Infertility is defined as the inability to conceive after 1 year with appropriately timed coitus without the use of contraception. It is said to be primary if no conception has ever occurred, and secondary, if there has been a pregnancy whatever the outcome.

INCIDENCE

Infertility affects almost 15% of couples, with the risk increasing for women after 35 years of age.

FACTORS AFFECTING FERTILITY

Female Factors

- Problems of ovulation:
    - Ovarian abnormalities such as hypogonadism (Turner's syndrome), radiation, chemotherapy and use of oral contraceptives
    - Hormonal abnormalities: Irregularities in the hypothalamic-pituitary-ovarian axis, which alter the hormonal balance needed for ovulation
    - Poor general health, inadequate nutrition, stress and excessive exercise affecting ovulation.
- Tubal structural problems:
    - Obstruction or narrowing of the tube
    - Blockage resulting from congenital defects, infections or endometriosis
    - Scarring can result from organisms such as *Neisseria gonorrhea, Chlamydia, trachomatis, Mycoplasma* and *Mycobacterium*
    - Infection and adhesion following laparoscopy or appendectomy.
- Structural problems of the uterus:
    - Fibroid tumors obstructing the fallopian tubes or interfering with implantation
    - Inadequate endometrium—thin endometrium due to inadequate hormone production or Asherman's syndrome
    - Endometriosis
    - Abnormal uterine division such as bicornuate, unicornuate or septate uterus.
- Structural problems of the vagina and cervix:
    - Imperforate hymen
    - Irregularly shaped uterus, tubes or cavities
    - Congenital anomalies.
- Hostile mucus and antisperm antibodies in mucus
- Infection causing vaginismus or dyspareunia.

Male Factors

- Endocrine disorders: Dysfunction of hypothalamus, pituitary, adrenals and thyroid
- Systemic diseases: Diabetes mellitus, renal failure, celiac disease
- Testicular disorders: Trauma, environmental factors (high temperature):
  - Congenital (hydrocele, undescended testes)
  - Acquired (varicocele, tight clothing)
  - Occupational (long distance truck driving).
- Anticancer medications
- Obstruction or absence of seminal ducts due to infection, trauma or congenital anomalies
- Impaired secretions from prostate or seminal vesicles due to infection or metabolic disorders
- Ineffective delivery:
  - Ejaculatory dysfunction
  - Physical disability
  - Physical anomalies such as hypospadias, epispadias or retrograde ejaculation.

Unexpected Infertility

For approximately 10% of infertile couples no specific causative problem can be identified.

ASSESSMENT OF THE INFERTILE COUPLE

History

Female History

- Age
- Fertility history: Duration, prior contraception, abortion
- Menstrual history: Age of menarche, characteristics of menses
- Medical history: Laparoscopy, appendectomy, D and C
- Medications: Oral contraceptives, antibiotics, Retin A
- Occupation: Exposure to radiation, toxic drugs
- Personal and sexual habits: Alcohol or drug use, smoking, obesity, frequency and timing of intercourse.

Male History

- Fertility history: Age, frequency of intercourse difficulties such as erection and ejaculation
- Medical history: Major diseases, mumps in childhood, diseases of genital tract, sexually transmitted diseases (STDs)
- Surgical history: Hernia repair, prostate surgery
- Medications
- Occupation: Prolonged sitting that affects spermatogenesis, exposure to radiation, chemicals, and gases
- Personal and sexual habits: Use of alcohol or street drugs, smoking, wearing tight underwear, frequency of ejaculation (frequent ejaculation reduces sperm count).

Physical Examination

Female

- Secondary sexual characteristics such as breast development, facial and genital hair distribution, and presence of acne
- Palpation of thyroid for enlargement or nodules
- Breast evaluation for development and discharge
- Surgical scars on abdomen indicating adhesions
- Examination of genitalia for anatomic abnormalities and infection
- Pelvic examination and Pap smear
- Blood tests: Blood type, Rh antibodies, immunity to measles.

Male

- Presence of secondary sexual characteristics and genital abnormalities
- Undescended testes or absence of vas deferens
- Varicocele or abnormal blood vessels in scrotum.

Specific Investigations of Females

Female

- Cervical mucus test: Clear, copious and stretchy at ovulation and shows a ferning pattern when dried on a glass slide

- Ovulation prediction kit: A urine test to predict ovulation based on luteinizing hormone (LH)
- Basal body temperature (BBT)—considered less accurate
- Ultrasound scanning: Detects ripening Graafian follicle and thickening of endometrium
- Hormonal assays: Series of tests shows fluctuations in circulating estrogens, progesterone, follicle-stimulating hormone (FSH) and LH.

Male

- Semen analysis: Volume, viscosity, pH, motility, morphology and count are determined
- Agglutination test: Occurs due to antisperm antibodies or infection
- Testicular biopsy to determine if sperms are produced
- Chromosome studies to detect presence of Klinefelter's syndrome (XXY), which causes infertility
- Blood tests for hormone levels: Which suggest possibilities for treatment
- Postcoital test: Cervical mucus aspirated and tested within 6 hours of intercourse for its quality for sperm penetration

Management of Infertility

Couple

- Counseling to both partners
- Instructions to maintain normal body weight, and to correct coital problems
- Instructions to reduce smoking and consumption of alcohol.

Female

Correction of the cause found:
- Anovulation:
    - Induction of ovulation using psychotherapy and medications such as clomifene.
- Medical and hormonal problems:
    - Specific hormones and medications.
- Polycystic ovarian disease (PCOD):
    - Wedge resection
    - Laparoscopic ovarian diathermy.

- Tubal and peritoneal factors:
  - Tuboplasty
  - Cannulation of the tube.
- Endometriosis:
  - Hormonal treatment
  - Diathermy, laser vaporization or dissection of the endometriomas.
- Immunological factors (antisperm antibodies):
  - Cortisone PO
  - Intrauterine insemination.
- Surgical corrective measures:
  - Myomectomy of submucous fibroids
  - Metroplasty (removal of septum)
  - Adhesiolysis with insertion of intrauterine contraceptive device (IUCD)
  - Enlargement of vaginal introitus or removal of vaginal septum (for dyspareunia)
  - Cauterization or amputation of the cervix for congenital elongation of cervix
  - Ventrosuspension operation for correction of retroversion of uterus
  - Cannulation of the tube for tubal obstruction.
- Adjuvant therapy:
  - Hydrotubation
  - Antibiotics and hydrocortisone.

Male

Treatment for the male is indicated in:
- Extreme oligospermia
- Azoospermia
- Low volume ejaculate
- Impotence.

Measures to Improve Spermatogenesis

- General:
  - Improvement of general health
  - Reduction of weight in obese

- Avoidance of tight and warm undergarments and cold scrotal bath at least twice a day for 5 minutes each time
- Avoidance of too frequent intercourse.
- Administration of vitamin E, C, B_{12} and folic acid to improve spermatogenesis and to reduce the toxic-free radicals released by abnormal sperm leukocytes present in the semen
- Medications to treat hypogonadism:
  - Clomifene citrate (Clomid)
  - Human chorionic gonadotropin (hCG)
  - Testosterone
  - Dexamethasone in men with antisperm antibodies
  - Phenylephrine in case of retrograde ejaculation
  - Artificial insemination in case of genetic abnormality.
- Surgical treatment:
  - Vasoepididymostomy or vaso-vasoanastomosis for obstruction in vas deferens
  - Correction of varicocele or hydrocele
  - Orchidopexy in case of undescended testes.
- Psychosexual therapy and Viagra for erectile dysfunction
- Assisted reproductive technology (ART) (For details refer to chapter 13, page 79).

UNEXPLAINED INFERTILITY

Unexplained infertility refers to couples who have undergone a complete infertility work up and in whom no abnormality has been detected and still remains infertile. About 4 out of 10 such couples become pregnant within 3 years without having any specific treatment.

TREATMENT

Because of spontaneous cure rate such couples are asked to wait for some time and then to go for assisted reproductive technologies.

COMBINED FACTOR

In the management of infertility, it is important that both partners should be treated for the faults detected simultaneously and one after the other.

75. INSTRUMENTS IN OBSTETRICS AND GYNECOLOGY

Medical instruments are various types of objects such as tools, apparatuses and machines that are used on humans for medical purposes. This may include diagnosis, therapy or surgery. Healthcare professionals use these instruments in order to effectively treat patients.

SPONGE HOLDING FORCEPS (Fig. 75.1)

Specifications and Uses

- A heavy metal instrument 23–75 cm in length
- Shafts are thin and blades are fenestrated
- Has a catch-lock, which gives firmness, while holding any material
- Has ring-shaped tips, which may be serrated or smooth
- Used for cleaning the operative field
- Used for swabbing or packing body cavities like vagina
- Can be used to catch hold of soft organs such as ovary and cervix in pregnancy
- Can be substituted in the place of an ovum forceps
- Used for deep moping to clear the area during surgery.

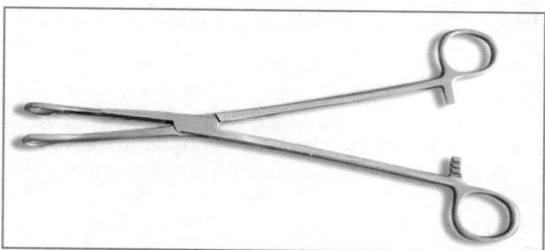

Fig. 75.1: Sponge holding forceps.

KOCHER'S HEMOSTATIC FORCEPS (Figs. 75.2A and B)

Specifications and Uses

- A strong, straight metal instrument
- Has a catch-lock to bring the blades together for locking
- Inner surface of both blades are transversely serrated
- It may be straight or curved
- Single toothed at distal end
- Used to catch the edges of the incision while suturing skin
- Used for artificial rupture membranes
- Used to clamp the umbilical cord.

HEMOSTAT (ARTERY FORCEPS) (Figs. 75.3A and B)

Specifications and Uses

- Artery forceps may be small or mosquito, straight or curved, strong metal instrument

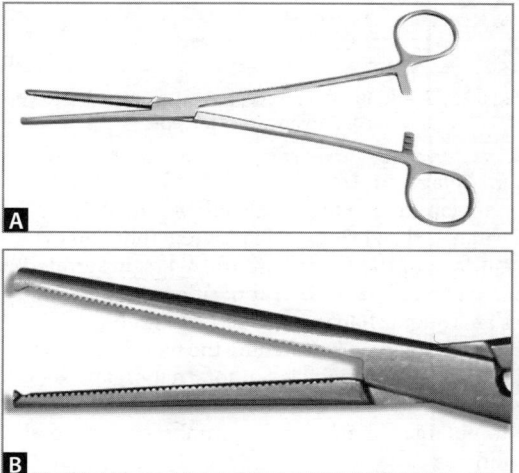

Figs. 75.2A and B: A. Kocher's forceps; **B.** View of the toothed tips.

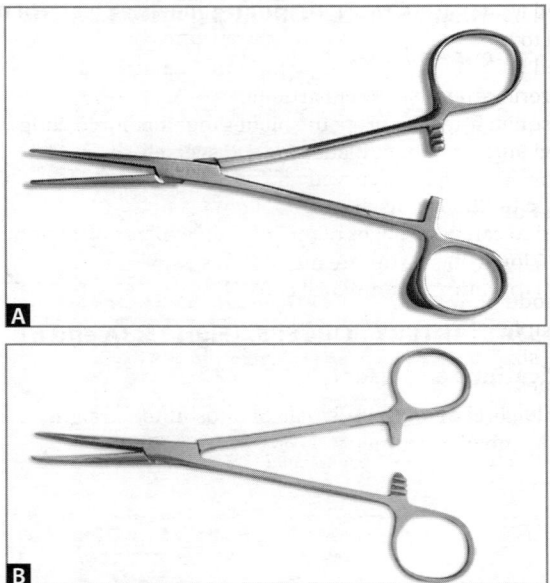

Figs. 75.3A and B: Artery forceps. **A.** Straight artery forceps; **B.** Curved artery forceps.

- Medium or large in size
- Blades are tapering to the distal end, but blunt
- Has a catch-lock to bring the blades together and to lock it
- Inner surface of the blades are transversely serrated and when locked, the blades are well in apposition
- Blades are roughly half the size of the handle
- Used to stop bleeding by catching the blood vessel
- Used as a clamp for pedicles of internal organs such as kidney, spleen, ligaments of uterus, etc.
- Used to enlarge the opening of an abscess in the absence of a sinus forceps
- Can be used to substitute a needle holder
- Used to hold the incised edges of skin and fascia

- Used to hold the free ends of sutures at the beginning of suturing and to hold the cut ends of tension sutures before tying
- Used to hold the tape of abdominal pads or sponges during surgeries to prevent them missing in the cavity
- Mosquito forceps are used to hold the small bleeding points
- Used for blunt dissection by holding swabs.

Ovum Forceps (Figs. 75.4A and B)

Specifications and Uses

- A moderately heavy metal instrument having cupped blades with linear fenestrations
- The size and type of blades can hold a reasonable amount of tissues in between with good grip
- The length is about 30 cm

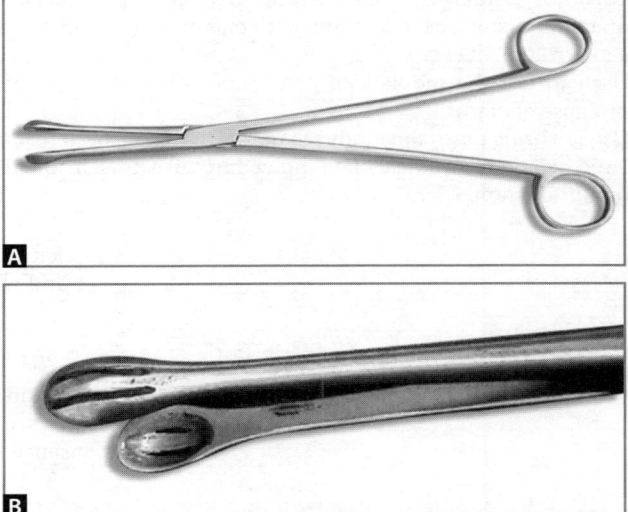

Figs. 75.4A and B: A. Ovum forceps; **B.** Ovum holding tip of the forceps.

- Used for removing products of conception from the uterus in incomplete abortion
- Used to remove any foreign body from the uterine cavity, e.g. intrauterine device when threads are broken
- Used to remove any retained placental bits or membrane pieces from the uterus after delivery.

Vulsellum Forceps (Fig. 75.5)

Specifications and Uses

- An average sized metal instrument resembling forceps at the distal end
- The proximal end has a lock for fixing and distal end has multiple sharp teeth for firm grip
- The curvature of blades helps to retract the anterior vaginal wall when the instrument is pulled up after holding the cervical lip for better visualization
- Used for holding the anterior or posterior lip of cervix in operations such as dilatation and curettage (D and C) and cauterization of cervix
- Used to test the mobility of cervix and laxity of ligaments in prolapse of uterus
- Used to bring down the fundus of uterus in vaginal hysterectomy
- Used to hold the cervical lip for procedures like tubal insufflation or introduction of laminaria tent.

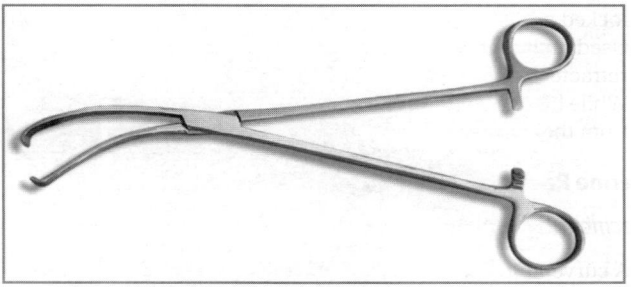

Fig. 75.5: Vulsellum forceps.

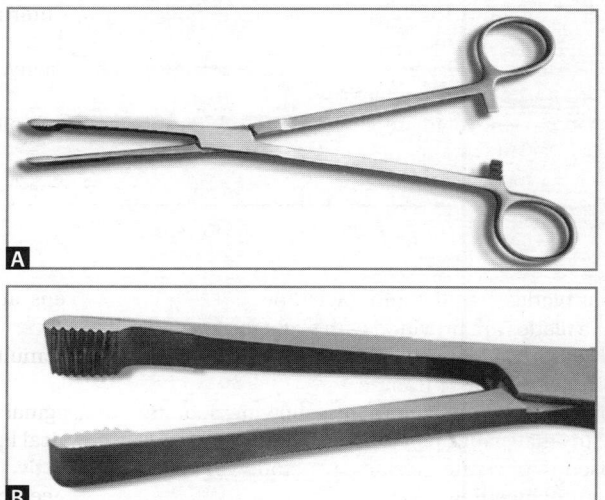

Figs. 75.6A and B: A. Green Armytage forceps; **B.** View of the tip of the forceps.

Green Armytage Forceps (Figs. 75.6A and B)

Specifications and Uses

- A metal instrument resembling any other forceps except for triangular blades with serrated edges
- Has small space between the blades, even when the forceps is locked and fully closed
- Used in lower segment cesarean section (LSCS) to hold the retracted edges of the uterine wall for easy stitching
- While holding the edges it acts as a hemostat to decrease bleeding from the incision.

Uterine Packing Forceps/Uterine Dressing Forceps (Fig. 75.7)

Specifications and Uses

- A curved forceps about 35 cm in length, the curvature corresponding to axis of birth canal for easy packing

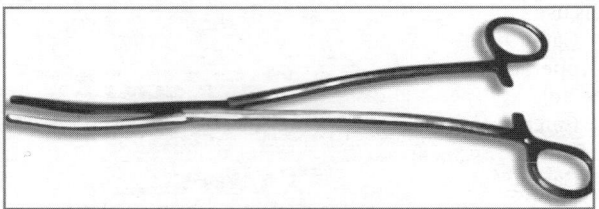

Fig. 75.7: Uterine packing forceps.

- Has blades, handles and finger bows
- The blades are provided with slight groves on inner surfaces
- Used for vaginal packing to control bleeding from lacerations in birth canal due to trauma
- Used to swab uterine cavity following dilatation and evacuation with small gauze pieces.
- Used to pack the uterine cavity following D and C or delivery to control bleeding.
- Used for application of drug into the uterine cavity.

Allis Tissue Forceps (Fig. 75.8)

Specifications and Uses

- An instrument with straight blades and catch-lock
- Have sharp teeth at the tip, with interlock on closing
- The tips are slightly curved or angulated for better grip of tissues

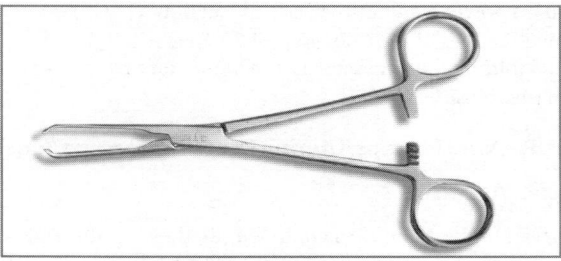

Fig. 75.8: Allis tissue forceps.

- It is used to:
  - Catch hold of the anterior lip of the cervix during D and C operation
  - Hold the apex of the episiotomy wound during repair
  - Catch hold of the torn ends of the sphincter ani prior to suturing in repair of complete perineal tear
  - Catch hold of the margins and angles of the uterine flaps in LSCS after delivery of the baby
  - Hold thinner structures such as skin, deep fascia and layers of rectus sheath.

Tenaculum Forceps (Fig. 75.9)

Specifications and Uses

- An instrument resembling Vulsellum forceps except there is a single tooth at the distal end
- Used to hold the tissues at one point only so as to minimise bleeding
- Used to hold the anterior lip of cervix transversely, while doing Rubin's test in order to fit the cannula airtight in the cervix.

Laminaria Tent Introducing Forceps

Specifications and Uses

- A metal instrument with a handle and lock
- Almost similar to uterine dressing forceps

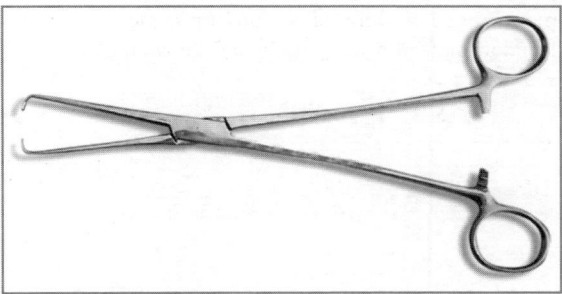

Fig. 75.9: Tenaculum forceps.

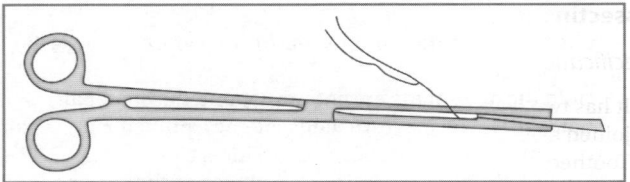

Fig. 75.10: Laminaria Tent introducing forceps.

- Has a grove on either blade to catch the Laminaria Tent
- Used to hold and introduce the Laminaria Tent conveniently into the cervix.

Laminaria Tent

Specifications and Uses

- It is dehydrated, compressed, Chinese seaweed
- It is sterilised by keeping it immersed in absolute alcohol
- Tents are about 7–10 cm in length, with an eye at one end, and a thread hanging through the eye of each tent
- The thread attached to the tent facilitates easy removal
- Laminaria Tents (more than one) are introduced into the cervical canal and kept for 12–24 hours.
- The tent being hygroscopic swells up by absorbing fluid from cervix causing slow dilatation of cervical canal.
- Used for dilating cervical canal in cases of spasmodic dysmenorrhoea, and for expulsion of products of conception in MTP, incomplete abortion and hydatidiform mole.

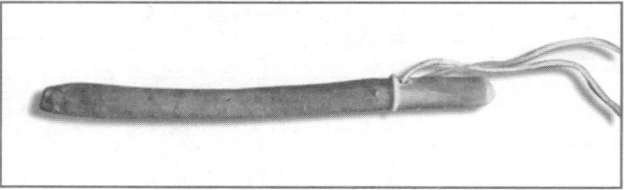

Fig. 75.11: Laminaria Tent.

Dissecting Forceps

Specifications and Uses

- It has two equal, flat shafts with a sharp curve at the middle and joined at the proximal end
- Toothed dissecting forceps has tooth in the inner surface of the distal end
- On pressing the shafts, the pointed tips are well apposed so that they do not slip against each other
- The outer surface of shafts is made rough and irregular to get a firm grip while holding in the hand
- Plain dissecting forceps are used to hold delicate structures like peritoneum, vessels, bowel wall, etc. for suturing and to lift swabs and gauze pieces for dressing
- Toothed dissecting forceps are used to hold tough structures like skin or fascia while suturing
- It is used to lift the knots of sutures while removing them after the wounds are healed. It is used to dissect soft, friable tissues.

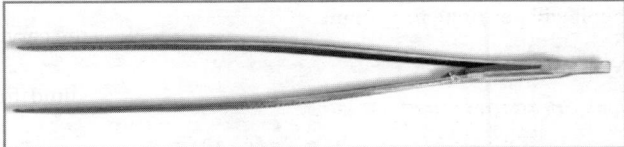

Fig. 75.12A: Non-toothed dissecting forceps.

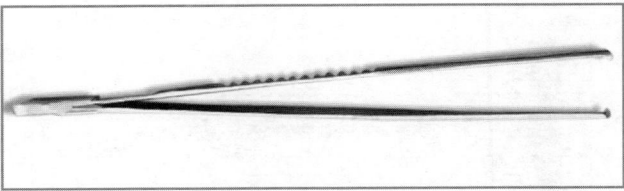

Fig. 75.12B: Toothed dissecting forceps.

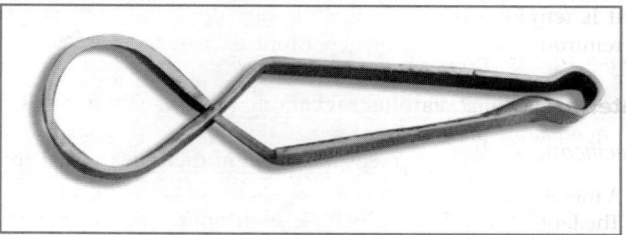

Fig. 75.13: Doyen's Towel clip.

Doyen's Towel Clip

Specifications and Uses

- It is a light and strong metal instrument
- It has a catch-lock to fix the grip of drapes
- The tips are sharply pointed for better grasping
- Used to fix drapes in order to expose only the required area
- Used to fix tubing such as suction tubes to drapes preventing displacement
- It can be used as tongue holding forceps in emergency situations, but it will perforate the tongue.

Doyen's Retractor

Specifications and Uses

- It is a metal instrument with flat solid blade on one end and a long handle
- Used to retract pelvic organs during cesarean section

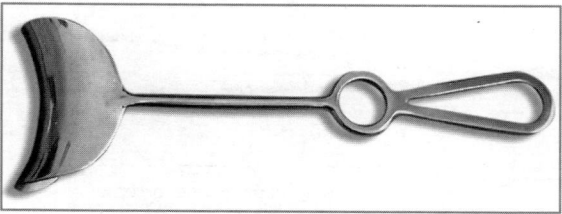

Fig. 75.14: Doyen's retractor.

- It is temporarily taken off while delivering the baby and then reintroduced till toileting of peritoneal cavity is done.

Anterior Vaginal Wall Retractor

Specifications and Uses

- A metal instrument with two oval shaped and fenestrated ends
- The fenestrated end has transverse serrations
- The oval shaped ends are connected at an angle of 45° to both ends of the shaft
- It is used with Sim's speculum to retract the anterior vaginal wall for exposing the cervix and anterior fornix.

Kelly's Deep Retractor

Specifications and Uses

- A large metal retractor with a broad and slightly curved blade
- Handle is long and end is curved like a hook, which provides better grip
- This type of retractor is available in various sizes
- It is used for retracting intra-abdominal viscera like liver and spleen during surgeries like cholecystectomy
- Smaller size retractor is used to retract the bladder walls in intravesical operations
- It is used to retract pelvic structures during surgery of appendix, caecum, etc. to prevent injury to pelvic organs.

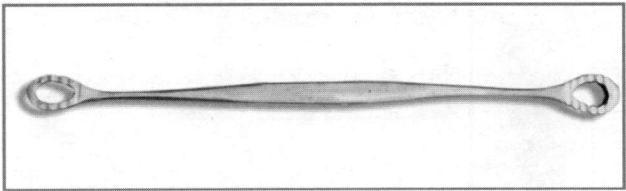

Fig. 75.15: Anterior vaginal wall retractor.

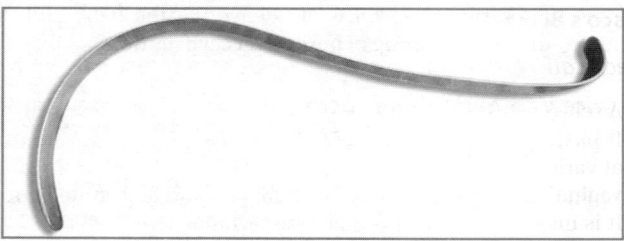

Fig. 75.16: Kelly's deep retractor.

Sim's Double Bladed Vaginal Speculum

Specifications and Uses

- A moderately heavy metal instrument
- It has two thick blades of unequal breadths to facilitate introduction according to the size of vagina
- It is used to:
  - Toilet the vagina following delivery
  - Visualise any injured site on the cervix or vagina
  - Inspect the cervix to exclude any local lesion causing bleeding in suspected cases of abortion, APH or PPH.
- Used in operations of the cervix and vagina in lithotomy position
- Used in D and C and D and E surgery
- Used for taking biopsy from genital tract and for cauterisation of erosions of cervix.

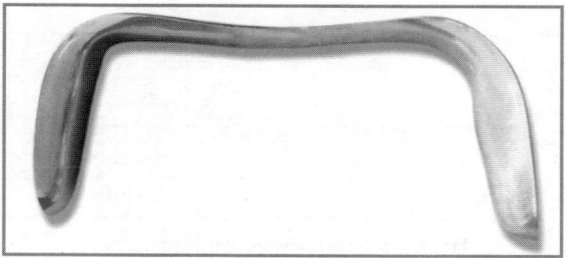

Fig. 75.17: Sim's double bladed vaginal speculum.

Cusco's Bivalved Speculum

Specifications and Uses

- A self-retaining speculum with a special screw arrangement
- It has two blades, which can be opened laterally and adjusted, at various angles by adjusting the screw after introducing in the vagina
- It is introduced into the vagina with its blades closed in vertical position and then made horizontal, opened and locked in position. It can be closed and rotated further and opened again to see other sides of vagina after locking in required position
- Can be used without any assistance
- Used to visualise or inspect vagina and cervix
- Can be used without bringing the patient to the edge of bed
- Used in insertion of intrauterine contraceptive device
- Used to reach into the cervix to apply medications, to take swabs for culture and sensitivity, to get biopsy specimens and to do electrocautery in the cervix.

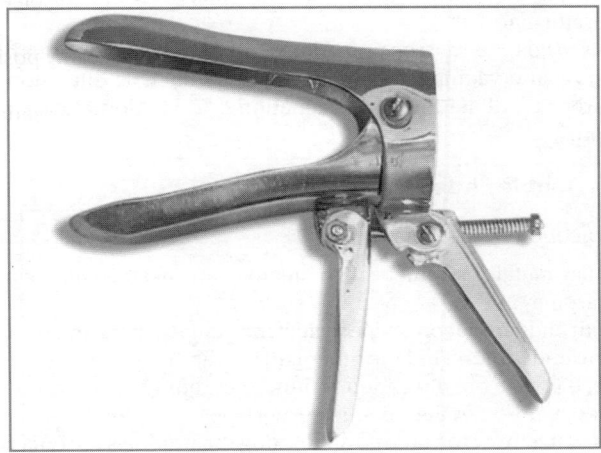

Fig. 75.18: Cusco's bivalved speculum.

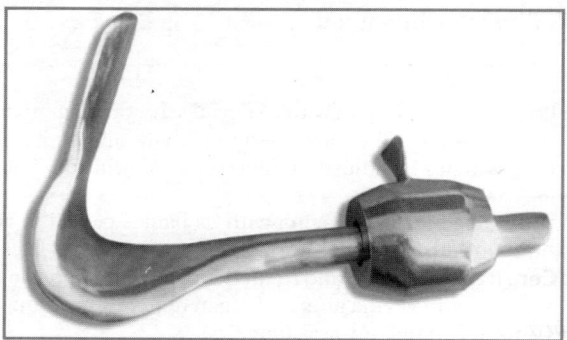

Fig. 75.19: Auvard's weighted vaginal speculum.

Auvard's Weighted Vaginal Speculum

Specifications and Uses

- It is weighted vaginal speculum for retaining
- The weight is due to the metal weight attached to the handle
- There is a channel in the handle for collection of discharges and curette material
- It is used to retract the posterior vaginal wall in operations of the cervix and vagina in lithotomy position such as dilatation and curettage, dilatation and evacuation or dilatation and insufflation.

Sim's Double Ended Uterine Curette

Specifications and Uses

- A flat metal instrument with small spoon-like arrangement for scarping
- Both ends are spoon-shaped with fenestrations in the middle
- One end is blunt and the other end is sharp for curetting
- Used to take out the endometrium by curetting the uterine cavity for diagnostic or therapeutic purpose
- Used to empty the uterus by curetting the products of conception in incomplete or missed abortion.

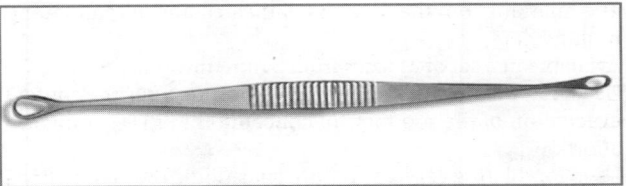

Fig. 75.20: Uterine curette.

Das's Cervical Dilators

Specifications and Uses

- Heavy metal instruments of gradually increasing sizes
- Has smooth, round body and tip having two different sizes in a single dilator

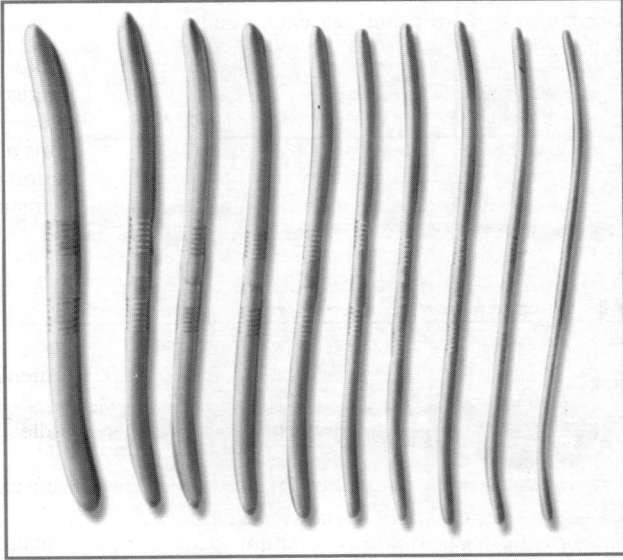

Fig. 75.21: Das's dilators.

- The marking on the dilators indicates the circumference in millimeters
- Available in a set of 24 sizes from 2 mm upwards
- Used for dilating the cervix for curetting uterine contents in evacuation of the products of conception in MTP or incomplete abortion
- Used for dilating cervix to relieve spasmodic dysmenorrhoea.

Flushing Curette

Specifications and Uses

- A curette with small spoon-like arrangement at one end for scraping
- The stem of the curette is hollow for the passage of any fluid to the interior of the spoon-like end
- To the other end (proximal), rubber tubing can be attached from a reservoir to pass fluids through the hollow area to the curetting end, which is blunt
- Used to wash out the uterine cavity, usually with warm antiseptic solution.

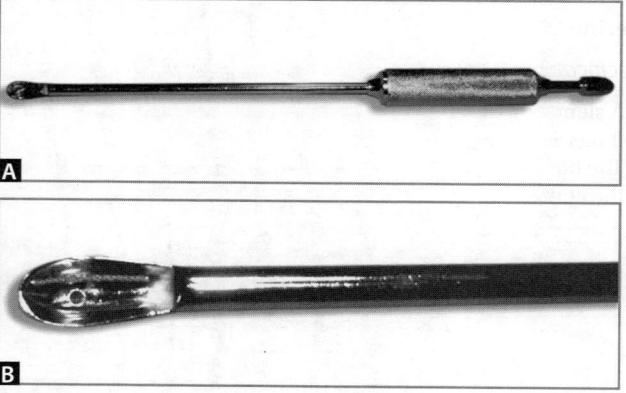

Figs. 75.22A and B: A. Flushing curette; **B.** View of the tip of the curette.

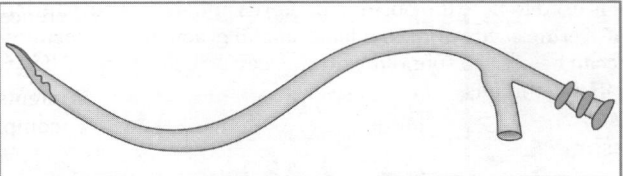

Fig. 75.23: Drew-Smythe catheter.

Drew-Smythe Catheter (Membrane Perforator)

Specifications and Uses

- It is a S-shaped, double curved metal catheter with a blunt stilet
- It has two openings—one inlet and one outlet, and double tube—one inner tube and one outer tube
- It is used for high rupture of membranes in hydramnios
- It allows controlled escape of liquor amni through it
- It can be passed between the membranes and uterus some length before puncturing
- The high rupture of membranes accomplished preserves the dilating effect of bag of waters and reduces the chances of infection and prolapse of the cord.

Uterine Sound

Specifications and Uses

- A slender, graduated, malleable metallic instrument
- It has an olive pointed tip and a broad handle
- The body is graduated and it can be used as a first dilator to dilate the cervix

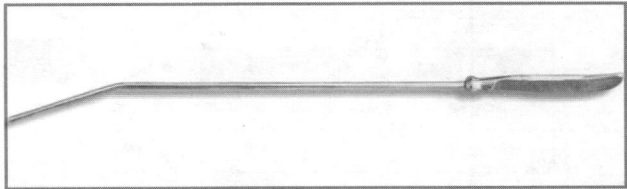

Fig. 75.24: Uterine sound.

474 Manual of Midwifery and Gynecological Nursing

- It is used to note the position of uterus and to measure the length of uterine cavity prior to dilatation and evacuation procedure
- It can be used to sound the uterine cavity to locate the IUCD with missing threads.

Scissors

Specification and Uses

- Scissors are used for blunt or sharp dissection

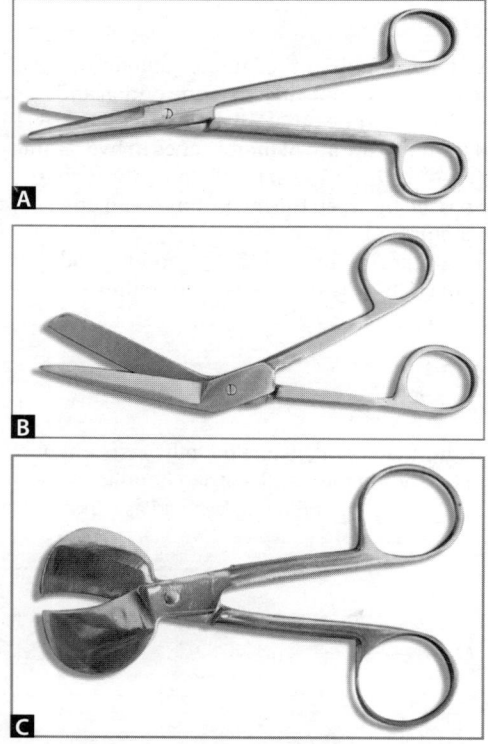

Figs. 75.25A to C: Scissors. **A.** Straight Mayo scissors; **B.** Episiotomy scissors. **C.** Umbilical cord cutting scissors.

- Straight or curved Mayo scissors, which are very smooth at the ends, are sued to cut the tissues and internal organs so that adjacent tissues are protected while using
- Episiotomy scissors are used for cutting the perineum to enlarge the vaginal opening to deliver the fetal head
- Umbilical cord cutting scissors with broad rounded end are used for cutting umbilical cord.

Bulb Syringe

Specifications and Uses

- A rubber bulb with elongated tip
- Used to remove secretions from mouth and nostrils of neonates following delivery of head.

Mucus Sucker

Specifications and Uses

- A plastic device with graduated barrel and tubes
- Used to suck secretions from oropharynx and hypopharynx of neonates following birth, prior to the attempt of respiration.

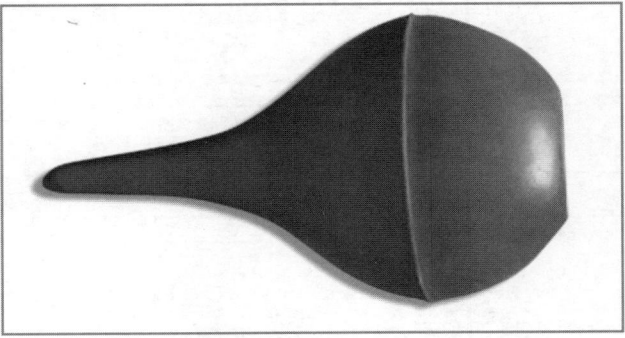

Fig. 75.26: Bulb syringe.

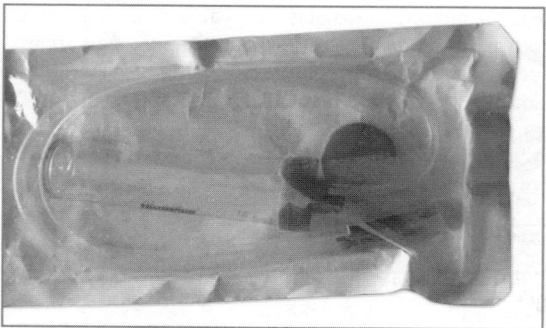

Fig. 75.27: Mucus sucker.

CORD CLAMP

Specifications and Uses

- A plastic device fused to clamp the umbilical cord
- It is kept in place until the cord dries and falls off. The clamp falls off with the detached cord stump.

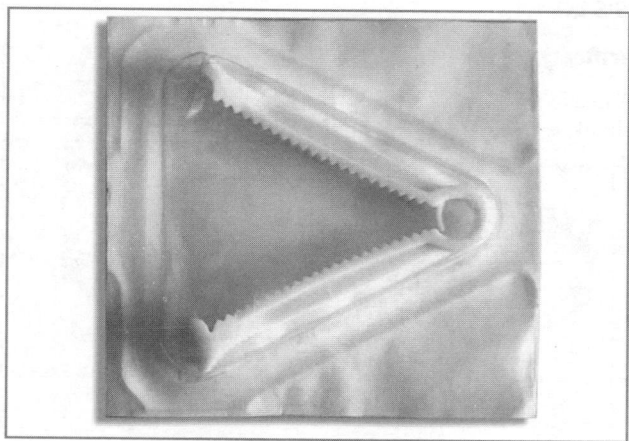

Fig. 75.28: Disposable cord clamp.

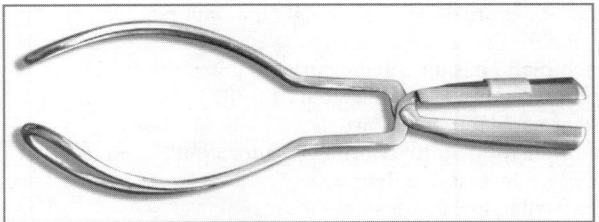

Fig. 75.29: Wrigley's forceps.

Wrigley's Outlet Forceps

Specifications and Uses

- A metal instrument in two pieces (halves) articulated by lock
- Each piece has a handle, lock, shaft and a fenestrated expanded blade
- The fenestrated portion of the blade allows good grip of the fetal head
- It is used to deliver the fetal head presenting at the pelvic outlet
- Delivery of the head is accomplished by extending it.

DAS'S LONG CURVED OBSTETRIC FORCEPS

Specifications and Uses

- A heavy metal instrument about 37 cm long. Its parts are blade, shank, lock and handle

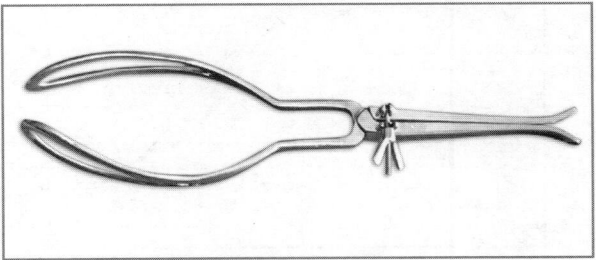

Fig. 75.30: Long curved forceps.

- The blades are named left or right in relation to maternal pelvis in which they lie when applied
- Each blade has a cephalic curve to grasp the fetal head without compression and a pelvic curve to fit the curve on the axis of pelvic canal (curve of Carus)
- In order to lock the two halves after application, the left blade needs to be inserted first
- It is used in low forceps operation.

AXIS TRACTION DEVICES

Specifications and Uses

- Axis traction devices includes two axis traction rods (right and left) and a traction handle

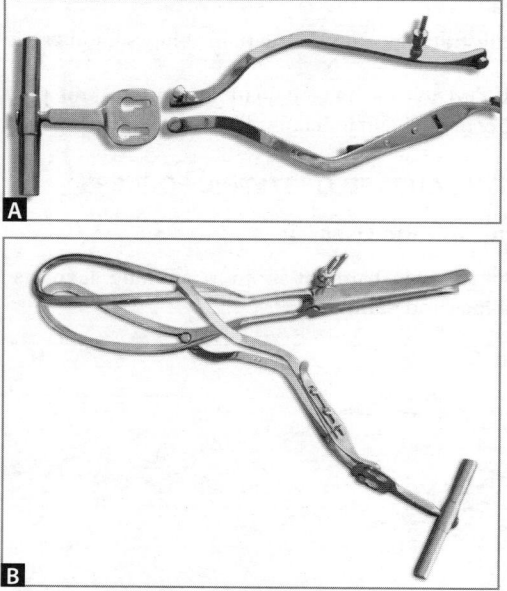

Figs. 75.31A and B: A. Axis traction devices; **B.** Long curved forceps with axis traction device.

- The rods are assembled in the blades of long curved obstetric forceps prior to introduction and lastly the handle is attached to the rods
- The devices are required (used) where; much force is necessary for traction as in midforceps operation
- It provides traction in the correct axis of pelvic curve and as such less force is necessary to deliver the head.

KIELLAND'S FORCEPS

Specifications and Uses

- Kielland's forceps is a long, almost straight (very slight pelvic curve) obstetric forceps with a sliding lock
- Usually used as rotation forceps in deep transverse arrest of occipitoposterior position of the head
- Facilitates grasping and correction of an asynclitic head because of its sliding lock.

VENTOUSE CUP WITH TRACTION DEVICE/VACUUM EXTRACTOR

Specifications and Uses

- An instrumental device designed to assist delivery by creating a vacuum between it and the fetal scalp
- The bell-shaped cups are of four sizes (30, 40, 50 and 60 mm)
- The cups have metallic plates at their apex. Each cup has a traction tube (rubber tube through which the traction chain passes) and a traction bar

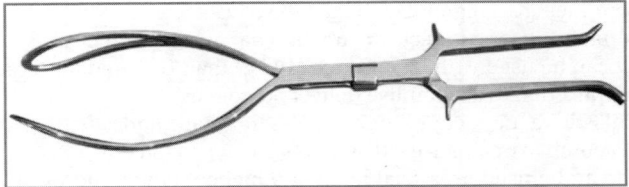

Fig. 75.32: Kielland's forceps.

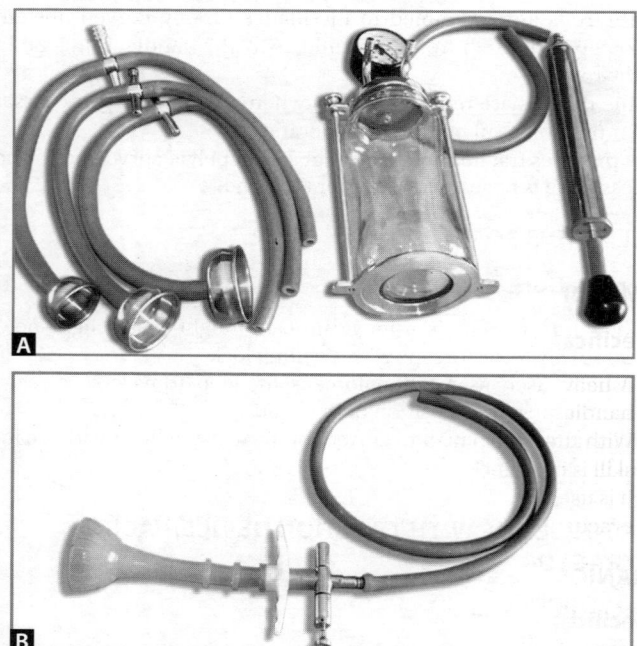

Figs. 75.33A and B: Components of vacuum extractor. **A.** Metal suction cups with metal chain, vacuum bottle and vacuum pump and tube; **B.** Silastic vacuum cup.

- The traction device is used with a vacuum pump
- It is used in the operation of vacuum extraction of the fetal head
- The cup is to be fitted to the scalp of the fore coming head by producing a 'chignon' with the help of vacuum
- A manometer connects the traction bar and suction bottle
- It can be used with lesser force (10 kg) than required for forceps application to accomplish delivery of the head
- Silastic vacuum cups are softer, less traumatic and safer to use
- Vacuum extractor is used as an alternative to forceps
- It can be used on a fetal head at a higher station and not well-rotated.

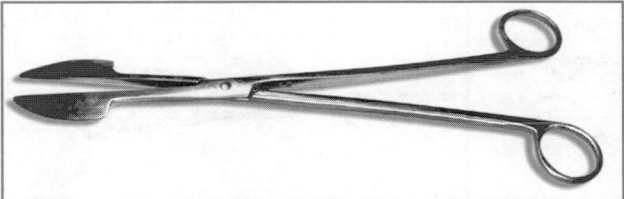

Fig. 75.34: Simpson's perforator.

SIMPSON'S PERFORATOR

Specifications and Uses

- A heavy metal instrument with spear-shaped sharp blades and handles with ridges
- With the blades closed, it is introduced into the vagina and fetal skill is perforated using rotary movements
- It is used to churn the brain matter before withdrawal, to facilitate evacuation of brain matter.

CRANIOCLAST

Specifications and Uses

- A heavy metal instrument with two blades. One blade is solid and the other fenestrated
- Used to compress the head following perforation
- The solid blade is introduced inside the cranium and the fenestrated blade outside for compression and extraction by traction.

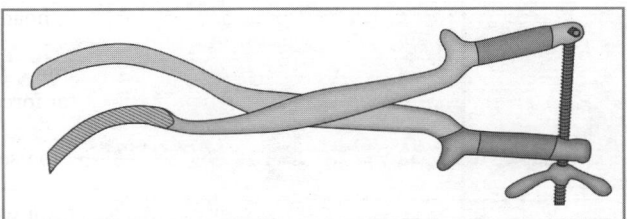

Fig. 75.35: Cranioclast.

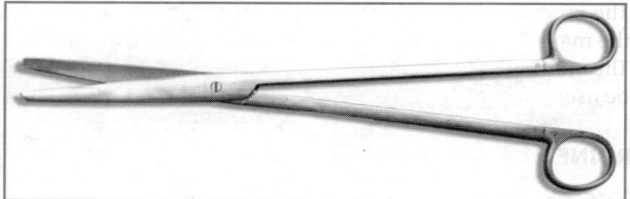

Fig. 75.36: Embryotomy scissors.

EMBRYOTOMY SCISSORS

Specifications and Uses

- A heavy scissors used in destructive operation
- It is used to cut the thoracic cage or the abdominal wall during evisceration or to cut the remnant of the soft tissue of neck behind, during decapitation or in cleidotomy or spondylotomy operation
- With this instrument, only the tissues of the baby are cut.

BREECH HOOK AND CROCHET

Specifications and Uses

- A metal instrument, which has curves at both ends. One end is acutely curved (the crochet) and the other gradually bent (breech hook)
- The hook is used to give traction to groin of a dead baby, when breech is impacted at the outlet

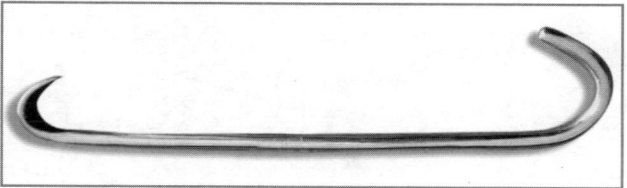

Fig. 75.37: Breech hook and crochet.

- The crochet is used to deliver the decapitated head by hooking the mandible through mouth or through a hole in the skull
- The middle portion is ridged to act as a handle and both ends may be used.

JARDINE'S DECAPITATION HOOK

Specifications and Uses

- This instrument has a handle and a head
- It is used in decapitation operation in neglected transverse lie or in impacted shoulder presentation, where the fetal neck is accessible per vagina
- The hook with knife is used to serve both the vertebral column and soft tissue. In locked twins where disengagement is impossible, it is used to perform decapitation to save the second twin
- It is used in rare cases of double-headed fetus to facilitate extraction.

COMBINED CRANIOCLAST AND CEPHALOTRIBE

Specifications and Uses

- The instrument consists of three parts, which can be adjusted and locked by a screw
- The central piece is placed within the skull through the opening made by a perforator
- The other two blades are almost straight without any pelvic curve
- They are placed externally over the skull and brought together by a butterfly screw prior to extraction of a dead fetus.

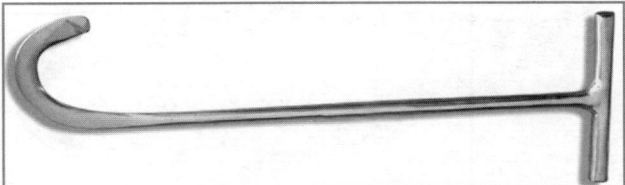

Fig. 75.38: Decapitation hook.

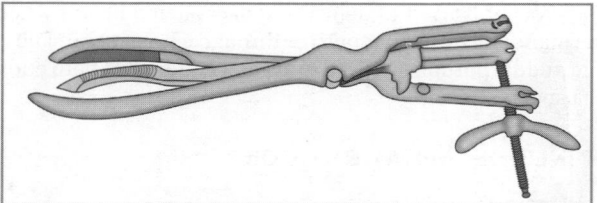

Fig. 75.39: Cranioclast and cephalotribe.

EXTERNAL PELVIMETER

Specifications and Uses

- A metal instrument with a joint at one end and a graduated bar
- Used to determine the external pelvic measurements
- Used to measure fundal height from symphysis pubis.

PINARD'S STETHOSCOPE/FETOSCOPE

Specifications and Uses

- A light, aluminum instrument
- It has an open abdominal end and an aural end
- When used to listen to fetal heart tones, it should be held firmly at right angle to the point on abdominal wall
- While listening to the fetal heart tones, the fetoscope should not be touched by hand.

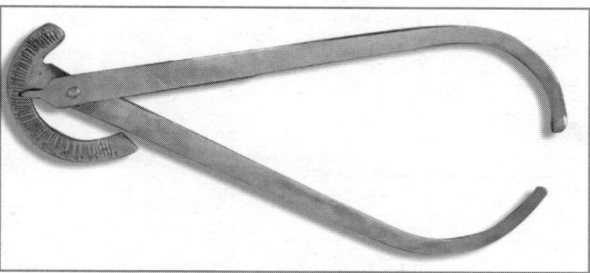

Fig. 75.40: Pelvimeter.

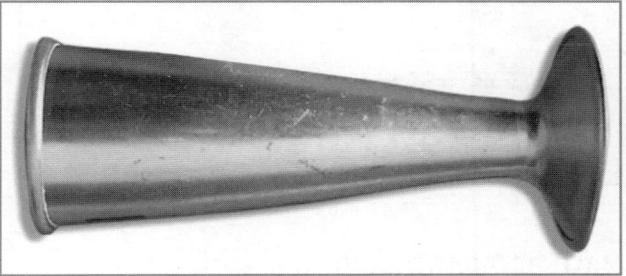

Fig. 75.41: Fetoscope.

NEEDLE HOLDER

Specifications and Uses

- The instrument has long handles and small blades and resembles an artery forceps
- The blades have cross serrations
- It has a groove for catching the needle on its inner surface
- It may be straight or curved
- Used to hold the needle for suturing
- Straight type is used for holding needles, while suturing a surface; curved type is used to work at depth or inside the cavity.

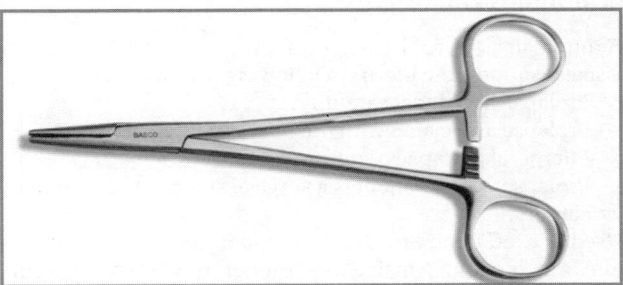

Fig. 75.42: Needle holder.

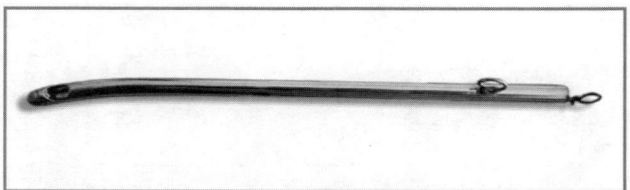

Fig. 75.43: Female metal catheter.

FEMALE METAL CATHETER

Specifications and Uses

- A hollow, metallic tube, which may be straight or curved, tapering at the tip with an opening in the side and a ring at the base
- Used to evacuate the bladder in labor when rubber or flexible catheter cannot be inserted into the bladder
- Used to differentiate between a vesicovaginal fistula and an urethrovaginal fistula
- Used to ascertain the lower limit of the bladder before operations for genital prolapse
- Used only when other softer catheters cannot be used or when urethra is obstructed. Gentle manipulation is needed; as it can cause injury.

RING PESSARY

Specifications and Uses

- A round, flexible, rubber instrument
- Used to support the uterus in following conditions:
  - Prolapse in older age group
  - Prolapse associated with pregnancy
  - Puerperal prolapse or retroversion
  - Prolapse, when patient is a surgical risk or refuses to undergo surgery.
- Used as a temporary measure to support uterus
- The watch spring, inside the rubber ring of the instrument stretches the vaginal walls, which can thus act as a better support.

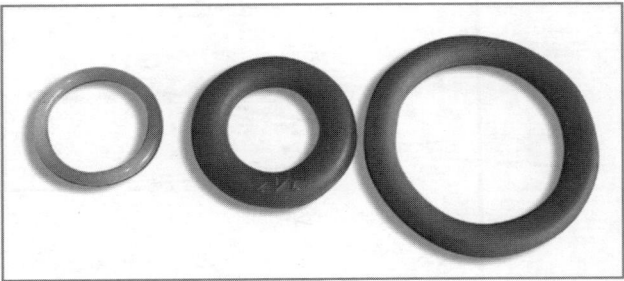

Fig. 75.44: Ring pessary.

HODGE-SMITH PESSARY

Specifications and Uses

- A rubber or plastic device shaped as ring with one end broader
- Used to support uterus in the following conditions:
  - Symptom-producing, mobile, uncomplicated retroverted uterus
  - Retroverted uterus in puerperal period
  - Retroverted gravid uterus upto 24th week of gestation.

BABCOCK TISSUE FORCEPS

Specifications and Uses

- A light and delicate instrument
- It is a non-traumatising type of tissue forceps

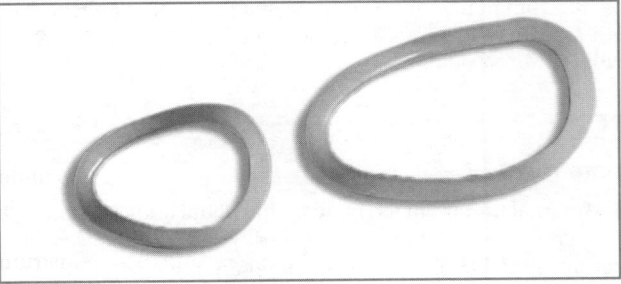

Fig. 75.45: Hodge-Smith pessary.

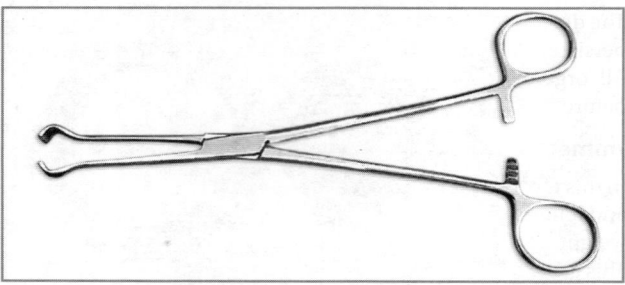

Fig. 75.46: Babcocks tissue forceps.

- The blades are curved and fenestrated
- Tips of the blades are in the form of transverse bars with transverse serrations on its inner aspects
- It is used to hold soft and delicate tissues such as fallopian tubes, ureters, appendix and gut wall as in gastrostomy, and colostomy
- It can be used as a hemostat when the bleeder is difficult to pinpoint. The whole chunk of tissue is held with Babcock forceps to cause temporary hemostasis.

76. INTRAUTERINE GROWTH RESTRICTION (RETARDATION)

Intrauterie growith restriction (IUGR) refers to infants born at or below the 10th percentile at birth on standardized graphs in weight, length and head circumference are considered as having retarded growth.

TYPES

Symmetric IUGR

- The ratio of the size of the head to that of the body is often normal
- The growth restriction occurs early in pregnancy caused by chromosomal aberration, congenital anomaly, viral infection or idiopathic

- The defect occurs in the first trimester of pregnancy and there is a persistently slow rate of growth, and a reduction in absolute size
- All organs are affected equally and usually becomes evident before 32 weeks of gestation.

Asymmetric IUGR

- In this type of IUGR, the measurements of the head circumference and length are in a higher percentile than is the measurement for weight
- This growth pattern occurs later in pregnancy and may be caused by placental insufficiency, maternal malnutrition or other extrinsic factors such as maternal hypertension
- These infants appear wasted
- There is high association with fetal distress, meconium aspiration, asphyxia and neonatal hypoglycemia
- Hypoxia is probably the common denominator in this type of growth retardation
- All organs are not affected to the same extent (asymmetrical)
- Oligohydramnios is often associated with IUGR.

FACTORS ASSOCIATED WITH IUGR

Fetal Factors

- Congenital infection
- Congenital malformations such as anencephaly, gastrointestinal atresia, renal agenesis and some cardiovascular defects
- Chromosomal abnormalities such as trisomy 13 (Patau's syndrome), trisomy 18 (Edward's syndrome) or trisomy 21 (Down's syndrome)
- Inborn errors of metabolism such as transient neonatal diabetes, galactosemia, and phenylketonuria.

Maternal Factors

- Maternal hypoxemia due to sickle cell disease, cardiovascular disease or living in high altitude
- Short maternal stature, young maternal age, low socioeconomic status, primiparity and grand multiparity
- Maternal exposure to teratogenic agents such as alcohol, cigarette smoke and anticonvulsant medications.

Placental Factors

- Decreased placental functioning due to minor abruption of placenta, placental infarctions, small placenta, post-term pregnancy and multiple pregnancy
- Placental insufficiency due to maternal vascular disease, hypertension and diabetes
- Intrinsic placental conditions such as poor implantation site, malformations, e.g. circumvalate placenta.

DIAGNOSIS

Because of the high perinatal mortality, early diagnosis is important:
- History of medical and obstetric problems
- Weight gain in pregnancy
- Uterine fundal height
- Fetal kick count
- Ultrasonography
- Doppler waveform analysis to assess resistance of blood flow
- Ponderal index to assess fetal malnutrition.

MANAGEMENT

Antepartum

- Identify patients at high risk
- Differentiate IUGR fetus from those that are small, but healthy
- Establish adequate methods of fetal surveillance and deliver them under optimal conditions
- Induction of labor by artificial rupture of membranes and infusion of oxytocin as appropriate, if cervix is favorable
- When cervix is unfavorable, prostaglandin to ripen the cervix followed by ARM and infusion of oxytocin
- Cesarean section if immediate delivery is necessary.

Intrapartum

- Delivery in hospital with specialized high-risk facilities
- Continuous electronic fetal monitoring

- Neonatologist to attend the birth regardless of the modality of delivery
- Delivery as atraumatic as possible.

COMPLICATIONS

- Asphyxia and acidosis in the perinatal period
- Meconium aspiration syndrome
- Hypoxic-ischemic encephalopathy
- Metabolic alterations: Hypoglycemia, hypocalcemia, hyperglycemia and hypothermia
- Infections
- Problems related to congenital malformations, e.g. neural tube defects, trisomy 18 or 21.

77. INTRAUTERINE TAMPONADE USING BAKRI BALLOON

The Bakri balloon is a medical device invented by Dr. Younes Bakri, a French obstetrician in 1992 for the treatment of obstetric hemorrhage during cesarean delivery. Later it was used to manage hemorrhage from lower uterine segment due to placenta previa and placenta accreta. As per WHO recommendations, the use of intrauterine balloon tamponade (UBT) is recommended for treatment of postpartum hemorrhage (PPH) due to uterine atony, if the woman does not respond to uterotonics.

DEFINITION

Bakri balloon insertion is a procedure used for temporary control or reduction of postpartum hemorrhage when conservative management of uterine bleeding is warranted after bleeding from genital tract laceration and retained products of conception have been excluded.

DESCRIPTION OF THE BAKRI BALLOON

The device consists of a 24 French, 54 cm long silicon catheter that contains a large central lumen and a balloon around it at the proximal end below the tip **(Figs. 77.1 and 77.2)**.

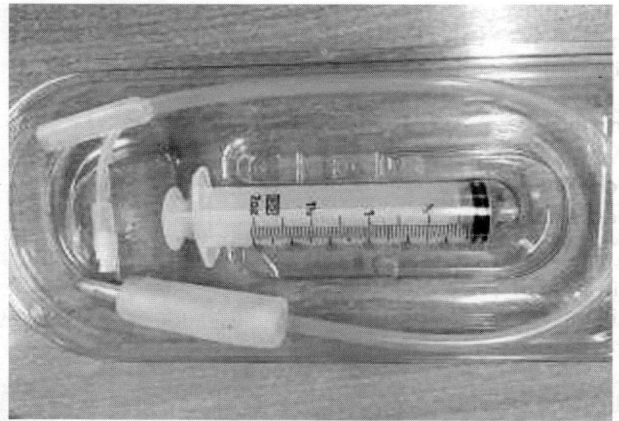

Fig. 77.1: Bakri balloon.

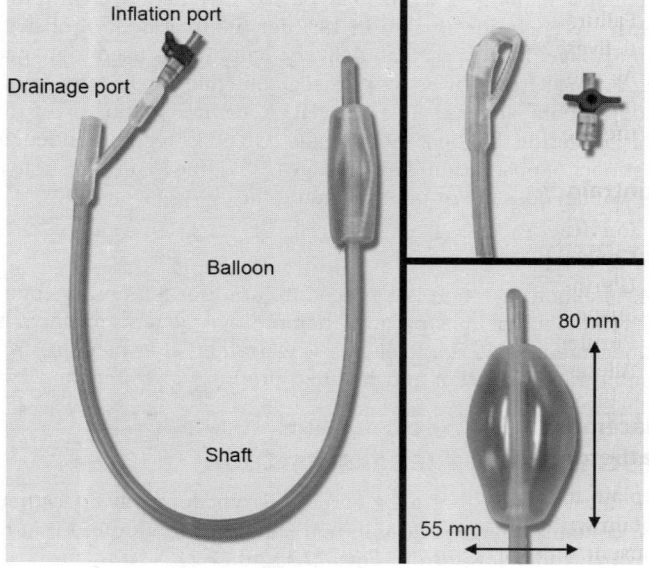

Fig. 77.2: Parts of Bakri balloon.

The collapsed balloon is inserted in to the uterus. When filled with the fluid, the balloon adapts to the configuration of the uterine cavity to tamponade endometrial bleeding. The central lumen of the catheter allows drainage and aids to monitor ongoing bleeding above the level of the balloon.

Mechanism of Action of the Balloon in the Control of Bleeding

The balloon is believed to act by exerting inward to outward pressure against the uterine wall resulting in a reduction in persistent capillary and venous bleeding from the endometrium and the myometrium.

Indications for Balloon Use

- For temporary control or reduction of PPH when conservative management of bleeding is warranted
- Failure to cause sustained control of hemorrhage after vaginal delivery, secondary to uterine atony
- As a temporary measure to decrease hemorrhage while waiting and preparing for other definitive treatment such as abdominal uterine surgery or uterine artery embolization.

Contraindications

- Cervical cancer
- Congenital uterine anomaly
- Uterine cavity distorting pathology (leiomyomas)
- Suspected uterine rupture
- Purulent infection of vagina, cervix or uterus
- Allergy to silicone material

Placement of Bakri Balloon in the Uterus/Insertion of the Catheter (Fig. 77.3)

Explain to patient about PPH, which is a medical emergency and obtain written consent if patient is alert, and if not a quick verbal consent. Inform family members about the need for immediate intervention

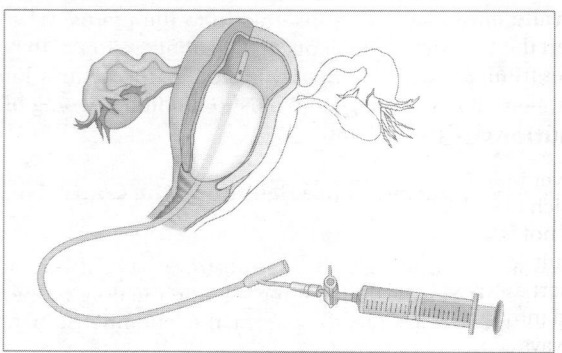

Fig. 77.3: Bakri Balloon inserted in the uterus and inflated.

- Assess the patient's vital signs, blood loss and general condition to exclude possible development of shock
- Place the patient in lithotomy position, drape and clean the perineum with antiseptic solution to avoid infection
- Insert a Foly's catheter to empty the bladder
- Cleanse vagina and cervix with povidone iodine to maintain asepsis
- Assist the doctor who will inspect the uterine cavity and visualize the cervix
- The deflated balloon is then inserted in to the uterine cavity under ultrasound guidance, making sure that the entire portion of the balloon passes the cervical canal above the internal os
- Once the placement is confirmed, the balloon will be inflated with the recommended amount of 500 ml of sterile normal saline. A vaginal pack may be placed if needed to maximize the effect of tamponade

Transabdominal Placement Post-cesarean Delivery

- The balloon is inserted through the uterine incision to the cervix and then into the vagina
- The uterine incision is then closed, taking special care not to damage the balloon by the suture needle.

An alternative approach used is to close the uterus first and then to insert the balloon from the vagina and inflate it while the surgeon watches from above.

Precautions

- Never inflate the balloon with air, carbon dioxide or any other gas which may cause complications.
- Do not fill the balloon with more than 500 mL. Overinflation may result in the balloon getting displaced in to the vagina
- Insert and leave a Foley's catheter in the bladder to collect urine and monitor urine output
- Always confirm proper placement of the balloon using an ultrasound after inflating it to the predetermined volume.

Post Procedural Care

- Connect the drainage port of the balloon to a collection bag to monitor hemostasis
- Monitor the patient for signs of increased bleeding and uterine cramping
- The device should not be kept indwelling for more than 24 hours
- Closely monitor bleeding, fundal height and vital signs of the patient
- After 6 hours and up to 24 hours, if the patient is stable with no virginal bleeding and her fundal height is at the same level. Start to slowly remove the fluid from the balloon
- Use antibiotics if recommended to avoid the risk of iatrogenic infection
- Use of oxytocin or other uterotonics such as Mehtylergometrine and prostaglandins are generally recommended.

78. INVERSION OF UTERUS

Inversion is a condition where the uterus becomes turned inside out, with the fundus prolapsing through the cervix.

CAUSES

- Acute inversion: Following childbirth
- Chronic inversion: Partial inversion not noticed or taken care of after childbirth
- Submucous myomatous polyp arising from the fundus causing traction effect
- Fundal fibroma with infiltration into myometrium leading to softening of the wall
- Senile inversion following high amputation of cervix.

TYPES

- Incomplete—the fundus protrudes through the cervix and lies inside vagina
- Complete—whole of the uterus including the cervix are inverted.

SIGNS AND SYMPTOMS: CHRONIC AND ACUTE

Chronic Inversion of Uterus

- Sensation of something coming down
- Irregular vaginal bleeding
- Offensive vaginal discharge
- The protruding mass will appear globular with no opening in the leading part
- Tumor may be present at the bottom.

Diagnosis

- Vaginal examination
- Rectal examination
- Sound test—measuring uterine cavity using uterine sound
- Examination under general anesthesia.

With inversions secondary to a fibroid polyp or sarcoma and when the inversion is incomplete, the diagnosis is more difficult.

Management of Chronic Inversion

- General measures—improvement of general conditions and treatments of sepsis if present

- Definitive treatment—rectification by surgery:
  - Correction of inversion by cutting and removing a portion; correcting the inversion and repairing the incised uterine wall. The procedure is done either abdominally (Haultain's operation) or vaginally (Spinelli's operation)
  - Hysterectomy—removal of uterus for older women, those who completed their families or with associated complications.

Acute Inversion of Uterus

Acute inversion occurs in the third stage of labor. It is usually considered as a serious complication of labor.

Causes

- Excessive traction on cord in third stage of labor to deliver placenta
- Combining cord traction and fundal pressure to deliver placenta
- Use of fundal pressure, while the uterus is atonic
- Use of undue traction on a pathologically adherent placenta (placenta accrete)
- Short umbilical cord
- Sudden emptying of a distended uterus.

Manifestations

- Hemorrhage in third stage to the range of 800–1,800 mL
- In cases of adherent placenta bleeding may be minimal
- Sudden onset of pain due to stretching of peritoneal nerves and pulling of ovaries downwards with the fundus
- Fundus not palpable per abdomen
- Uterus may not be visible at introitus, if inversion is incomplete. It may be felt on vaginal examination.

Management

Immediate management is required in acute inversion:
- Summon immediate medical help
- Attempt to replace the fundus by pushing it with the palm of hand along the direction of the vagina towards the posterior fornix
- Administer intravenous fluids and blood if required

- If placenta is still attached, do not attempt to remove it. Administration of medication is required to relax the cervical constriction ring if one is detected. This may be followed by attempt to remove the placenta and replacement of uterus
- Information to mother, spouse and family, and emotional support through out
- Assessment of vital signs, bleeding and level of consciousness through out.

79. JAUNDICE IN NEONATE

Jaundice or hyperbilirubinemia is an excess of bilirubin in blood, which causes yellow discoloration of the neonate's skin, mucous membranes and sclera.

MECHANISM OF JAUNDICE

- Increased production of bilirubin:
  - Increased red cells destruction due to shorter life span of the excess red blood cells (RBC) (80 days)
  - Inadequate production of enzyme from the liver, (glucuronyl transference) which normally converts unconjugated bilirubin to soluble bilirubin
  - Reduced conversion of bilirubin to urobilinogen by intestinal bacterial flora resulting in absorption of more bilirubin back into the circulation.
- Delayed clearance of bilirubin by the Liver:
  - Biliary atresia or choledocal cyst. Bile does not pass into the bowel in normal quantities and the stool is pale.

TYPES

Physiological Jaundice

- Most common type of jaundice
- Occurs in most preterm babies and some full-term babies
- Appears on the 2nd day in term babies peaking on 5th or 6th day
- Maximum bilirubin level reaches 12 mg/dL (normal value 1.8 mg/dL)

- Peak level reaches on 5th or 6th day in preterm babies and clears by 2–3 weeks
- Cause is immaturity of liver
- Jaundice is exaggerated in prematurity, hypoxia, narcotic and barbiturate use and cephalhematoma
- No specific treatment is needed
- Careful observation and more fluids are needed
- Use of phenobarbitone and phototherapy are indicated; if bilirubin level reaches critical level.

Pathological Jaundice

- Jaundice appears within 24 hours of birth.
- Bilirubin level increases at the rate of 0.5 mg/100 mL per hour.
- Absolute bilirubin level reaches more than 15 mg/100 mL.
- Jaundice in a sick baby manifests with lethargy, temperature instability, poor feeding and apnea.
- Jaundice persists after 8 days in a term infant and 14 days in a preterm infant.
- Common causes are blood group incompatibility specifically ABO and Rh incompatibility.
- Other less common causes are maternal or fetal infections, swallowed maternal blood, fetal enzyme deficiencies (G6PD), fetal enclosed hemorrhage (e.g. cephalhematoma or bruising), fetal polycythemia and fetal hypothyroidism.

Specific Conditions Causing Pathological Jaundice

Rhesus incompatibility: Incompatibility arises when the mother is Rhesus (Rh)-negative and carries a fetus that is Rh positive. Isoimmunization occurs, when fetal blood cells escape and pass through the placenta into the maternal circulation. The woman may form protective antibodies against the fetal blood cells (maternal sensitization). Usually the woman becomes sensitized during the first pregnancy, but does not form enough antibodies to adversely affect the infant. During subsequent pregnancies, antibodies form rapidly, resulting in lysis or destruction of fetal blood cells.

ABO incompatibility: Occurs as a result of the mother and fetus having different blood groups. The mixing of maternal and fetal blood leads to hemolysis of fetal blood cells. ABO incompatibility is the most common and mildest type of hemolytic disease. The incompatibility, occurs when the fetal blood type is A, B or AB and the mother's blood type is O.

Kernicterus: A possible complication of pathologic jaundice is kernicterus also termed as 'bilirubin encephalopathy'. There is excess accumulation of unbound, unconjugated bilirubin, which is deposited in brain tissues, particularly the basal ganglia. The excess bilirubin crosses the blood-brain barrier, causing yellow staining of the brain tissue, similar to its effect on the skin. In a term neonate, when the total serum bilirubin exceeds 25 mg/dL, the risk for kernicterus increases. Premature and sick neonates are at risk for kernicterus at much lower serum bilirubin levels. Early signs include lethargy, poor feeding, temperature instability, hypotonia and high-pitched cry. Permanent neurologic complications are possible and include ataxia, opisthotonos, deafness and mental retardation.

Erythroblastosis fetalis: It is a condition in which there is vast destruction of fetal red cells by maternal antibodies (in Rh compatibility) resulting in fetal anemia and hyperbilirubinemia. The destruction of fetal blood cells may be so severe that a marked hemolytic anemia develops. Fetal death or birth of an infant with hydrops fetalis may result.

Hydrops fetalis is the most severe form of fetal hemolytic disease—there is severe anemia resulting in hypoxia, cardiac decompenzation and hepatosplenomegaly. The signs of Rh incompatibility such as jaundice, pallor and enlargement of liver and spleen appear within 4–5 hours of birth and peaks when the newborn is 3–4 days old.

MANAGEMENT

The goal of management is to keep the serum bilirubin below neurotoxic levels are:

Phototherapy

Phototherapy is the use of ultraviolet light in the treatment of jaundice in the newborn. It works by encouraging the liver to excrete bile in the form of unconjugated bilirubin. Blue or fluorescent bulbs are commonly used in phototherapy. Prolonged exposure to ultraviolet light may cause retinal damage; therefore, it is important to keep the infant's eyes shielded with eye patches when under the light.

The adverse effects of using phototherapy includes dermal rash, dehydration, thrombocytopenia, hypocalcemia, secretary diarrhea and 'bronze baby' syndrome.

Care of the baby undergoing phototherapy includes close monitoring of body temperature, fluid and electrolyte balance, and checking of serum bilirubin level at intervals.

Exchange Transfusion

An exchange transfusion is used when phototherapy is ineffective and the bilirubin level is rising. Exchange transfusion lowers the bilirubin level by 50–60%. During transfusion, the neonate's antibodycoated red cells and excess bilirubin are removed and replaced by donor blood that contains non coated RBCs. Only small amounts of infant's blood are removed and replaced at a time. The procedure is repeated until the infant's total blood volume has been diluted with fresh blood.

The nurse must be alert for the following complications during transfusion—bradycardia, arrhythmias, infection, thrombosis, hypocalcemia and fluid overload.

80. LABOR—STAGE I

The first stage of labor is the stage of dilation of the cervix and begins with regular rhythmic contractions of the uterus and culminates in complete dilatation of the cervix.

PHASES OF STAGE I

Stage I is further explained in three phases:
- **Latent phase or the first phase of stage I:** It begins with the onset of true labor and ends with the cervix dilated 4 cm. The phase averages approximately 8–10 hours, upto 20 hours for nulliparas and 3–6 hours, upto 14 hours, for multiparas.
- Active phase: It is the second phase in which contractions increase to moderate intensity and the cervix dilates from

4 to 8 cm. The client becomes more involved and focused on the labor process. This phase lasts approximately 3–4 hours in the nullipara and 1–2 hours, in the multipara.

- Transition phase: This is the most intense of the three phases lasting an average of 2–3 hours in nulliparas and 1 hour in multiparas. The cervix dilates 8–10 cm as the fetus descends approximately 1 cm per hour in nulliparas and 2 cm per hour in multiparas.

PHYSIOLOGICAL PROCESSES IN THE FIRST STAGE OF LABOR

- **Fundal dominance:** Each contraction starts in the fundus near one of the cornua and spreads across and downwards.
- **Polarity:** A neuromuscular harmony prevails between the two poles or segments of uterus through out labor. The upper pole contracts stronger and retracts to expel the fetus, the lower pole contracts slightly and dilates to allow expulsion to occur.
- **Formation of retraction ring:** A ridge forms between the upper and lower uterine segments, which gradually rises as the upper segment contracts and retracts, and the lower segment thins out to accommodate the descending fetus. Once the cervix is fully dilated and the fetus can leave the uterus, the retraction ring rises no further.
- **Cervical effacement:** The thinning of cervix and shortening of cervical canal occurs.
- **Cervical dilatation:** Enlargement of external cervical os from an orifice of a few millimeters to an opening large enough for the baby to pass through takes place.
- **Ripening of the cervix:** The cervical tissues soften to butter soft consistency after certain number of contractions.

MANAGEMENT OF CLIENT IN THE FIRST STAGE OF LABOR

- Admission to labor and delivery unit
- History and physical examinations
- Perineal preparation
- Enema, if in early first stage and membranes are intact
- Hydration: IV fluids

- Ambulation and position of comfort
- Monitoring maternal physiological changes, vital signs, urinary output, gastric motility and hematological changes
- Monitoring of fetal well-being:
  - Fetal lie, presentation, position and variety
  - Fetal adaptation to pelvis
  - Fetal heart rate (FHR) and pattern.

NURSING PROCESS

Assessment

Latent Phase

- Client may be excited or anxious
- Regular contractions, increasing in frequency, duration and severity occur
- Contractions are mild to moderate, 10–20 minutes apart, progressing to 5–7 minutes apart, lasting 15–20 seconds, progressing to 30–40 seconds
- Fetal heart tones best heard below level of umbilicus (in vertex presentation)
- Membranes may or may not have ruptured
- Cervix dilates from 0–4 cm
- Fetus may be at station −1 to 0 in primigravidas or 0 to +2 cm in multigravida
- Scant vaginal discharge, may be pink or brownish mucus (show) or may consist of mucous plug.

Active Phase

- Client may show evidence of fatigue
- Contractions are moderate, occurring every 2.5–5 minutes and lasting 45–60 seconds
- Fetal heart tones detected slightly below umbilicus
- The FHR variability can be noted in response to contractions and fetal movement
- Cervix dilates from approximately 4–8 cm
- Moderate amount of bloodshow
- Fetus descends from 11–12 cm below ischial spines.

Transition Phase

- Nausea or vomiting may occur
- Strong uterine contractions occurring every 2–3 minutes and lasting 60+ seconds
- Intense level of discomfort in abdominal and sacral area
- May become very restless or fearful
- May report being 'too hot' tingling sensation of finger tips, toes and face
- Leg tremors and diaphoresis may occur
- The FHT heard just above symphysis pubis
- Cervix dilates 8–10 cm
- Fetus descends 12–14 cm
- Copious amount of bloody show.

Nursing Diagnosis

- Risk for anxiety
- Deficient knowledge regarding progress of labor and available options
- Risk for deficient fluid volume
- Risk for maternal infection
- Risk for fetal injury
- Acute pain
- Risk for ineffective individual coping.

Expected Outcomes

The client will:
- Verbalize anxiety reduced to manageable level
- Verbalize understanding of physiologic and psychologic changes and demonstrate appropriate breathing and relaxation techniques
- Demonstrate adequate hydration
- Be free of signs of infection
- Display FHR within normal limits
- Report minimized discomfort and rest between contractions
- Identify effective coping skills and activities to maintain control.

Nursing Interventions

1. **Reporting anxiety at a manageable level:**
   - Provide continuous support as indicated
   - Orient client to environment, staff and procedures
   - Provide information about physiologic and psychologic changes in labor
   - Assess level and cause of anxiety, and preparedness for childbirth
   - Monitor uterine contractile pattern
   - Encourage to verbalize feelings, concerns and fears
   - Demonstrate breathing and relaxation methods, provide comfort measures
   - Monitor blood pressure (BP) and pulse as indicated
   - Provide privacy and respect for modesty, use draping during vaginal examination.

2. **Verbalizing, understanding of physiological changes and practicing appropriate techniques:**
   - Assess client's expectations and knowledge level regarding birth process
   - Provide information about procedures (fetal monitoring, vaginal examinations) and normal progression of labor. Teach and review pushing positions for stage II
   - Obtain informed consent for invasive procedures (e.g. episiotomy, internal monitoring). Explain usual procedures and possible risks.

3. **Maintaining adequate hydration:**
   - Monitor intake and output. Encourage to empty bladder every 1½–2 hours. Note urine specific gravity
   - Monitor temperature every 4 hours and more frequently; if elevated, monitor FHR as indicated
   - Assess skin turgor and production of mucus
   - Provide clear fluids as permitted and mouth care as appropriate
   - Administer parenteral fluids, as indicated
   - Monitor hematocrit level.

4. **Mother staying free of infection:**
   - Explain importance of demonstrate good hand washing
   - Use aseptic technique during vaginal examination

- Provide/Encourage perineal care as indicated and change underpad/Linen when wet
- Assess vaginal secretions and amniotic fluid after rupture of membranes
- Monitor temperature, pulse and respirations and white blood cells (WBC) count as indicated
- Provide oral and parenteral fluids, as indicated
- Carry out perineal preparation as appropriate
- Administer cleansing enema; if indicated
- Administer prophylactic antibiotic IV; if indicated
- Administer oxytocin infusion as indicated
- Obtain blood culture; if symptoms of sepsis are present.

5. **Fetus displaying FHR within normal limits:**
   - Perform Leopold's maneuvers to determine fetal position, lie and presentation
   - Obtain baseline FHR and evaluate frequently per protocol. Note FHR variability and periodic changes in response to uterine contractions
   - Note progress of labor
   - Note FHR when membranes rupture, reassess periodically per protocol
   - Assess for visible cord prolapse at vaginal introitus
   - If present, calm patient, elevate hips (elevated Sim's position) or help assume knee-chest position and push presenting part off cord and hold off while summoning help
   - Check cord for pulsations; wrap cord in sterile gauze soaked in saline
   - Monitor FHR, note presence of bradycardia or sinusoidal pattern
   - Position client in lateral recumbent position
   - Turn off oxytocin if infusing, and increase plain IV solution
   - Administer oxygen via face mask
   - Collaborative interventions: Prepare for surgical intervention as indicated.

6. **Reporting minimized discomfort:**
   - Assess degree of discomfort through verbal and nonverbal cues

- Assist in use of appropriate breathing and relaxation techniques and abdominal effleurage
- Assist with comfort measures (e.g. back rubs, sacral pressure, back rest, mouth care repositioning, perineal care, and linen changes)
- Encourage to void every 1-2 hours; palpate above symphysis pubis to determine distension
- Provide information about available analgesics, usual response and side effects
- Time and record the frequency, intensity and duration of uterine contractility pattern per protocol
- Assess nature and amount of vaginal show, cervical dilation, effacement, fetal station and fetal descend
- Assess BP and pulse every 1-2 minutes after regional injection for first 15 minutes, then every 10-15 minutes for the remainder of labor.
- Collaborative interventions: As follows:
  - Administer analgesic such as stadol or demerol if indicated/ordered
  - Administer oxygen and increase plain fluid intake if systolic pressure falls below 100 mm Hg
  - Administer emergency medications as indicated [e.g. naloxone (Narcan)].

7. **Engaging in activities to maintain control:**
   - Ascertain client's understanding and expectations of the labor process
   - Encourage verbalization of feelings
   - Reinforce use of positive coping mechanisms and relaxation techniques
   - Note withdrawn behavior
   - Demonstrate behaviors and techniques client can use for pain control and relaxation
   - Provide positive reinforcement for efforts. Use touch and smoothing words of encouragement.

81. LABOR—STAGE II

Stage II of labor, the stage of expulsion begins with full dilation of cervix (10 cm) and ends with the birth of the newborn.

FEATURES OF STAGE II LABOR

- Contractions occur 1.5–2 minutes apart, lasting 60–90 seconds
- The average fetal descend is 1 cm per hour for nulliparas and 2 cm or more for multiparas
- Maternal efforts to bear down occur involuntarily during contractions
- May have fecal discharge, while bearing down
- Bladder distension may be present
- May report burning/stretching sensation of perineum
- Legs may tremble during pushing efforts
- BP may rise 5–10 mm Hg in between contractions
- Respiratory rate increases
- Diaphoresis often present
- Fetal bradycardia may appear as early decelerations on electronic monitor during contractions due to head compression
- Cervix is fully dilated and 100% effaced
- Increased amount of vaginal bloody show
- Rectal/Perineal bulging with fetal descend
- Membranes may rupture at this point; if still intact
- Increased expulsion of amniotic fluid during contractions
- Crowning occurs; caput is visible just before birth in vertex presentations.

MECHANISM OF NORMAL LABOR

The mechanisms of labor are the positional movements that the fetus undergoes to accommodate itself to the maternal pelvis. This is necessary for the full term fetus to negotiate its way through the pelvis to be born.

When the fetus presents in left or right occipitoanterior position, the way the fetus is normally situated are as follows:

- The lie is longitudinal
- The presentation is cephalic
- The position is right or left occipitoanterior

- The attitude is one of flexion
- The denominator is vertex
- The presenting part is the posterior part of the anterior parietal bone.

Positional Movements (Figs. 81.1A to G)

- Engagement
- Descend (occurs through out)
- Flexion
- Internal rotation of the head
- Crowning
- Birth of the head by extension
- Restitution
- Internal rotation of the shoulders and simultaneous external rotation of the head
- Birth of shoulders and body by lateral flexion.

Summary of Mechanisms of Labor in Left Occiput Anterior Position (LOA)

- Engagement: It takes place with the sagittal suture of the fetal head in the right oblique and the biparietal diameter in the opposite diameter (left oblique). The occiput points to left iliopectineal eminence and sinciput to the right sacroiliac joint
- Descend: It occurs through out
- Flexion: Increases and the engaging diameter suboccipitofrontal 10 cm changes to suboccipito bregmatic 9.5 cm
- **Internal rotation of the head:** It takes place as the occiput turns oneeighth of a circle (45°) anteriorly (to the right). The sagittal suture comes to the anteroposterior diameter of the maternal pelvis
- **Crowning:** It occurs next, as the occiput escapes under the symphysis pubis and the biparietal diameter stretches the vulval outlet without recession of the head between contractions
- **Birth of the head by extension:** The head is born by extension pivoting on the suboccipital region around the pubic bone. The sinciput, face and chin sweep the perineum, and are born by a movement of flexion
- **Restitution:** The occiput turns one eighth of a circle (45°) towards the side from which it started (mother's left in LOA) and the twist

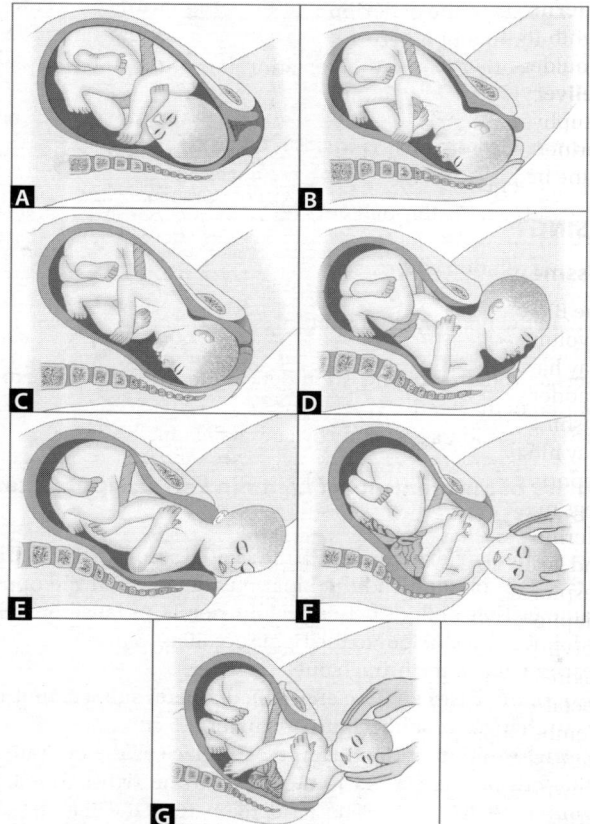

Figs. 81.1A to G: Mechanisms of labor. **A.** Engagement descend flexcon; **B.** Internal solation; **C.** Extension begining; **D.** External complete; **E.** External rotation; **F.** External rotation; **G.** Lateral flexion (expulsion).

on the neck that occurred during internal rotation of the head gets undone
- **Internal rotation of shoulders:** The anterior shoulder reaches the pelvic floor and rotates forward to lie under the symphysis pubis

- **External rotation of the head:** The occiput rotates further one eighth to the mother's left simultaneously as internal rotation of shoulders occur
- **Delivery of the body:** The anterior shoulder escapes under the symphysis pubis and the posterior shoulder passes over the perineum, remainder of the body is born by lateral flexion as the spine bends sideways through the curved birth canal.

NURSING PROCESS

Assessment

- The BP may rise 5–10 mm Hg in between contractions
- Involuntary urge to defecate/push with contractions occur
- May have fecal discharge, while bearing down
- Bladder distension may be present, with urine expressed during pushing efforts
- May moan/groan during contractions
- Reports of burning or stretching sensation of the perineum
- Legs may tremble during pushing efforts
- Uterine contractions become strong, occurring 1–2 minute apart and lasting 60–90 seconds
- Respiratory rate increases
- Diaphoresis often present
- Cervix becomes fully dilated (10 cm) and 100% effaced
- Vaginal bloody show increases
- Rectal/perineal bulging occurs with fetal descend
- Membranes may rupture at this point if still intact
- Increased expulsion of amniotic fluid during contractions
- Crowning occurs and caput becomes visible just before birth in vertex presentations.

Nursing Diagnosis

- Acute pain
- Cardiac output fluctuation
- Risk for impaired fetal gas exchange
- Risk for impaired skin/tissue integrity
- Risk for maternal infection
- Risk for fetal injury.

Expected Outcomes

The client will:
- Rest between contractions
- Maintain vital signs appropriate for second stage of labor
- Remain free of preventable lacerations
- Stay free of infections.

Fetus will:
- Remain free of variable or late decelerations with FHR within normal limits
- Stay free of preventable trauma or other complications.

Nursing Interventions

1. **Resting between contractions:**
    - Identify discomforts and its sources
    - Provide comfort measures, such as mouth care, perineal care, back massage, clean, dry linen and underpads
    - Review information about type of regional analgesia/anesthesia available, specific to the delivery setting
    - Provide informations and support related to progress of labor
    - Encourage client to manage efforts to bear down with spontaneous rather than sustained, pushing during contractions. Stress importance of using abdominal muscles and relaxing pelvic floor
    - Observe for perineal and rectal bulging, opening of vaginal introitus and changes in fetal station
    - Assist client to assume optimal position for bearing down (e.g. semi-Fowler's position). Assess effectiveness of bearing down efforts
    - Encourage client to relax all muscles and rest between contractions
    - Monitor maternal BP and pulse, and FHR
    - Assess bladder fullness. Catheterize between contractions; if distension is noted and the client is unable to void
    - Assist as needed with administration of local anesthetic just before episiotomy, if done.

2. **Maintaining maternal vital signs and FHR within normal limits:**
   - Monitor BP and pulse every 15 minutes. Note amount and concentration of urine output, test for albuminuria
   - Instruct client to push only when she feels the urge to do so. Avoid forced pushing
   - Encourage client to inhale and exhale during bearing down efforts, using an open glottis technique and holding breath no longer than 5 seconds at a time
   - Monitor FHR after every contraction or bearing down effort
   - Monitor BP and pulse immediately after administration of anesthesia if used and repeat until client is stable, e.g. epidural or subarachnoid block
   - Regulate intravenous (IV) infusion as indicated and decrease the rate of oxytocin; if necessary.
3. **Staying free of preventable lacerations:**
   - Assist client with proper positioning, breathing and efforts to relax
   - Ensure that client relaxes perineal floor, while using abdominal muscles in pushing
   - Monitor safety and support legs, especially; if epidural catheter is in place
   - Lift legs simultaneously, if leg supports/stirrups are used and place feet and legs properly in low position, supporting feet
   - Assess for bladder fullness, catheterize prior to delivery as appropriate
   - Assist as needed with hand maneuvers, apply pressure to fetal chin through maternal perineum, while exerting pressure on the occiput with the other hand (reduces trauma to maternal tissues)
   - Assist with midline or mediolateral episiotomy
   - Maintain accurate delivery records of location of episiotomy and/or laceration. Record type and timing of forceps if used.
4. **Staying free of infection:**
   - Provide perineal care per protocol, using medical asepsis
   - Remove fecal contaminants expelled during pushing, change linen and underpad as needed
   - Note date and time of rupture of membranes

- Perform vaginal examination only when absolutely necessary, using aseptic technique
- Monitor temperature, pulse and white blood cell (WBC) count as indicated
- Use surgical asepsis in preparing equipment. Clean perineum with sterile water and soap or surgical disinfectant just prior to delivery
- Collaborative intervention: As follows:
  - Administer antibiotics as indicated
  - Provide aseptic conditions for delivery.

5. **Fetal condition remaining within normal limits:**
   - Position client in lateral recumbent or upright position or turn to side as indicated
   - Avoid placing client in dorsal recumbent position
   - Determine fetal station, presentation and position. If fetus is in occiput posterior position, place client on her side
   - Assess client's breathing pattern. Note reports of tingling sensation of face or hands, dizziness or carpopedal spasms (indicating alkalosis or acidosis)
   - Have client breathe into cupped hands or small paper bag as indicated
   - Monitor client for fruity breathe odor
   - Encourage client to inhale and exhale every 10–20 seconds during bearing down efforts
   - Assess FHR during and after each contraction or pushing effort
   - Note short and long-term FHR variability
   - Perform sterile vaginal examination feeling for cord prolapse, if present, lift vertex off cord
   - Collaborative intervention: As follows:
     - Assist as needed with intermittent fetal scalp blood sampling, if done
     - Prepare for surgical intervention if spontaneous vaginal or low forceps delivery is not immediately possible after approximately 30 min, and fetal pH is 7.20 or less.

6. **Fetus staying free of preventable trauma or other complications:**
   - Assess fetal position, station and presentation
   - Monitor labor progress and rate of fetal descend

- Assess amount of amniotic fluid expelled at the time membranes rupture and then during contractions
- Note color of amniotic fluid
- Transfer to delivery room as appropriate when multipara is 8 cm dilated and vertex is visible at the introitus in nullipara
- Remain with client and monitor pushing efforts as head emerges. Instruct client to pant during process
- Maintain record of events
- Collaborative intervention: Prepare for instrumental delivery or surgical intervention, if indicated.

82. LABOR—STAGE III

Stage III of labor begins with the birth of the baby and is completed with placental separation and expulsion. Third stage lasts from 1 to 30 minutes, with an average length of 3-4 minutes in the nullipara and 4-5 minutes in the multipara, this stage is the shortest. Careful management and monitoring are necessary to prevent short- and long-term negative outcomes.

PLACENTAL SEPARATION AND EXPULSION

Separation of the Placenta

- Results from abrupt reduction in size of the uterine cavity
- Decrease in the area of placental attachment, due to the process of retraction of uterine muscle
- Separation of the placenta from the spongiosa layer of the decidua occurs
- Separation begins at the center; so that a retroplacental clot is formed
- The retroplacental clot facilitates completion of the separation.

Descend of the Placenta

After separation, the placenta descends into the lower uterine segment and into the upper vaginal vault causing the following clinical signs of separation:
- Sudden trickle or gush of blood
- Lengthening of the umbilical cord visible at the vaginal introitus

- Change in the shape of the uterus from a circular to globular
- Level of uterine fundus rises in the abdomen.

Expulsion of the Placenta (Figs. 82.1A and B)

Schultz Mechanism of Placental Expulsion

- Delivery of the placenta with the fetal side presenting
- Occurs when separation begins at the center with retroplacental clot formation.

Duncan Mechanism of Placental Expulsion

- Delivery of the placenta with the maternal side presenting
- Occurs when separation begins at the margin or periphery of the placenta
- Placenta descends sideways and amniotic sac trails behind placenta.

CARE OF THE MOTHER IN THE THIRD STAGE OF LABOR

- Guard the uterus: Keep anyone from massaging it prior to placental separation
- Do not pull on the umbilical cord before the placenta separates or with uncontracted uterus

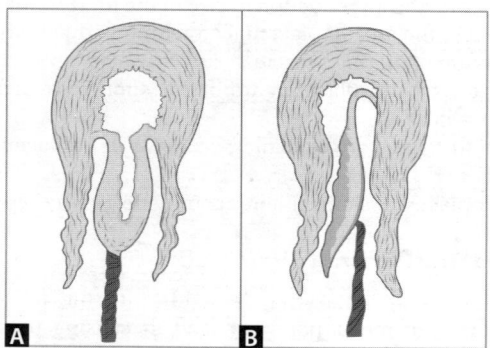

Figs. 82.1A and B: Methods of placental expulsion. **A.** Schultz method; **B.** Matthew's duncan method.

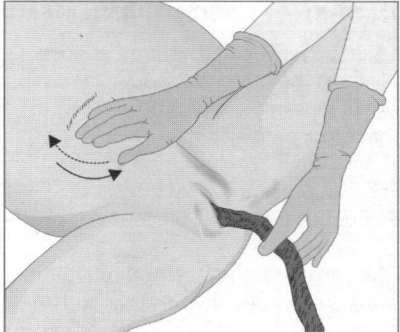

Fig. 82.2: Controlled cord traction (Brandt-Andrew method).

- Do not try to deliver the placenta prior to its complete separation
- Wait for the natural process to occur and do not interfere.

Delivery of Placenta and Membranes (Fig. 82.2)

Expectant Management

- A hand is placed over the fundus to feel the signs of placental separation, the state of uterine activity (contraction and relaxation) and any collection of blood in the uterine cavity
- When the features of placental separation and it is descend into the lower uterine segment are confirmed, the client is asked to bear down simultaneously with the hardening of the uterus.

Expression by Fundal Pressure

- Four fingers of one hand are placed behind the fundus and the thumb in front of the uterus to use as a piston
- Gentle rub on the fundus to make the uterus contract
- Pushing downwards and backwards till the placenta passes through the introitus
- Membranes follow the placenta immediately and are delivered with the placenta normally.

EXAMINATION OF THE PLACENTA AND MEMBRANES

Examination should be performed as soon as possible after delivery. Remove any clots from the maternal surface and replace any broken cotyledons before beginning examination. Items to look for are:
- Infarctions that are recent or old
- Localized calcifications
- Completeness with presence of all lobes
- Blood vessels denoting normal placenta or presence of succenturiate lobe
- Insertion of the cord—whether central or lateral
- Number of umbilical vessels—two arteries and one vein are normal.

NURSING PROCESS

Assessment

- Behaviors may range from excitement to fatigue
- The BP increases as cardiac output increases; then returns to normal levels shortly thereafter
- Hypotension may occur in response to change in cardiac output
- Normal blood loss is less than 500 mL
- May complain of leg/body tremors, chills or leg cramps
- Extension of episiotomy or birth canal lacerations may be present
- Dark vaginal bleeding as a trickle occurs as the placenta separates from the endometrium, usually within 3–5 minutes after delivery of the neonate
- Umbilical cord lengthens at vaginal introitus
- Uterus changes from discoid to globular shape and rises in abdomen.

Nursing Diagnosis

- Acute pain
- Risk for deficient fluid volume
- Risk for maternal injury.

Expected Outcomes

The client will:
- Verbalize management or reduction of pain

- Maintain BP, heart rate, pulse and blood loss within normal limits
- Be free of injury.

Nursing Interventions

1. **Managing pain:**
   - Assist with use of breathing techniques during surgical repair as appropriate
   - Apply ice bags to perineum after delivery (reduces edema and produces local comfort)
   - Change wet clothing and bedding
   - Provide a warm blanket.
2. **Maintaining vital signs and blood loss within normal limits:**
   - Instruct client to push with contractions, help direct attention toward bearing down (bearing down helps separation and expulsion of placenta)
   - Assess vital signs before and after administering oxytocin
   - Palpate uterus, note ballooning (suggests uterine relaxation and bleeding into uterine cavity)
   - Monitor for signs of excess fluid loss or shock (e.g. check BP, pulse, sensorium, skin color and temperature)
   - Place infant at client's breast; if she plans to breastfeed
   - Massage uterus gently after placental expulsion
   - Record time and mechanism of placental separation (Schultz mechanism or Duncan's mechanism)
   - Inspect maternal and fetal surfaces of placenta. Note size, cord insertion, intactness, vascular changes or calcification
   - Obtain and record information related to inspection of uterus and placenta for retained placental fragments
   - Administer fluids through parenteral route
   - Collaborative interventions: As follows:
     - Administer oxytocin through intramascular (IM) route or dilute intravenous (IV) drip in electrolyte solution as indicated
     - Assist with repair of cervix, vagina and episiotomy extension.
3. **Being free of injury:**
   - Palpate uterus, note 'ballooning' of uterus and massage gently

- Gently massage uterus after placental expulsion
- Clean vulva and perineum with sterile water and antiseptic solution; apply perineal pad
- Remove client's legs simultaneously from leg supports; if used
- Assist in transfer from delivery bed to recovery bed as appropriate
- Obtain sample of cord blood; send to laboratory for blood typing of newborn and banking as desired
- Assist with episiotomy repair as necessary.

83. LACTATION

Lactation is a complex physiologic process under neuroendocrine control. It is the biologic completion of the reproductive cycle. Starting at about 16 weeks gestation the breasts develop and prepare for full lactation. In the 1st few postpartal hours and days the breasts respond to hormones and the stimulation of the infant's sucking to produce and release milk.

PHYSIOLOGY OF LACTATION

The physiological basis of lactation is divided into four phases:
- Mammogenesis or preparation of breasts
- Lactogenesis or initiation of milk secretion
- Galectokinesis or ejection of milk
- Galectopoiesis or maintenance of established milk secretion.

Mammogenesis

Pregnancy is associated with a remarkable growth of both ductal and lobulo-alveolar system. During lactation, the breast tissue is characterized by large numbers of alveoli. After lactation when, milk is no longer removed from the breast by the infant, the alveoli gradually collapse and adipose tissue increases.

Lactogenesis

Complex nervous and endocrine factors are involved in the establishment of milk production in the first 2–5 days postpartum.

Childbirth results in a rapid decrease in estrogen and progesterone, and an increase in prolactin secretion. Prolactin from the pituitary gland triggers milk production by stimulating the alveolar cells of the breast. Prolactin levels increase in response to tactile stimulation of the breast and sucking by the infant.

Galactokinesis

Discharge of milk from mammary glands depends not only on the suction exerted by the baby during suckling, but also on the contractile mechanism, which expresses the milk from the alveoli into the ducts. The milk ejection is inhibited by factors such as pain, breast engorgement or adverse psychic condition.

Galactopoiesis

Prolactin is the most important galactopoietic hormone. For maintenance of effective and continuous lactation, suckling is essential as it causes release of prolactin. Milk pressure reduces the rate of production and hence periodic breastfeeding is necessary to relieve the pressure, which in turn maintains the secretion.

LET-DOWN REFLEX AND MILK EJECTION

The infant's sucking also stimulates the release of oxytocin, the hormone produced by posterior pituitary that stimulates uterine contractions and release of milk from the mammary glands. Oxytocin increases the contractility of the myoepithelial cells that line the walls of the mammary ducts, resulting in the let-down reflex. The let-down reflex is the ejection of milk from the breast and milk flow toward the nipple triggered by nipple stimulation or emotional response to the infant.

COLOSTRUM

Colostrum is the thin fluid present in the breast from pregnancy into the early postpartal period. It is deep yellow serous fluid, alkaline in reaction. It has a higher specific gravity, high protein, vitamin A, sodium and chloride content, but has lower carbohydrate, fat and potassium

Table 83.1: Percentage composition of colostrum and breast milk.

	Protein	Fat	Carbohydrates	Water
Colostrum	8.6	2.3	3.2	86
Breast milk	1.2	3.2	7.5	87

than the breast milk. It contains antibodies [immunoglobulin A (IgA), immunoglobulin G (IgG), immunoglobulin M (IgM)] and humoral factors (lactoferrin), which provide immunological defence to the newborn. It has laxative action on the baby, because of large fat globules. The percentage composition of colostrum and breast milk is shown in **Table 83.1**.

ESTABLISHMENT OF MILK SUPPLY

The supply of breast milk is based on demand and the best way to increase breast milk supply is for the infant to demand more by nursing more often. Therefore, supplemental feeding to be discouraged and night feeding to be encouraged. Exclusive breastfeeding with feeding every 2–3 hours during the first 3–4 weeks to be explained to mothers. Signs of adequate intake include 8–10 wet diapers in 24 hours, frequent stooling, steady weight gain and contentment after breastfeeding. The stools from breastfed infants are golden yellow, sweet smelling and loose or liquid in consistency. Breastfed infants usually regain their birth weight by 14 days of age, and then gain approximately 15 gm/day in the first 6 months of life. Birth weight is usually doubled by approximately 5 months of age.

PROMOTING SUCCESSFUL BREASTFEEDING

In order to promote successful breastfeeding mothers need to be taught the techniques of correct breastfeeding:
- Find a comfortable position before beginning; so that she can relax, while feeding and experience the let-down reflex
- Position her and infant, so that both are comfortable, and the breast is supported

- Cup her breast in one hand with all four fingers underneath and the thumb on top without touching the areola, and support the baby's head with the other hand
- Initiate rooting reflex by touching the baby's lips with her nipple
- Ensure that the infant latches on to the entire areola, not just the end of the nipple forming solid suction
- When sucking is over remove the baby from breast by inserting a finger into the corner of the sucking baby's mouth to break the suction, which will facilitate removal without damage to the nipple
- Start each feed on alternate breast to ensure emptying of both breasts
- After removal, burp the baby on mother's shoulder or by placing the baby face down across the lap. Burping may also be done by holding the baby upright on the mother's lap.

WHO/UNICEF 'Ten Steps to Successful Breastfeeding'

Hospitals that are willing to adopt 10 specific steps are known 'Baby-Friendly hospitals'. These 10 steps are as follows:

1. Have a written breastfeeding policy that is routinely communicated to all healthcare staff.
2. Train all healthcare staff in the skills necessary to implement this policy.
3. Inform all pregnant women about the benefits and management of breastfeeding.
4. Help mothers initiate breastfeeding within a half hour of birth.
5. Show mothers how to breastfeed and maintain lactation, even when separated from their infants.
6. Newborn infants must not be given any food or drink other than breast milk, unless medically indicated.
7. Practice rooming-in and allow mothers and infants to remain together 24 hours a day.
8. Encourage breastfeeding on demand.
9. Give no pacifiers or artificial teats.
10. Foster the establishment of breastfeeding support groups and refer mothers on discharge from the hospital or clinic.

INFANT ASSESSMENT FOR INSUFFICIENT LACTATION

Possible signs of insufficient lactation in the exclusively breastfeeding infant in the 1st month after birth:
- Low urination pattern: At least six wet diapers is the norm
- Low stooling frequency: At least three greenish-yellow, seedy, soft stools is the norm
- Very irritable or sleepy infant, nursing less than 7 times a day
- Weight loss of more than 10% of the birth weight or continued weight loss after day 10 of life.

BENEFITS OF BREASTFEEDING

To Mother

- Lactational amenorrhea, which promotes longer period of decreased fertility
- Earlier involution of the uterus to its prepregnant state due to increased uterine contraction from oxytocin stimulation
- Increased feelings of maternal well-being, a psychological advantage
- Increased mother-infant attachment from early and continuous contact
- Delayed ovulation and natural birth control
- Weight loss after delivery because of the greater expenditure of energy
- Less expensive than formula feeding.

To baby

- Breast milk is nutritionally superior to formula milk
- Breast milk contains immunoglobulins, enzymes, and leukocytes to protect against infections
- Breast milk is easily available at a perfect temperature and with no preparation
- Breast milk may reduce allergies
- Breastfeeding promotes the development of facial and jaw muscles
- Breast milk reduces the risk of bacterial contamination.

NATURAL VARIATIONS IN COMPOSITION OF HUMAN MILK

Milk composition changes as the infant nurses at each feeding:
- Transitional milk is produced at end of colostrum production and immediately before mature milk comes into breast
- Foremilk is the thin, watery breast milk; secreted at the beginning of a feeding. Foremilk is low in calories, but high in water-soluble vitamins
- Hindmilk is the thick, high-fat breast milk secreted at the end of a feeding. It is ejected approximately 10–15 minutes after the initial 'let-down' and has the highest concentration of calories. Hindmilk is thicker in appearance than the foremilk owing to its higher fat content essential for the infant's proper growth and development
- Mature milk is breast milk that contains 10% solids for energy and growth.

84. LOW BIRTH WEIGHT BABY

DEFINITION

Lowbirth weight baby is one whose birth weight is less than 2,500 grams irrespective the gestational age. Very lowbirth weight infants weigh 1,500 grams or less and extremely lowbirth weight infants weigh 1,000 grams or less.

Lowbirth weight babies are again classified into two groups correlating both the birth weight and gestational age:
- Preterm: The growth potential is normal and is appropriate for the gestational period (10th to 90th percentile).
- Small for gestational age (SGA): An infant who has not achieved genetic growth potential. Other terms used interchangeably with SGA are dysmaturity, fetal growth restriction (FGR) and intrauterine growth restriction (IUGR).

The term IUGR is used for infants who are at less than the 10th percentile at birth on standardized graphs in weight, length and head circumference:
- Preterm baby (detailed in Chapter 80)
- SGA in term infant.

CLINICAL APPEARANCE

- Baby is long and thin with a disproportionately large head
- Dry and peeling skin
- Abundant palmar and plantar creases
- Facial features similar to worried old men
- Active and often hungry
- Length of body and occipitofrontal head diameters are normal for gestational age.
  *Babies of multiple gestation and those with growth stunted in utero are SGA, but growth retardation is symmetrical.

CAUSES OF SGA

- Maternal disease such as hypertensive disorders, which lead to poor placental perfusion, reduced availability of nutrients or placental transfer of inappropriate substances, which have a teratogenic effects such as nicotine, alcohol, cocaine or infective agents.
- Extremes of maternal age, i.e. at end of the childbearing spectrum, socioeconomic factors, parity and the number of fetuses in utero.

MANAGEMENT AT BIRTH AND IN THE NEONATAL PERIOD

- At the time of delivery, care should be taken to ensure that the baby is dried and wrapped in warm blankets.
- Early and frequent feedings to be given to meet the nutritional needs of the baby; who has been starved in utero.
- Nurse the baby in thermoneutral environment, as baby is susceptible to hypothermia and loss of brown fat.
- Baby's skin to be kept clean and dry to prevent infection, skin massage using emollients offers additional benefits.

85. MATERNAL PELVIS

The maternal pelvis or female pelvis is adapted for childbearing. It is a bony canal through which the fetus passes during the process of birth.

FUNCTIONS OF THE PELVIS

- Pelvis allows movement of the body, especially walking and running
- Permits to sit and kneel
- Transmits the weight of trunk to legs acting as bridge between femurs
- Takes the weight of the sitting body on to the ischial tuberosities
- Affords protection to the pelvic organs and abdominal contents
- The sacrum transmits the cauda equina and distributes the nerves to various parts of the pelvis.

BONES OF PELVIS (Fig. 85.1)

Pelvis consists of two innominate bones, a sacrum, and coccyx:

Sacrum

- Formed by fusion of five vertebrae, wedge-shaped.
- Sacroiliac joints: Articulation of sacrum with the innominate bones.
- Lumbosacral joint: Articulation with the fifth lumbar vertebra.
- Sacral promontory: Anteroposterior edge of the first sacral vertebra.
- Shape of pelvic side: Concave.

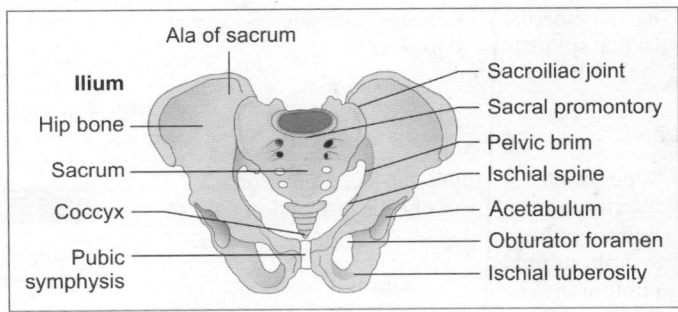

Fig. 85.1: Female pelvis—anterior view.

- Sacral foramina (eight in number, four on either side).
- Hollow of sacrum.

Coccyx

- Formed with four fused vertebrae forming a small triangular bone.

Formation of Innominate Bones

It is placed laterally and are formed by fusion of three bones—ilium, ischium and pubis.

Ilium

- Iliac crest—upper boarder.
- Anterior superior iliac spine.
- Anterior inferior iliac spine.
- Posterior superior iliac spine—prominence on posterior side.
- Posterior inferior iliac spine.
- Iliac fossa: Concave anterior surface.
- Iliopectineal eminence.
- Two fifth of acetabulum.
- Iliac fossa.

Ischium

- Thick lower part of innominate bone
- Ischial tuberosity—large prominence
- Ischial spine: Inward projection
- Two fifth of acetabulum.

Pubis

- Superior ramus: Upper oar-like projection
- Inferior ramus: Lower oar-like projection
- Body of pubis
- Symphysis pubis
- Pubic arch
- Obturator foramen (upper border)
- One fifth of acetabulum.

Greater sciatic notch: Curve that extends from posterior inferior iliac spine upto ischial spine.

Lesser sciatic notch: Between the ischial spine and ischial tuberosity.

PELVIC JOINTS AND LIGAMENTS

Joints

One symphysis pubis, two sacroiliac joints and a one sacrococcygeal joint:
- Symphysis pubis: Formed at the junction of two pubic bones, united by a pad of cartilage
- Sacroiliac joints: Joins sacrum to ilium on each side
- Sacrococcygeal joint: Base of the coccyx articulates with the sacrum.

Ligaments (Fig. 85.2)

- Interpubic ligaments at the symphysis pubis
- Sacroliac ligaments
- Sacrotuberous ligaments
- Sacrospinous ligaments.

DIVISIONS OF PELVIS

False Pelvis

The part of the pelvis lying above the pelvic brim.

Boundaries

Lumbar vertebrae posteriorly, iliac fossa laterally and anterior abdominal wall anteriorly.

True Pelvis

The part of pelvis lying below the pelvic brim, through which the fetus passes during birth. The parts are inlet, cavity and outlet.

Inlet/Brim

Landmarks of the brim are:
- Sacral promontory
- Sacral ala/wing

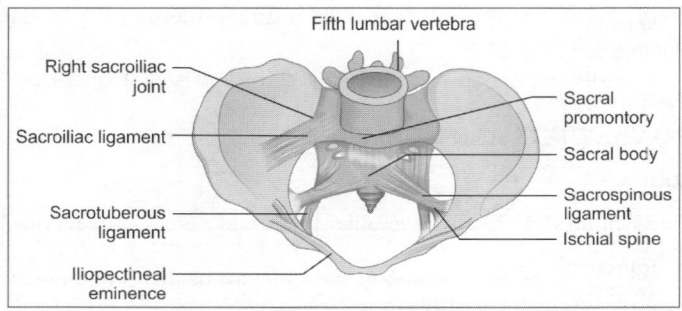

Fig. 85.2: Pelvic ligaments.

- Sacroiliac joint
- Ileopectineal line
- Ileopectineal eminence
- Superior ramus of the pubic bone
- Upper inner boarder of the body of pubic bone
- Upper inner boarder of the symphysis pubis.

Diameters of pelvic brim (Fig. 85.3)

Anteroposterior diameters

- Anatomical conjugate (12 cm) from the sacral promontory to the uppermost point of the symphysis pubis.
- Obstetrical conjugate (11 cm) from the sacral promontory to the posterior boarder of the upper surface (represents the available space for passage of the fetus).
- Diagonal conjugate (12–13 cm) from the sacral promontory to the lower boarder of the symphysis pubis.

Oblique diameter (12 cm): From one sacroiliac joint to the ileopectineal eminence on the opposite side of the pelvis.

Transverse diameters (13 cm): Measured between the points furthest apart on the ileopectineal lines.

Sacrocotyloid (9–9.5 cm): Measured from sacral promontory to the ileopectineal eminence on each side.

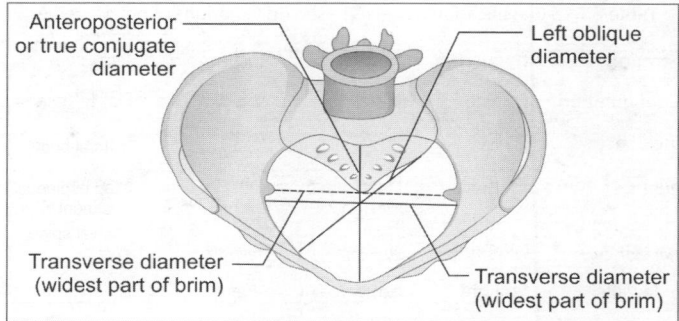

Fig. 85.3: Diameters of pelvic brim.

Pelvic Cavity (12 cm Circular in Shape)

Extends from the brim above to the outlet below. Anterior wall is formed by symphysis and depth is 4 cm. Posterior wall is formed by curve of sacrum and length is 12 cm. All diameters are considered to be 12 cm.

Pelvic Outlet

Anteroposterior diameter (13 cm): From the lower border to the symphysis pubis to the sacrococcygeal joint.

Transverse diameter (10–11 cm): Distance between the two ischial spines.

Oblique diameter (12 cm): Measured between obturator foramen and sacropinous ligament.

CLASSIFICATION OF PELVIS (Table 85.1)

The pelvis is classified into four types based on the shape of the brim; namely gynaecoid, android, anthropoid and platypelloid.

86. MECONIUM ASPIRATION SYNDROME

Meconium aspiration syndrome (MAS) is caused by aspiration of meconiumstained liquor during birth and is associated with asphyxia and post-term delivery.

Table 85.1: Classification of pelvis based on variations of pelvic shapes.

Features	Gynaecoid	Android	Anthropoid	Platypelloid
Configuration	Female	Male	Ape-like	Flat female
Incidence	50%	20%	25%	5%
Shape of brim	Rounded	Heart or wedge	Long oval	Transverse oval
Foreplevis	Generous	Narrow	Narrow	Wide
Sidewalls	Straight	Convergent	Divergent	Divergent
Ischial spines	Blunt	Prominent	Blunt	Blunt
Sciatic notch	Rounded	Narrow	Wide	Wide
Subpubic angle	90°	< 90°	> 90°	> 90°

FEATURES AND MANAGEMENT

Clinical Features

- Seen in term and post-term babies particularly in the intrauterine growth restricted group
- Signs of respiratory distress ranging from mild to severe
- Chest may appear barrel-shaped or hyperinflated
- Yellow-green staining of the skin and nail beds
- Chest X-ray showing hyperinflation of lungs and atelectasis.

Management

- Immediate suction of the oropharynx and endotracheal intubation and suction of the larynx
- Mechanical ventilation
- Intravenous antibiotics
- Chest physiotherapy.

Complications

Pneumothorax and pulmonary hypertension are possible.

87. MEDICAL TERMINATION OF PREGNANCY

DEFINITION

Deliberate induction of abortion by a registered medical practitioner in the interest of mother's health and life.

MTP ACT

In India the abortion law was legalized in 1971 by the 'Medical Termination of Pregnancy (MTP) Act'. The act came into force in 1972. The provisions of the act were revised in 1975.

Provisions of the MTP Act

- The continuation of pregnancy would involve serious risk of life or grave injury to the physical or mental health of the pregnant woman
- Eugenic consideration: When there are risks of the child being born with serious congenital disorders or being born with serious mental or physical handicaps
- Social indications: When the pregnancy is caused by rape, both in cases of major and minor girls, and in mentally imbalanced women
- Pregnancy caused as a result of failure of a contraceptive.

Indications for Termination under MTP Act

To save the life of the mother (Therapeutic or medical termination):
- Severe cardiac decompensation, which responds poorly to treatment
- Chronic glomerulonephritis
- Uncontrolled hypertension
- Diabetes with complications of retinopathy or nephropathy
- Certain psychiatric disorders
- Intractable hyperemesis gravidarum
- Cervical or breast malignancy
- Teratogenic drugs or exposure to radiation in early pregnancy
- Rubella infection in the first trimester.

Recommendations

- A registered medical practitioner is qualified to perform an MTP if:
  - One has assisted in at least 25 MTP in an authorised center
  - One has 6 months house surgeon training in obstetrics and gynecology

    One has diploma or degree in obstetrics and gynecology.
- Termination can only be performed in hospitals established or maintained by the government or places approved by the government
- Pregnancy can only be terminated on the written consent of the woman. Husband's consent is not required
- Pregnancy in a minor girl (below 18 years) or lunatic cannot be terminated without written consent of parents or legal guardians
- Termination is permitted up to 20 weeks of pregnancy. When pregnancy exceeds 12 weeks, opinion of two medical practitioners is required
- The abortion has to be performed confidentially and to be reported to the Director of Health Services of the State in the prescribed form.

METHODS OF TERMINATION

First Trimester (up to 12 Weeks)

- Menstrual regulation
- Suction evacuation and/or curettage
- Dilatation and evacuation: Rapid method or slow method
- Prostaglandin
- Mifepristone
- Methotrexate.

Second Trimester

- Intrauterine instillation of hypertonic solutions:
  - Intra-amniotic: 20% saline, 40% urea, mannitol
  - Extra-amniotic: Abdominal route is generally used than the vaginal route.
- Prostaglandins (used intramuscularly, as vaginal suppository, extra or intra-amniotic)

- Oxytocin infusion: Usually used along with one of the above methods
- Hysterotomy: Abdominal route is generally used than the vaginal route.

COMPLICATIONS OF MTP

Complications of MTP are three to five times higher in midtrimester terminations as compared to first trimester MTP:
- Anesthesia: Drug reactions, allergies, circulatory collapse, seizures, cardiac damage, fluid overload, embolism
- Cervical dilation: Cervical laceration, cervical tear, hemorrhage, future infertility, future cervical incompetence
- Incomplete evacuation leading to heavy bleeding, cramping, rise of temperature and uterine tenderness
- Sustained temperature over 38.6°C (101.5°F)
- Uterine perforation
- Uterine atony
- Postabortal hematometra
- Other complications that are uncommon:
  - Amniotic fluid embolism, uncontrolled bleeding, undiagnosed twin, undiagnosed molar pregnancy.
- Long-term complications (quite uncommon):
  - Repeated miscarriage due to cervical incompetence
  - Infertility as a result of pelvic infection
  - Psychiatric disorders and sexual dysfunction.

88. MENOPAUSE

DEFINITION

Permanent physiologic cessation of menstruation at the end of reproductive life due to loss of ovarian follicular activity is called menopause. It is the point of time when last and final menstruation occurs.

Climacteric is the phase of aging process during which a woman passes from the reproductive to the non-reproductive stage. This phase covers 5–10 years on each side of menopause, premenopause and postmenopause.

Age of menopause: 45–55 years; average being 50 years.

CHANGES INVOLVED

Endocrinology of Climacteric and Menopause

- There is significant fall in the level of serum estradiol in the climacteric period and after menopause
- The secretion of both follice-stimulating hormone (FSH) end and luteinizing hormone (LH) are increased due to absent negative feedback effect of estradiol and inhibition or due to enhanced responsiveness of pituitary to gondotropin-releasing hormone (GnRH)
- Rise in FSH is about 10–20 fold and LH about three fold
- During menopause there is fall in the level of prolactin and inhibitin
- Ultimately, there are no more follicles responsive to gonadotrophins. Estradiol production drops and endometrial growth stops resulting in absence of menstruation
- The sustained level of estrogens may cause endometrial hyperplasia and clinical manifestations of menstrual abnormalities prior to menopause
- The remaining follicles become resistant to gonadotropins, and estradiol production drops resulting in absence of endometrial growth and menstruation.

Organ Changes

Genitourinary System

- Ovaries shrink in size, become wrinkled and white. Thinning of cortex and abundance of stromal cells occur
- Fallopian tubes show features of atrophy. The muscle coat becomes thinner, the cilia disappear and the plicae become less prominent
- The uterus becomes smaller, endometrium becomes thin and atrophic. The cervical secretion becomes scanty
- The vagina becomes narrower due to gradual loss of elasticity. The rugae progressively flatten. There is no glycogen and Doderlein's bacillus is absent. The vaginal pH becomes alkaline
- The vulva shows features of atrophy. The labia become flattened and the pubic hair becomes scantier resulting in a narrow introitus

- Bladder and urethra: The epithelium becomes thin and is more prone to damage and infection
- Loss of muscle tone leads to pelvic relaxation, uterine descent and anatomic changes in the urethra and neck of the bladder.

Breasts

Fat gets reabsorbed and the glands atrophy. The nipples decrease in size resulting in breasts becoming flat and pendulous.

Bone Metabolism

Following menopause, there is loss of bone mass by about 3–5% per year due to deficiency of estrogen, leading to osteoporosis.

Cardiovascular system

Deficiency of estrogen increases the risk of cardiovascular disease because of loss of its function of decreasing HDL cholesterol and antioxidant property.

Menstruation Pattern Prior to Menopause

Any of the following patterns may be observed prior to menopause:
- Abrupt cessation of menstruation (rare)
- Gradual decrease in both amount and duration
- Irregular, with or without excessive bleeding.

MENOPAUSAL SYMPTOMS

Apart from cessation of menstruation some women experience additional symptoms though others may not experience any symptom.

Vasomotor Symptoms

The characteristic symptom of menopause is 'hot flush'. It is characterized by sudden feeling of heat followed by profuse sweating with extraneous vasodilatation.

Genital and Urinary Symptoms

Atrophy of epithelium of vagina, urinary bladder and urethra causes dyspareunia; vaginal infections, dryness, pruritus, and leukorrhea.

Urinary symptoms include urgency, dysuria, stress incontinence and frequent urinary tract infections.

Psychological Symptoms

Estrogen deficiency is associated with decreased sexual desire. There may be psychological changes such as increased anxiety, headache, insomnia, irritability, dysphasia and depression. Dementia, mood swings and inability to concentrate are also seen.

Osteoporosis

It occurs in postmenopausal women due to estrogen loss, deficiency of calcium and vitamin D or hereditary. Osteoporosis may lead to back pain, loss of height and kyphosis and fracture of bones. Fracture may involve vertebral body, femoral neck or distal forearm.

Cardiovascular and Cerebrovascular Effects

Risks of ischemic heart disease, coronary artery disease, and stroke are increased due to atherosclerotic changes, vasoconstriction and thrombus formation.

DIAGNOSIS AND MANAGEMENT OF MENOPAUSE

Diagnosis

- Cessation of menstruation for 12 consecutive months during climacteric
- Occurrence of hot flushes and night sweats
- Features of low estrogen on vaginal cytology
- Serum estradiol: :ess than 20 pg/mL
- Serum FSH and LH > 40 mLU/mL at one week interval for 3 times.

Management

- Counseling: Adequate explanation to every woman with symptoms. Those who have artificial and early menopause due to bilateral oophorectomy or radiation may require more reassurance

- Non-hormonal treatment:
  - Nutritious diet—balanced with protein and calcium
  - Supplementary calcium—total daily requirement of calcium is 1.5 g
  - Exercise—walking, jogging and weight bearing exercises.
- To follow healthy life styles, health promotion and regular health screening
- Supplementation with vitamin D 400–800 IU/day
- Cessation of smoking and alcohol
- Hormone replacement therapy (HRT)—replacement of estrogen and progestin are prescribed for women with premature ovarian failure, gonadal dysgenesis and surgical or radiation menopause.

ABNORMAL MENOPAUSE

Premature Menopause

- Occurs at or below the age of 40
- Treatment by substitution therapy is usually followed.

Delayed Menopause

- Does not occur beyond 55 years of age
- Detailed investigation for any pelvic pathology and appropriate treatment is indicated.

Artificial Menopause

- Permanent cessation of ovarian function as a result of surgical removal of ovaries or by radiation.

NURSING MANAGEMENT

- Encourage women to view menopause as a natural change resulting in freedom from symptoms related to menses
- Discuss measures to improve general health
- Educate women that:
  - Sexual urges will continue and that they can retain their usual response to sex long after menopause
  - Life styles, health promotion and health screening are important to continue.

89. MINOR DISORDERS OF PREGNANCY

Discomforts experienced by women following conception, which are not of serious nature, but may become serious if they escalate, are termed as minor disorders of pregnancy.

CAUSES OF MINOR DISORDERS

- Hormonal changes
- Accommodation changes
- Metabolic changes
- Postural changes.

SYSTEMWISE CLASSIFICATION OF MINOR DISORDERS AND MANAGEMENT

Digestive System

Nausea and Vomiting

- Presents between 4 and 16 weeks
- Occurs due to increased level of human chorionic gonadotropin (HCG)
- Other hormonal contributors are estrogen and progesterone
- Vomiting may occur at any time in the day
- Aggravated by smell of cooking food.

Management and advice

- Six small meals per day and light snacks instead of three large ones
- Carbohydrate snacks at bedtime and before rising to prevent hypoglycemia
- Eat dry, unsalted crackers before rising in the morning to prevent nausea resulting from an empty stomach
- Avoid greasy or spicy food that irritates stomach and reduces gastric motility
- Avoid cooking odors that predispose to nausea
- Reduce intake of carbonated beverages
- Take frequent walks outside in fresh air
- Take iron pills and vitamins only after meals to avoid irritating stomach

- Separate food and fluid intake by half hour to avoid distending stomach
- Avoid very cold fluids and food at meal times
- Seek medical help if vomiting continues and becomes severe.

Heartburn

Burning sensation in the mediastinal region due to reflux of gastric contents into oesophagus as the cardiac sphincter becomes relaxed from the effect of progesterone:
- Heartburn becomes more troublesome at about 30–40 weeks.

Management and advice
- Avoid bending over while doing household chores
- Encourage taking small meals, which are digested easily
- Sleep with more pillows and on right semi-reclining position
- Seek physician's help if heartburn persists.

Excessive Salivation (Ptyalism)

- Often accompanies heartburn
- Occurs from 8 weeks gestation

Management: It is by explanation and attentive listening.

Pica

Mother craves for certain foods or unnatural substances such as coal.

Management: Seek medical advice if the substance craved is potentially harmful to the fetus.

Constipation

Relaxation and decreased peristalsis of the gut caused by progesterone causes constipation.

Management and advice
- Increase intake of water, fresh fruits, vegetables and whole meal foods in the diet
- Take a glass of warm water in the morning before tea or breakfast
- Encourage exercise especially walking
- Take bulk increasing agents.

Musculoskeletal System

Backache

Occurs due to changing center of gravity as the fetus grows, and softening of ligaments due to the effects of hormone.

Management: Reassurance and instructions regarding posture such as avoiding high-heeled shoes help.

Cramp

Occurs possibly due to ischemia or results from changes in pH or electrolyte status.

Management: Instructions include to:
- Dorsiflex the foot
- Raise the foot end of the bed about 25 cm
- Make gentle leg movements whilst in a warm bath
- Take vitamin B complex and calcium.

Genitourinary System

Frequency of micturition

Occurs in the early weeks of pregnancy and latter weeks pregnancy.

Management: Reassurance that the problem will subside as the uterus rises into the abdomen after the 12th week.

Leukorrhea

Increased white, non-irritant vaginal discharge in pregnancy.

Management
- Attention to personal hygiene
- Use of cotton underwear and avoiding tights
- Using mild cream after washing with plain water twice a day.

Circulatory System

Fainting

In early pregnancy, fainting occurs due to vasodilatation under the influence of progesterone.

Management
- Avoid long periods of standing
- Sit or lie down quickly if feeling of faint occurs.

Later in pregnancy, feeling of faint may occur, while lying flat on back.

Instructions
- Turn quickly on to one side.

Varicosities

Valves of the dilated veins become inefficient resulting in varicosities. Varicose veins may occur in the legs, anus (hemorrhoids) and vulva.

Management
- Exercising the calf muscles by rising on to the toes or making circling movements with the ankles
- Resting with legs elevated
- Wearing support tights after resting or before rising
- Avoidance of constipation by fiber in the diet and adequate fluids to reduce hemorrhoids
- Topical applications to reduce discomfort
- Using sanitary pad for support in case of vaginal varicosities.

Skin

Pigmentation

Darkening of areola of breasts, linea nigra and chloasma occur in pregnancy.

Management: Reassurance that these will diminish after delivery.

Generalized Itching

Itching starting from abdomen occurs sometimes.

Management: Use of local applications if prescribed. Antihistamines if prescribed. Reassurance that it would subside after delivery.

Nervous System

Carpal Tunnel Syndrome

Numbness and feeling 'pins and needles' in fingers and hands, usually in the morning hours.

Management

- Wearing a splint at night with the hand resting on two or three pillows
- Diuretics if prescribed for edema.

Insomnia

Sleep disturbance occurs due to frequency of micturition, fetal movement, bad dreams or fears.

Recommendations: Mother to lie down and rest in the morning and when she can sleep easily. Reassurance that such difficulties are normal.

DISORDERS THAT CAN TURN TO BE MAJOR PROBLEMS AND REQUIRE IMMEDIATE CARE

- Vaginal bleeding
- Reduced fetal movements
- Frontal or recurring headaches
- Sudden development of edema
- Rupture of membranes
- Premature onset of contractions
- Epigastric pain
- Increased anxiety.

90. MINOR DISORDERS OF NEWBORN

Minor disorders are most common among newborns. Neglecting the minor health problem is one of the factors contributing to the newborn morbidity and mortality.

Table 90.1: Minor disorders of newborn.

Sr. No.	Minor problem	Treatment
1.	**Erythema toxicum (Newborn rash)** Skin rashes consisting of small, red, flat or raised lesions seen on chest, abdomen, back and buttocks of newborn **(Fig. 90.1)**	No specific treatment needed. It will disappear within first two weeks

Contd...

Contd...

Sr. No.	Minor problem	Treatment
2.	**Milia** Yellow, pin-point size lesions seen on the bridge of the nose, chin or cheeks. These are distended sebaceous glands in the skin	The lesions will disappear after few weeks. No treatment needed
3.	**Telangiectic nevi (Stork bite/angel kisses)** Dilation of capillary vessels and minute arteries; seen at the nape of neck, extending over to the lower occipital area, between the eyebrows, on upper eyelids and around the nose **(Fig. 90.2)**	The lesion blanches when pressed and gradually fades when the baby grows.
4.	**Mongolian spots** Aggregations of melanin rich dark cells. Purple or bluish dark areas of discoloration mostly present over the sacrum and coccygeal area of a large percentage and seen over back, buttocks, and extremities **(Fig. 90.3)**	No treatment needed. The discoloration disappears as the child grows
5.	**Nevus flammeus (Port-wine stain)** Smooth, flat, superficial angioma (dilated blood vessels) that vary in size from a few millimeters to an area that covers most of the face and neck **(Fig. 90.4)**	These do not fade with time
6.	**Epstein epithelial pearls** Small epithelial inclusion cysts. These appear as whitish spots on the hard palate or along the alveolar ridge **(Fig. 90.5)**	No treatment is required
7.	**Bednar's aphthae** Small ulcers on mucous membrane, usually located in hard palate posteriorly and generally bilateral. May be caused by rigorous sucking	Condition will disappear by itself

Contd...

Contd...

Sr. No.	Minor problem	Treatment
8.	**Conjunctivitis (Sticky eyes)** Eyes red with purulent exudates. Eyelids are swollen. Onset occurs within 24 hours of birth and lasts for about 24 days. It may occur due to silver nitrate drops instilled after birth or bacterial conjunctivitis	Cleaning the eyelids with cotton balls soaked in warm saline solution and use of erythromycin (0.5%) every 6 hours for 7–10 days will cure the condition
9.	**Stuffy nose** Mouth breathing and excessive air swallowing which in turn may lead to abdominal distension and vomiting	The nostrils may be cleaned with cotton soaked with normal saline
10.	**Napkin rash (ammonium dermatitis)** The perianal skin becomes red, indurated and excoriated due to the dermatitis. More common in artificially fed babies	Frequent care and attention to the napkin area and changing of napkin at regular intervals
11.	**Perianal dermatitis** Seen around the anal opening. Occurs due to the alkalinity of the stool and is common in artificially fed babies	Use of lactose instead of glucose in feed
12.	**Oral thrush** It manifests as white patches with erythematous margins distributed over tongue and buccal mucosa. The patches of thrush are adherent and they often bleed if attempted to remove **(Fig. 90.6)**	Local application of 0.5% aqueous solution of gentian violet or nystatin suspension (100,000 units/mL) applied to each side of mouth with a cotton tipped swab 3–4 times a day is effective
13.	**Congenital hydrocele** Collection of fluid in the testicular structure. This is due to hormone withdrawal	No specific treatment is needed. It will usually disappear. Incision and drainage can be done

Contd...

Minor Disorders of Newborn

Contd...

Sr. No.	Minor problem	Treatment
14.	**Genital crisis** This include mastitis neonatorum, hydrocele, vaginal bleeding, and vaginal mucoidal secretions due to withdrawal of maternal hormone after birth	It does not need any treatment. It will disappear with local aseptic cleaning of genitalia. If breast engorgement is present, there is no need to squeeze or to express milk

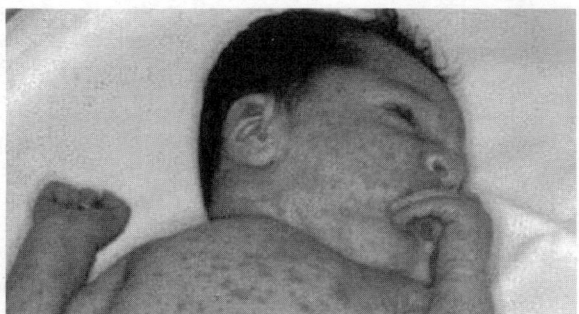

Fig. 90.1: Erythema toxcum neonatorum.

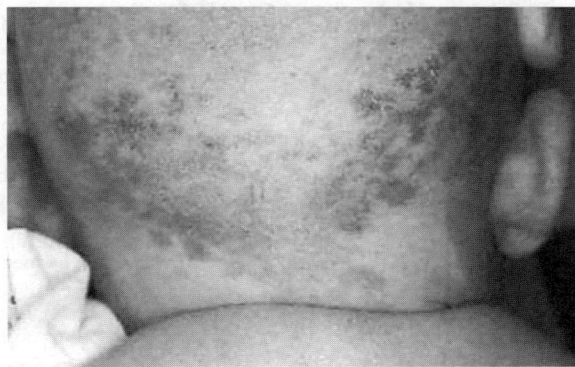

Fig. 90.2: Telangiectasia/stork bite in newborn.

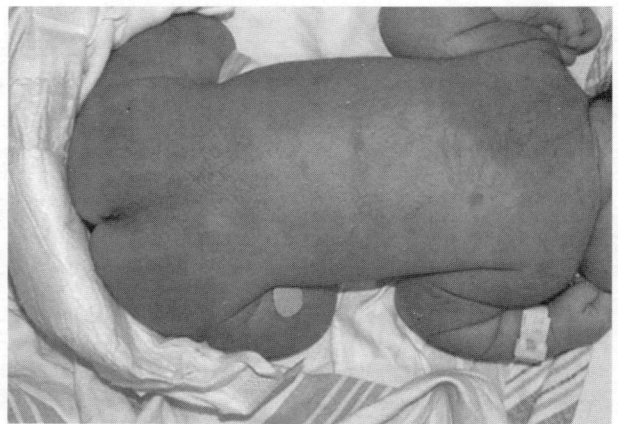

Fig. 90.3: Mongolian spots.

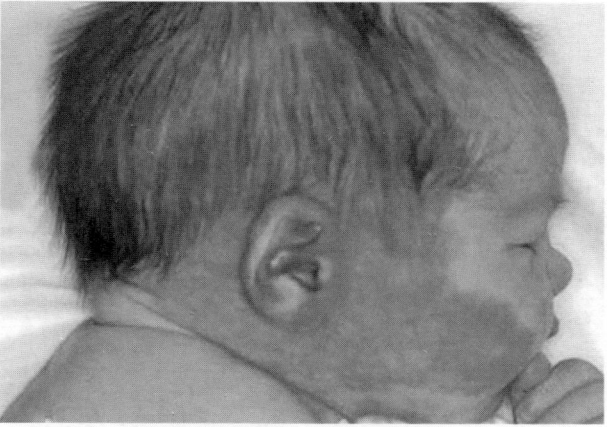

Fig. 90.4: Nevus flammeus/Portwine stain

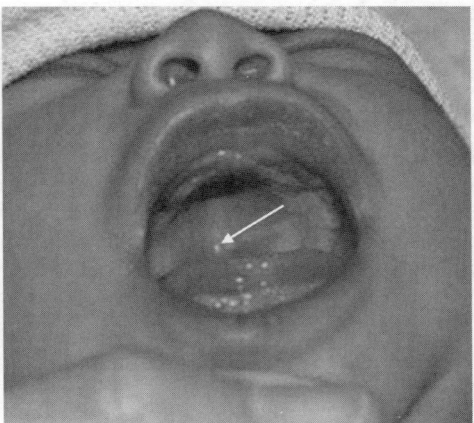

Fig. 90.5: Epstein pearls.

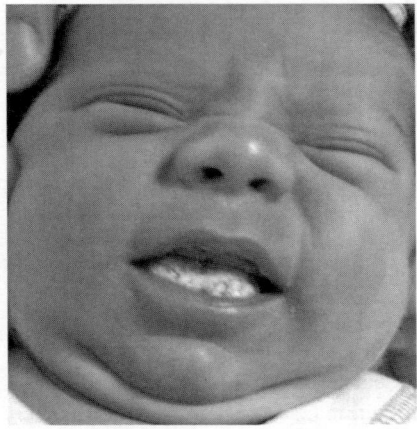

Fig. 90.6: Oral thrush.

91. MINOR SURGERIES IN GYNECOLOGICAL PATIENTS

DILATION OF CERVIX

An operation to dilate the cervix, in some cases external os only is dilated and is some others the canal and internal os need to be dilated. Dilatation is done by graduated cervical dilators. When the internal os is be dilated, position of the uterus is confirmed by introducing a uterine sound prior to introducing the dilators.

Indications

- Prior to hysteroscopy
- Prior to introduction of uterine curette and insertion of intrautedrine contraceptive device (IUCD), radium or laminaria tent
- Spasmodic dysmenorrhea
- Prior to amputation of the cervix incase prolapse of uterus with elongation of cervix.

DILATATION AND CURETTAGE (D&C)

An operative procedure in which dilatation of the cervical canal followed by uterine curettage is done.

Indications

Diagnostic

- Infertility
- Dysfunctional uterine bleeding (DUB)
- Pathologic dysmenorrhea
- Endometrial tuberculosis
- Endometrial carcinoma
- Postmenopausal bleeding
- Chorion epithelioma.

Therapeutic

- Dysfunctional uterine bleeding
- Endometrial polyp

- Removal of IUCD
- Incomplete abortion.

Combined

- Dysfunctional uterine bleeding
- Endometrial polyp.

Procedure

- Patient's urinary bladder to be emptied
- General anesthesia or paracervical block is generally given
- Patient is placed in lithotomy position
- Local antiseptic cleansing and draping are done
- Bimanual examination is performed
- Posterior vaginal wall speculum is introduced
- Anterior lip of cervix is held with an Allis tissue forceps
- A uterine sound is introduced to note the position and length of uterine cavity
- Cervical canal is dilated with graduated dilators, while steadying the uterus by traction of the vulsellum
- After the desired dilatation, the uterine cavity is curetted from fundus down to internal os
- Curetting is done with sharp curette for benign lesions and blunt curette for malignant lesions
- Vulsellum and speculum are then removed and the curetted material is sent for histological examination.

Care of Patient After D&C

- Observation for 3–4 hours
- May go home after anesthetic effect wears off.

Possible Complications

Immediate

- Injury to cervix
- Uterine perforation
- Infection.

Remote

- Cervical incompetence
- Uterine synechia (adhesion) resulting in secondary amenorrhea.

DILATATION AND INSUFFLATION

The procedure includes dilatation of the cervix and introduction of air or carbon dioxide (CO_2) into the uterine cavity to know the patency of the fallopian tubes. It is also known as Rubin test.

Indications

- To note the tubal patency in case of infertility
- Following tuboplasty operation.

Timing of Procedure

It should be done in the first half of the cycle, between 8th and 12th day.

Procedure

Procedure steps up to cervical dilatation are similar to D and C operation. After the desired dilatation of the cervix, the insufflation cannula with a "Y" rubber tube is introduced into the cervical canal. CO2 is introduced and pressure in the manometer is raised gradually by pressing the rubber bulb. As the pressure in the manometer is watched by the operator, the assistant auscultates over the flanks for any sound.

Positive Test (Tubes Patent)

- A hissing sound is audible on the flanks due to exit of air through the abdominal ostium
- Drop in the manometer reading
- Patient may complain of shoulder pain on sitting due to irritation of the diaphragm by air and the pain sensation carried by phrenic nerve.

If the test is negative—no hissing sound is audible on the flanks, the test may be repeated in the same sitting. After the test is completed, the cannula, vulsellum and the speculum are taken off.

Complications

- Complications due to the use of instruments are same as that of D and C operation
- Rupture of the tube, if the tube is blocked and the pressure is raised beyond 200 mm Hg
- Flaring up of pre-existing infection.

CERVICAL BIOPSY

Cervical biopsy is the process of removing tissue from the patient's cervix for diagnostic examination.

Types of Cervical Biopsies

Punch Biopsy

Removal of a cylindrical specimen by means of a punch biopsy forceps. Cusco's bivalve speculum is used for steadying cervix and specimen is taken from the suspected area of cervix.

Wedge Biopsy

Excision of a cuneiform specimen from a definite and visible growth. Generally an area nearer the edge is selected. Posterior vaginal wall speculum and Allis forceps are used for holding the cervix and with a scalpel a wedge of tissue is cut. Hemostasis may be achieved by gauze packing or by sutures.

Cone Biopsy (Conization)

Removal of a cone of the cervix, which includes entire squamocolumnar junction, stroma with glands and endocervical mucous membrane. Conization is done for diagnostic and therapeutic purposes in cases of suspected malignant lesions.

Procedure of Obtaining Cone Biopsy

1. The procedure is usually done with conventional knife (cold knife cone) or CO_2 laser used as knife under colposcopic guidance.

2. For cold knife technique the procedure is done under general anesthesia.
3. After cutting and removing the cone, endocervical and uterine curettage is done if indicated.
4. Cone margins are repaired with hemostatic sutures. The excised tissue is then sent for histological examination. If laser method is chosen; the procedure can be done in the outpatient unit under local anesthesia. Tissue damage and blood loss and postoperative pain are less with this technique. Cone biopsy can be performed with a procedure called loop electrosurgical excision procedure (LEEP), which uses a laser beam.

Management Following Cone Biopsy

- A patient who has received anesthesia for cone biopsy is advised to rest for 24 hours after the procedure
- Vaginal packing is kept for 24 hours. Any bleeding after removal needs to be reported
- Sexual intercourse to be avoided until complete healing is verified at follow-up
- Complications
- Secondary hemorrhage
- Cervical stenosis
- Infertility
- Diminished cervical mucus
- Cervical incompetence
- Mid-trimester abortion or preterm labor.

THERMAL CAUTERIZATION

This is an operation whereby the eroded area of the cervix is destroyed either by thermocoagulation or red hot cauterisation.

Indication

Cervical ectopy (congenital malposition) with discharge.

Anesthesia

- No anesthesia for superficial cauterisation
- General anesthesia for deeper or extensive cauterisation.

Procedure

Lower part of the cervix is dilated by one or two small dilators. The eroded area is cauterised by cautery point. The cauterised area is smeared with antibiotic ointment. Healing takes place by 6–8 weeks. There may be serosanguineous discharge for about 2–3 weeks.

CRYOSURGERY

This is an operation using freezing temperature (achieved by liquid nitrogen or carbon dioxide in an instrument) to destroy tissue.

Indications

- Benign cervical lesions such as cervical intraepithelial neoplasia (CIN), condyloma accuminata, leukoplakia, etc.
- To arrest bleeding in carcinoma cervix as a palliative measure
- To remove vault granulation tissue.

Procedure

The cryosurgery probe is applied to the cervix and freezing activated. When 4–5 mm area of tissue beyond the edge of the probe is obtained, the freezing is stopped. The probe is then thawed (temperature raised about freezing point) and removed. The application to the cervix freezes the tissue to a depth of about 3 mm.

Advantages

- Anesthesia is not required
- Precise destruction of tissue is possible
- No secondary hemorrhage
- Cervical stenosis is rare.

Drawbacks

- Cramping and occasional fainting may occur due to vasovagal response
- Watery discharge for few weeks after the procedure. Complete healing may take place in 2–3 weeks.

PERINEOPLASTY

Perineoplasty is plastic surgery of the perineum wherein reconstruction of the narrow vaginal introitus is done to make it adequate for sexual function.

Indications

- Congenitally small introitus
- Rigid perineal body
- Rigid hymeneal ring
- Narrowed introitus following perineorrhaphy or episiotomy repair.

Procedure

- A longitudinal incision is made in the midline from above the fourchette down through the skin and perineal body
- The divided perineal muscles are sutured transversely to make the introitus wider.

AMPUTATION OF CERVIX

Amputation is an operative procedure whereby a part of the lower cervix is excised.

Indications

- Congenital elongation of cervix
- Hypertrophied cervix following chronic cervicitis.

Procedure

- A circumferential incision is made around the cervix and vaginal mucosa is separated from the stroma of the cervix

- A cone-shaped amputation is done
- Cut margins and raw surfaces of the cervix are sutured.

Complications

- Hemorrhage
- Sepsis
- Cervical stenosis
- Cervical incompetency leading to mid-trimester abortion
- Cervical dystocia during labor.

92. MULTIFETAL PREGNANCY

Presence of more than one fetus in the gravid uterus is described as multifetal pregnancy or multiple pregnancy. About 1.5% of all births are multiple gestations.

TYPES OF MULTIFETAL PREGNANCIES

- Twins: 1:90–100
- Triplets: 1:8,000–10,000
- Quadruplets: 1:700,000–1,000,000.

TYPES OF TWIN PREGNANCY

1. **Binovular: Dichorionic diamniotic:**
   - Develop from two separate ova, which may or may not come from the same ovary
   - There are two separate and distinct placentae
   - Each develop from separate ova and separate spermatozoa liberated during the same menstrual cycle.
2. **Uniovular: Monochorionic diamniotic:**
   - A single ovum after fertilization undergoes division to form two embryos
   - They are always of the same sex
   - The arrangement of genes in the chromosomes is identical.
3. **Fetus papyraceous:** One fetus perishes early in pregnancy and is retained until term:
   - The small fetus is discovered compressed flat on the membranes.

4. **Conjoined twins or Siamese twins.**
5. **Super fecundation:** Fertilization of two different ova at different intermenstrual periods. It is only a theoretical possibility.

ETIOLOGY

- Often unknown
- Common in pregnancies following ovulation induction for infertility treatment
- Heredity: Runs in certain families.

FETAL PRESENTATIONS

Various combinations of fetal presentations are seen in clinical practice (**Fig. 92.1**).
- Vertex and vertex 45%
- Vertex and breech 37%
- Breech and breech 10%
- Vertex and transverse 5%
- Breech and transverse 2%
- Transverse and transverse 0.5%.

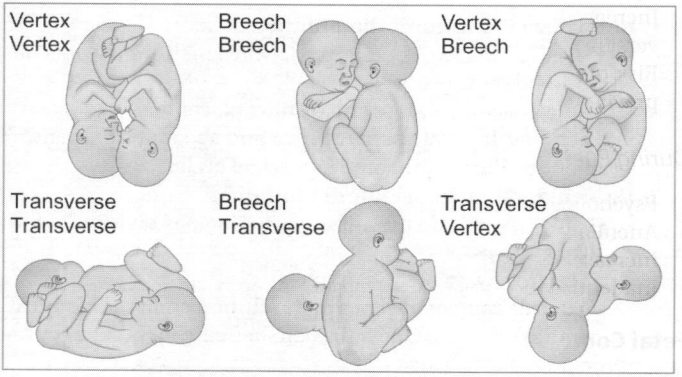

Fig. 92.1: Possible fetal presentations of twin fetus.

COMPLICATIONS IN PREGNANCY AND LABOR

In multiple pregnancy, generally all pregnancy complications are aggravated.

Maternal Complications

During Pregnancy

- Hyperemesis
- Increased pressure symptoms:
  - Shortness of breath
  - Abdominal tightness and discomfort
  - Edema of legs
  - Dyspnea
  - Hemorrhoids and varicose veins.
- Increased risk of preterm labor
- Pregnancy-induced hypertension (25%)
- Polyhydramnios 10%
- Placenta previa
- Accidental hemorrhage
- Anemia.

During Labor

- Prolonged labor
- Increased operative delivery (forceps, cesarean section, internal version)
- Risk of PPH due to uterine atony, retained placenta or placenta previa.

During Puerperium

- Psychological stress
- Anemia
- Increased risk of infections of genital and urinary tracts
- Inadequate lactation.

Fetal Complications

- Twin to twin transfusion in monochorionic twin pregnancies
- Discordant growth

- Prematurity
- Premature rupture of membranes and cord prolapse
- Intrauterine growth retardation
- Intrauterine hypoxia due to:
  - Premature separation of placenta
  - Cord prolapse
  - Breech delivery or extraction
  - Birth trauma.
- Fetal abnormalities:
  - Conjoined twins.
  - Acardiac formation.
  - Fetus-in-fetu.
  - Vanishing twin.
- Malpresentations
- Monoamniotic twins
- Locked twins
- Delay in birth of second twin
- Premature expulsion of placenta.

DIAGNOSIS OF TWIN PREGNANCY

History

- Family history of twins
- Maternal age over 35 years
- Pregnancy following treatment for infertility
- Excessive nausea and vomiting in early pregnancy
- Size of abdomen bigger than expected
- Fetal heart rate audible in two separate areas with difference of at least 10 bpm.

Examination

- Uterus larger than expected for the period of amenorrhea
- Palpation of at least three distinct separate poles (two heads and a breech)
- Two fetal heart sounds auscultated distinctly by two observers at the same time with a difference of at least 10 bpm
- Palpation of multiple fetal parts.

Ultrasound Scan

- Two separate gestational sacs can be detected as early as 6th to 7th week
- Separate fetal bodies can be identified from 12th week.

MANAGEMENT

Antenatal

- Early diagnosis by routine ultrasound examination
- Advice on frequent rest periods, early maternity leave for working women and restricting travel
- Diet adequate in calories and proteins, supplementary iron and vitamins
- Ultrasound screening at 18–20 weeks to detect fetal anomalies
- More frequent prenatal visits
- Admission to hospital between 30 and 36 weeks.

Management of Labor

- Induction of labor at term in view of the possibilities of placental insufficiency
- Delivery must always be in a hospital with an anesthetist and pediatrician present during delivery
- Delivery of the first twin is the same as in any case with a generous episiotomy
- For delivery of second twin:
    - External cephalic version, if the lie is transverse or oblique
    - Surgical rupture of forewaters
    - Await for 10 minutes for spontaneous delivery
    - Syntocinon infusion if uterine inertia is diagnosed
    - Vacuum extraction or breech extraction depending on the presentation may be carried out.

If at any stage there is evidence of fetal distress, intrapartum bleeding or cord prolapse delivery should be effected at once by operative method.

Cesarean section: An elective cesarean section is considered in a twin pregnancy in the following circumstances:

- Severe pregnancy induced hypertension
- Bad obstetric history
- Long history of infertility
- Elderly patient
- Preterm delivery at 33–34 weeks
- If the leading twin presents by breech.

Management of Third Stage and Puerperium

- Prevention of PPH
- Treatment of anemia
- Psychological support
- Family planning counseling.

MORBIDITY AND MORTALITY IN MULTIFETAL PREGNANCY

Maternal Morbidity

- Preeclampsia
- Primary postpartum hemorrhage (PPH)
- Sepsis.

Fetal Morbidity

- Congenital defects
- Prematurity
- Twin to twin transfusion and discordant growth
- Placental insufficiency
- Traumatic delivery and birth injury

POSTNATAL CARE

Care of Babies

Immediately After Birth

- Ensure that both babies have clear airways
- Maintain body temperature
- Ensure gentle handling
- Apply identification bracelets and have mother cuddle her babies if condition permits

- Transfer babies to neonatal unit if required
- Encourage breastfeeding either simultaneously or separately
- Top up feedings if the babies are preterm, or small for dates
- Expressed breast milk to be given if the babies are not able to suck adequately at the breast
- Feeding to be nasogastric, orogastric or cup feeding if sucking and swallowing reflexes are poor
- Encourage and involve mother in feeding and care
- Monitor weight gain
- Monitor blood glucose levels and prevent hypoglycemia
- Teach mother measures to prevent infection such as washing hands before handling babies and after changing their nappies.

Care of Mother

- Explain that involution may be slower because of increased bulk of uterus
- Offer analgesics for after pains and night sedatives for adequate rest
- Encourage high calorie, high protein diet and additional snacks if hungry between meals
- Instruct in postnatal exercises to improve the tone of abdominal muscles and pelvic floor
- Provide support and encourage to care for two babies.

93. NATIONAL FAMILY WELFARE PROGRAMS

India launched the national family welfare program (NFWP) in 1951. The objective of the program was to reduce the birthrate to the extent necessary to stabilise the population at a level consistent with the requirement of national economy.

The family welfare program in India is recognized as a priority area and is being implemented as a 100% centrally sponsored program. With the targets and plans in various five year plans, the following aspects of the program have been implemented:

- Reduction of birth rate
- Reduction of maternal morbidity and mortality
- Increase of couple protection rate
- Increase of life expectancy.

Box 93.1: Schemes and programs.

- Reproductive and child health program (RCH)
- Janani Suraksha Yojana
- Vandemataram scheme
- Safe abortion services
- National rural health mission (NRHM)
- Integrated child development scheme (ICDS).

The main components of the present programs of family welfare programs are maternal health, child health and population control/stabilization. The schemes and programs for implementing the family welfare program are listed in **Box 93.1**.

REPRODUCTIVE AND CHILD HEALTH PROGRAM

The objective of the RCH program was to provide quality, integrated and sustainable primary health care services to women in the reproductive age group and children with special focus on family planning and immunization.

Essential Components of RCH Program

- Prevention and management of unwanted pregnancy
- Services for mothers during pregnancy, childbirth and postpartum period
- Child survival services for newborns and infants
- Management of reproductive tract infections (RTI) and sexually transmitted diseases
- Establishment of an effective referral system
- Reproductive services for adolescent health
- Health services including counseling on sexuality and family life.

Services Included in the Program for Mothers and Children

Essential Care for all Mothers and Children

- Registration by 12th to 16th week of pregnancy
- Antenatal check-up at least three times during pregnancy

- Tetanus toxoid to all women as early as possible during pregnancy with two doses at one month interval
- Iron and folic acid tablets daily for 100 days. Women with clinical signs of anemia to receive 2 tablets daily for 100 days
- Deworming with Mebendazole during 2nd or 3rd trimester in areas where hookworm infestation is common
- Safe and clean delivery services
- Preparation of women for exclusive breastfeeding and timely weaning
- Postpartum care, including advices and services for limiting, and spacing births.

Early Detection of Complications

- Clinical examination to detect anemia
- Referral and transportation to the nearest hospital of women with hemorrhage or complications
- Referral of all women identified as having pregnancy-induced hypertension (BP > 140/90 mm Hg and weight gain > 3 kg/month)
- Referral of all women who develop signs of infection following delivery or abortion
- Transfer of women in labor for more than 12 hours to the nearest hospital that has facilities for cesarean delivery.

Emergency Care to Those Who Need It

- Early identification of obstetric emergencies
- Initial management of emergencies and transfer to referral hospital without delay using the fastest available mode of transport.

Care to Women in the Reproductive Age Group

- Counseling on:
  - Optimal timing and spacing of birth
  - Small family norm
  - Use and choice of contraceptives
  - Prevention of sexually transmitted diseases and reproductive tract infections
  - Importance of girl child.

- Information on availability of:
  - Medical termination of pregnancy (MTP) services
  - Intrauterine contraceptive device (IUCD) and sterilization services.
- Family planning services:
  - Condom distribution
  - Oral contraceptive dispensing
  - IUCD services.
- Recognition and referral of clients with sexually transmitted diseases and reproductive tract infections.

Provision of Clean and Safe Delivery Practices at the Community Level

- Creation of awareness about the need for clean and safe deliveries
- Deliveries by trained personnel
- Provision of disposable delivery kits for deliveries
- Promotion of institutional deliveries
- Early identification and referral of high-risk cases.

Newborn Care

- Weighing all newborns at birth. Normal weight 2,500–2,800 g. Referral of newborns weighing > 2,000 g
- Resuscitation of asphyxiated newborns using mucus sucker or breathing as required
- Prevention of hypothermia
- Breastfeeding within 1 hour of birth
- Referral of newborns who show signs of illness
- Education of mother on newborn to care and feeding.

Immunization

Infants

- Bacillus Calmette–Guérin (BCG) one dose at birth
- Diphtheria, pertussis, tetanus (DPT): Three doses, beginning at 6th week and at monthly interval
- Polio: '0' dose at birth for all institutional deliveries and 3 doses at one month interval

- Measles: One dose at completion of 9 months
- Vitamin A: First dose of 100,000 IU along with measles vaccination.

Children 1–3 years
- DPT
- OPV booster doses at 16th–18th month
- Vitamin A:
  - Second dose 200,000 IU at 16th–18th month
  - Third to fifth doses 200,000 IU each at 6 monthly intervals.

Children 3–5 years:
- Iron and folic acid (smaller dose) for children with signs of anemia
- Treatment for worm infestation with Mebendazole.

Prevention of Deaths Due to Diarrheal Diseases

- Corrective management
- Teaching mothers to increase body fluid with oral rehydration solution (ORS) and normal feeding.

Prevention of Deaths Due to Pneumonia

- Correct management of all cases of acute respiratory infections
- Referral of children with severe pneumonia or severe illness.

RCH Phase II

RCH phase II began in April 2005. The focus of the program was to reduce maternal and child morbidity and mortality with emphasis on rural health care. The major strategies of the second phase of RCH are:

Essential Obstetric Care

1. **Institutional delivery:** In order to promote institutional deliveries it is envisaged that 50% of the primary health centers (PHCs) and all the community health centers (CHCs) would be made operational as 24 hour delivery centers in a phased manner by 2010. Basic emergency obstetric care, essential

newborn care and basic newborn resuscitation services will be provided in these centers round the clock.
2. **Skilled attendance at delivery:** Guidelines for conducting normal delivery and management of obstetric complications at PHC and CHC for medical officers and for skilled attendance at birth for auxiliary nurse midwives (ANM) and lady health visitors (LHVs) have been formulated and disseminated to the states.
3. **Policy decisions regarding use of drugs and interventions:** ANMs, LHVs and staff nurses (SNs) have now been permitted to use certain drugs in specific emergency situations to reduce maternal mortality. They have also been permitted to carry out certain emergency interventions when the life of the mother is at stake.

Emergency Obstetric Care

The first referral units (FRU) will be made operational/functional with following services on a 24 hour basis:
- 24 hour delivery services including normal and assisted deliveries
- Emergency obstetric care including surgical interventions such as cesarean sections:
  - Newborn care
  - Emergency care of sick newborns
  - Full range of family planning services including laparoscopic services
  - Safe abortion services
  - Treatment for sexually transmitted infections and respiratory tract infections
  - Blood storage facility
  - Essential laboratory services
  - Referral (transport) services.
- In order to perform full range of FRU functions a health facility must have:
  - Minimum bed strength of 20–30
  - Fully functional operation theater
  - Fully functional labor room with well-equipped care area
  - A functional laboratory and blood storage facility

- 24 hour water and electricity supply
- Arrangements for waste disposal
- Ambulance facility.

Strengthening Referral System

In order to improve referral linkage practiced in RCH Phase-I, new initiatives were added:
- Training of MBBS doctors in lifesaving anesthetic skills for emergency obstetric care
- Setting up of blood storage centers at FRUs according to Government of India guidelines
- Janani Suraksha Yojana: The national maternity benefit scheme has been modified into a new scheme called Janani Suraksha Yojana.

JANANI SURAKSHA YOJANA

This program was launched on 12th April 2005. The objectives of the scheme are: reducing maternal mortality and infant mortality, through encouraging delivery at health institutions and focusing at institutional care among women below poverty line families.

Salient Features of the Janani Suraksha Yojana

It is a 100% centrally sponsored scheme. Benefit of cash assistance with institutional care during antenatal, delivery and postpartum care to all women both rural and urban, belonging to below poverty line households and aged 19 years or above, up to first two live births. In ten low performing states, the cash benefit will be extended up to the third child, if the mother chooses to undergo sterilization in the health facility where she delivered. The accredited social health activist (ASHA) will be responsible for making institutional care available. She would also be responsible for escorting the pregnant woman to the health center.

The cash assistance for availing sterilization services will be ₹1,400 for mothers in rural areas of low performing states and ₹1,200 for mothers in urban area. All women including those from SC and ST families delivering in government institutions or accredited private institutions are eligible for cash assistance. Women from rural areas of high performing states get ₹700, while those from urban areas get ₹600.

The Yojana gives cash assistance of ₹250 for transportation of women to the nearest health center for delivery. The women get a subsidy of ₹1,500 for cesarean deliveries and management of obstetric complications. According to the government report of 2008, in the years 2006–2008 about 28.11 lakhs pregnant women received benefits from this scheme, out which 18.72 lakh had institutional deliveries.

VANDEMATARAM SCHEME

This is a voluntary scheme wherein any obstetric or gynecology specialist, maternity home or nursing home lady doctor or MBBS doctor can volunteer herself/himself for providing safe motherhood services. The enrolled doctor will display 'Vandemataram logo' at the clinic. Iron and folic acid tablets, oral pills, TT injections, etc. will be provided by the respective District Medical Officers (DMO) to the 'Vandemataram doctors or clinics' for distribution to beneficiaries. The cases needing special care and treatment can be referred to the government hospitals that have been advised to take due care of such patients coming with Vandemataram cards.

SAFE ABORTION SERVICES

In India abortion is a major cause of maternal morbidity and mortality and accounts for nearly 8.9% of maternal deaths. Majority of abortions take place outside authorized health services and/or by unauthorized and unskilled persons. Under RCH Phase II, following facilities are provided.

Medical Method of Abortion

Termination of early pregnancy with drugs—Mifepristone (RU486) followed by misoprostol; Currently, the use of these two drugs are recommended up to 7 weeks (49 days) of amenorrhea in a facility with provision for safe abortion services and blood transfusion. Termination of pregnancy using these two drugs is offered to women under the preview of the MTP Act, 1971.

Manual Vacuum Aspiration

Manual vacuum aspiration (MVA) is a safe and simple technique for termination of early pregnancy and is feasible to be used in primary health centers or comparable facilities, thereby increasing the access to safe abortion services.

All the below listed interventions included in RCH phase I will continue in the phase II implementation period:

- Appointing additional public health nurses, ANMs, anesthetists, and safe motherhood consultants
- Providing 24 hours delivery services at PHCs and CHCs
- Providing referral transport and integrated financial package
- Conducting RCH camps and training of Dais
- Implementing interventions for newborn care and child health [Immunization, control of acute respiratory infection (ARI) and diarrhea, vitamin A and iron supplementation, etc.]

NATIONAL RURAL HEALTH MISSION (NRHM)

The Government of India launched National Rural Health Mission (NRHM) on 5th April 2005 for a period of 7 years (2005–2012) in order to improve the quality of life of its citizens. The mission seeks to improve the health care delivery system. It is operational in the whole country with special focus on North East states.

The main aim of NRHM is to provide accessible, accountable, effective and reliable PHC and to bridge the gap in rural health care through creation of a cadre of ASHA, and strengthening the services of sub-centers, PHCs and CHCs.

Goals to be Achieved by NRHM

At National Level

- Reduction of infant mortality rate to 30/1,000 live births
- Reduction of maternal mortality rate to 100/100,000
- Reduction of total fertility
- Reduction of mortality rates of Malaria, Filaria, Dengue, Kala-azar and Japanese encephalitis
- Reduction of prevalence rates of Leprosy and Tuberculosis
- Upgrading CHCs to Indian Public Health standards

- Increasing first referral units from less than 20–75%
- Engaging 250,000 female ASHA.

At Community Level

- Availing trained community level workers at village level with a drug kit for general ailments
- Provision of immunization, antenatal and postnatal check ups, and services-related to health of mother and child including nutrition at anganwadi level
- Availing of generic drugs for common ailments at sub-center level
- Providing good hospital care through assured availability of doctors, drugs and quality services at PHC and CHC level
- Improved access to universal immunization
- Improved facilities for institutional deliveries
- Availability of assured health care at reduced financial risk
- Improved outreach services through mobile medical units at district level
- Provision of household toilets.

Plan of Implementation of NRHM

Implementation of the NRHM program will be through ASHAs and ANMs.

Selection of ASHA

ASHA must be a resident of the village: A woman (married/widowed/divorced) preferably in the age group of 25–45 years with formal education up to eight class, having communication skills and leadership qualities. The general norm will be one ASHA for 1,000 populations. In tribal, hilly and desert areas, the norm could be relaxed to one ASHA per habitation. The selected ASHAs will be trained to carry out specific responsibilities.

Roles and Responsibilities of ASHA

The ASHA will function as a health activist in the community and carry out the following responsibilities:

1. Take steps to create awareness and provide information on health determinants such as nutrition, basic sanitation and hygienic practices, healthy living and the need for utilisation of existing health and family welfare services.
2. Counsel women on birth preparedness, safe delivery, breastfeeding, complementary feeding, immunization, contraception and prevention of common infections including reproductive tract infections and sexually transmitted infections.
3. Mobilise community in accessing health related services available at the anganwadi, sub-center, and PHC such as immunization, antenatal check-up, postnatal check-up, supplementary nutrition, sanitation and other services being provided by the government.
4. Identify women in families below poverty line (BPL) as beneficiaries of the scheme (NRHM) and assist them to obtain BPL registration.
5. Ensure that the JSY card is filled up at least 16–20 weeks prior to delivery.
6. Work with the village health and sanitation committee of the Gram Panchayat to develop comprehensive village health plan.
7. Arrange escort/accompany pregnant women and children requiring treatment/admission to the nearest preidentified health facility (subcenter or PHC).
8. Provide primary medical care for minor ailments such as fever, diarrhea and first aid for minor injuries.
9. Be a provider of 'directly observed treatment short-course' (DOTS) under national tuberculosis control program.
10. Will act as a direct depot holder for essential provisions like oral rehydration solution (ORS), iron and folic acid tablets, chloroquin, disposable delivery kits, oral pills and condoms and keep a medicine kit with AYUSH and allopathic formulations recommended by the technical/expert advisory group of the government.
11. Ensure registration of births and deaths in her village, any unusual health problems or disease outbreaks in the community.
12. Promote construction of household toilets under total sanitation campaign.

Role and Integration with ANM

The ANM will guide ASHA in performing her functions through activities such as:
- Holding weekly/fortnightly meetings to discuss activities
- Acting as resource person for training of ASHA
- Guiding ASHA regarding arrangement for outreach programs
- Participating and guiding ASHA in organising health days in anganwadi center
- Utilising ASHA to motivate pregnant women to go to the sub-center for check-ups, take full course of iron and folic acid tablets and tetanus toxoid injections.

The ANMs will inform ASHA on date, time and place for initial and periodic training schedule and also ensure that ASHA gets the compensation for performance and TA/DA for attending training.

INTEGRATED CHILD DEVELOPMENT SERVICES

The ICDS scheme is one of the world's largest and most unique programs for early child development, which was launched on 2nd October 1975, to break the vicious cycle of malnutrition, morbidity, reduced learning capacity and morbidity. This program adopts a multisectoral approach to child well-being incorporating health education and nutrition interventions and is implemented through a network or anganwadi centers at the community level. Malnutrition is fought through interventions targeted at unmarried adolescent girls, pregnant women, mothers and children up to 6 years.

Objectives of the Scheme

- To improve the nutritional and health status of children in the agegroup 0–6 years
- To lay the foundation for proper psychological, physical and social development of children
- To reduce the incidence of mortality, morbidity, malnutrition and school dropout
- To achieve effective coordination of policy and implementation amongst the various departments to promote child development

- To enhance the capability of the mother to look after the normal health and nutritional needs of the child through proper nutrition and health education.

Key Services Provided Through ICDS

- Supplementary feeding
- Immunization
- Health check-up
- Micronutrient supplementation
- Preschool education for 3-6 years old
- Nutrition and health education
- Referral services.

Supplementary nutrition service includes growth monitoring, prophylaxis against vitamin A deficiency and control of nutritional anemia. All families in the community are surveyed to identify children below the age of 6, pregnant and nursing mothers. They are given supplementary nutritional support for 300 days in 1 year. The program aims to bridge the caloric gap between the national recommended and average intake of children and women in low income and disadvantaged groups.

Children below the age of three are weighed once a month and children below 3-6 years are weighed quarterly. Growth rate and nutritional status are assessed and malnourished children are given supplementary feeding and referred to medical centers.

Immunization of pregnant women against tetanus is undertaken towards reducing maternal and neonatal mortality. Vaccination of infants and children for six vaccine preventable diseases such as poliomyelitis, diphtheria, pertussis, tetanus, tuberculosis and measles are also included.

Health check-ups are offered to children up to 6 years, and expectant and nursing mothers. The services are provided by anganwadi workers and PHC staff and include weight checking, immunization, management of malnutrition, treatment of diarrhea, deworming and distribution of simple medicines. Through the 1.4 million anganwadi centers, the education component of the ICDS program is implemented. The early learning provides foundation for cumulative, life-long learning and development. This also contributes to universalization of primary education. Providing to children the necessary preparation for primary schooling, nutrition, and health education are key elements of the work of anganwadi workers. Capacity building of women, especially in the age group of 15–45 years is a long-term goal to be achieved.

ICDS Team

The ICDS team comprises the anganwadi workers, anganwadi helper, supervisors, child development project officers (CDPOs) and district program officers (DPOs). Anganwadi workers are ladies selected from the local communities and as such community-based front line workers of the ICDS program. The health teams include medical officers, ANMs and ASHAs as functionaries of ICDS to provide different services.

94. NEONATAL INTENSIVE CARE UNIT

INTRODUCTION

Neonatal Intensive Care Unit (NICU) is a very specialized unit where critically ill neonates are cared to reduce the neonatal morbidity and mortality. NICU specializes in the care of ill and premature newborn infants.

CRITERIA FOR ADMISSION OF NEONATES IN NICU

Indications for admission to the neonatal ICU are:
- Low birth weight 2000 gms or less
- Large babies more than 4 Kg
- Birth asphyxia (Apgar score less than or equal to 6)
- Meconium aspiration syndrome
  If symptomatic/thick meconium seen in Lab test
- Severe jaundice
- Infants of diabetic mothers
- Neonatal sepsis
- Neonatal convulsions
- Severe congenital malformation/congenital heart disease
- Immediate surgery required

- Unstable heart rate and respiratory rate requiring cardio-respiratory monitoring
- Need for exchange blood transfusion
- Premature rupture of membranes/foul smelling liquor.

BABIES WHO NEED SPECIAL CARE IN NICU

Most babies admitted to NICU are premature (born before 37 weeks of pregnancy), have low birth weight (less than 2500 gm.) or have medical conditions that require special care. Twins and other multiples often are admitted to the NICU, as they tend to be born earlier and are smaller than single birth babies (**Fig. 94.1**).

High-risk factors that can place the babies as high-risk and needing admission in NICU:
- Maternal factors
  - Age younger than 16 or older than 40 years
  - Drug or alcohol abuse
  - Diabetes
  - Hypertension
  - Bleeding
  - Sexually transmitted diseases
  - Multiple pregnancy
- Delivery factors
  - Fetal distress/birth asphyxia
  - Breech delivery
  - Meconium stained amniotic fluid
  - Nuchal cord
  - Forceps/cesarean delivery
- Baby factors
  - Pre or post-term deliveries (less than 37 weeks or more than 42 weeks)
  - Birth weight less than 2500 grams or over 4000 grams.
  - Resuscitation in the delivery room
  - Birth defects
  - Respiratory distress such as grunting or apnea
  - Infections such as herpes, group B streptococci, chlamydia
  - Seizures
  - Hypoglycemia

- Hypoxia
- Needing blood transfusion.

LEVELS OF NICU

Level- 1

Nurseries that care for healthy, full term babies. They are able to stabilize faster and be ready for transfer to special care nurseries.

Level- 2

Nurseries that have Infants who are moderately ill with problems that are expected to resolve rapidly and are recovering from serious illnesses.

Level- 3, NICU capable of caring for very small or very sick newborn babies. Small and ill babies are nursed in isolettes/incubators **(Fig. 94.1)**. Nursery is staffed with a variety of staff on site including neonatologists, neonatal nurses, and respiratory therapists who are available for 24 hours a day. Baby's care-givers in NICU include:

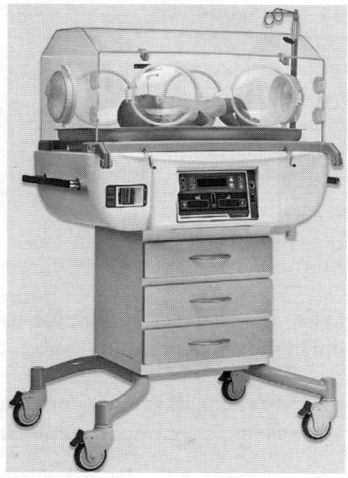

Fig. 94.1: Incubator for care of babies in NICU.

- Doctors: Neonatologists, Pediatricians
- Nurses: Staff nurses, Nurse in-charge
- Other health care professionals such as pharmacist, and group of developmental team (paramedical staff).

GOALS OF NEONATAL INTENSIVE CARE UNIT

The goals of NICU are:
- To improve the condition of the critically ill neonate keeping in mind the survival of the neonate so as to reduce the neonatal morbidity and mortality.
- To provide continuing in-service training to medical and nursing personnel in the care of ill newborns.
- To maintain the function of the pulmonary, cardiovascular, renal and nervous systems.
- To monitor the heart rate, body temperature and blood pressure by non-invasive techniques.
- To measure the oxygen concentration of the blood by using oxygen analyzers.
- To administer precise amounts of fluids and minute quantities of drugs through IV infusion pumps.

PREPARATION AND MAINTENANCE OF THE UNIT

- Warm incubator 33–36°C.
- Adequate light source.
- Resuscitation and treatment trolley stocked and ready for use any time.
- All patient records like History, Treatment, Diet sheet, Nursing care and Flowcharts.
- Oxygen and suction apparatus ready to available.
- Vital sign monitors.
- Specific equipment as indicated by diagnosis.

HISTORY AND EXAMINATION

Maternal history, paternal history, previous obstetric history of mother, details of present pregnancy, labor, delivery and Apgar score should be obtained and recorded.

ON ADMISSION

- Inform the neonatologist.
- Resuscitate the infant as necessary and maintain warmth.
- Check the infant's identification label.
- Quickly examine the infant from head to toe for any abnormalities if the baby's condition permits.
- Record weight, length and head circumference as soon as possible.
- Transfer to warm environment as soon as possible.
- Check the baby's temperature; normal range of body temperature is 36°C – 37°C, heart rate, respiration, color and activity.
- Explain to parents and take over from the transferring unit staff.
- Record following information in the baby's clinical chart:

Birth history in progress sheet, oxygen level in flow sheet, hydration status in fluid balance sheet and the condition on admission to NICU in the Nurses record.

A. Infection Control in Neonatal Intensive Care Units (NICU)

A neonatal intensive care unit, is a unit specializing in the care of ill and premature newborn infants. NICU has health care providers who have special training, and equipment to give best possible care to neonates.

Most babies admitted to NICU are preterm (born before 37 weeks of gestation) or have health condition that requires special care. Neonates in NICU receive care in a safe, controlled environment. An incubator helps provide the baby with constant body temperature. These babies are given high-calorie nutrition, intravenous hydration and other therapies based on their specific condition. Babies with mild respiratory distress syndrome (RDS) are treated with oxygen therapy as well as placed in a ventilator. Hypoglycemia in babies born to diabetic mothers and those with any infection are treated appropriately in NICU. Twins, triplets and other multiples are often admitted in NICU.

A difficult birth can cause decreased supply of oxygen and blood and such babies are managed in ICU. Sepsis is more likely in babies born earlier than full term. Protocols for care and maintenance of the unit are detailed in the following sessions.

Newborn care is one of the important areas of concern and need special attention in all respects of the units design, layout, staffing, policies and practice. Newborn babies especially premature infants are susceptible to blood borne infections. Babies in NICU often have immature immune system. They are exposed to many different caregivers and may have multiple blood tests. The approach towards prevention of neonatal sepsis is multidisciplinary comprising of neonatologists, hospital administrators, nursing staff and engineers. Microbes enter the NICU via visitors and healthcare workers (HCWs) and proliferate in susceptible sites. They spread in the neonates via contaminated articles and contaminated hands of HCWs. Once the babies are colonized, the organisms then enter through the umbilical cord, and skin during procedures, such as venous access, parenteral fluids, feeds, intubation and suctioning of endotracheal tubes.

In order to reduce or minimize morbidity and mortality in NICU babies, several measures are recommend by the Center for Disease Control (CDC).

1. **Prevent entry of microbes into NICU.**

   Clean the immediate environment: Organisms from labor room, resuscitation room environment and maternal vaginal flora can colonize the newborn skin. This can be prevented by the following clean measures.
   - Clean the mother's perineum
   - Clean the delivery surface
   - Clean the cord and cutting instruments
   - Ensure clean cord care
   - Ensure that nothing unclean is introduced into mother's vagina.

   Equipment for resuscitation in the 'baby receiving' area should be regularly cleaned and articles autoclaved.

2. **Standardize the NICU design.**

   Location of NICU should have a controlled access. Each infant space has to be a minimum of 120 sq. ft. clear floor space excluding the handwashing area and corridor. There should be a minimum of 4 feet between two infant beds.

3. **Airborne infection isolation room**

   An airborne infection isolation room should be available with following facilities.

- A hands-free handwashing station for hand hygiene.
- An area for gowning and storage of clean materials near the entrance to the NICU.
- According to the American Institute of Architecture (AIA) guidelines, the NICU and isolation room using exhaust to the exterior should have a minimum of six air exchanges per hour (AEH).

4. **Handwashing station**

   Every infant bed should be within 20 ft. of a hands-free handwashing station. Handwashing sink should be large enough to control splashing. Pictorial handwashing instructions should be provided. There should be space for soap and towel dispensers. Non-absorbent wall material should be used around the sink to prevent the growth of mold.

5. **Hand hygiene (Fig. 94.2)**

   The Center for Disease Control (CDC) recommends handwashing before and after contact with every infant for 20

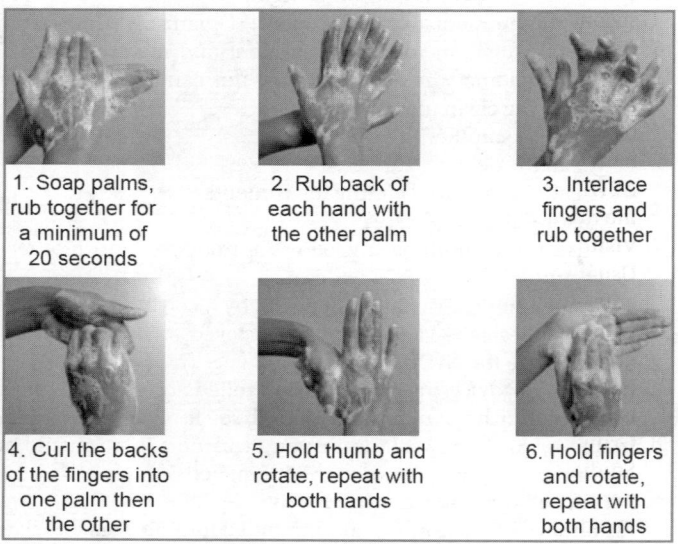

Fig. 94.2: Handwashing steps.

seconds, and 40–60 seconds of handwashing before entering the NICU. CDC recommended handwashing steps for infection control must be followed, which are:
- No wrist watch, no bracelet and no rings on fingers.
- Turn on water wet hands, and apply antimicrobial soap
- Wash palms of hands
- Wash between fingers at back of hands
- Wash between fingers palm to palm
- Wash palm area
- Pay particular attention to thumb area and thumb joint
- Wash fingertips paying particular attention to thumb area and thumb joint
- Wash fingertips paying particular attention to fingernails
- Rinse under running water
- Turn off water without contamination
- Wipe from fingertips to wrist
- Discard paper towel in garbage bin.

Each of the action should take 5 seconds, taking a total of 30 seconds.

6. **Use of alcohol-based hand rubs (ABHR)**

   Alcohol based hand rubs can be used as hand hygiene agents if hands are not visibly dirty or contaminated. Alcohol rubs may be used in between patient examination. At least 2-3 mL. of hand rubs should be applied over surface of palms and fingers. ABHRs are not useful after touching an infected patient or when the hands are soiled.

7. **Visitors policy**

   Usually microbes enter into NICU through personnel who enter into NICU and hence restriction entry is a must. People with active infection (respiratory, mucocutaneous, and gastrointestinal) and children should not be allowed inside NICU. Infected and out-born infants should be managed in the isolation room. NICU should be a "cell phone free' zone.

8. **Growing to reduce nosocomial infection**

   Studies have shown no reduction of infection during gowning period as compared to no gowning. The focus should be more on adequate handwashing by all hospital personnel and visitors before handling neonates.

Table 94.1: Housekeeping measures for NICU.

Daily cleaning.	
Incubators, warmers, infusion pumps, phototherapy units, mattresses, pulse-oxymeter, monitors, oxygen hoods, ventilators, CPAP machines and telephones.	Dry dusting followed by cleaning using a moist wipe.
Suction bottles, humidifier, chambers of CPAP.	Change and fill with distilled water
Bag and mask	Immerse in 2% Bacillocid for 6-8 hours after dismantling and cleaning with running water
Incubator, Radiant Warmers	Clean with 2% Bacillocid if not occupied by an infant
Laryngoscopes, masks, stethoscopes, measuring tapes, thermometers, B.P. Cuff, temperature and SpO_2 probes, flash lights	Wipe with alcohol after each use
Walls, floors, wash basins	Clean with phenol or Lysol or 2% bacillocid or 0.5% chlorine (for walls only) in each shift
Dust bins, buckets for waste	Empty in each shift and clean with soap and water
Weekly cleaning:	
Ventilators and CPAP circuits	Change with a new circuit
Window air conditioners	Surfaces and filters with soap and water
Procedure sets	Use disposable sets where possible. Autoclave after every use and keep ready the sets
Refrigerators	Sorted and cleaned once a week. Use separate fridge for milk and lab samples

9. **Jewelry and fingernails policy**

Healthcare workers should not wear artificial finger nails or extenders while having contact with neonates, and natural nails should be kept short.

10. **Measures to prevent proliferation of microbes in NICU**

 In order to prevent proliferation of microbes, in the NICU good housekeeping measures are to be followed. Avoid wet areas inside the NICU. A dry and clean NICU is unlikely to harbor microbes. Details of housekeeping routines and waste disposal are described below.

 Feeding utensils such as feeding paladai/katori should be cleaned and boiled for 15 minutes after each feeding.

11. **Waste segregation protocol adopted in India (Fig. 94.2 and 94.3).**

12. **Prevention of cross contamination**

 In order to prevent spread of infection from proliferation sites to baby and from one baby to another, the following steps are important.
 - Nurse to patient ratio: All neonatal intensive and high dependency care units should have appropriate number of neonatal nurses. Recommended ratio is 1:1, if baby has multidrug resistant microbes, 1:2 if babies have similar organism or susceptible organism, 1:3, if babies are already on adequate antibiotics cover.

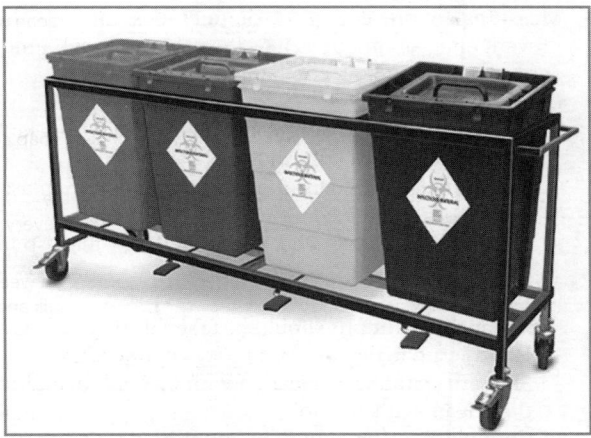

Fig. 94.3: Color coded bins for segregation of waste.

Table 94.2: Color coded bins for segregation of waste.

Black drums/ bins	Needles without syringes, blades, sharps and all metal articles
Yellow drums/bins (Disposal by incineration)	Infectious waste, bandages, gauze, cotton or any other things in contact with body fluids human body parts placenta
Blue drums/ bins	All types of glass bottles and articles, outdated and discarded medicines
Red drums/bins Made non-infectious by autoclaving and disposed by shredding	Plastic waste, such as catheters, infected syringes, tubings, IV bottles.

- Use of disposables: Ample disposables are needed for each baby. A baby kit containing a stethoscope, measuring tape, thermometer and a flash light in a sterile container should be available at each bed. All articles used for the baby such as syringes, suction catheter, gloves and antibiotic vials should be disposable. Do not keep articles such as files, X-ray films and pens on the baby cot.
- Measures to prevent entry of microbes into the infant: Prevent entry of microbes into the infant through umbilical cord, skin and into the circulation.
- Cord care
  - Careful application of adhesive tapes and take precautions during removal of adhesive.
  - Use skin friendly Duropore instead of Dynaplast and micropore.
  - Bath should be avoided in hospitals, instead sponging may be done.
- Precautions during procedures
  - Aseptic precautions should be taken during procedures.
  - Hand scrub to be done prior to each procedure.
  - Skin area should be cleaned with alcohol, betadine and then again with alcohol.
  - Cannulation sites should be monitored daily for signs of thrombophlebitis.

- Catheters should be removed as soon as the baby's condition is stabilized.
- Feeding of breast milk/breastfeeding/formula feeding
  Encourage use of colostrum and expressed breast milk
  Mother's entry into NICU and pumping of milk to ensure adequate breast milk for the infant to be encouraged
  If the infant needs formula feed, reconstituted formula at right temperature is recommended.

Infection Control Protocols

Prevention of nosocomial infections is the prime responsibility of all individuals. Therefore infection control protocols should be in place. Every hospital should have an infection control committee in place with the goals to review and approve promptly.
- Programmes of activity for surveillance and prevention
- Epidemiological surveillance data and identify areas for interventions.
- Ensure appropriate staff training in infection control and safety
- Provide input into investigation of epidemics.

The morbidity and mortality of neonates can be significantly reduced by instituting strict infection control strategies. Prevention of entry of microbes to NICU can be achieved by clean environment, hand hygiene and conducive infrastructure. Curtailing proliferation of microbes in NICU can be successful by daily and weekly maintenance of equipment like incubators, warmers, syringes, pumps, ventilator filters, circuits and bag and mask. Efficient biomedical waste disposal is important. Early breastfeeding, use of colostrum and early discharge plan are important in prevention of neonatal morbidity. The role of hospital management and an efficient infection control committee play an important role in prevention of infection, related to neonatal morbidity and mortality.

B. Records and Reports in Neonatal Intensive Care Unit

Neonatal intensive care unit (NICU) is a very specialized unit where critically ill neonates are treated and cared to reduce the neonatal morbidity and mortality. All professional persons need to be accountable for the performance of their duties and nursing being a profession, nurses need to record their work in completion. Every ICU keeps several records and reports. Records are administrative tools used to classify and prevent duplication of the information. Reports are document forms which include conclusions or findings based on facts or recommendations concerning the patient. The ICU nurse has to be highly skilled today due to technological advances and complex care of the critically ill patients or neonates. Documentation and care required are complex and time consuming activities.

Purpose of Documentation in ICU

Documentation in the ICU is carried out for a number of reasons. It ensures continuity of care and provides up-to-date patient status. It fulfills hospital policies which furnish the legal aspects of 'duty of care'.

Principles of Record Keeping

- Since the clinical records is a legal document, it is essential that they should be written clearly, accurately, appropriately and legibly.
- All entries should be signed by the individual who writes them.
- Care to be taken not to make any errors in the records. If anything is crossed out, it should be dated and initialed.
- All records should be written with black ink or typed for better legibility.
- Records should be written in chronological order as to date and time. When recording medications and treatments, enter exact time and date when they are carried out.
- Records should be written continuously with no blank spaces. If any space is left out, it should be crossed out, dated and signed.
- Lengthy corrections of records are to be written as amendments.
- Each page of the record should be properly identified with the patient's name, age, IP Number. OP Number. Date, etc.
- Use only standard abbreviations.

Importance of Records

The records form a permanent account of a patient's illness. Their clarity and accuracy is paramount for effective communication between healthcare professionals and patients. Maintenance of good records ensures that a patient's or neonate's assessed needs are met comprehensively.

- Records should be truthful, brief and complete. It should include all the services carried out or care given to the patient from day-to-day and results of treatment or nursing activity.
- Records are to be factual, consistent and accurate.
- Provide current information of the care given and condition of the infant.
- Document clearly in such a way that the text cannot be erased.

Types of NICU Records

Every ICU maintains complete patient record. This will contain the bio-data of the patient/neonate, diagnosis, mothers health and obstetric history, type of delivery, findings of neonatal assessment (APGAR score), resuscitation information if done, treatments and medications given, progress notes and summary made at the time of discharge or transfer to NICU.

- **Nurses' notes:**
  - Large parts of patient's records are filled by the nurse.
  - Nurses' notes are a record of treatments and nursing measures carried out by the nurse, their effects and observations made on the patient. Avoid bulky reports containing unnecessary and irrelevant materials.
  - Observation of the baby is continuous and it is impossible for the nurse to record all the observations. Observations should be specific and objective as possible.
- **Doctors' order sheet:** The doctors' orders (prescriptions) regarding medications, investigations and nutrition supply.
- **Graphic charts of TPR:**
  - On this, the neonate's temperature, heart rate and respirations are written in a graphic form so that any slight deviation from the normal can be noted at a glance.
  - Other information such as heart rate, respirations, number of bowel movements, body weight, name and date of any surgery performed, etc., are recorded in the chart according to the hospital policy.

- **Intake and output chart:**
  Babies on intravenous fluids, enteric feeds, vomiting, diarrhea, etc., should have intake-output maintained.
- **Registers:**
  To maintain the statistics, every NICU maintains certain registers in order to register admissions, discharges, and operations, census, etc. It is the nurses' responsibility to maintain those registers up-to-date. Other registers include:
  - Register with entries of laboratory examinations, biochemistry, hematology reports, etc.
  - Diet sheet entries.
  - Consent forms of parents for anesthesia and operations.

Nurses' Responsibility for Care of Patient Records

- Records are kept under the safe custody of the nurse in each unit or department,
- No individual sheet is separated from the complete record.
- Records are to be kept in a place not accessible to patients or visitors.
- No stranger is ever permitted to read patient records.
- Patients' records are not to be handed over to legal advisors without the written permission of the administration.
- All hospital personnel are legally and ethically obliged to keep in confidence all the information provided in the records.
- All records are to be handled carefully to avoid damage.
- All records are filed according to the hospital policy, so that they can be traced easily. It may be arranged alphabetically or numerically with index cards.
- All records are identified with the bio data of the patient such as name, age, unit, bed number, IP number, OP number, diagnosis, etc.

Reports

A report is a document that presents information in an organized format for a specific audience and purpose. Although summaries of reports may be delivered orally, complete reports are almost always in the form of written documents.

Reports in Patient Care Units

Incident Reports

An ancient is an unfavorable event that affects patient or staff safety. Typical health care incidents are related to physical injuries, medical error, equipment failure or patient care anything that enlargers a patient's or staff's safety is called an incident in the medical system.

The principle regarding errors is that "to err is human, to cover up is unforgivable, and to fail to learn is inexcusable". The process of collecting incident data and presenting it properly is known as "incident reporting in healthcare system with incident reporting, an emerging problem is highlighted in a non-blaming way to provide a catalyst for changing the factors contributing to the error. Designated staff with authority to file a report or staff who has witnessed an incident firsthand, usually file the incident. Usually, nurses or other hospital staff who has witnessed an incident report within 24 to 48 hours after the incident occurred.

A Situation for Incident Reporting

While injecting an IV pain medication, the nurse misread the label and administered a heavier dosage than prescribed, which increased the patient's blood pressure level. In this situation, it is necessary to fill in the incident report. Simply because an unexpected event occurred and lead to harm. It does not matter how severe or minor the incident is, it is essential to report all such incidents.

Purpose of Incident Reports

Incident reports provide valuable information to hospital administration. They capture data required to highlight necessary measures to improve the overall safety and quality of services of the hospital. An accurate incident report serves multiple purposes such as:
    a. Root cause identification
    b. Policy and process improvements
    c. Clinical risk management
    d. Continuous quality improvement
    e. Better training and continuous learning

1. **Types of incident reports**
   - Clinical incidents
     Unpleasant and unplanned event that causes or can causes physical harm to a patient.
     Example:
     – A patient falls out of bed while sleeping.
     – A patient brutally scratched a nursed while she was taking his temperature.
     – Nurse mislabeled the medicine box while storing it.
   - Near miss incidents
     An error or unsafe condition is caught before it reaches the patient.
     Example:
     A patient attempts to leave the hospital facility before discharge, but the security guard stopped him and brought him back to the ward.
   - Work place incidents
     Example:
     Patient or next of kin abuses a care provider verbally or physically leading to unsafe work conditions.

   Most hospitals have incident reporting forms available in all units and departments in which details cab be entered and forwarded to administration through proper channel.

2. **Day and Night Reports**
   In hospitals nurses provide patient care around the clock and to prepare bedside shift reports. These are written reports, tape recorded report or verbal face-to-face report conducted in a private setting, and face-to-face beside patients (handoff). The reports are verbal or written communication of data regarding the clients' health status needs, treatments, outcomes and responses. Reporting facilitates clinical decision making, continuity of care and coordination among health team members, particularly nursing personnel. Day and night reports are used at change of duty shifts.

3. **Transfer Report**
   Patients will be frequently transferred from one unit to another to receive different levels of care. When giving transfer request the nurse should include the following information.

Transfer reports contain the following information
- Client's name, age, primary doctor and medical diagnosis.
- Summary of medical progress up to the time of transfer.
- Current health status-physical and psycho-social.
- Current nursing diagnosis or problems and care plans.
- Any critical assessment or "interventions" to be completed shortly.
- Needs of any special equipment.

Admission to the neonatal intensive care unit often happens when a baby is in critical condition and needs the care in an incubator. Mostly neonates go to NICU from labor rooms, Operation Theater or referred and transferred from another hospital. Premature and critically ill babies are placed in NICU. Information in NICU records include ICU treatment, medications, visitation by specialists, daily health status and progress made. NICU records of the neonate provide the nurse a basis for analyzing the needs of the baby in terms of what has been done, what is being done and what needs to done. Nursing records of the neonate must be maintained correctly and accurately and safeguarded carefully according to the agency policies as well as in accordance with the legal and ethical standards. Reports are oral or written exchange of information shared between care givers or health personnel in a number of days.

Different kinds of reports are prepared to meet specific purpose in the unit. An organized account of an event, unit activities or requirements in the unit for patient care are prepared for oral presentation or written and submitted to personnel in authority.

95. NEWBORN ASSESSMENT

Assessment of the newborn is done during and after the transition period of 4–6 hours of life. The nurse determines that the infant is physiologically stable by skilled examination and assessment of the infant's general appearance (skin), thermoregulatory effort and different body systems.

Assessment of the Skin

The skin of all babies to be examined for the following:

- Pallor (pale, mottled appearance indicating poor perfusion)
- Plethora (beetroot color indicating excess of circulating red blood cells)
- Cyanosis: Central cyanosis always requires immediate attention
- Jaundice: Early jaundice is abnormal
- Skin rashes such as milia, miliaria, petechiae, Mongolian blue spots, bruising and erythema toxicum
- Infectious lesions, e.g. thrush, herpes simplex virus, umbilical sepsis and bullous impetigo.

Respiratory System

Respiration to be counted by watching the lower chest and abdomen rise and fall for a full minute. Rate of respiration will vary between levels of activity. The chest should expand symmetrically. Abnormalities to look for include the following:
- Unilateral chest expansion and diminished breath sounds on one side
- Tychypnea (rate above 60/min)
- Retraction (inspiratory pulling in of the chest wall above and below the sternum or between the ribs)
- Nasal flaring
- Grunting; an abnormal expiratory sound
- Apnea; cessation of breathing for 20 seconds or more.

Body Temperature

The normal body temperature range for term infants is 36.5–37°C rectally (core temperature):
1. Hypothermia: A core temperature below 36° is termed as hypothermia, which can indicate respiratory distress, hypoglycemia, and sepsis.
2. Hyperthermia: An axillary temperature above 37.5° C is considered hyperthermia. The usual hyperthermia is due to overheating of the environment, but it can also be a sign of sepsis, brain injury or drug therapy.

Cardiovascular System

The normal heart rate of a term newborn is 120–160 bpm and of a preterm infant is 130–170 bpm.

Cardiovascular dysfunction should be suspected in infants who present with lethargy and breathlessness during feeding. Other signs include slowness with feeds, pale at times or fast labored breathing.

Infants who appear breathless with little or no rib recession and no grunting may have heart disease. Presence of a murmur heard on routine examination may be suggestive of an underlying cardiac lesion.

Central Nervous System

Abnormal postures such as neck retraction, frog-like postures, hyperextension or hyperflexion of limbs, jittery or abnormal involuntary movements, high-pitched or weak cry when assessed indicate neurological impairment.

Genitalia and Anus

The genitalia should be examined for sex determination and any abnormalities such as ambiguous genitalia or undescended testes. Patency of anus should be checked using a rectal thermometer or rubber catheter.

Limbs and Digits

Length and movement of limbs are checked and the digits counted and separated to ensure that webbing is not present. Normal flexion and rotation of wrists and ankle joints are confirmed.

Spine

With the baby lying prone, the back should be inspected and palpated to detect any swellings, dimples or hairy patches, which may signify occult spinal defect.

Measurements

The baby's head circumference, chest circumference, length and weight are measured and recorded.

Examination by the Pediatrician

All newborn babies are examined by the pediatrician within the first 24 hours. In addition to the general appearance of the baby, color, activity, response to handling and specific examinations are done:

- *Neurological assessment:* Baby's reflex responses are elicited in order to establish normality of the neurological system (refer to Chapter 79 for details on reflexes)
- *Auscultation:* Heart and lung sounds are checked
- *Palpation:* Abdominal organs and femoral pulses are palpated
- *Hips:* Examinations to detect developmental dysplacia of hips are done using Ortolani's test or Barlow's test.

Behavior

After birth, there is distinct pattern of normal behavior. During the first hour of life, the newborn appears alert and interested in his/her surrounding. Will cry lustily and is keen and eager to feed. Following this activity, the baby will sleep for 2–4 hours.

The vital signs of temperature, heart rate and respiration will be within normal range. After sleeping, the baby will wake up, begin rooting for food and have a strong suck and swallow reflex (refer to Chapter 98 for newborn reflexes).

96. NEWBORN CARE

Newborn care includes both initial care and general care:
1. Initial care:
    - As the baby's head is born, excess mucus may be wiped gently from his/her mouth, taking care not to touch the nares to avoid stimulation and reflex inhalation
    - Oral and endotracheal suction are done when indicated
    - As the body is delivered, the baby is drawn up towards and onto the mothers' abdomen and quickly covered with warm blanket
    - The time of birth and sex of baby are noted and recorded
    - If necessary, the airway is cleared with a mucus extractor or soft suction catheter attached to low pressure (10 cm water), oropharynx first and then nasopharynx
    - The umbilical cord is divided (cut) between two clamps applied approximately 8–10 cm from the abdomen

- The nursery nurse receives the infant into a baby blanket or towel and places him/her into a radiant warmer
- The mouth and nose are again cleared with a suction bulb if needed
- The infant is then thoroughly dried and wrapped in warm blanket after removing the wet towel
- While drying the infant, respiratory effort, color and muscle tone are observed
- Heart rate and respiratory rate are counted
- Apgar score is assigned at 1 and 5 minutes after birth
- After a period of rest in the warmer, or in his/her mother's arms, the baby is transferred to the ward with his mother; The care at this stage include:
    - Replacing the initial cord clamp with a disposable plastic clamp, 2–3 cm from the umbilicus
    - Administering vitamin K, 1 mg IM
    - Instillation of prophylactic eyedrops.
- A head-to-toe physical assessment is done to determine the infant's health status:
    - General inspection: For position; flexed or not
    - Skin: Dry or cracking
    - Heart auscultation for rate and rhythm
    - Lungs for expansion and breath sounds
    - Blood pressure
    - Axillary body temperature
    - Head-to-toe length, head and chest circumference
    - Head for molding and suture lines
    - Face for symmetry, birth marks, milia and nevi over the forehead and eyelids
    - Mouth for natal teeth abnormalities of the hard and soft palate and tongue
    - Femoral and brachial pulses
    - Hip for any dislocation
    - Genitalia for descend of testes and location of urethral meatus

- Spine and skin on the back for alignment, breaks in skin, moles, birth marks or markers along the spinal column
- Reflexes for maturity of the neurological system such as rooting and sucking reflex, tonic neck or fencing reflex, grasp reflex
- Moro reflex, head lag or traction reflex.

The baby should remain with his/her mother whenever both are in good condition.

2. General care:
   - The nurse receiving the baby from the delivery room nurse should verify the baby's name, sex, date and time of birth on both name bands and transfer them to the cot card; the name bands should remain on the baby until his/her discharge
   - During the first few hours after birth, the midwife should observe the baby's color, breathing and umbilical cord; temperature to be monitored and mother assisted with breastfeeding
   - Ongoing and daily care should include:
     - Positioning the baby in cot on his/her side after feeding, with a mucus extractor readily available to prevent airway obstruction
     - Dressing and wrapping the baby adequately to prevent hypothermia
     - Using individual articles for the baby and ensuring proper hand hygiene by personnel handling the baby to prevent infection
     - Skin care: First bath after the baby's condition is stable, and cleansing of face, skin flexures and napkin area once or twice daily is recommended; cord to be cleansed with alcohol swab and kept dry.
   - Vaccination and immunization are given according to the policy, e.g. bacillus Calmette–Guérin (BCG) vaccination during the early neonatal period, followed by hepatitis B and polio vaccines
   - Daily examination of the baby to include:
     - Noting the baby's posture, color and respirations.
     - Jaundice may be noted from the 3rd day

- Palpation of the head for assessment of the anterior fontanelle for its level, resolution of caput succedaneum, molding and cephalhematoma
- Inspection of eyes and mouth for signs of infection
- Response to handling and mother's voice
- Inspection of skin for rashes, septic spots, excoriation or abrasions
- Examination of umbilical cord base for redness
- Checking of body temperature in the axilla
- Observation of the stools for constipation, watery stools and excoriation, and frequency of passing stools and urine
- Presence of breast engorgement and pseudomenstruation
- Daily weight to assess the normal loss in the first 3 days (less than 10%)
- Recording the findings in the baby's record.

Nursing Process

Assessment

- Wakeful hours may be 2–3 hours for first several days
- Sleep hours average 20 hours per day
- Apical pulse 120–160 bpm, while awake, 80–100 bpm, while sleeping and upto 180 bpm while crying
- Heart murmur present during transition periods
- Blood pressure 60/40 to 80/45 mm Hg
- Abdomen soft, active bowel sounds present
- Urine colorless or pale yellow, with 6–10 wet diapers/24 hours
- Passage of meconium stool within 24–48 hours
- Mean weight 2,500–4,000 grams
- Weight loss 5–10% initially
- Mouth: Scant saliva, natal teeth may be present
- Head: Circumference 32–37 cm, fontanelles soft and flat, caput succedaneum may be present
- Neurological: Reflexes present
- Absence of jitteriness, lethargy, hypotonia and paresis

- Breathing diaphragmatic and abdominal
- Chest circumference approximately 30–35 cm
- Skin temperature 36–36.5°C (96.8–97.7°F) by axilla
- Acrocyanosis may be present for several days
- Extremities: Normal range of motion
- Genitalia:
  - Male: Testes descended, scrotum covered with rugae, phimosis common
  - Female: Labia may be slightly reddened or edematous; white mucos or bloody discharge may be present.

Diagnostic Studies

- White blood cell (WBC) 18,000/mm^3 (decline occurs in sepsis)
- Hemoglobin (Hb) 15–20 g/dL
- Hematocrit (Hct) 43–61%
- Total (bilirubin) 6 mg/dL.

Nursing Diagnosis

1. Risk for imbalanced body temperature.
2. Risk for impaired gas exchange.
3. Risk for imblanced nutrition: less than body requirements.
4. Risk for infection.
5. Risk for constipation.
6. Deficient knowledge regarding infant care (for parent).

Expected Outcomes

Neonate will be:
1. Free of cold stress or hyperthermia.
2. Free of signs of respiratory distress.
3. Display weight loss of 5–10% or less of body weight by time of discharge.
4. Free from signs of infection.
5. Pass meconium stool within 48 hours after birth.

6. Mother demonstrates behaviors to meet physiological and emotional needs of newborn.

Nursing Interventions

1. Newborn remaining free of cold stress or hypothermia:
   - Provide adequate clothing considering the neonate's weight and gestational age, e.g. swaddle wrapping in warm blanket and hat for head
   - Monitor body temperature hourly/per protocol during stabilization period
   - Assess respiratory rate, note any tachypnea
   - Postpone initial bath until body temperature is stable and reaches 36.5°C (97.7°F)
   - Bathe neonate rapidly, exposing only a portion of the body at a time and drying each part immediately
   - Note signs of cold stress such as irritability, pallor mottling, respiratory distress, tremors, jitteriness, lethargy and cool skin
   - Assess for signs of hyperthermia such as increased restlessness, perspiration that begins on head or face and proceed to chest, apnea or seizure
   - Note signs of dehydration, e.g. poor skin turgor, delayed voiding, dry mucous membranes, elevated temperature and sunken fontanelles
   - Initiate early breastfeeding.
2. Remaining free of signs of respiratory distress:
   - Review prenatal and intrapartum events, noting risk factors that could have contributed to excess lung fluid
   - Assess respiratory rate, effort and normal breathing patterns
   - Suction nasopharynx as needed, note color, amount and character of regurgitated mucus
   - Position newborn on side with rolled towel for support at back
   - Auscultate breath sounds and record equality and clarity

- Assess newborn for presence, location and degree of cyanosis
- Monitor newborn for signs of hypothermia or hyperthermia
- Note symmetery of chest movement
- Auscultate heart sounds and note presence of murmurs.

  *Administer supplemental oxygen as indicated by the newborn's condition.

  *Determine Rh factor and ABO blood group of newborn and mother.

  *Assess Hb and Hct levels if done.

  *Denotes collaborative interventions.

3. Maintaining body weight and blood glucose levels within normal limits:
   - Note mother's prenatal history for possible stressors impacting on neonates glucose stores, e.g. pregnancy-induced hypertension (PIH), cardiac or renal disorders
   - Review intrapartal records for Apgar scores and condition at birth
   - Reduce physical stressors such as cold stress or excessive exposure to radiant warmers
   - Observe newborn for tremors, irritability, tachypnea, diaphoresis, cyanosis, pallor and seizure activity
   - Monitor for ruddiness; note elevated Hb/Hct levels (Hb > 20 g/dL; Hct > 60%)
   - Auscultate bowel sounds and presence of rooting and sucking behaviors
   - Encourage demand feeding and note frequency, amount/length of feeding
   - Monitor color, concentration and frequency of voidings
   - Observe newborn for indications of feeding problems such as regurgitation, abdominal distension or refusal to feed.

4. Newborn remaining free from signs of infection:
   - Review maternal risk factors that predispose infant to infection, which may be acquired transplacentally or at delivery
   - Determine newborn's gestational age to assess the status of passive immunity
   - Monitor vital signs including skin temperature
   - Scrub and wash hands before and after handling infant

- Teach parents and siblings, proper handwashing technique to use before handling infant
- Monitor parents, personnel and visitors with infections, illnesses or skin lesions who need to limit contact with newborn
- Maintain individual equipment and supplies for each newborn
- Instruct mother to inspect skin daily for rashes or interruption in skin integrity
- Recommend use of mild soaps and avoiding excessive rubbing
- Assess cord and skin area at the base of cord daily for redness or discharge
- Facilitate drying through exposure to air by folding diaper below and T-shirt above the cord stump
- Inspect newborn's mouth for white plaque on oral mucosa, gums and tongue; distinguish between white patches of thrush and milk curds
- Note lowered temperature, jaundice, respiratory symptoms or visible lesions
- Isolate newborn, if indicated.
  *Administer hepatitis B vaccine per institution's policy.
  *Monitor laboratory studies, as indicated, e.g. WBC count, cultures of lesions, blood cultures.
  *Apply nystatin (Mycostatin) to mouth for candidiasis infection.
  *Administer topical, oral or parenteral antibiotics as indicated.
  *Denotes collaborative interventions.

5. Pass meconium stool within 48 hours after birth:
   - Review intrapartal record of indications of passage of meconium, e.g. hypoxia
   - Auscultate bowel sounds
   - Take rectal temperature: Insert soft rubber catheter into anus with caution
   - Monitor frequency and amount/length of feeding, frequency of voiding, skin turgor and status of fontanelles and weight
   - Encourage early feeding
   - Note passage of first meconium

- Record frequency, color, consistency and odor of stools
- Assess abdomen for constant or intermittent distension
- Observe for motility, disturbance associated with constipation, vomiting, fluid and electrolyte imbalances.
  *Assist with diagnostic studies, e.g. radiological studies.
  *Transfer to neonatal intensive care unit (NICU) if indicated.
  *Denotes collaborative interventions.

6. Demonstrating appropriate behaviors to meet the needs of newborn:
   - Appraise parent's understanding of infant's physiological needs and adaptation to extrauterine life
   - Discuss newborn behavior such as wakefulness, mucus regurgitation, gagging and passage of first meconium stool
   - Perform newborn assessment in presence of parent as appropriate and provide information about normal characteristics and variations
   - Discuss and demonstrate normal newborn reflexes and review ages at which each reflex disappears
   - Discuss different types of cries that the neonate may use to communicate; demonstrate consoling measures
   - Provide information about ways to minimize or prevent excessive heat loss or overheating
   - Discuss newborn's usual sleep patterns and ways of promoting sleep
   - Demonstrate and supervise infant care activities related to feeding and holding, bathing, diapering and clothing
   - Discuss feeding techniques, frequency and burping
   - Instruct mother regarding positioning of newborn after feeding and demonstrate use of bulb syringe
   - Instruct regarding use of diapers, recognition of rashes and appropriate treatment
   - Emphasize infants need for follow-up care and timely immunizations
   - Discuss signs of jaundice and when to contact the pediatrician
   - Discuss manifestations of illness and infection and times at which physician to be contacted.

97. NON-STRESS TEST

A non-stress test (NST) is the evaluation of fetal heart rate in response to an increase in either spontaneous or stimulated fetal activity. It is a noninvasive method that combines detection of fetal heart rate accelerations and presence of spontaneous or evoked fetal movement.

Timing and Indications

Non-stress testing can be reliably performed after 28 weeks gestation. In the healthy fetus with a functional central nervous system (CNS), 90% of fetal body movements are associated with accelerations in fetal heart rate.

Some common indications for NST are:
- Suspected postmaturity
- Maternal diabetes mellitus
- Maternal hypertension
- Suspected or documented intrauterine growth restriction (IUGR)
- History of previous stillbirth
- Decreasing fetal movement
- Severe maternal anemia
- Chronic renal disease
- Isoimmunization
- Sickle cell disease
- High-risk antepartal conditions such as premature rupture of fetal membranes or preterm labor.

Patient Preparation

- The woman's blood pressure is taken and recorded
- Ensure that she has eaten food, as the fetus moves more after their mothers have eaten
- Have the woman empty her bladder
- Have her lie in reclining position with a lateral tilt to avoid supine hypotension
- The monitoring devices (tocodynamometer for measuring uterine pressure and fetal heart sensor for fetal heart detection)

are placed on the abdomen and held in place by elastic belts. An event button is given to mother with instructions to depress it to mark episodes of fetal movements on the monitor strip.

Procedure

The fetal heart rate is detected and recorded in the monitor strip. The event button and tocotransducer documents the fetal movements and intermittent changes in uterine pressure. The test usually is completed in 20–30 minutes, but may take longer if the fetus is in a sleep state. The criteria for a reactive (normal) NST are two accelerations in a 20-minute test period and a normal baseline fetal heart rate. A nonreactive test result is the absence of accelerations during the test period. A third result is an inconclusive or equivocal test result. This is the finding of less than two accelerations in 20-minutes test window or accelerations that do not meet the criteria of an amplitude increase of 15 beats per minute for duration of 15 seconds, or a poor quality recording that is inadequate for interpretation.

When the NST is reactive, it is highly predictive of fetal health and well-being. Repeat NSTs are done twice weekly and the pregnancy is continued if results remain reassuring. When the NST is inconclusive or equivocal, either the NST is repeated within 12–24 hours or a contraction stress test (CST) or a biophysical profile to further evaluate fetal well-being may be ordered.

98. NURSING DIAGNOSIS

Nursing diagnosis is a statement made by the nurse that addresses the focus of nursing care to be provided to a patient. The diagnosis reflect an issue or state of health to direct care planning that falls within the nurse's scope of practice.

The nurse serves as a diagnostician through the use of nursing diagnosis. This dynamic process involves comprehensive clinical decision-making derived from data collection. The most pressing needs that the nurse can manage are discovered through assessment findings by employing sound diagnostic reasoning. A diagnosis encompasses an individualized approach to the patient's unique situation, personal preferences and needs by striving to direct the remaining components of the nursing process, which are planning, intervention (implementation) and evaluation. Most patient care and educational facilities require nurses and nursing students to use North American Nursing Diagnosis Association (NANDA)-approved diagnoses and supporting terminology in their clinical documentation. Included in the nursing diagnosis is a diagnosis label, related factors and defining characteristics. Relevant and well-prepared nursing diagnoses improve the quality of thought process for prioritization in order to gauge the most vital care to be given. Use of nursing diagnosis assists nurses in understanding the client's problems and promotes patient-focused care rather than medical or nursing-focused care.

The process of nursing diagnosis development enables the nurse to focus care on the most vital needs that are conducive to optimal patient outcomes. Nursing diagnoses can be applied to any setting in which the nurse provides care to a patient, family, or community. Learning to correctly identify the priority nursing diagnosis or diagnoses is beneficial in implementing the steps of nursing process and in the development or critical thinking. The types of nursing diagnoses are actual, at-risk, healthpromotion and syndrome diagnosis. The list of nursing diagnoses prepared and revised every four years by the NANDA serves as guidelines for making comprehensive and need-based nursing care plans for mothers and newborns as well as individuals with health problems.

NURSING DIAGNOSIS TAXONOMY II

Taxonomy II for nursing diagnosis contains 13 domains and 47 classes *(Image via: Wikipedia.com)*
- **Domain 1. Health Promotion**
    - Class 1. Health awareness
    - Class 2. Health management
- **Domain 2. Nutrition**
    - Class 1. Ingestion
    - Class 2. Digestion
    - Class 3. Absorption
    - Class 4. Metabolism
    - Class 5. Hydration

- **Domain 3. Elimination and Exchange**
  - Class 1. Urinary function
  - Class 2. Gastrointestinal function
  - Class 3. Integumentary function
  - Class 4. Respiratory function
- **Domain 4. Activity/Rest**
  - Class 1. Sleep/Rest
  - Class 2. Activity/Exercise
  - Class 3. Energy balance
  - Class 4. Cardiovascular/Pulmonary responses
  - Class 5. Self-care
- **Domain 5. Perception/Cognition**
  - Class 1. Attention
  - Class 2. Orientation
  - Class 3. Sensation/Perception
  - Class 4. Cognition
  - Class 5. Communication
- **Domain 6. Self-Perception**
  - Class 1. Self-concept
  - Class 2. Self-esteem
  - Class 3. Body image
- **Domain 7. Role relationship**
  - Class 1. Caregiving roles
  - Class 2. Family relationships
  - Class 3. Role performance
- **Domain 8. Sexuality**
  - Class 1. Sexual identity
  - Class 2. Sexual function
  - Class 3. Reproduction
- **Domain 9. Coping/stress tolerance**
  - Class 1. Post-trauma responses
  - Class 2. Coping responses
  - Class 3. Neurobehavioral stress
- **Domain 10. Life principles**
  - Class 1. Values
  - Class 2. Beliefs
  - Class 3. Value/Belief/Action congruence

- **Domain 11. Safety/Protection**
  - Class 1. Infection
  - Class 2. Physical injury
  - Class 3. Violence
  - Class 4. Environmental hazards
  - Class 5. Defensive processes
  - Class 6. Thermoregulation
- **Domain 12. Comfort**
  - Class 1. Physical comfort
  - Class 2. Environmental comfort
  - Class 3. Social comfort
- **Domain 13. Growth/Development**
  - Class 1. Growth
  - Class 2. Development

New 'NANDA' Nursing Diagnosis List

In this edition of NANDA nursing diagnosis list (2018-2020), 17 new nursing diagnoses were approved and introduced. These new approved nursing diagnoses are:

1. Readiness for enhanced health literacy
2. Ineffective adolescent eating dynamics
3. Ineffective child eating dynamics
4. Ineffective infant eating dynamics
5. Risk for metabolic imbalance syndrome
6. Imbalanced energy field
7. Risk for unstable blood pressure
8. Risk for complicated immigration transition
9. Neonatal abstinence syndrome
10. Acute substance withdrawal syndrome
11. Risk for acute substance withdrawal syndrome
12. Risk for surgical site infection
13. Risk for dry mouth
14. Risk for venous thromboembolism
15. Risk for female genital mutilation
16. Risk for occupational injury
17. Risk for ineffective thermoregulation

Approved NANDA Nursing Diagnosis List 2018-2020

Domain 1. Health promotion

Class 1. Health awareness
- Decreased diversional activity engagement (Nursing care plan)
- Readiness for enhanced health literacy
- Sedentary lifestyle (Nursing care plan)

Class 2. Health management
- Frail elderly syndrome (Nursing care plan)
- Risk for frail elderly syndrome
- Deficient community health
- Risk-prone health behavior
- Ineffective health maintenance (Nursing care plan)
- Ineffective health management
- Readiness for enhanced health management
- Ineffective family health management
- Ineffective protection.

Domain 2. Nutrition

Class 1. Ingestion
Imbalanced nutrition: Less than body requirements (Nursing care plan).
- Readiness for enhanced nutrition
- Insufficient breast milk production
- Ineffective breastfeeding (Nursing care plan)
- Interrupted breastfeeding (Nursing care plan)
- Readiness for enhanced breastfeeding
- Ineffective adolescent eating dynamics
- Ineffective child eating dynamics
- Ineffective infant feeding dynamics
- Ineffective infant feeding pattern (Nursing care plan)
- Obesity
- Overweight
- Risk for overweight
- Impaired swallowing (Nursing care plan)

Class 2. Digestion
This class does not currently contain any diagnoses.
Class 3. Absorption
This class does not currently contain any diagnoses.

Class 4. Metabolism
- Risk for unstable blood glucose level (Nursing care plan)
- Neonatal hyperbilirubinemia
- Risk for neonatal hyperbilirubinemia
- Risk for impaired liver function
- Risk for metabolic imbalance syndrome

Class 5. Hydration
- Risk for electrolyte imbalance
- Risk for imbalanced fluid volume
- Deficient fluid volume (Nursing care plan)
- Risk for deficient fluid volume
- Excess fluid volume (Nursing care plan)

Domain 3. Elimination and Exchange

Class 1. Urinary function
- Impaired urinary elimination
- Functional urinary incontinence
- Overflow urinary incontinence
- Reflex urinary incontinence
- Stress urinary incontinence
- Urge urinary incontinence
- Risk for urge urinary incontinence
- Urinary retention

Class 2. Gastrointestinal function
- Constipation (Nursing care plan)
- Risk for constipation
- Perceived constipation
- Chronic functional constipation
- Risk for chronic functional constipation
- Diarrhea
- Dysfunctional gastrointestinal motility

- Risk for dysfunctional gastrointestinal motility
- Bowel incontinence

Class 3. Integumentary function
This class does not currently contain any diagnoses

Class 4. Respiratory function
Impaired gas exchange

Domain 4. Activity/Rest

Class 1. Sleep/Rest
- Insomnia sleep deprivation
- Readiness for enhanced sleep
- Disturbed sleep pattern

Class 2. Activity/Exercise
- Risk for disuse syndrome
- Impaired bed mobility
- Impaired physical mobility
- Impaired wheelchair mobility
- Impaired sitting
- Impaired standing
- Impaired transfer ability
- Impaired walking

Class 3. Energy balance
- Imbalanced energy field
- Fatigue
- Wandering

Class 4. Cardiovascular/Pulmonary responses
- Activity intolerance
- Risk for activity intolerance
- Ineffective breathing pattern
- Decreased cardiac output
- Risk for decreased cardiac output
- Impaired spontaneous ventilation
- Risk for unstable blood pressure
- Risk for decreased cardiac tissue perfusion
- Risk for ineffective cerebral tissue perfusion
- Ineffective peripheral tissue perfusion

- Risk for ineffective peripheral tissue perfusion
- Dysfunctional ventilatory weaning response

Class 5. Self-care
- Impaired home maintenance
- Bathing self-care deficit
- Dressing self-care deficit
- Feeding self-care deficit
- Toileting self-care deficit
- Readiness for enhanced self-care
- Self-neglect

Domain 5. Perception/Cognition

Class 1. Attention
Unilateral neglect

Class 2. Orientation
This class does not currently contain any diagnoses

Class 3. Sensation/Perception
This class does not currently contain any diagnoses

Class 4. Cognition
- Acute confusion
- Risk for acute confusion
- Chronic confusion
- Labile emotional control
- Ineffective impulse control
- Deficient knowledge
- Readiness for enhanced knowledge, impaired memory

Class 5. Communication
Readiness for enhanced communication, impaired verbal communication

Domain 6. Self-perception

Class 1. Self-concept
- Hopelessness
- Readiness for enhanced hope
- Risk for compromised human dignity

- Disturbed personal identity
- Risk for disturbed personal identity
- Readiness for enhanced self-concept

Class 2. Self-esteem
- Chronic low self-esteem
- Risk for chronic low self-esteem
- Situational low self-esteem
- Risk for situational low self-esteem

Class 3. Body image
Disturbed body image

Domain 7. Role Relationship

Class 1. Caregiving roles
- Caregiver role strain
- Risk for caregiver role strain
- Impaired parenting
- Risk for impaired parenting
- Readiness for enhanced parenting

Class 2. Family relationships
- Risk for impaired attachment
- Dysfunctional family processes
- Interrupted family processes
- Readiness for enhanced family processes

Class 3. Role performance
- Ineffective relationship
- Risk for ineffective relationship
- Readiness for enhanced relationship
- Parental role conflict
- Ineffective role performance
- Impaired social interaction

Domain 8. Sexuality

Class 1. Sexual identity
This class does not currently contain any diagnoses

Class 2. Sexual function
- Sexual dysfunction
- Ineffective sexuality pattern

Class 3. Reproduction
- Ineffective childbearing process
- Risk for ineffective childbearing process
- Readiness for enhanced childbearing process
- Risk for disturbed maternal-fetal dyad

Domain 9. Coping/Stress Tolerance

Class 1. Post-trauma responses
- Risk for complicated immigration transition
- Post-trauma syndrome
- Risk for post-trauma syndrome
- Rape-trauma syndrome
- Relocation stress syndrome
- Risk for relocation stress syndrome

Class 2. Coping responses
- Ineffective activity planning
- Risk for ineffective activity planning
- Anxiety (Nursing care plan)
- Defensive coping
- Ineffective coping
- Readiness for enhanced coping
- Ineffective community coping
- Readiness for enhanced community coping
- Compromised family coping
- Disabled family coping
- Readiness for enhanced family coping
- Death anxiety
- Ineffective denial
- Fear
- Grieving
- Complicated grieving
- Risk for complicated grieving

- Impaired mood regulation
- Powerlessness
- Risk for powerlessness
- Readiness for enhanced power
- Impaired resilience
- Risk for impaired resilience
- Readiness for enhanced resilience
- Chronic sorrow
- Stress overload

Class 3. Neurobehavioral stress
- Acute substance withdrawal syndrome
- Risk for acute substance withdrawal syndrome
- Autonomic dysreflexia
- Risk for autonomic dysreflexia
- Decreased intracranial adaptive capacity
- Neonatal abstinence syndrome
- Disorganized infant behavior
- Risk for disorganized infant behavior
- Readiness for enhanced organized infant behavior

Domain 10. Life Principles

Class 1. Values
This class does not currently contain any diagnoses

Class 2. Beliefs
Readiness for enhanced spiritual well-being

Class 3. Value/belief/action congruence
- Readiness for enhanced decision-making
- Decisional conflict
- Impaired emancipated decision-making
- Risk for impaired emancipated decision-making
- Readiness for enhanced emancipated decision-making
- Moral distress
- Impaired religiosity
- Risk for impaired religiosity
- Readiness for enhanced religiosity
- Spiritual distress
- Risk for spiritual distress

Domain 11. Safety/Protection

Class 1. Infection
- Risk for infection
- Risk for surgical site infection

Class 2. Physical injury
- Ineffective airway clearance
- Risk for aspiration
- Risk for bleeding (Nursing care plan)
- Impaired dentition
- Risk for dry eye
- Risk for dry mouth
- Risk for falls
- Risk for corneal injury
- Risk for injury
- Risk for urinary tract injury
- Risk for perioperative positioning injury
- Risk for thermal injury
- Impaired oral mucous membrane integrity
- Risk for impaired oral mucous membrane integrity
- Risk for peripheral neurovascular dysfunction
- Risk for physical trauma
- Risk for vascular trauma
- Risk for pressure ulcer
- Risk for shock
- Impaired skin integrity (Nursing care plan)
- Risk for impaired skin integrity
- Risk for sudden infant death
- Risk for suffocation
- Delayed surgical recovery
- Risk for delayed surgical recovery
- Impaired tissue integrity
- Risk for impaired tissue integrity
- Risk for venous thromboembolism

Class 3. Violence
- Risk for female genital mutilation
- Risk for other-directed violence
- Risk for self-directed violence

- Self-mutilation
- Risk for self-mutilation
- Risk for suicide

Class 4. Environmental hazards
- Contamination
- Risk for contamination
- Risk for occupational injury
- Risk for poisoning

Class 5. Defensive processes
- Risk for adverse reaction to iodinated contrast media
- Risk for allergy reaction
- Latex allergy reaction
- Risk for latex allergy reaction

Class 6. Thermoregulation
- Hyperthermia
- Hypothermia
- Risk for hypothermia
- Risk for perioperative hypothermia
- Ineffective thermoregulation
- Risk for ineffective thermoregulation

Domain 12. Comfort

Class 1. Physical comfort
- Impaired comfort
- Readiness for enhanced comfort
- Nausea
- Acute pain
- Chronic pain
- Chronic pain syndrome
- Labor pain

Class 2. Environmental comfort
- Impaired comfort
- Readiness for enhanced comfort

Class 3. Social comfort
- Impaired comfort
- Readiness for enhanced comfort

- Risk for loneliness
- Social isolation

Domain 13. Growth/Development

Class 1. Growth
This class does not currently contain any diagnoses

Class 2. Development
Risk for delayed development

99. NURSING CARE OF NEWBORN IN INCUBATOR/ISOLETTE

Preterm babies and small babies require to be nursed in an incubator to maintain their body temperature. The infant's environment inside the incubator must be modified to minimize heat loss by employing following measures:
- Place incubator away from external wall and windows and away from drafts
- Prewarm incubators before placing the infant in it
- Use warm blankets for wrapping the infant
- Avoid opening the incubator unnecessarily
- Use plastic sleeves on the portholes when caring for the baby
- It is used until infants can maintain normal body temperature themselves
- Warmed air is circulated inside the incubator to provide heat
- Humidity may be added if required
- Portholes and doors of the incubator must remain closed as much as possible to prevent heat loss every time they are opened
- On removal from incubator, the infant should be wrapped in warmed blankets and head covering should be used
- To retain heat inside the incubator, the door should be closed while the infant is out of it.

Clothing the Baby

- Keep infants in incubators swaddled
- Keep the baby's head covered preferably with a woolen or knit hat
- Replace wet blankets immediately with dry, warmed ones.

Monitoring Temperature

- Monitor body temperature using a mercury thermometer in the axilla
- Alternatively a skin probe may be used with or without attachment to servocontrol.

Positioning the Baby

- Encouraging the baby to assume a flexed position by the use of rolled blankets, which will also reduce heat loss.

Preventing Infection

- Meticulous handwashing using bactericidal soaps and antiseptic solutions and drying the hands properly are to be practiced by all care givers
- Minimize the number of people handling the baby to minimize the risk of cross infection
- Use disposable articles for the baby as much as possible
- Keep articles for individual babies
- Wash and dry any reusable articles used for the baby immediately after use.

Skin Care

- Keep the baby socially clean by removing milk or vomit debris
- Clean and dry the napkin area
- Bathe the baby occasionally in a quick manner without overexposure.

Visiting

- Avoid anyone with a known or obvious infection visiting the baby
- Visits and care by parents to be encouraged after educating them about measures to prevent spread of infection such as handwashing.

Weaning to an Open Crib

Infants who weigh about 1,500 grams, who have consistent weight gain for 5 days, who have no medical complications and who are tolerating enteral feedings are gradually weaned from external heat:

- Preparation of infants for moving to open cribs should begin early
- When stable, an infant can be dressed in a shirt, diaper and hat while in the incubator
- The incubator temperature is usually decreased gradually
- If the infant's temperature remains stable, the process continues the next day
- When the infant is ready for transfer to an open crib, double wrapping with warm blankets at first help to insulate body heat
- The temperature is assessed at gradually increasing intervals until the infant is on a routine schedule
- If the temperature does not rise to normal, the infant is returned to the incubator
- Nurses should observe the infant carefully during the first few days after transfer to an open crib
- Signs that indicate inadequate thermoregulation include decreased weight gain, poor feeding or increased requirement for oxygen.

100. OBSTRUCTED LABOR

Definition

Obstructed labor is one where in spite of good uterine contractions, the progressive descent of the presenting part is arrested due to mechanical obstruction.

Incidence

The prevalence is about 1–2% in developing countries.

Causes

Maternal conditions
- Contracted pelvis and cephalopelvic disproportion
- Pelvic tumors, uterine fibroids and ovarian tumors
- Tumors of pelvic bones, rectum or bladder
- Pelvic kidney
- Constriction ring of the uterus
- Non-gravid horn of a bicornuate uterus below the presenting part.

Fetal Conditions

- Macrosomia
- Malpresentations: Brow presentation, transverse or oblique lie, compound presentation
- Locked twins
- Malformations of the fetus: Hydrocephalus, fetal ascites, fetal abdominal tumors and conjoined twins.

Course of Labor

- Labor in patients with mechanical obstruction is characterized by strong uterine contractions
- Primigravidae often respond to obstruction by developing inefficient uterine action (hypotonic uterine inertia)
- Multigravidae develop excessive strong contractions in an attempt to overcome the obstruction
- This may lead to tonic contractions of the uterus causing retraction ring (Bandl's ring)
- Untreated or neglected obstruction leads to fetal death, overdistension of the lower uterine segment and rupture of the uterus.

Clinical Features

Early detection of possible obstruction in labor is imperative:
- The membranes usually rupture early as the presenting part is poorly applied to the lower segment and cervix
- As the cervix dilates, it hangs like a loose curtain below the presenting part
- In vertex presentation, large caput succedaneum often forms and the fetal head becomes extremely molded
- The patient gradually becomes anxious and exhausted; maternal pulse rate and respiration increases; quantity of urine diminishes and it becomes highly colored; ketone bodies appear in urine, metabolic acidosis and ketosis develops
- There is retraction of placental site leading to fetal hypoxia (fetal distress) and liquor is frequently stained with meconium

- Secondary uterine inertia develops in primigravidae; over-distension of lower segment and threatened rupture is seen in multigravidae
- Repeated internal examination may cause infection
- Postpartum hemorrhage is common
- Soft tissues of the pelvis become avascular and necrotic as they get compressed between the head and bony pelvis. This result in sloughing off of the tissues in 10 days resulting in vesicovaginal fistula.

Diagnosis

- Partograph will help to identify impending obstruction early
- On general examination, the patient is exhausted, dehydrated, often infected and with ketoacidosis
- On abdominal examination:
  - Retraction ring (Bandl's ring) as seen and felt between the contracted upper segment and stretched lower segment
  - Fetal heart sounds may show evidence of fetal distress and may become absent.
- On vaginal examination:
  - Vulva is usually swollen and edematous vagina is hot, dry with offensive, purulent discharge
  - The cervix is almost fully dilated
  - The presenting part is extremely molded and jammed in the pelvis; there is usually large caput formation
- In advanced obstructed labor:
  - The uterus is found molded to the shape of the baby
  - The uterus feels hard all the time and is tender on palpation
  - In such a case fetal heart sounds may be absent.

Management

General measures

- Assessment of the general condition of the patient
- Investigations: Blood group and Rh typing, hemoglobin and routine examination of urine

- Intravenous infusion to correct dehydration and sodium bicarbonate to correct acidosis
- Broad spectrum antibiotics
- Self-retaining Foley's catheter to monitor urinary output.

Specific Management

- Cesarean section is the procedure of choice in obstructed labor
- Laparotomy is done when there is suspicion of ruptured uterus
- In the presence of rupture, hysterectomy is the method of management
- Destructive operations may be the management in rural obstetrics.

Complications

1. **Maternal:**
   - Trauma to bladder as a result of pressure from fetal head during labor or during delivery
   - Vesicovaginal fistula
   - Urinary incontinence due to prolonged pressure causing necrosis
   - Intrauterine infection due to prolonged rupture of membranes
   - Rupture of uterus in case of neglected obstruction causing thinning of lower uterine segment
   - Possible death of mother and fetus resulting from hemorrhage after rupture of uterus
   - Psychological problems following the traumatic experience.
2. **Fetal:**
   - Intrauterine asphyxia causing permanent brain damage if born alive
   - Ascending infection and meconium aspiration causing neonatal pneumonia
   - Fresh stillbirth.

Nursing Diagnoses

Numbers 33, 69, 78, 81 and 100 in appendix.

101. OCCIPITOPOSTERIOR POSITION

Occipitoposterior positions are the most common type of malpositions of the occiput.

Causes

- The direct cause is often unknown
- Associated with an abnormally shaped pelvis, e.g. android pelvis.

Diagnosis

- The position is frequently diagnosed late in labor
- It remains undiagnosed until there is delay in the first or second stage of labor.

Abdominal Examination

- On inspection there is a saucer-shaped depression at or just below the umbilicus
- On palpation:
  - Limbs are felt with unusual ease and on both sides of the midline
  - Back may be difficult to locate
  - Prominent sincipital end of the head is directed forwards; both sinciput and occiput are at the same level because the head is partly deflexed.
- Position of the fetal heart sounds are laterally placed near the flanks.

Vaginal Examination

- The anterior fontanelle is felt with ease when the head is more deflexed
- When the head is less deflexed, both anterior and posterior fontanelles are felt
- When well-flexed, posterior fontanelle is felt
- Caput succedaneum may be present making palpation of sutures difficult.

Possible Course and Outcome of Labor

- Long anterior rotation of the occiput (three eighth of a circle) resulting in normal delivery as occiput anterior
- Incomplete anterior rotation causing vertex to be arrested in transverse diameter, termed as deep transverse arrest
- Non-rotation causing the vertex arrested in oblique occipito-posterior position
- Malrotation:
  - Sinciput touches the pelvic floor first, anterior rotation of the sinciput occurs causing the occiput to be at the sacral hallow (occipitosacral position)
  - Favorable outcome: Spontaneous delivery as face to pubis
  - Unfavorable outcome: Direct occipitoposterior arrest.

Management

Possible outcomes of an occipitoposterior position are:
1. Spontaneous delivery after trial of labor.
2. Rotation of the head and forceps delivery:
   - Manual rotation and forceps extraction
   - Forceps rotation and extraction
   - Vacuum extraction
   - Cesarean section.
3. Cesarean section.
4. Conversion to face presentation.

Spontaneous Delivery

Spontaneous delivery is the most common outcome. With good uterine contractions, flexion and descend occurs so that the occiput rotates three eighth of a circle and delivery occurs as in right/left occipitoanterior position.

With a short of posterior rotation, the occiput descends along the sacral curve, the sinciput fixes under the pubic arch. Further descend occurs with good uterine contractions, occiput is born by flexion followed by birth of sinciput by extension of the head. This step is described as face to pubes delivery.

Rotation and Forceps Delivery

After assessing the station and position of head, size of the fetus, maternal pelvis and pattern of uterine contractions, manual rotation and extraction by forceps or ventouse is done. Rotation with forceps and extraction with forceps or ventouse may also be done.

Cesarean Section in the Following Situations

- Severe PIH
- Elderly primigravidity
- Post CS pregnancy
- IUGR
- Large baby (≥ 4 kg)
- Prolonged labor
- Fetal distress
- Arrest of labor
- Failed trial forceps.

Conversion to Face Presentation

When the head is deflexed at the onset of labor, extension occasionally occurs instead of flexion. If extension is complete, a face presentation results. Delivery is effected as in face presentation.

Complications Associated with Occipitoposterior Positions

- Obstructed labor when the head remains deflexed or partially extended and becomes impacted in the pelvis
- Maternal trauma from forceps delivery
- Neonatal trauma from instrumental delivery
- Cord prolapse
- Cerebral hemorrhage.

102. OXYTOCIN CHALLENGE TEST

Oxytocin challenge test (OCT) or contraction stress test (CST) is performed on a patient lying in semi-Fowler or left lateral recumbent position with the FHR and tocodynamic leads attached to the monitor.

A baseline reading is obtained for 15 minutes. If spontaneous uterine activity does not occur at the rate of three in 10 minutes, a stimulating oxytocin at 0.5 milliunits/minute is commenced and progressively increased until a uterine contraction pattern of three contractions lasting for at least 40 seconds in 10 minutes is attained.

Close monitoring is essential to avoid hyperstimulation, which is indicated by contractions that exceed five per 10 minutes or pains lasting longer than 90 seconds.

Results of the Test

- Negative: No late decelerations present through out the duration of the test
- Positive: Late decelerations present with at least 50% of the contractions in the absence of excessive contractions or presence of decelerations prior to achieving adequate uterine stimulation
- Suspicious: Inconsistent appearance of lake decelerations
- Unsatisfactory: When the tracing is not satisfactory or satisfactory uterine stimulation has failed to achieve three sustained contractions every 10 minutes.

Advantages of OCT

- Provides early warning of fetal compromise as compared to NST test
- Lower false positive rates as compared to the NST test.

Disadvantages of OCT

- Time consuming, requires close supervision
- Patient discomfort as compared to the biophysical test
- Risk of onset of preterm labor and rarely fetal demise
- Requires hospitalization.

103. PARTOGRAPH

DESCRIPTION

The partograph is a graphical presentation of the progress of labor and of fetal and maternal condition during labor. It is the best tool to detect whether labor is progressing normally or abnormally and to warn if there are signs of fetal distress or if the mother's vital signs deviate from the normal range.

PURPOSES

- To record the clinical observations accurately during the period of labor.
- To monitor the progress of labor and to organize the need for action at the appropriate time for timely referral.
- To interpret the recorded partograph and to identify any deviation from normal.
- To monitor the well-being of mother as she goes through labor.
- To clearly identify the different stages of labor for providing appropriate attention and care.

PRINCIPAL FEATURES

- The partograph is a valuable tool to assess the progress of labor.
- Partograph is useful to detect deviations from normal such as abnormal progress, fetal distress, or maternal exhaustion.
- The partograph is designed for recording maternal identification data, fetal heart rate, color of amniotic fluid, moulding of the fetal skull, cervical dilatation, fetal descend, uterine contractions, whether oxygen was administered or intravenous fluids were given, maternal vital signs and urine output.
- Partograph reading to be started when labor is in active stage (4 cm cervical dilation or above).
- Cervical dilatation, descend of the fetal head and uterine contractions are used in assessing the progress of labor. About 1 cm/hour cervical dilation and 1 cm descend in 4 hours indicate good progress in active first stage.
- Fetal heart rate and uterine contractions are recorded every 30 minutes if they are in the normal range. Assess cervical dilatation, fetal descend, color of amniotic fluid (if membranes have ruptured) and the degree of moulding or caput every 4 hours.
- Perform a digital vaginal examination immediately if the membranes rupture and gush of amniotic fluid comes out while the woman is in any stage of labor.

- Fetal heart rate below 120/minute or above 160/minute for more than 10 minutes is an urgent indication to inform the physician unless labor is progressing too fast.
- Immediate reference to physician is required in cases where the cervical dilatation mark crosses the Alert line, moulding is +3 with poor progress of labor and if amniotic fluid is lightly stained in latent first stage or moderately stained in active first stage or thick amniotic fluid in any stage of labor.
- The latent phase of labor should last no longer than 8 hours.

Components of the Partograph

- **Identification section:** This portion of the partograph at the top, to write the name and age of the mother, her 'gravida', 'para' status, her hospital registration number, the date and time when she was first attended for delivery and the time, the fetal membranes ruptured.
- **The graph section:** The features of the fetus and mother are to be recorded in different areas of the chart. This includes the graph to record **Fetal Heart Rate,** initially and then every 30 minutes. The scale for fetal heart rate covers the range from 80 to 200 beats per minute. In the second stage of labor, if the liquor contains thick green or black meconium, the fetal heart rate is counted and recorded every five minutes. Each square for fetal heart on the partograph represents 30 minutes.
- **Liquor and moulding:** The rows placed below the heart rate section are to record liquor (amniotic fluid) if the membranes have ruptured and the moulding of fetal skull. The status of liquor is recorded using certain letters of the alphabet.

    I: intact membranes
    A: membranes have ruptured and liquor is absent
    C: clear liquor
    B: blood stained liquor
    M1: lightly meconium stained
    M2: little bit thick meconium stained
    M3: very thick liquor with meconium which has soup-like appearance

    The color of liquor should be recorded every four hours.
    For partograph see **Figure 103.1**.

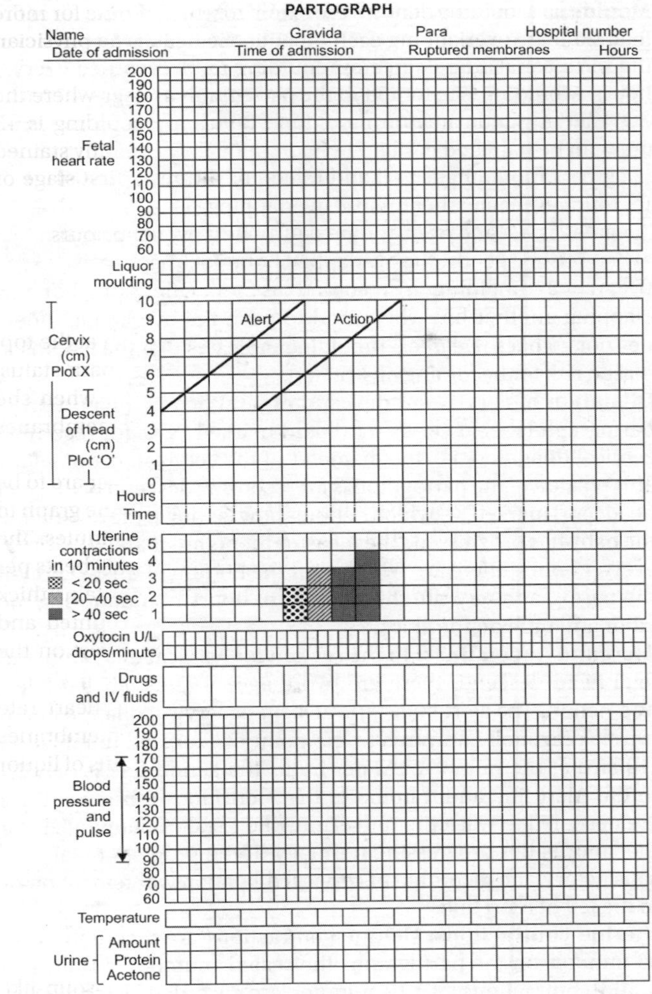

Fig. 103.1: WHO model partograph.
Source: Opoku. Research Journal of Women's Health. 2015.
www.hoajonline.com

- **Moulding:** Moulding denotes the extent to which the bones of the fetal skull are overlapping each other as the head is forced down the birth canal. The degree of moulding to be recorded every 4 hours. Moulding is recorded in the partograph as degrees 1 to 3.

    'O' marking indicates no moulding. Bones are separated and sutures can be palpated easily.

    Degree 1 moulding is '+1' and refers to; sutures apposed, skull bones touching each other but not overlapping.

    Degree 2 is '+2' and refers to; one skull bone is overlapping another, but when pushed gently, the overlapped bone goes back easily.

    Degree 3 moulding is recorded as '+3'. One skull bone is overlapping another but when tried to push the overlapped bone, it does not go back. Degree 3 moulding indicates that the labor is at increased risk for becoming obstructed.

- **Dilatation of cervix and descend of fetal head:** The portion of partograph labeled cervix (cm), and marked 'X' is for recording cervical dilatation, i.e. the diameter of the cervix in centimeters. This portion of the partograph is for recording descend of the fetal head (cm) marked 'O' which denotes how far down the birth canal the baby has progressed. The measurements are marked 'X' or 'O' every 4 hours. There are two rows at the bottom of this section of the partograph to write the number of hours of monitoring the labor and time on the clock.

- **Alert and Action lines:** In the section for cervical dilatation and fetal head descend, there are two diagonal lines labeled 'Alert and Action'. The alert line starts at 4 cm of cervical dilation and it travels diagonally upwards to the point of expected full dilation (10 cm) at the rate of 1 cm per hour. The action line is parallel to the Alert line and 4 hours to the Alert Line. These two lines are designed to warn the nurse/midwife to take action quickly if the labor is not progressing normally. If the progress of labor is satisfactory, the recording of cervical dilatation will remain on or to the left of Alert line.

- **Uterine contractions:** Uterine contractions are recorded every 30 minutes on the partograph. The scale is numbered from 1 to 5 and contractions per 10 minutes are recorded. Each square represents one contraction so that if two contractions are felt in

ten minutes, two squares need to be shaded. On each shaded square, the duration of each contraction is entered by using the symbols shown below:
- Dots represent mild contractions of less than 20 seconds duration.
- Diagonal lines indicate moderate contractions of 20–40 seconds duration
- Solid shading represents strong contractions of longer than 40 seconds duration.

- **Oxytocin:** There are two rows for recording administration of oxytocin during labor and the amount given
- **Drugs and IV fluids:** Medications and intravenous fluids given to the mother are recorded in these columns
- **Maternal well-being:** Maternal well-being is assessed by measuring the mother's vital signs; blood pressure, pulse, temperature and urine output. Pulse is recorded every 30 minutes and temperature every 2 hours. Urine output is recorded every time urine is passed. Any deviation from normal needs to be informed the physician.

104. PELVIC INFLAMMATORY DISEASE

DEFINITION

Pelvic inflammatory disease (PID) is defined as a spectrum of infection and inflammation of the upper genital tract organs typically involving the endometrium, fallopian tubes, ovaries, pelvic peritoneum and surrounding structures. PID is caused by microorganisms colonizing the endocervix ascending to the endometrium and fallopian tubes.

FACTORS INFLUENCING PID

Risk Factors

- Menstruating teenagers
- Multiple sexual partners
- Previous history of acute PID
- Intrauterine contraceptive device (IUCD) users.

Protective Factors

- Use of barrier methods of contraception along with spermicidal gel, which are bactericidal and virucidal
- Oral contraceptives—as they produce thick cervical mucus and decrease the duration of menstruation
- Life with monogamous partner
- Pregnancy
- Menopause
- Azoospermia or vasectomy for spouse.

MICROBIOLOGY

The PID is usually a polymicrobial ascending infection caused by sexually transmitted microorganism. Commonly found organisms are Neisseria gonorrhoeae, Chlamydia trachomatis and Mycoplasma hominis. Organisms normally found in the vagina are seen almost always associated and include nonhaemolytic *streptococcus*, Escherichia coli (E. coli), group B Streptococcus and Staphylococcus. Anaerobic bacteria are also seen.

MODE OF INFECTION

- Ascend of bacteria from lower to upper genital tract facilitated by sexual contact
- Reflux of menstrual blood along with gonococci into the fallopian tube
- Lymphatic spread to tube
- Organism from colon such as E. coli.

PATHOLOGICAL CHANGES

Involvement of the tube is almost always bilateral. The pathological process begins in the endosalpinx. There is destruction of cells, cilia and inflammatory reactions. Depending on the virulence of the organism hydrosalpinx or pyosalpinx may develop with the abdominal ostium of the tube closed and inflammatory adhesions. In some cases, the exudate pours through the abdominal ostium to produce pelvic peritonitis and pelvic abscess or may affect the ovary producing ovarian or tubo-ovarian abscess.

CLINICAL FEATURES

In acute PID, symptoms usually appear at and immediately following the menses:
- Bilateral and lower abdominal pain
- Fever, lassitude and headache
- Irregular and excessive vaginal bleeding
- Abnormal vaginal discharge, which becomes purulent and/or copious
- Pain in the right hypochondrium if there is perihepatitis
- Nausea and vomiting.
- Dyspareunia
- Temperature elevation beyond 38.3°C
- Tenderness on palpation of lower abdominal quadrants
- Congested external urethral meatus or openings of Bartholin glands on vaginal examination
- Congested cervix with purulent discharge from the canal on speculum examination
- Bilateral tenderness, thickening or definite mass on fornix palpation

DIAGNOSIS

Presence of Signs and Symptoms

- Laboratory test findings: Raised C-reactive protein and/or erythrocyte sedimentation rate (ESR)
- Positive test for Gonorrhoea or Chlamydia trachomatis
- Histopathologic evidence of endometritis on biopsy
- Sonographic evidence of tubo-ovarian pathology (abscess)
- Laparoscopic evidence of PID.

TREATMENT

Preventive

- Education on safe sex to prevent sexually transmitted infection
- Liberal use of contraceptives
- Routine screening of high-risk population.

Measures to Prevent Reinfection

- Education to avoid reinfection and the potential hazards of it
- Warning against multiple sexual partners

- Encourage use of condoms
- Effective treatment of sexual partners.

Definitive

- Antibiotic therapy—broad spectrum coverage initially, followed by specific antibiotic depending on the culture and sensitivity report
- Bedrest in cases of severe infection
- Restriction of oral feeding and IV therapy for correction of dehydration and acidosis
- Surgery, if patient has generalized peritonitis, pelvic abscess or tuboovarian abscess.

FOLLOW-UP

- Repeat smears and cultures after 7 days following full course of treatment
- Repeated tests (culture) following each menstrual period until it becomes negative for three consecutive reports.

NURSING IMPLICATIONS

Nursing Assessment

Nursing assessment for genital infections includes assessment for risk, symptoms, medical history, gynecologic history and lifestyle behaviors. Physical assessment focuses on data and specimen collection to aid diagnosis of specific infection.

Nursing Diagnoses

Nursing diagnoses are formulated after diagnosis of infection. Applicable nursing diagnosis may include the following:
- Pain related to infection
- Fear related to the diagnosis
- Deficient knowledge related to the experience regarding the disorder.

Nursing Plans

Nursing plans include specific actions; the client completes to achieve the highest level of wellness possible. Sample goals may include the following:

- Takes prescribed medications correctly
- Returns to the healthcare facility as scheduled for follow-up assessment of infection status
- Notifies physician of any failure of symptoms to improve as expected or adverse effects of prescribed medications
- Adopts recommended change in lifestyle behavior to prevent recurrent infection
- Comprehends health promotion counseling.

Nursing Interventions

Nursing interventions include teaching, counseling for prevention and explaining prescribed medications. Women who had infection with sexually transmitted organisms will require counseling to get the spouse treated and to use barrier contraceptives until both test negative for the organism.

105. PHYSIOLOGICAL CHANGES IN PREGNANCY

Numerous physiological changes occur in a woman's body during pregnancy. Changes in some systems are caused by the effects of specific hormones. These changes enable the mother to nurture the fetus, prepare her body for labor and prepare her breasts for lactation. All bodily systems are affected to a varying extent.

REPRODUCTIVE SYSTEM

Uterus

After conception, the uterus develops to provide a nutritive and protective environment for the fetus to develop and grow:
- Decidua becomes thicker, richer and more vascular in the upper segment and less vascular, and thinner in the lower segment
- Muscle fibers in the myometrium grow up to 15–20 times their nonpregnant length
- Hypertrophy (increase in size) and hyperplasia (increase in number) of the muscle fibers occur due to the effect of estrogen and progesterone
- Weight of the uterus increases from 50 to 100 g in non-pregnant state to 750 to 1200 g at term depending on parity

- Size increases from 7.5 × 5.0 × 2.5 cm to 30 × 23 × 20 cm
- Irregular and painless contractions known as Braxton Hicks contractions occur, which facilitate the formation of lower uterine segment
- Perimetrium, which is a layer of the peritoneum forms the uterovesical pouch anteriorly and the pouch of Douglas posteriorly
- The double folds of perimetrium (broad ligament) become longer and wider as the uterus enlarges
- The blood supply to the uterus increases to about 750 mL/minute at term to meet the needs of the functioning placenta
- Shape of the uterus changes to globular to accommodate the growing fetus, placenta, liquor and the walls of the uterus become progressively thin as pregnancy advances
- At 20 weeks the fundus of the uterus may be palpated at or just below the umbilicus
- At 30 weeks fundus can be palpated midway between the umbilicus and the xiphisternum
- At 38th weeks, the fundus reaches the level of xiphisternum
- A reduction in fundal height known as lightening may occur at the end of pregnancy, when the fetus sinks into the lower pole of the uterus. In primigravida this occurs as the fetus descends into the pelvis and the head becomes engaged. In multiparous women descend often does not occur until labor begins.

Cervix

- The cervix protects the fetus during its development by remaining firmly closed and by providing resistance to pressure from above, when the mother is in upright position
- The mucus produced by the endocervical cells becomes thicker and more viscous during pregnancy. This thickened mucus plug forms the cervical plug called the operculum
- Late in pregnancy, the cervix becomes softer and more distensible under hormonal control and in readiness for the onset of labor
- Effacement or taking up of the cervix occurs in primigravida during the last 2 weeks of pregnancy and in multigravida when labor begins.

Vagina

The muscle layer hypertrophies and the capacity of the vagina increases. The surrounding connective tissues allow the vagina to become more elastic enabling it to dilate during the second stage of labor to accommodate the passage of the baby.

CARDIOVASCULAR SYSTEM

Heart

The heart muscle hypertrophies, particularly in the left ventricle leading to enlargement of the heart. The growing uterus pushes the heart upwards and to the left. Heart sounds are changed, systolic and other murmurs occur.

Cardiac Output

- Heart rate and stroke volume increase resulting in increased cardiac output
- The heart rate increases about 15 beats per minute. The stroke volume rises from about 64 to 71 mL.
- The cardiac output increases by 40% above pre-pregnancy values by 12th week and by 50% by the 34th week.

Blood Pressure

- Systolic pressure remains almost constant, while diastolic pressure drops slightly in the first trimester
- Changes in blood pressure (BP) cause fainting in midtrimester and supine hypotension in later pregnancy
- Poor venous return in late pregnancy and increased pressure in the veins of the legs, vulva, rectum and pelvis can lead to edema in the lower legs, varicose veins and hemorrhoids.

Hematologic System

Principal hematological changes occurring during normal pregnancy are tabulated in **Table 105.1**.

Table 105.1: Principal hematological changes during normal pregnancy.

	Nonpregnant	Pregnancy near term
Blood volume (mL)	4,000	5,500 at 34 week
Plasma volume (mL)	2,500	3,750 at 34 week
Red cell volume (mL)	1,400	1,650 at 34 week
Hemoglobin	12–13 g/dL	10.5–11.0 g/dL
Hematocrit	38%	32%
Leucocyte count	7,000–9,000/mm^3	12,000–15,000 mm^3
Fibrinogen	200–300 mg%	400–600 mg%

- Blood volume increases beginning at about 10 weeks gestation and until about 30-34 weeks. A higher circulating volume is required to:
    - Provide extra blood flow for placental perfusion
    - Provide extra metabolic needs of the fetus
    - Provide extra perfusion of kidneys and other organs
    - Counter balance the effects of increased arterial and venous capacity
    - Compensate for blood loss at delivery.
- Plasma volume increases corresponding to the increase in blood volume
- The red cell mass increases as a result of increased production and the total increase may be up to 30%, when iron supplementation is given
- As the increase in plasma volume is much greater than that of the red cell mass, hemodilution occurs at around 32-34 weeks and the effect is reduced packed cell volume, which is referred to as physiological anemia
- Iron absorption doubles in pregnancy to meet the demands of growing maternal blood volumes, tissue mass and fetal needs
- There is normal increase in the white blood cell counts from 9,000 to about 12,000 cu mm and further increases upto 15,000 cu mm during labor. A moderate leukocytosis of 15,000-18,000 cu mm is commonly observed in the postpartum period

- Changes in coagulation profile are seen during pregnancy. The platelet count is generally normal, however, the platelet survival time gets shortened
- Plasminogen levels increase concomitantly with fibrinogen levels, causing an equilibration between clotting and lysing activity. Hypercoagulability of pregnancy is caused by venous stasis in the pelvis and lower limbs.

RESPIRATORY SYSTEM

Certain anatomical changes take place during pregnancy. The lower ribs flare out resulting in increase in subcostal angle and there is also increase in transverse diameter of the chest. The diaphragm is raised by about 4 cm.

Functional Changes

- Hyperemia and congestion of upper respiratory tract predisposing to phlegm, sinusitis and epistaxis
- There is marginal increase in respiratory rate. The tidal volume and minute ventilation increase by 30–40%. The functional 'reserve capacity' and 'inspiratory reserve volume' may diminish by 20%
- Alteration in blood gases occurs, PO_2 increases above 100 mm Hg, PCO_2 decreases to 27–32 mm Hg, the pH remains normal
- Dyspnoea is a common symptom during pregnancy for 60–70% of women. The low pCO_2 and the elevation of the diaphragm contribute the sense of dyspnoea
- Maternal hyperventilation occurs as a protective measure to prevent exposure of fetus to excessive levels of CO_2.

ENDOCRINE CHANGES AND ALTERED METABOLISM

- Thyroid gland enlarges in size. Total T_4 rises, but the levels of free T_3 and T_4 are unaffected, maintaining the euthyroid state. Increase in pulse rate, warm skin and increased hair loss, which are normal findings in pregnancy, mimic altered thyroid function
- Suprarenals: There is increase in levels of corticosteroid-binding globulin and also total, and free cortisol
- Pancreas: Exaggerated fasting hypoglycemia and starvation ketosis are common. To overcome symptomatic hypoglycemia,

pregnant women are advised to consume small frequent meals. Insulin resistance increases with advancing pregnancy due to insulin antagonism by human placental lactogen
- There is maternal weight gain during pregnancy. The average weight gain of 10–15 kg is the result of growth of uterus and its contents, increased breast tissue, fluid retention and rise in circulating blood volume. There is also an increase in deposition of fat and proteins. Carbohydrate intolerance during pregnancy may lead to a diabetic state in some non-diabetic women, which reverses after delivery.

BREASTS AND INTEGUMENTARY SYSTEM

- Estrogen produces ductal proliferation and progesterone causes alveolar growth resulting in breast enlargement to meet expected lactational demands
- Early in pregnancy, the woman experiences breast discomfort and the heaviness continues throughout pregnancy
- As pregnancy advances, there is enlargement of breasts, areolae and nipples. Montgomery tubercles appear and clear secretion can be expressed from breasts
- Skin shows increased pigmentation especially in the nipples, areolae, axillae, umbilicus, linea nigra and perineum. This is the result of an increase in levels of melanocyte-stimulating hormone, estrogen and progesterone.

DIGESTIVE SYSTEM

- About 70% of women experience nausea and vomiting during early pregnancy. In small number of women, this vomiting leads to dehydration and metabolic acidosis resulting in a condition called hyperemesis gravidarum
- High levels of circulating progesterone during pregnancy produces relaxation of smooth muscles leading to sluggish peristalsis. This causes delayed emptying of stomach, relaxation of esophageal sphincter causing gastroesophageal reflux and esophagitis
- Delayed small bowel transit and increased water reabsorption cause constipation and passage of hard stools

- Changes in hepatic function are reflected in the increased levels of alkaline phosphatase, fibrinogen, steroid binding globulins, cholesterol and lipids
- In the oral cavity, the gum hypertrophies and becomes softer leading to a tendency to bleed. Tooth decay occurs more easily possibly due to increased acidic salivation

URINARY SYSTEM

- There are significant changes in the urinary tract and renal function
- The kidneys enlarge in size. As a result of dilation due to the effect of maternal progesterone, the capacity of the renal pelvis and ureters increases from 15 to 75 mL. The tone of ureters and the bladder is reduced, thus stasis of urine is common, predisposing the pregnant woman to urinary tract infection
- As a result of increased cardiac output and diminished renovasuclar resistance, renal perfusion and glomerular filtration increases. There is a lowering of renal threshold for glucose resulting in physiologic glycosuria in euglycemic women
- As a result of increased glomerular filtration and enhanced renal clearance, the serum levels of urea nitrogen and creatinine reduce
- Salt and water metabolism are affected by circulating steroid hormones resulting in sodium retention
- The urinary bladder shows marked congestion and hypertrophy of muscles of bladder wall. Frequency of micturition occurs during first 12 weeks as the enlarging uterus in the pelvis rests on the bladder. It may occur in the third trimester during engagement of the presenting part of the fetus. Stress incontinence may occur causing discomfort to the woman.

NERVOUS SYSTEM

The nervous system is in a more excitable condition in pregnant women. Temperamental changes are frequently noticed. Mood changes and symptoms of psychosis may develop in those with a family history. Hemodynamic changes occur during pregnancy due to neurohormonal responses to pregnancy. Nitric oxide and prostaglandins are vasodilators that may be responsible for the observed drop in peripheral resistance and for changes in uterine and renal blood flow.

Activation of the sympathetic nervous system typically occurs in response to decrease in periphearl vascular resistance and arterial pressure. Overactivity of the autonomic nervous system and renin-angiotensin systems and impairment in production or activity of vasodilators such as nitric oxide and prostaglandins have all been implicated in the pathogenesis of preeclampsia (Silversides, Coleman).

106. PHYSICAL EXAMINATION OF NEWBORN

Once the newborn enters the nursery, the nurse conducts a complete head-to-toe physical assessment to determine the infant's health status. A general inspection is done first to identify abnormalities:

- A normal newborn assumes a flexed position (hands and legs flexed)
- Skin is inspected for color and texture. A full-term newborn may display signs of skin dryness and cracking. Acrocyanosis may be present in the hands and feet, but should diminish
- The newborn's heart is auscultated for rate and rhythm
- The lungs are auscultated to ensure expansion of both lungs and equal breath sounds
- The newborn's first blood pressure (BP) measurement is taken followed by axillary body temperature
- The newborn is weighed and amount of lanugo estimated
- Head-to-toe length is measured
- Head circumference [frontal-occipital circumference (FOC)] is measured and fontanelles are assessed
- Chest circumference and abdominal circumference are measured
- Head is inspected for moulding and suture lines are palpated
- Face is then inspected for symmetry, birth marks, milia and nevi (stork bites) over the forehead and eyelids
- The amount of cartilage in the ear is assessed
- The mouth is inspected for natal teeth and abnormalities of the hard and soft palates, and the tongue
- Femoral and brachial pulses are palpated
- Ortolani's maneuver is done to check for hip dislocation

- The genitalia of the male baby is inspected for descend of the testes and presence of rugae and female genitalia for development of labia and clitoris
- The spine and skin on the back are then inspected for alignment, brakes in skin, birth marks or markers along the spinal column
- Plantar surfaces of the feet are assessed for creases.

During the examination, the nurse will check certain reflexes. The presence of these reflexes suggest maturity of the neonatal neurological system.

Newborn Reflexes (Figs. 106.1A to I)

Examination of a newborn includes checking the various reflexes. A newborn baby is equipped with a wide range of reflex activities, the presence of which at varying ages provides indication of the normality of the neurological and musculoskeletal systems. During the examination of newborn, the nurse will check these reflexes:

1. Rooting reflex **(Fig. 106.1A)**.

   The infant turns his head and opens his mouth when the perioral area is stimulated. The corner of the baby's mouth, the upper lip, and the lower lip are touched in turn with a finger. Upon this stimulation, the head turns towards the stimulated side, the mouth opens, and the tongue moves to the point of stimulation. Rooting reflex is elicited when the baby is awake and alert.

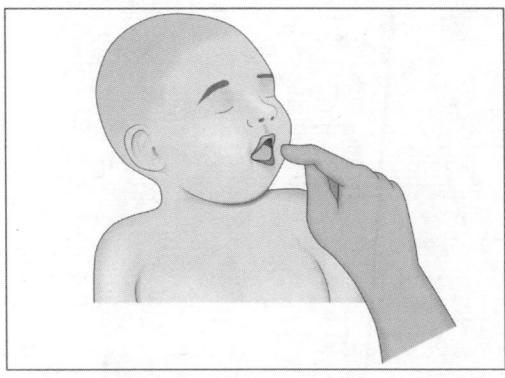

Fig. 106.1A: Rooting reflex.

2. Sucking and swallowing reflex **(Fig. 106.1B)**.
   If the examiner's index figure is placed in he infant's mouth, rhythmical sucking movements will be felt. Sucking is often intense and less regular during the first 3–4 days. Poor sucking is often the first indication of problems such as sepsis.
3. Blink reflex.
   In order to elicit this reflex, a bright light is shone suddenly at the infant's eyes. Normally a quick closure of the eyes and a slight dorsal flexion of the head occur. With impaired light perception, this reflex is absent.
4. Corneal reflex.
   When the eyes are open, the cornea is touched lightly with a piece of cotton with care to avoid touching eyelids or lashes. Normally, the eyes close. The absence of this response denotes lesions of the 5th cranial nerve.
5. Tonic neck reflex **(Fig. 106.1C)**.
   The infant is placed on his or her back and head is turned to one side. The arm and leg on the same side extend and the opposite arm and leg flex, thus the infant assumes a fencing position. If the head is turned to the opposite side, the same reaction should occur. This responses may be present for 2 or 3 months. If persists longer, it usually indicates neurological dysfunction.

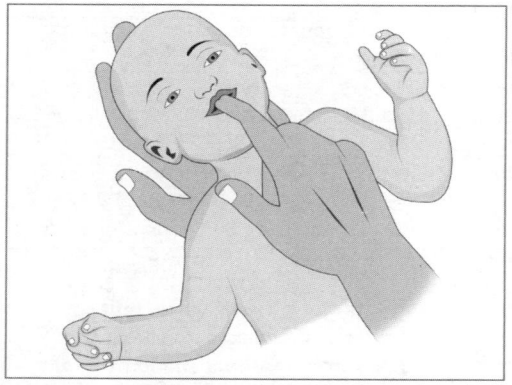

Fig. 106.1B: Sucking and swallowing reflex.

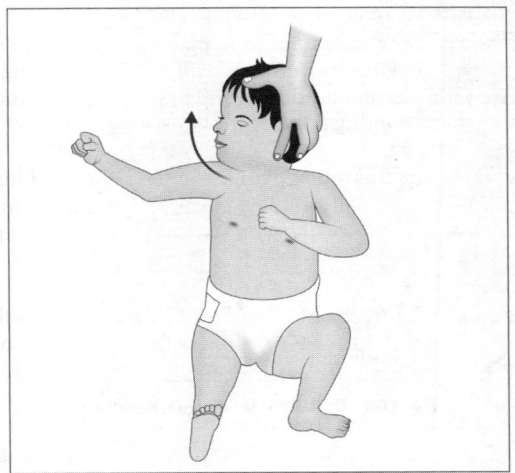

Fig. 106.1C: Tonic neck reflex.

6. Palmar reflex or Grasp reflex **(Fig. 106.1D)**.

   With the baby in supine and the head in midline, the finger of the examiner or a thin object such as a pencil is placed in the baby's hand. The newborn shows palmar reflex by wrapping the palm and the fingers around it. Normally there should be flexion of all he fingers around the examiner's flinger. This reflex diminishes, weakens and disappears after three months. Absence of this reflex is found in newborns with brain damage.

7. Traction response or Head lag reflex **(Fig. 106.1E)**.

   When pulled upright by the wrists to a sitting position, the head will lag initially, then right itself momentarily before falling forward on to the chest.

8. Plantar reflex **(Fig. 106.1F)**.

   The examiner's thumb or a thin such as pencil is pressed against the ball of the infant's foot. There will be reflexion of all toes.

9. Moro reflex or Embracing reflex **(FIg. 106.1G)**.

   This reflex occurs in response to a sudden stimulus. Acceptable ways to elicit a Moro reflex include the following:

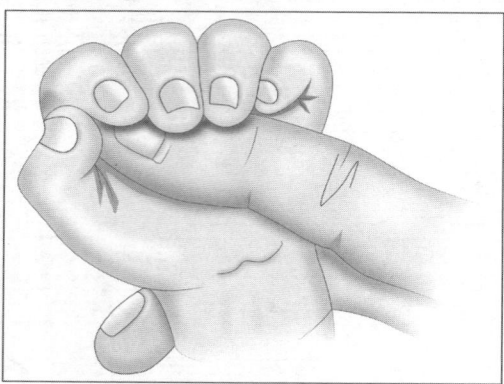

Fig. 106.1D: Palmar reflex (Grasp reflex).

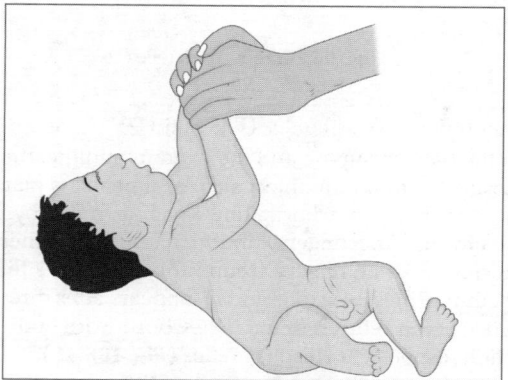

Fig. 106.1E: Traction response.

- Holding the baby at 45° angles and then permitting the head to drop 1 or 2 cm
- The examining table is struck near the head of the baby
- The table is jarred suddenly
- A loud noise or hand clap is made.

In response to the stimulus, the newborn responds by extending his hands and fanning the fingers, sometimes

Physical Examination of Newborn

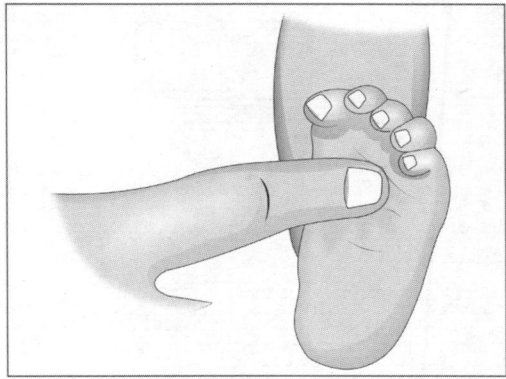

Fig. 106.1F: Plantar reflex.

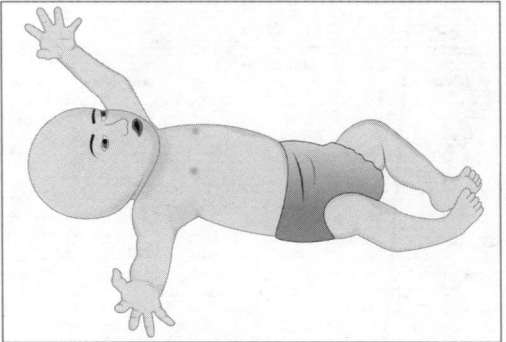

Fig. 106.1G: Moro reflex.

accopmanied by a tremor. The arms then flex and embrace the chest. A similar response may be seen in the legs, which following extension, flex on to the abdomen. The reflex is symmetrical and is present for the first 8 weeks of life. Absence of moro reflex may indicate brain damage or immaturity. Persistence of the reflex beyond the age of six months is suggestive of mental retardation.

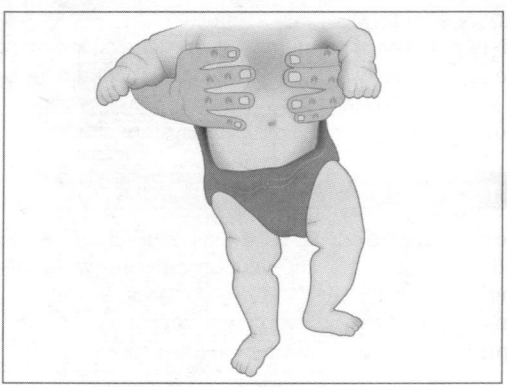

Fig. 106.1H: Stepping reflex.

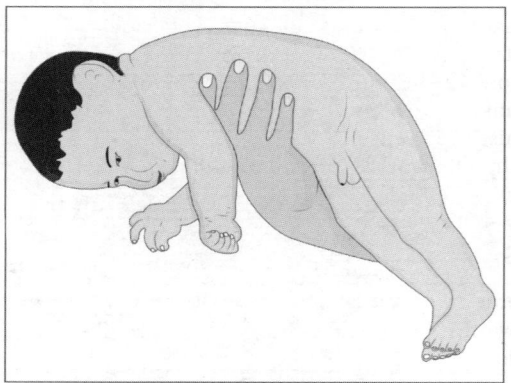

Fig. 106.1I: Ventral suspension.

10. Walking or Stepping reflex **(Fig. 106.1H)**.
    The baby is held erect so that the sole of the foot touches a flat surface. This should stimulate a stepping or dancing movement with both legs. This reflex is present at birth and gradually disappears after 3–4 weeks.

11. Ventral suspension **(Fig. 106.1I)**.
    When held prone, suspended over the examiner's arm, the baby shortly holds his head level with his body and flexes his limbs.

12. Incurvation of trunk or peres reflex.
    Hold the baby suspended ventrally and stroke the sides of spine alternatively. The baby would turn his pelvis to the side stimulated. This response disappears in one month. No response indicates central nervous system deficit.

107. POLYCYSTIC OVARY SYNDROME

Polycystic ovary syndrome (PCOS) is a complex endocrine disorder associated with long-term anovulation and an excess of androgen circulating in the blood. The syndrome is characterized by formation of cysts in the ovaries. PCOS is the leading cause of amenorrhea in young reproductive age group women (20–30%).

CLINICAL FEATURES

- Increasing obesity, especially central obesity
- Menstrual abnormalities in the form of oligomenorrhea, amenorrhea or dysfunctional uterine bleeding
- Infertility
- Hirsutism and acne
- Acanthosis nigricans (thickened and pigmented skin) over nape of neck, inner thighs and axilla.

CAUSES

The disorder is characterised by excessive androgen production by the ovaries, which interfere with reproductive, endocrine and metabolic functions.

The syndrome begins with an imbalance of luteinizing hormone (LH) and follicle stimulating hormone (FSH). LH is seen elevated and FSH low to normal.

The result of hormonal imbalance is continued follicular development, elevated estrogen levels, anovulation and multiple cysts.

DIAGNOSTIC MEASURES

Diagnosis is based on the presence of any two of the following three criteria:

- Oligo and/or anovulation
- Hyperandrogenism
- Polycystic ovaries.

Investigations

- **Sonography:** Transvaginal sonography will show enlarged ovaries with peripherally arranged cysts
- **Serum values:**
  - LH level is elevated and LH: FSH ratio is elevated (> 3:1)
  - Raised level of estradiol and estrogen
  - Reduced level of sex hormone binding globulin (SHBG)
  - Raised serum testosterone (> 150 ng/dL)
  - Raised fasting insulin levels
  - Raised level of prolactin.
- **Laparoscopy:** Bilateral polycystic ovaries.

POSSIBLE LATE SEQUELAE

- Risk of developing diabetes mellitus due to insulin resistance (15%)
- Risk of developing endometrial carcinoma due to persistently elevated level of estrogens
- Risk of hypertension and cardiovascular disease due to abnormal lipid profile (dyslipidaemia)
- Postmenopausal breast cancer.

MANAGEMENT

Management of PCOS needs to be individualized. It depends on her presenting symptoms such as menstrual disorder, infertility, obesity, hirsutism or combined symptoms.

Medical Management

- Correction of biochemical abnormalities with combination oral pills, GnRH agonists and Medroxyprogesterone (provera)
- For patients wanting pregnancy: Ovulation induction by giving clomiphene citrate with or without dexamethasone or bromocripine

- For patients with hyperinsulinaemia, metformin is given with clomiphene.

Surgical Management

Surgical treatment is indicated for those resistant to medical therapy. Endoscopic cauterisation or CO_2 Laser vaporisation of multiple cysts is usually done.

NURSING PROCESS

Nursing Assessment

Nursing assessment for pelvic conditions involves assessing risk factors, presenting symptoms and medical, and gynecological history. Data from physical assessment, laboratory tests and diagnostic procedures are considered.

Nursing Diagnoses

Nursing diagnoses are formulated based on assessment data and findings. Applicable nursing diagnoses may include:
- Pain related to pelvic condition
- Fear related to procedures and treatment
- Anxiety related to effects of condition or treatment
- Anxiety related to future childbearing
- Deficient knowledge regarding specific pelvic condition.

Nursing Care Plans

Nursing care plans include specific actions that the client will complete to achieve the highest level of wellness. Goals for the client may be that she will:
- Develop strategies for coping with pain
- Reduce stress and promote wellness by following exercise regimens
- Consume recommended food to control obesity and maintain optimum body weight
- Return to physician for follow-up care

- Notify physician of response to therapy and improvement or lack of it
- Be informed about the choices of medical management and expected outcomes of therapy.

Nursing Interventions

Nursing interventions include education about the condition, specific procedures, expected outcomes of therapy and providing emotional support.

108. POSTPARTUM CARE

Postpartum care involves care of the mother and her newborn. With the concept of rooming-in, where the infant remains in the mother's room, at her bedside, education about self-care and newborn care is integrated during the nurse's daily physical care of the couplet. Purposes of hospitalization and care after birth are:
- To identify maternal and neonatal complications
- To provide professional assistance at a time when the mother is likely to need supportive care.

An organized method should be followed when examining the postpartum client. For a consistent quality approach, the acronym BUBBLE-HE can be used. BUBBLE-HE stands for Breasts, Uterus, Bladder, Bowel, Lochia, Episiotomy, Homan's sign and Emotional support.

BREASTS

- On palpation after delivery, breasts usually are soft, warm and contain only small amount of colostrum. The nipples should be intact without redness, tenderness, cracks or blisters
- Breast engorgement, which may begin as tingling sensation may appear from 2 to 4 days following delivery
- Breasts should be inspected for presence of inverted nipples, cracks, blisters, fissures and palpated for fullness and tenderness.

UTERUS

- Immediately after delivery, the uterus begins the process of involution or reduction in size
- It generally takes 6 weeks for complete physiological involution and return of the reproductive system to its non-pregnant state
- The uterus diminishes in size and weight, and anatomic location back into the pelvis
- Level of fundus:
    - Immediately after delivery: At level or one or two fingers below the umbilicus
    - 12 hours after delivery: Approximately 1 cm above or below the umbilicus
    - After the first postpartum day: Descends about 1–2 cm (one finger breadth) each day.
- Fundus becomes nonpalpable on or about 9 days postpartum as it descends into the pelvis
- If bleeding continues despite fundal message and oxytocin administration, other reasons are determined and pharmacologic agents such as methylergonovine (Methergine) may be given intramuscularly (IM)
- When Methergine is contraindicated (high BP), prostaglandin preparation (Hemabate) is given
- For abdominal pain or after pains, which occur usually up to 3 days after delivery, analgesics may be given according to physician's order.

BLADDER

- When the client cannot urinate and the bladder remains distended, straight catheterization is done
- In the immediate postpartum period, urinary distension, incomplete emptying and residual urine may occur due to edematous perineum, pain, reflex spasms, and bladder desensitization. Early ambulation and comfort facilitates urination. Urination within 6 hours of at least 300 mL with complete emptying of bladder is appropriate.

BOWELS AND GASTROINTESTINAL SYSTEM

- Client's appetite typically will return to normal, immediately after delivery; if there are no complications from anesthesia, regular food may be resumed; a diet high in protein and iron facilitates tissue healing and restores iron levels
- Bowel pattern should remain unchanged after vaginal delivery, with a bowel movement normally occurring 2 or 3 days postpartum
- Drinking 6–8 glasses of fluids daily and eating a high-fiber diet should be encouraged
- When constipation is severe, administering an analgesic and stool softener before ambulation may assist in facilitating a bowel movement
- If large painful hemorrhoids cause problems, topical anesthetic medications help.

LOCHIA

The uterine discharge of blood, mucus, and tissue after childbirth is called lochia. Lochia rubra, which is of bright-red color is present for first 3 days. Lochia serosa, which is watery, pink or brown-tinged and light in amount occurs for 4–10 days. Lochia alba, a whitish-yellow creamy discharge occurs from 10 to 14/17 days:

- The amount of lochia varies with position changes, but should continually decrease through out the first 4–6 weeks postpartum
- Lochia with a reddish color that persists after 2 weeks of delivery may indicate subinvolution of the placental site or retained placental parts
- Assessing the fundus for firmness and involution, and lochia for amount and characteristics should be the daily nursing intervention in the 1st week following delivery. Lochia has a characteristic menstrual-like musky or fleshy smell. A foul-smelling discharge, along with other indicators, such as fever and uterine tenderness may suggest an infection such as endometritis.

EPISIOTOMY

- Using a good light source the episiotomy wound should be inspected; the redness, edema, echymosis, discharge and

approximation (REEDA) scoring scale can be used when assessing the episiotomy
- Immediately after delivery, the vagina appears edematous, bruised, stretchable and may gape at the introitus. By 4th week, the vaginal rugae return. Always remaining slightly larger than in the prepregnant state, the vagina returns to its prepregnant state by 6–8 weeks postpartum.

Extremities

- Assessment of the extremities should include examination of varicosities, deep tendon reflexes (DTRs), tenderness and presence of edema or nodular areas on the legs. DTRs should be no greater than +1 or +2. Brisk DTRs (+3 to + 4) are suggestive of pregnancy-induced hypertension (PIH). Pretibial or pedal edema may be present, especially in client with PIH
- Pain, erythema or local swelling on the legs especially the calves, may signify thrombophlebitis
- In clients who had spinal or epidural anesthesia, legs should be assessed for sensation and mobility. With appropriate assistance, the client should be able to move her toes and lift her buttocks off the bed within 2–4 hours after discontinuation of the anesthesia.

HOMAN'S SIGN

Homan's sign may be assessed by one of the two following methods:
- Have the woman keep her leg flat on the bed; place one hand on the knee, applying gentle pressure to keep the leg straight; place the other hand on her foot, gently flexing the foot towards the body (dorsiflexion)
- Have the woman slightly bend her knees. With your hand under the knee (popliteal region) and placing the foot flat on the bed, flex the foot towards the body.

The feeling of calf pain on flexion in either foot is a positive sign of thrombophlebitis. Using both hands on either side of the leg, the calf should be palpated for warmth and tenderness, and along the vein for nodules. The ankle and pretibial area must be checked for edema.

EMOTIONAL STATUS

The nurse should continually assess the mother for appropriate responses to her infant. Many times the client experiences a sense of elation immediately after the birth of her baby. She is excited and relieved that labor is finally over. She may also be exhausted and need sleep and rest to restore her body to health. After the taking-in phase, the mother's attainment of parental role, infant care and family concern should begin and that should be assessed by the nurse.

OTHER ASSESSMENTS

In addition to the basic postpartum assessments, other important body systems need to be examined.

Hemodynamic Status

- A complete blood count (CBC) may show marked leukocytosis, predominantly neutrophils both during and after delivery. The leukocyte count may increase during labor and may remain elevated for the first 2 days
- Hemoglobin, hematocrit and erythrocyte levels may fluctuate during the first postpartum days. Immediately after delivery, the hematocrit begins to rise and by 4–5 days, it returns to normal values. Cardiac output remains increased for at least 48 hours after delivery.

Integumentary System

Skin discoloration that appeared during pregnancy (chloasma) usually disappears by the end of pregnancy. The hyperpigmentaion of the areola and linea nigra may be permanent. The striae on her breasts, thighs and abdomen eventually fade to a pale color, but may never completely disappear.

Profuse perspiration especially at night is normal during the first week as the body rids itself of excess fluid from pregnancy. Women who suffered from pruritic urticarial rash will have regression of this in 1–2 weeks after delivery. There may be hair loss for the first 2 months after delivery.

Musculoskeletal System

Abdominal muscles relax and become flaccid after delivery. Some degree of muscle separation, called diastasis recti may be noticed along the center, while palpating the abdomen and fundus. Following multiple gestation, macrosomia and hydramnios, muscle tone do not fully return to prepregnant state.

ACTIVITY

Many mothers complain of fatigue after childbirth. They require time to recuperate and recover from the effects of labor and delivery. Once the woman is stable, she should be encouraged to ambulate often. Early ambulation helps to reduce the problem of consitpation and incidence of bladder infection, deep vein thrombosis and pulmonary embolism. Women who deliver vaginally often are able to ambulate to the restroom within few hours of delivery.

When the mother is very tired or has received an epidural or analgesics that may cause drowsiness, she may not have the ability to stand or walk independently. Before rising from bed, she should be assessed for dizziness and motor weakness from weak knees or legs. Ask the client how she feels when she rises from a recumbent position and if she is able to stand without assistance. When necessary, she should be offered the use of a wheelchair. When getting up from bed for the first time, the nurse should accompany her because she may experience orhostatic hypotension and be at risk of falling.

EXERCISES (Figs. 108.1A to F)

A woman who has had an uncomplicated vaginal delivery needs to begin moderate exercises soon after she feels recovered. She may perform mild stretching and flexing of muscles, especially abdominal muscles, which may relieve tension and muscle strain. Care should be exercised because joints do not stabilize until 6–8 weeks postpartum. Some of the safe exercises include Kegel exercise, deep breathing and pelvic tilts. These exercises support the organs, protect the back, improve posture and improve physical appearance. Exercising too much and too soon may result in an increase in bright red vaginal blood flow. The mother must not lift anything heavier than her baby for at least 2 weeks after childbirth. She should avoid climbing stairs for about 2–3 weeks.

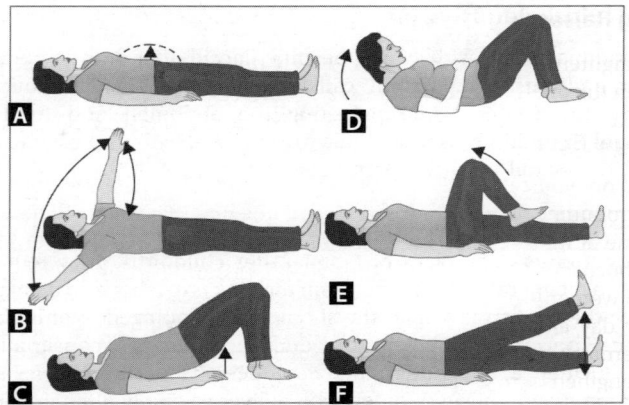

Figs. 108.1A to F: Postpartum exercises. **A.** Deep breathing; **B.** Arm raises; **C.** Pelvic tilt; **D.** Head raises; **E.** Knee flexes; **F.** Leg raises.

Deep Breathing (Fig. 108.1A)

Breathe deeply, expanding your abdominal muscles; then slowly exhale, tightening your abdominal muscles.

Arm Raises (Fig. 108.1B)

Place your arms at right angles to your body. Slowly raise them, touch your hands together then slowly lower your arms.

Pelvic Tilt (Fig. 108.1C)

Place your arms at your sides and your feet flat on the floor. Tighten abdominal and buttock muscles, press back into floor, then tilt pelvis towards ceiling.

Head Raises (Fig. 108.1D)

Lie with your knees flexed and feet flat on the floor. Contract your buttocks and tilt your head.

Knee Flexes (Fig. 108.1E)

Flex one knee toward your abdomen; lower foot towards the floor, then straighten your leg. Repeat same with the other leg.

Leg Raises (Fig. 108.1F)

Straighten legs and point toes. Slowly raise then lower one leg and then the other using your abdominal muscles.

Kegel Exercise

Lie on your back with both knees bend. Contract the muscles surrounding the vagina and anus and hold for 5 seconds as if holding urine at midstream, then slowly release. Kegel exercises contract the pubococcygeus muscle (the muscle supporting the pelvic organs) and the woman repeats the exercise 10 times and about 8–10 repetitions per day along with other exercises, spaced out during the day. By alternately contracting and relaxing these muscles, the exercise strengthens the pelvic muscles.

NURSING PROCESS

Assessment

- Fatigue and decreased energy level
- Insomnia
- Diaphoretic episodes during night
- Diuresis between days 2 and 5
- Perineal soreness from stretching and sutures if episiotomy/laceration is present
- Uterus between one finger breadth above to two finger breadths below umbilicus at 12 hours following delivery, descends one finger breadth daily thereafter
- Lochia rubra for 2–3 days progressing to lochia serosa
- Production of colostrum in first 48 hours progressing to mature milk by days 3.

Nursing Diagnoses

- Acute pain/Discomfort
- Deficient knowledge regarding breastfeeding
- Risk for injury
- Risk for infection
- Impaired urinary elimination
- Risk for deficient fluid volume

- Risk for constipation
- Disturbed sleep pattern
- Deficient knowledge regarding infant care.

Expected Outcomes

The client will:
- Verbalise lessening of discomfort
- Demonstrate effective techniques of breastfeeding
- Be free of complications
- Be free of infection and have normal lochial flow and character
- Void unassisted within 6-8 hours after delivery and empty bladder with each void
- Remain normotensive with fluid intake and urine output appropriately balanced
- Resume optimal bowel habits within 4 days after delivery
- Identify adjustments to accommodate changes required by demands of new family member in order to get adequate rest and sleep
- Perform necessary activities correctly and explain reasons for the actions.

Nursing Interventions

1. **Verbalizing lessening of discomfort:**
    - Determine presence, location and nature of discomfort; review labor and delivery record
    - Inspect perineum and episiotomy repair (note edema, ecchymosis, tenderness, purulent exudate or loss of approximation)
    - Apply ice pack to perineum, especially during the first 24 hours of delivery
    - Encourage use of moist heat (e.g. sitz bath) for 20 minutes, 3-4 times daily after the first 24 hours
    - Recommend sitting with gluteal muscles contracted over episiotomy repair
    - Assess uterine tenderness, determine presence and frequency/intensity of afterpains
    - Suggest client to lie prone with pillow under abdomen

- Inspect breast and nipple tissue; assess for presence of engorgement and/or cracked nipples
- Encourage wearing supportive bra
- Provide information regarding applying heat to breasts before feedings, positioning the infant properly and expressing milk manually
- Suggest to initiate feedings on non-tender nipple for several feedings in succession if only one nipple is sore or crakced
- Assess client for bladder fullness; implement measures to facilitate voiding. Instruct client in use of Kegel exercise
- Collaborative interventions:
  - Administer mild analgesic 30–60 minutes prior to brest-feeding; for non-lactating client, administer analgesics every 3–4 hours for breast engorgement and afterpains
  - Provide topical ointment for perineum (for episiotomy pain or hemorrhoidal discomfort).

2. **Practicing effective techniques of breastfeeding:**
   - Assess client's knowledge and previous experience with breastfeeding
   - Provide information about physiology and benefits of breastfeeding, nipple and breast care
   - Demonstrate and review breastfeeding techniques including latching on and removal from breast (note positioning of infant during feeding and length of feedings)
   - Assess client's nipples; recommend that client inspect nipples after each feeding
   - Encourage client to air-dry nipples for 20–30 min after feedings. Instruct to avoid use of soap on nipples.

3. **Remaining free of complications:**
   - Review hemoglobin (Hb) level and blood loss at delivery, note signs of anemia
   - Encourage early ambulation and exercise as appropriate following delivery
   - Assist with initial ambulation; provide adequate supervision in shower or sitz bath
   - Have client sit on floor or chair with head between legs or have her lie down in a flat position, if she feels faint. Use ammonia slat if available

- Assess client for hyperreflexia, epigastric pain, headache or visual disturbances. Maintain seizure precautions and quiet environment as indicated
- Note effects of $MgSO_4$ if administrated
- Inspect lower extremities for signs of thrombophlebitis (e.g. redness, warmth and tenderness). Note presence or absence of Homan's Sign
- Administer Rho(D) immune globulin (RhIg) IM, within 72 hours postpartum as indicated.

4. **Being free of infection and having normal lochial flow:**
   - Assess prenatal and intranatal records, noting frequency of vaginal examination, premature rupture of membranes (PROM), prolonged labor, lacerations or retained placenta
   - Monitor temperature and pulse; note signs of chills, anorexia or malaise
   - Assess location and contractility of uterus, note involutional changes or presence of uterine tenderness
   - Note color, amount and odor of lochial discharge and progression from rubra to serosa
   - Evaluate condition of nipples, noting presence of cracks, redness or tenderness. Review proper care and feeding techniques
   - Inspect site of episiotomy/laceration repair every shift
   - Note frequency and amount of voidings
   - Assess for signs of urinary tract infection
   - Encourage to take perineal care three to four times daily or after voiding/defecation
   - Demonstrate and encourage use of careful handwashing technique and appropriate disposal of soiled underpads
   - Assess client's nutritional status. Provide information about selecting foods high in protein, vitamin C and iron
   - Encourage to increase fluid intake to 2,000 mL/day
   - Promote rest and sleep
   - Assess white blood cell (WBC) count, Hb and hematocrit (Hct)
   - Collaborative interventions:
     - Administer iron preparations and vitamin supplements as necessary
     - Administer Methergine every 3–4 hours as appropriate

- Assist with or obtain cultures from vagina, serum and site of episiotomy repair as indicated
- Encourage client to apply antibiotic creams to perineum, as indicated
- Administer antibiotics based on culture report
- Teach client regarding possible complications and follow-up care.

5. **Maintaining optimal urinary output:**
   - Assess fluid intake and urine output, note intrapartal intake and output and length of labor
   - Monitor fundal height and location and amount of lochial flow
   - Note presence of edema or laceration/episiotomy and type of anesthesia used
   - Encourage voiding within 6–8 hours postpartum and every 4 hours thereafter
   - Instruct client to use Kegel exercise daily
   - Encourage drinking 6–8 glasses of fluid per day
   - Assess for signs of urinary tract infection (UTI) such as burning, increased frequency and cloudy urine
   - Collaborative interventions:
     - Catheterize using straight or indwelling catheter as indicated
     - Obtain urine specimen for laboratory test if client has symptoms of UTI
     - Monitor laboratory test results, such as blood urea nitrogen (BUN) and 24 hours urine for total protein, creatinine clearance and uric acid as indicated.

6. **Remaining normotensive with balanced intake and output:**
   - Note fluid loss at delivery, review intrapartal history
   - Evaluate location and contractility of uterine fundus, amount of vaginal lochia and condition of perineum every 2 hours for first 8 hours as appropriate, then every 8 hours for the remainder of hospitalization
   - Gently massage fundus if uterus is boggy
   - Note presence of thirst, provide liquids as tolerated
   - Evaluate status of bladder, promote emptying if bladder is full
   - Monitor temperature, pulse and BP as indicated

- Evaluate fluid intake and urine output during intravenous (IV) infusion or until normal voiding patterns are re-established
- Monitor filling of breasts and milk supply if lactating
- Collaborative interventions:
    - Replace fluid loss with IV infusion containing electrolytes
    - Administer Methergine parenterally or synthetic oxytocin preparations (Syntocinon/Pitocin) IM/IV
    - Assess BP before administering and withhold if BP is elevated
    - Review prenatal Hb/Hct levels; note blood loss at delivery and obtain postpartal Hb/Hct as indicated.

7. **Resuming optimal bowel habits:**
   - Auscultate for presence of bowel sounds, determine normal evacuation habits
   - Provide appropriate dietary information regarding importance of roughage, increased fluids and the attempt to establish normal evacuation pattern
   - Encourage increase in activity level and ambulation as tolerated
   - Assess episiotomy: Note presence of laceration and degree of tissue involvement.
   - Collaborative interventions: Administer stool softeners suppositories, enemas or laxatives as indicated.

8. **Accommodating changes required by demands of newborn for improved rest and sleep:**
   - Assess level of fatigue and need for rest. Note length of labor and type of delivery
   - Determine factors interfering with rest and sleeping periods
   - Encourage verbalization about birth experience, provide quiet environment
   - Provide information about needs for rest and sleep following discharge
   - Provide information about effects of fatigue and anxiety on milk supply
   - Assess home environment, availability of assistance and presence of siblings and other family members.

- Provide guidance on ways to plan activities and rest periods according to individual family situation.
9. **Performing infant care and self-care activities appropriately:**
    - Assess client's readiness and motivation for learning
    - Assist client in identifying needs
    - Provide information about role of a progressive postpartal exercise program
    - Provide information about perineal care and hygiene, normal progression of lochial discharge, needs for rest and sleep and role changes
    - Have client demonstrate the material learned when appropriate
    - Discuss sexuality needs and plans for contraception. Provide information about available and feasible methods
    - Explain importance of postpartal examination 4–6 weeks following delivery
    - Discuss normal physical and psychological changes and needs associated with postnatal period.

109. POSTDATED PREGNANCY/POST-TERM PREGNANCY

DEFINITION

Post-term pregnancy is one that has lasted 42 weeks (294 days) or more.

INCIDENCE

About 6–8% of pregnancies go beyond 42 weeks.

FACTORS ASSOCIATED WITH POST-TERM PREGNANCIES

- Hereditary: Postmaturity often runs in the family and often manifests in consecutive pregnancies in the same individual
- High standard of living with sedentary habits
- Congenital malformations such as anencephaly, fetal osteogenesis imperfecta
- Elderly primigravida or elderly multigravida.

TYPES OF POST-TERM GESTATION

- Placental function is unaffected:
  - The fetus continues to grow
  - The baby is often macrosomic
  - Cephalopelvic disproportion and shoulder dystocia occur frequently
  - Accounts for 90% of post-term pregnancies.
- Placenta is dysmature and its function is adversely affected:
  - The prognosis of the fetus is guarded
  - Accounts for about 10% of post-term pregnancies.

PATHOPHYSIOLOGY

Inadequacy of placental function and reduction in its reserve capacity renders the fetus vulnerable to hypoxia. The post-term neonate who is a victim of a dysmature placenta may reveal the following characteristics:

- Early features:
  - Dry parchment-like skin, which shows wrinkling and peeling
  - Long fingernails, and lack of subcutaneous fat
  - A thin, long infant that appears malnourished.
- Intermediate stage:
  - The infant passes meconium, which stains the membranes, placenta and fetal skin.
- Advanced stage:
  - Amniotic fluid, placental membranes and fetal skin are markedly stained and appear yellow.
- Amniotic fluid is found to be scanty.

FETAL COMPLICATIONS

- Intrapartum fetal distress from cord compression due to oligohydramnios or placental insufficiency
- Meconium aspiration syndrome when thick meconium is present in amniotic fluid
- Fetal trauma especially in those complicated by fetal macrosomia
- Fetal dysmaturity causing the neonate to be born with a low Apgar score.

DIAGNOSIS

- Menstrual history: Last menstrual period (LMP)
- Clinical findings:
  - Weight stationary or even falling weight after term
  - Abdominal girth diminishing after term
  - Feeling of hard bones through the cervix or fornix
  - Uterus feels full of fetus as liquor amni diminishes
  - Sonographic assessment of crown-rump length (CRL), biparietal diameter (BPD) and femur length (FL)
  - Cardiotocography (non-stress test) twice weekly
  - Amniotic fluid measurement
  - Doppler ultrasound of umbilical artery to assess uteroplacental blood flow.

MANAGEMENT

- Elective induction of labor. Timing between 10 and 14 days:
  - If cervix is favorable (ripe), induction is done by stripping of membranes or by low rupture of membranes.
- If liquor is clear, oxytocin infusion is added. If liquor is thickly meconium stained, cesarean section is recommended.
  - If cervix is unripe, it is made favorable with prostaglandin E_2 (PGE_2) gel. This is followed by low rupture of membranes. Oxytocin infusion is added when required.
- Elective cesarean section is indicated:
  - When postmaturity is associated with complicating factors such as contracted pelvis, postcesarean pregnancy, malpresentation, elderly primigravida, etc.
  - In the presence of associated medical complications, which are likely to produce placental insufficiency, e.g. PET, history of bleeding during pregnancy or diabetes.

Care During Labor

- Continuous monitoring of fetal heart rate (FHR)
- Assess fetal scalp blood pH as and when required
- Make facilities available for prompt intervention
- Beware of shoulder dystocia in suspected case of fetal macrosomia.

110. POSTNATAL ASSESSMENT (POSTDELIVERY ASSESSMENT)

Following delivery/childbirth, the maternal organs begin the task of readjusting to the non-pregnant state. Careful observations are to be made and recorded.

The woman remains in the labor area for about 2 hours for observation during the recovery period and transferred to the postpartum ward when the condition becomes stable.

Assessment of the postnatal client includes checking the uterus, lochia, perineum, bladder, blood pressure, heart rate, temperature, psychosocial status and pain.

UTERUS

- Uterus is assessed every 15 minutes for 1st hour
- Woman is positioned supine with legs crossed
- Position of the fundus is noted in relation to the umbilicus and recorded as centimeters above or below the umbilicus. During the fourth stage fundus is usually at the level of the umbilicus
- Placement of the uterus in relation to the midline and consistency are noted
- If fundus is not firm (boggy), it is massaged gently in a circular motion, until the uterus contracts and becomes firm
- Clots are expelled at this time by applying gentle, but firm pressure downward on the fundus, while observing the perineum for amount and size of expelled clots
- If repeated massage is required, bladder fullness must be checked and bladder emptied. With a full bladder, uterus remains at or above the level of umbilicus and displaced to one side.

LOCHIA

- Lochia is monitored every 15 minutes for the 1st hour and findings are recorded
- The amount, color and presence of clots are noted. Estimation of lochia as standardized by Jacobson (1985):
    - Scant: Blood on perineal pad less than 2 inches in 1 hour
    - Light: Blood, less than 4 inches in 1 hour

- Moderate: Less than 6 inches stain
- Heavy: A saturated perineal pad in 1 hour.
- Continuous bleeding in the presence of a well-contracted uterus indicates soft tissue damage.

PERINEUM

- Perineum is observed every 15 minutes for the 1st hour to assess the episiotomy site or laceration repair to ensure that it is intact and for edema, bleeding and hematoma
- Ice packs provide comfort and prevent swelling.

BLADDER

- Difficulty in voiding spontaneously occurs owing to bruising of the meatus or the effects of epidural anesthesia
- Bladder must be assessed for filling every 15 minutes during the 1st hour
- When the mother's vital signs are stable and the effects of sedation and anesthesia are worn out, she may be assisted to the bathroom to void or a bedpan offered
- Urine has to be measured and the time of voiding recorded
- If the woman is unable to void, even though the bladder is palpable, or the uterus is displaced, catheterization is necessary.

BLOOD PRESSURE

- Blood pressure is monitored every 15 minutes for the 1st hour or more frequently if the woman's condition warrants
- Under normal circumstances, pressure readings should return to prelabor levels within the 1st hour of vaginal delivery.

HEART RATE

- Pulse readings, rhythm and regularity are assessed every 15 minutes for the 1st hour; the pulse usually returns to prelabor rate within the 1st hour
- If the nurse detects tachycardia, dehydration or hypovolemia, infection should be ruled out.

TEMPERATURE

- A temperature reading is taken during the first hour. An increase up to 100.4°F is not unusual owing to the dehydrating effects of labor
- A higher temperature than this should be reported.

PSYCHOSOCIAL STATUS

- The mother may be emotionally and physically exhausted and at the same time elated and talkative
- Women often feel hungry immediately after delivery
- Food is usually withheld until after 1 hour as the gastrointestinal (GI) tract is still slowed from the hormones of labor.

PAIN

- Abdominal cramping or after pains may occur as the uterus contracts
- Oxytocin administration after delivery of the placenta also will stimulate uterine contractions
- Analgesics should be administered according to physician's order or hospital policy.

NURSING PROCESS

Assessment

- May appear energised or fatigued/exhausted, sleepy
- Pulse usually slow (50–70 beats per minute owing to vagal hypersensitivity)
- BP may be lower in response to analgesia/anesthesia or elevated in response to oxytocin administration or PIH
- Blood loss during delivery may be up to 400–500 mL
- Hemorrhoids may be present and protruding
- Bladder may be palpable over symphysis pubis if a catheter is not in place
- Diuresis may occur if IV fluids were administered during labor and delivery

Postnatal Assessment (Postdelivery Assessment)

- May report discomfort from various sources, e.g. afterpains, episiotomy repair, bladder fullness or feeling cold
- Slight temperature elevation may be there due to exertion and dehydration
- Uterine fundus firmly contracted and located at the level of the umbilicus
- Breasts soft with nipple erect.

Nursing Diagnoses

- Risk for deficient fluid volume
- Acute pain.

Expected Outcomes

The client will:
- Display stable vital signs within normal limits. Uterus firmly contracted and moderate lochial flow
- Verbalize reduction of discomfort/pain and display relaxed posture and facial expression.

Nursing Interventions

1. **Displaying normal vital signs, contracted uterus and moderate lochia:**
    - Place client in recumbent position
    - Assess intrapartal events, e.g. labor induced/augmented and length of third stage
    - Gently massage fundus if it is soft (boggy); use firm, steady, downward pressure on the fundus for expulsion of clots if required
    - Place infant at client's breast if client has chosen to breastfeed
    - Assess for bladder fullness above symphysis pubis. Notify physician if distension is noted and client is unable to void
    - Assess amount, color and nature of lochial flow every 15 minutes

- Assess BP and pulse every 15 minutes
- Assess perineum every 15 minutes per protocol noting condition of episiotomy/laceration repair if present for edema and eccymosis
- Review initial Hb and Hct levels, obtain stat levels as indicated
- Maintain IV infusion or insert saline lock as indicated
- Administer oxytocin intramuscularly/intravenously (IM/IV). Increase rate of IV oxytocin infusion per protocol if uterine bleeding persists.

2. **Reporting reduction of level of discomfort, displaying relaxed posture and facial expressions:**
   - Assess nature and degree of discomfort, type of delivery and nature of intrapartal events
   - Provide appropriate information about routine care in the postpartal period
   - Inspect episiotomy/laceration repair. Apply ice pack if required
   - Assess for leg or body tremors. Place warm blankets on client if required
   - Institute comfort measures such as mouth care, partial bath, clean dry linen and perineal care
   - Offer clear fluids as appropriate
   - Assess for bladder fullness by palpating above symphysis pubis and assist in voiding as required
   - Massage uterus gently as indicated; note presence and severity of afterpains
   - Encourage use of breathing and relaxation techniques
   - Position or reposition client as needed
   - Provide quiet environment and encourage rest between assessments
   - Collaborative intervention: Administer analgesics as needed.

111. PRECIPITATE LABOR

DEFINITION

Precipitate labor refers to a labor pattern that progresses rapidly and ends with delivery occurring in less than 3 hours after the onset of uterine activity.

CONTRIBUTORY FACTORS

- Maternal multiparous status
- Small fetus
- Relaxed pelvic and vaginal musculature
- History of rapid labors with previous deliveries.

RISKS OF PRECIPITATE LABOR AND DELIVERY

- Delivery out of asepsis
- Maternal soft tissue injuries
- Fetal injuries from rapid expulsion at delivery.

MANAGEMENT

- Readiness of the healthcare team for delivery, when the client has a history of rapid labor
- Medical induction of labor to ensure a hospital delivery and to increase the likelihood for a controlled delivery that minimizes the potential for maternal and fetal injuries.

NURSING CARE

Important nursing interventions include:
- Continuous assessment of maternal and fetal status
- Communicating to physician any change in status, maternal or fetal intolerance or signs of impending problems
- Teaching and reinforcing relaxation techniques
- Administering tocolytic medication as ordered
- Side-lying position to enhance placental blood flow and to reduce the effects of aortocaval compression
- Oxygen to the mother and adequate blood volume with non-additive intravenous fluids.

After Delivery

- Assessing uterine fundus for atony
- Checking perineum for hematoma or laceration
- Assessing neonate for soft tissue injuries
- Monitoring vital signs to ensure stability.

112. PREGNANCY-INDUCED HYPERTENSION

Hypertension develops as a result of the gravid state with no history of hypertension prior to pregnancy. Pregnancy-induced hypertension (PIH) includes preeclampsia and eclampsia.

PREECLAMPSIA

Development of hypertension in pregnancy together with proteinuria and/or generalized edema after 20 weeks of gestation.

Incidence

Average incidence is about 10%.

Predisposing Factors

- Elderly and young primigravida
- Family history of preeclampsia, eclampsia or hypertension
- Neglect of antenatal care
- Pregnancy complications such as hydatidiform mole, multiple pregnancy, polyhydramnios, rhesus (Rh) incompatibility
- Medical disorders—nephritis, diabetes
- Hereditary.

Diagnostic Criteria

- Rise of blood pressure to 140/90 mm Hg (a rise in systolic pressure of at least 30 mm Hg, or a rise in diastolic pressure of at least 15 mm Hg over the previously known blood pressure)
- Pitting edema over the ankles, swollen fingers, puffy eyelids, vulval edema and excessive weight gain > 0.5 kg/week
- Proteinuria: Presence of protein in urine is a late development and signifies worsening of the disease
- Headache in severe disease, as a warning sign of impending convulsion
- Epigastric pain due to stretching of the liver capsule by edema, which is a symptom of severe disease.

LABORATORY TEST FINDINGS

Degree of Severity

Mild Preeclampsia

- Diastolic blood pressure is above 90 mm Hg, but less than 110 mm Hg
- Systolic blood pressure is 30 mm Hg above the prepregnancy reading in early pregnancy
- The mean arterial pressure (MAP) exceeds 105 mm Hg.

Severe Preeclampsia

- Systolic blood pressure more than 160 mm Hg or diastolic blood pressure ≥ 110 mm Hg on at least two occasions at least 4 hours apart
- Proteinuria ≥ 5 g in 24 hours (3+ or 4+ on qualitative examination)
- Oliguria ≥ 400 mL in 24 hours
- Cerebral or visual disturbances
- Severe headache or epigastric pain.

MANAGEMENT OF PREECLAMPSIA AND ECLAMPSIA

- Prevention
- Treatment of mild preeclampsia
- Treatment of severe preeclampsia
- Treatment of eclampsia.

Prevention

- Low dose aspirin in dose of 50–100 mg/day inhibits the platelet enzyme and reverses the abnormal ratio of prostaglandins, thus retarding disease progress
- Dietary calcium supplements have been found effective in preventing preeclampsia.

Treatment of Mild PIH

- Hospitalization and monitoring of blood pressure, urine protein, and fetal status

- Bedrest preferably in left lateral position
- Diet: Adequate calorie (2,000 kcal/day) and protein intake. Salt is neither restricted nor forced.

Medications

- Continuation of iron, folic acid and calcium supplements
- Mild sedatives such as phenobarbitone or diazepam at bedtime
- Mild laxative if patient is constipated
- Antihypertensive medications such as nifedipine, labetalol or hydralazine, which do not have deleterious effects on uteroplacental blood flow are used.

Monitoring

- Blood pressure at least four times a day
- Urine albumin daily
- Body weight on alternate days
- Blood investigations for serum uric acid, creatinine and blood urea nitrogen weekly
- Urinary protein excretion in 24 hours specimen
- Fetal heart rate and fetal movement count daily
- Non-stress test weekly
- Ultrasonography to assess fetal growth every 7–14 days.

Indications for Definitive Treatment; Termination of Pregnancy

- Gestational age over 37 weeks
- Worsening of hypertension or proteinuria
- Impending eclampsia
- Placental abruption
- Onset of labor or ripe cervix.

If cervix is ripe (Bishop score more than 6), an amniotomy along with oxytocin is used to induce labor. If cervix is not ripe, local prostaglandin gel may be tried. If induction fails, cesarean section is performed.

Management in Labor

- Progress of labor is recorded on partogram
- Abdominal and vaginal examinations at regular intervals

- Bedrest in first stage of labor
- To cut short second stage with application of prophylactic forceps
- Methergine is contraindicated in third stage.

Treatment of Severe PIH

Mother and fetus are to be monitored with lot of care because of possible complications such as:
- Placental abruption
- HELLP syndrome
- Disseminated intravascular coagulation (DIC)
- Acute renal failure.

Expectant Management

This is considered when the gestational age is less than 34 weeks of pregnancy. The objectives of expectant management are:
- Prevention of convulsions
- Stabilization of blood pressure
- Maintenance of adequate urinary output
- Prevention of serious complications such as DIC. Some patients with severe preeclampsia require initial stabilization and delivery within 24 hours. Maternal indications for delivery or termination of pregnancy include:
  - Uncontrolled severe hypertension
  - Development of persistent, severe headache with visual symptoms and epigastric pain
  - Preterm labor, rupture of membranes
  - Fetal distress, severe oligohydramnios and severe intrauterine growth restriction (IUGR)
  - Attainment of 34 weeks gestation.

A delay in delivery of 48 hours in this situation increases the risk of intrauterine fetal death.

Intrapartum Management

Labor is best managed in a well-equipped hospital.

Anticonvulsants

Magnesium sulfate ($MgSO_4$) is administered by the Pritchard regimen. Serum magnesium level is maintained between 4 and

7 mg% and clinically according to patellar reflex, urinary output and respiratory rate.

Antihypertensives

Hydralazine is administered when the maternal diastolic blood pressure rises above 110 mm Hg. Sublingual nifedipine may be used until diastolic blood pressure is 100.

Monitoring

- Maternal:
  - Pulse, respiration and blood pressure every 15 minutes
  - Urine albumin and output (100 mL/3 h)
  - Magnesium level (4–6 mg%).
- Fetal:
  - Continuous electronic monitoring.
- Progress of labor:
  - Partogram to evaluate maternal and fetal parameters
  - Blood ready for use if postpartum hemorrhage (PPH) occurs.
- Induction of labor:
  - Patients over 34 weeks or with ripe cervix may be induced with oxytocin infusion or prostaglandins
- Monitoring in labor ward for a period of 24 hours after delivery
- $MgSO_4$ is continued for 24 hours after the time of delivery.

Treatment of Eclampsia

When there is occurance of convulsions in a patient with preeclampsia with no coincidental neurological disease, it is called eclampsia. Eclampsia may be antepartum (50%), intrapartum (25%), postpartum (25%) and rarely intercurrent (recovers from convulsion and pregnancy continues).

Phases of Eclamptic Seizure

Described in four phases:
- **Initial or prodromal phase:**
  - An aura, followed by convulsive movements that begin around mouth (30 seconds).
- **Tonic phase:**
  - The entire body becomes rigid, and opisthotonos, limbs flexed and hands clenched

- Ceases and tongue protrudes between teeth
- Cyanosis appears and eyeballs become fixed (20–30 seconds).
- **Clonic phase:**
  - Jerking movements appear starting from facial muscles to involve the entire body (muscle contraction and relaxation)
  - Frothing of sputum at the mouth and cyanosis appear
  - Duration (1–2 minutes).
- **Recovery/Stage of coma:**
  - Movements slowly subside, stertorous respirations then resumes and the patient passes into coma of variable duration
  - The fits are usually multiple. When it occurs in quick succession, it is called status eclampticus.

Management

General measures

- Patient to be nursed in:
  - Darkened, isolated room with minimum stimulation
  - Propping up the guard rails
  - Padded tongue depressor at bedside
  - Large-bore IV line
  - Urinary catheterization
  - Investigations such as complete blood count (CBC), platelet count, liver function tests, arterial blood gas (ABG), serum electrolytes, bleeding time, clotting time, prothrombin time (PT), partial thromboplastin time (PTT) and grouping
  - Crossmatching.
- Oxygenation
- Lateral position to facilitate drainage of secretions and to prevent aspiration
- Anticonvulsants—magnesium sulfate
- Delivery should be accomplished speedily and with as little trauma as possible (for more details on 'Management' refer Chapter 35).

HELLP SYNDROME

The HELLP syndrome (hemolysis, elevated liver enzymes and low platelet counts) is a rare complication of severe preeclampsia and may occur in 3–4% of patients with preeclampsia and eclampsia. Pathophysiology is similar to that of preeclampsia and include:

- Microvascular damage
- Platelet activation
- Vasospasm
- Periportal hemorrhage and fibrin deposits in liver.

Laboratory Findings

- Elevated bilirubin and lactate dehydrogenase > 600 IU/L
- Aspartate transaminase (AST) and alanine transaminase (ALT) levels of 200–700 IU/L
- Platelet count < 100,000/mL.

Management

- Daily monitoring of maternal platelet count and transaminase levels
- Prompt delivery under adequate supervision.

After delivery laboratory, abnormalities peak in the first 1–2 days and then return to normal within 3–11 days.

NURSING PROCESS

Assessment

- Persistent increase in BP over pregravid baseline > 30 mm Hg systolic and > 15 mm Hg diastolic
- Oliguria
- Weight gain of 1 kg in a week and edema
- Nausea and vomiting
- Dizziness and frontal headache
- Convulsion
- Epigastric pain
- Low platelet count < 100,000/mL^3
- Elevated serum creatinine
- Elevated liver enzymes
- Elevated uric acid > 5 mg/100 mL
- Proteinuria
- IUGR on ultrasonography.

Nursing Diagnoses

- Deficient fluid volume
- Decreased cardiac output
- Ineffective uteroplacental tissue perfusion
- Risk for maternal injury
- Deficient knowledge regarding condition, prognosis and treatment needs.

Expected Outcomes

The client will:
- Be free of signs of generalized edema and display Hct within normal limits
- Remain normotensive throughout the remainder of pregnancy
- Fetus will be full-term, appropriate for gestational age and display normal central nervous system (CNS) activity
- Display normal levels of clotting factors and liver enzymes
- Initiate lifestyle/behavior changes as indicated, based on knowledge of disease process and treatment plan.

Nursing Interventions

1. **Client staying free of generalized edema:**
   - Weigh client routinely—alternate days in hospital
   - Monitor location and degree of edema
   - Note change in Hct/Hb levels
   - Assess dietary intake of proteins and calories
   - Monitor intake and output, note color and specific gravity of urine
   - Test clean voided urine for protein
   - Monitor blood pressure and pulse
   - Place on strict regimen of bedrest and encourage left lateral position
   - Collaborative interventions:
     - Monitor serum uric acid, creatinine levels and blood urea nitrogen
     - Replace fluids either orally or parenterally as indicated.

2. **Remaining normotensive for the remainder of pregnancy:**
   - Monitor blood pressure and pulse
   - Note respiratory rate and assess for crackles, wheezes and dyspnea
   - **Collaborative interventions:**
     - Administer antihypertensive drugs such as hydralazine and nifedipine as ordered
     - Prepare for birth of fetus by cesarean section when severe PIH or eclamptic condition is present.
3. **Fetus remaining full-term and AGA:**
   - Identify factors affecting fetal activity
   - Provide information regarding assessment of fetal movements
   - Review signs of possible complications, which need to be identified for seeking timely medical attention
   - Monitor FHR manually or electronically if indicated
   - **Collaborative interventions:**
     - Assess fetal maturity from sonography and blood tests such as lecithin to sphingomyelin ratio and estriol levels
     - Administer corticosteroids as prescribed if severe PIH necessitates premature delivery
     - Evaluate fetal growth periodically
     - Note fetal response to medications such as $MgSO_4$, phenobarbitone and diazepam when used.
4. **Displaying normal liver enzymes and clotting factors:**
   - Assess for signs of CNS involvement such as headache, irritability and visual disturbances
   - Instruct client to promptly report signs and symptoms of CNS involvement
   - Note changes in level of consciousness
   - Assess for signs of impending eclampsia such as hyperactivity of deep tendon reflexes, ankle clonus, decreased pulse and respirations, epigastric pain, and oliguria (< 50 mL/h)
   - Institute measures to reduce likelihood of seizures such as quiet, dimly lit room, limited visitors and coordinated care, which promote rest

- Implement seizure precautions per protocol
- If seizure does occur:
  - Turn client on side
  - Insert airway/bite block when mouth is relaxed
  - Suction nasopharynx
  - Administer oxygen
  - Remove restrictive clothing
  - Document motor involvement, duration of seizure and post seizure behavior.
- Palpate uterine tenderness or rigidity and check for vaginal bleeding
- Monitor for signs and symptoms of labor
- Assess fetal well-being, noting FHR
- Monitor for signs of DIC such as epistaxis, GI bleeding and prolonged bleeding
- **Collaborative interventions:**
  - Administer $MgSO_4$ using infusion pump
  - Have calcium gluconate available for use if indicated
  - Administer diazepam if ordered
  - Monitor laboratory reports: PT, PTT, fibrin degradation products (FDP), sequential platelet count, bilirubin and peripheral smear
  - Prepare for cesarean birth if PIH is severe, placental functioning is compromised and cervix is not ripe or is not responsive to induction.

5. **Initiating lifestyle or behavior changes:**
   - Assess client's/couple's knowledge of the disease process
   - Provide information about the disease, implications for mother and fetus and the rationale for interventions, procedures and tests
   - Provide information about signs and symptoms indicating worsening of condition and when to notify physician
   - Keep client informed of health status, results of tests and fetal well-being
   - Provide information about taking adequate protein in diet and any restrictions.

113. PREMATURE RUPTURE OF MEMBRANES

DEFINITION

Rupture of membranes beyond 37th week, but before the onset of labor is called premature rupture of membranes (PROM). Preterm prelabor rupture of membranes (PPROM) occurs before 37 completed weeks of gestation, without the onset of spontaneous uterine activity resulting in cervical dilatation.

INCIDENCE

Incidence of premature rupture of membranes is 2–3%.

ETIOLOGY

- Poorly applied presenting part in unstable lie and other malpresentations
- Polyhydramnios with increase in hydrostatic pressure commonly with multiple pregnancy
- Incompetent cervix
- Traumatic:
  - External cephalic version
  - Amniocentesis.
- Weakness of the chorion and amnion:
  - Developmental
  - Inflammatory chorioamnionitis.

DIAGNOSIS

History: Discharge of clear fluid (liquor) vaginally.

Examination: Speculum examination shows liquor draining through cervical os. The smell is characteristically sweet and may be meconium stained.

INVESTIGATIONS

- Fern test—crystallization of liquor when dried on a slide
- Liquor may be examined for fetal squamae, hair and vernix

- Litmus test to distinguish liquor from urine, normal vaginal pH is 4.5, liquor pH is 7.

HAZARDS

Maternal

- Chorioamnionitis, which may be followed by systemic infection
- Oligohydramnios if prolonged leaking occurs.

Fetal

- Cord prolapse
- Premature labor often follows within next 10 days
- Intrauterine infection.

MANAGEMENT

Before 37 Weeks Gestation

- Bedrest and sedation
- Speculum examination:
  - To exclude cord prolapse
  - To confirm presence of liquor
  - To obtain cervical swab for bacteriology.
- Antibiotic therapy.

After 37 Weeks Gestation

- Exclude cord prolapse
- Oxytocin induction if there are no complications
- Cesarean section under antibiotic cover if induction is contraindicated.

114. PREMENSTRUAL SYNDROME

DEFINITION

Premenstrual syndrome (PMS) is a psychoneuroendocrine disorder of unknown etiology that occurs just prior to menstruation. There is cyclic appearance of several symptoms during the last 7–10 days of the onset menstrual cycle, which subside with the onset of menstrual flow. At least five of the following symptoms must have been present in most of the cycles over the past 1 year.

CLINICAL MANIFESTATIONS

- Depressed mood, hopelessness and self-depreciation
- Anxiety, tension, fearfulness
- Affective lability—mood swings
- Anger, irritability, interpersonal conflict
- Decreased energy
- Appetite changes or cravings
- Changes in sleep
- Feeling overwhelmed or out of control
- Physical symptoms such as breast tenderness, headache
- Dyspareunia, bloating
- Weight gain.

These symptoms should fulfill the following criteria:
- Not related to any organic lesion
- Occurs regularly during the luteal phase of each ovulatory menstrual cycle
- Severe enough to disturb the lifestyle of the woman
- Symptom-free period during the rest of the cycle.

PATHOPHYSIOLOGY

The exact cause is not known but following hypothesis is considered:
- Alteration in the level or ratio of estrogen and progesterone from the midluteal phase
- Neuroendocrine factors:
  - Decreased synthesis of serotonin in the luteal phase
  - Withdrawal of endorphins from central nervous system (CNS) during luteal phase.
- Psychological and psychosocial factors affecting behavior.

TREATMENT

No treatment for PMS has been validated by empirical studies. A number of lifestyle changes and other benign interventions are effective for some patients.

General

- Elimination of caffeine from the diet
- Avoidance of smoking, alcohol
- Regular exercise
- Regular meals and a nutritious diet
- Adequate sleep
- Relaxation techniques such as yoga, stress management and assurance.

Nonhormonal

- Tranquillizers or antidepressant drugs
- Pyridoxine
- Diuretics in the second half of the cycle
- Serotonin reuptake inhibitors such as fluoxetine.

Hormones

- Oral contraceptive pills to maintain a uniform hormonal milieu
- Progestogen
- Bromocriptine to relieve breast symptoms
- Gonadotropin-releasing hormone (GnRH) agonists to suppress gonadal steroids.

NURSING MANAGEMENT

- Encourage patient to set goals for reduction of symptoms such as mood swings, crying, binge eating and day-to-day stressors
- Teach positive coping measures, involve and encourage family members such as spouse or children for assistance and care
- Encourage use of exercise, meditation and creative activities to reduce stress
- Provide instructions about the desired effects of prescribed medications.

115. PRETERM BABY

DEFINITION

A baby born before 37 completed weeks of gestation calculating from the first day of last menstrual period.

CAUSES

- Maternal history of preterm birth, spontaneous abortion, incompetent cervix or other uterine anomalies
- Multiple gestation
- Infection
- Premature rupture of membranes
- Adolescent pregnancy
- Polyhydramnios
- Oligohydramnios
- Preeclampsia
- Placental insufficiency and rhesus disease
- Maternal habits such as cigarette smoking, substance abuse and poor diet.

PHYSICAL CHARACTERISTICS

- Relative to his/her size the preterm baby has a big head, small thoracic area and large abdomen
- Soft skull bones with wide sutures and large fontanels
- The head circumference disproportionately exceeds that of chest
- The skin is thin, red and shiny due to lack of subcutaneous fat, and covered by plentiful lanugo and vernix caseosa
- Muscle tone poor
- Plantar creases are not visible before 34 weeks
- The testicles are undescended, the labia majora are not in contact
- There is tendency of herniation
- The nails are not grown up to the fingertips.

COMPLICATIONS

- Asphyxia because of immaturity
- Hypothermia
- Pulmonary syndromes such as pulmonary edema, intraalveolar hemorrhage and respiratory distress syndrome.
- Cerebral hemorrhage
- Fetal shock following rough handling or rough resuscitation
- Heart failure

- Edema
- Infections such as bronchopneumonia, meningitis and gastroenteritis
- Jaundice because of hepatic insufficiency and inadequate excretion of bile
- Anemia due to lack of stored iron, hypofunction of bone marrow and excessive hemolysis
- Retrolental fibroplasias (retinopathy of prematurity).

MANAGEMENT OF THE PRETERM NEONATE

Immediate Management

- Cord to be clamped quickly to prevent hypervolemia and development of hyperbilirubinemia
- Cord length to be 10–12 cm for use if exchange transfusion is required
- Air passage to be cleared of mucus promptly
- Adequate oxygenation to be provided (not exceeding 35%)
- The baby should be wrapped including head in a sterile warm towel to prevent hypothermia and its sequelae such as hypoxia, hypoglycemia, and metabolic acidosis
- Injection of vitamin K to be given to prevent hemorrhagic problems.

Intensive Care

- Monitor body temperature at regular intervals to prevent hypothermia and hyperthermia the temperature should be maintained between 35.6° and 37.2°C (96–99°F)
- Smaller babies are to be nursed in incubator where temperature and humidity can be regulated
- Oxygen to be administered to tide over the initial cyanotic phase and later to maintain desirable level of saturation
- Prophylactic antibiotic therapy
- Nutrition: Gavage feeding or parenteral nutrition depending on the gestation age and vigor of the baby.

Nursing Care

- Temperature twice daily or according to institutional policy
- Weight every day to know if the newborn is over hydrated or under hydrated
- Constant observation and monitoring in the first 48 hours
- Visitation by mother
- Providing manually expressed breast milk to baby until able to suck and swallow
- Observer for signs of progress such as:
  - Color pink all the time
  - Smooth and regular breathing
  - Increasing vigor exhibited by limb movements and cry
  - Progressive gain in weight after the 1st week.
- Teach mother about the feeding to be continued, vitamin supplements, immunization and check-up.

116. PRETERM LABOR

Definition

A labor that begins spontaneously after the gestation of viability (24–28 weeks) and before 37 completed weeks of pregnancy.

Incidence

Of all pregnancies, 5–10% end in preterm labor.

Etiology

In many cases, no cause is found.

Pregnancy Factors

- Infections such as urinary tract infection (UTI)
- Antepartum hemorrhage
- Uterine overdistension, e.g. hydramnios
- Uterine anomalies, e.g. fibroids
- Past history of preterm labor

- Maternal illness, e.g. chronic illness or high fever
- Premature rupture of membranes
- Fetal growth retardation, e.g. in pregnancy-induced hypertension (PIH)
- Fetal anomalies, e.g. congenital malformations.

Epidemiologic Factors

- Maternal age: Extremes of reproductive age
- Poor nutrition
- Low socioeconomic status
- Tobacco consumption.

Psychological Factors

- Coitus: Release of prostaglandins
- Unwanted pregnancies.

Diagnosis

- Regular uterine contractions at intervals of 5–8 minutes
- Progressive dilatation and effacement of cervix:
  Cervical dilatation of > 2 cm.
  Cervical effacement of > 80%.
- Premature rupture of membranes
- Passage of blood and mucus (show)
- Low backache and pain about every 10 minutes
- Intestinal cramps with diarrhea at times.

Preventive Measures

In many cases there are no preventive measures:
- Good antenatal care and treatment of women with potential for placental insufficiency
- Timely rest for women with multiple pregnancy and polyhydramnios
- Shirodkar cervical sutures for women with history of cervical incompetence
- Conservative management for problem of rupture of membranes may allow the leak in the membranes to seal

- Treatment of rhesus (Rh) incompatibility
- Improvement of general health and nutritional status.

Management

Careful clinical evaluation of maternal and fetal condition is to be done including preliminary investigations:
- Ultrasound to ascertain:
  - Fetal number and congenital abnormalities
  - Fetal presentation
  - Estimated fetal weight
  - Placental site
  - Volume of the amniotic fluid
  - Fetal well-being by biophysical parameters.
- Sedation and hydration for 30–60 minutes
- Antibiotics if there is any infective pathology
- Corticosteroid therapy to enhance fetal maturity
- Tocolytics after excluding contraindications such as pulmonary or cardiac disease, intrauterine (IUGR), and premature rupture of membrane (PROM).

Labor and Delivery

Once preterm delivery appears inevitable, mode of delivery and expected neonatal outcome should be discussed with the patient and the husband.

During Labor and Monitor

- Uterine activity, cervical status and presentation of fetus
- Fetal heart sounds and characteristics by continuous electronic monitoring
- Maternal health.

Delivery

- Cesarean section if breech presentation
- Forceps or cesarean section according to standard obstetric indications
- Neonatologist in attendance.

Neonatal Outcome

Premature infants are likely to have a variety of problems in the neonatal period with the risk of complications being proportionate to the degree of prematurity.

The likely problems are:
- Maintenance of body temperature
- Oral feeding
- Risk for infection
- Maintenance of respiration.

Neonates will need to be managed in a neonatal intensive care unit.

117. PROLONGED LABOR

Definition

A labor is arbitrarily defined as being prolonged when its duration exceeds 18–24 hours in a primipara and 14 hours in a multipara.

Incidence

Prolonged labor is expected to occur in about 8% of all primigravidae and in about 2% of all multigravidae.

Causes of Prolonged Labor

First stage (failure of cervical dilation).
- Fault in power: Abnormal uterine contraction such as uterine inertia or incoordinate uterine contraction
- Fault in the passage: Contracted pelvis, cervical dystocia, pelvic tumor, or even full bladder
- Fault in the passenger: Malposition and malpresentation; congenital anomalies of the fetus such as hydrocephalus, deflexed head and minor degrees of disproportion.

Second stage (sluggish or non-descent of the presenting part).
- Fault in power: Uterine inertia, inability to bear down, epidural analgesia and constriction ring

- Fault in passage: Cephalopelvic disproportion, android pelvis, contracted pelvis, undue resistance of the pelvic floor due to spasm or scarring, soft tissue pelvic tumor
- Fault in the passenger: Malposition, malpresentation, big baby and congenital malformation of the baby.

Diagnosis

- Abnormal cervicograph on partograph denoting abnormal cervical dilation
- Prolonged latent phase (until cervical dilation of 3–4 cm)
- Prolonged active phase (cervical dilation from 4 to 10 cm)
- Secondary arrest of dilation (2 hours of arrest in cervical dilation is diagnostic)
- Sluggish or non-descent of the presenting part even after full dilatation of the cervix
- Variable degrees of molding and caput formation in cephalic presentation.

Dangers

Maternal

- Maternal exhaustion and shock
- Uterine atony and postpartum hemorrhage
- Soft tissue injury
- Infections and subin
- Puerperal sepsis.

Fetal

- Intrauterine hypoxia
- Low Apgar score at birth
- Infection after the rupture of membranes
- Intracranial stress and hemorrhage due to excessive molding
- Trauma from operative deliveries.

Management

First stage

- Monitoring fetal heart rate (FHR) and uterine action
- Amniotomy and/or oxytocin infusion

- Pain relief by injection or epidural anesthesia
- Cesarean section when vaginal delivery is unsafe.

Second stage
- Fetal heart rate monitoring
- Assisted vaginal delivery or cesarean delivery may be necessary when there is evidence of cephalopelvic disproportion.

118. PSYCHIATRIC DISORDERS DURING PREGNANCY

Mood and anxiety disorders are common in women during their childbearing years. Pregnancy and postpartum periods are considered to be relatively high-risk times for women with preexisting psychiatric illnesses, especially for depressive episodes. The prevalence of depression has been reported to be between 10 and 16% during pregnancy. For women with bipolar disorder, pregnancy and postpartum period have even higher risk. Rates of relapse are estimated at 30 to 50% during the postpartum period. The course of panic disorder can be variable with some studies reporting an improvement of symptoms and others reporting a worsening. In obsessive compulsive disorder, symptoms typically worsen during pregnancy. Some studies suggest an initial onset of symptoms during pregnancy. Special considerations are needed when psychotic disorders present during pregnancy.

STRESS AND PREGNANCY

Pregnancy either induces or exacerbates pre-existing stress and in turn stress seems to have a negative effect on pregnancy, especially in the first trimester. The period of greatest stress during pregnancy, the first trimester, is also the period of highest rate of pregnancy loss. According to records, in 17th and 18th centuries, medical profession had the belief that abortion occurred as a reaction to wrath, fear, grief, joy and even disagreeable odors.

MAJOR DEPRESSION IN PREGNANCY

Major depression is twice common in women than in men and frequently manifests during the childbearing years. Although pregnancy has traditionally been considered a time of emotional well-being for women conferring protection against psychiatric disorders, at least one prospective study describes rates of major and minor depression as approximately 10%. For women with past history of mood disorder, discontinuation of antidepressant medicines causes reappearance of clinically significant symptoms. It has been observed that in about one-third of depressed pregnant women, this represents the first episode of major depression.

Other risk factors of antenatal depression include marital discord or dissatisfaction, inadequate psychological supports, recent adverse life events, lower socio-economic status, and unwanted pregnancy. High rates of relapse occur after discontinuation of maintenance pharmacological treatment in non-gravid women. In women who have been diagnosed as having recurrent depression prior to conception and in whom antidepressant medications have been discontinued, rates of relapse can be up to 75% and can be seen frequently during the first trimester. Milder forms of depression during pregnancy can be missed. Pregnant women may have many clinical signs and symptoms overlapping with those seen in major depression (e.g. sleep and appetite disturbance, decreased libido and low energy). Some medical disorders commonly seen during pregnancy, such as anemia, gestational diabetes and thyroid dysfunction, may be associated with depressive symptoms and may complicate the diagnosis of depression during pregnancy. Clinical features that may support the diagnosis of major depression include loss of pleasure, feelings of guilt and hopelessness and suicidal thoughts. Suicidal ideation and self-injurious ideation are often reported; however, the risk of self-injurious or suicidal behavior appears to be low in the population of women who develop depression during pregnancy.

RISKS OF UNTREATED DEPRESSION IN THE MOTHER

The risks of untreated depression in the mother include:
- Risk of self-injurious or suicidal behavior.
- Inadequate self-care.
- Poor compliance with prenatal care.
- Decreased appetite and consequently lower than expected weight gain in pregnancy leading to negative pregnancy outcomes.

- Women with depression are also more likely to use either alcohol or illicit drugs, which are behaviors that further increase the risk to the fetus.
- Some studies suggests that maternal depression itself may adversely affect the developing fetus.

IMPACT OF MATERNAL DEPRESSION ON THE FAMILY

- Interpersonal difficulties.
- Disruption in mother-baby interactions and attachment affecting infant's development.
- Studies have also shown that depression during pregnancy significantly increases a woman's risk for post-partum depression.
- Antenatal depression thus have significant adverse effects that may extend beyond pregnancy and have more significant long-term effects on her psychological functioning.

BIPOLAR DISORDER

Pregnancy and especially the postpartum period are stressful periods for women and increases the risk of relapse for women with bipolar disorder. Bipolar disorder affects 0.5 – 1.5% of individuals. The typical age of onset is late adolescence or early adulthood, placing women at risk for episodes throughout their reproductive years. The presentation of a woman with bipolar disorder may resemble a depressive disorder, behavioral deregulation, or general medical disorders. It is important to access history of hypomania or mania when determining diagnosis in any woman presenting with psychological symptoms. Symptoms of post-partum psychosis tend to differ from the symptoms typically seen in bipolar mania. Therefore if postpartum psychosis is actually a manifestation of bipolar disorder, accurate diagnosis depends on knowledge of these differences.

ANXIETY DISORDER

Hormonal changes during pregnancy such as increased prolactin, oxytocin and cortisol may contribute to the suppression of stress response that occurs during this period. Studies have suggested that women with anxiety related to pregnancy may be at greater risk for postpartum depression.

PSYCHOTIC DISORDERS

Women with psychotic disorders are at an increased risk of obstetric complications. Recent studies have confirmed earlier findings of low fertility in women with schizophrenia. Psychotic relapse during pregnancy is rare, but women with a history of mood disorders (affective psychosis) are at a high risk for post-partum relapse.

TREATMENT OF PSYCHIATRIC DISORDERS DURING PREGNANCY

Specific Concerns

Psychotropic medications readily cross the placenta. Therefore following factors must be considered before starting psychotropic medications.
- Teratogenesis.
- Toxicity to the neonate.
- Neurobehavioral sequelae.
- Risk of medication discontinuation.
- Risk of no treatment.

Treatment of Specific Psychiatric Disorders

1. **Major depression**
   - **Psychotherapies**
     Interpersonal therapy (ITP).
     Interpersonal therapy is useful for four major problems with respect to human psychosocial functioning – grief, interpersonal disputes, role transitions, and interpersonal deficits. This treatment is needed considering the importance of interpersonal relationships in couples expecting a baby, and the significant role of transitions take place during pregnancy and subsequent to delivery. ITP is ideal for the treatment of the depressed pregnant women.
   - Antidepressant therapy
     Antidepressants during pregnancy are indicated for women whose symptoms interfere with maternal well-being and functioning. Medication choice depends on prior treatment

response. During pregnancy fluoxetine is usually the first line antidepressant choice. Other first line choices include nortriptyline and desipramine as they are less anticholinergic and therefore less likely to exacerbate orthostatic hypotension during pregnancy.

2. **Bipolar disorder**
   Special treatment options need to be considered due to the risk of fetal malformation when certain mood stabilizers are used during first trimester of pregnancy. Neurobehavioral teratogenicity and neonatal toxicity are also possible. Careful treatment management is necessary to reduce risks to the fetus/neonate and to effectively manage bipolar disorder in the mother.

3. **Anxiety disorders**
   Psychotherapy is found to be beneficial for panic disorder and obsessive compulsive disorder in both pregnant and non-pregnant women. Tapering of medication may be possible with adjunctive treatment with behavior therapy during pregnancy. For mild cases of OCD, pregnant women may do well with behavior techniques. However, moderate to severe symptoms may require maintenance pharmacological treatment.

   - Anxiolytics
     A slow taper of anti-panic medications over a period of two weeks may be possible in mild cases of panic disorder. However, maintenance medication may be necessary in patients with severe panic disorder. In such cases fluoxetine or a tricyclic antidepressant is a good treatment option. In patients who do not respond to their antidepressants, benzodiazepine may be considered. Clomipramine may also be considered but may aggravate orthostatic hypotension.

4. **Psychotic disorders**
   Neuroleptics should be considered as psychosis can be an obstetric and medical emergency.

119. PSYCHIATRIC DISORDERS IN PUERPERIUM

Several psychiatric disorders may arise in the postpartal period. These are classified as subclasses under mood disorders with a postpartum onset and include:

- Postpartum blues
- Postpartum depression (PPD)
- Postpartum psychosis (PPP).

Postpartum Blues

An adjustment reaction with a depressed mood occurring in 30–50% of new mothers. Blues typically occur in the early postpartum period, often within 10 days after delivery.

Etiology

- Hormonal levels after birth and adjustment to motherhood
- More common in primiparas.

Symptoms

- Feeling overwhelmed, tearful and fatigued
- Irritable, oversensitive and anxious
- Poor concentration or poor appetite
- Episodic tearfulness.

Management

- Adequate rest and family support
- Education of family to protect the mother and baby, if symptoms do not resolve quickly or serious symptoms appear.

Postpartum Depression

Postpartum depression affects 5–10% of women. The onset is slow and generally later than blues, often around 4th week postpartum and may occur any time within the 1st year.

Symptoms

- Depressed mood or loss of interest or pleasure
- Weight loss or gain
- Psychomotor agitation or retardation
- Fatigue and loss of energy

- Feelings of worthlessness
- Impaired concentration
- Intrusive thoughts of death or suicide
- Physically and mentally drained and exhausted.

Management

- Counseling and explanation
- Domestic help and extended family support
- Sedatives or tranquillisers for short time
- Resistant cases may be managed by a psychiatrist.

Postpartum Psychosis

Postpartum psychosis is the most serious psychiatric condition in the postpartum period. It occurs in one to two women per 1,000 births.

Symptoms

This condition generally appears after the 2nd week postpartum and include:

- Sleep and eating disturbances
- Agitation and confusion
- Difficulty remembering or concentrating
- Extreme mood lability
- Insomnia and irritability
- Delusions and hallucinations.

Risk Factors

- Previous history of postpartum psychosis
- History of bipolar or manic depressive disorders
- Family history of psychiatric disorders
- If not treated, may result in suicide or infanticide.

Treatment

- Antipsychotic medications
- Psychotherapy.

Prognosis

With proper treatment, majority of mothers may recover, however, there is high-risk for recurrence in subsequent pregnancies.

Nursing Implications

Most symptoms occur after discharge, therefore health teaching before going home should include instructions to family that development of depressive symptoms should prompt them to seek immediate treatment.

120. PUBERTY

Definition

Puberty is the period during which secondary sexual characteristics develop and the capability of sexual reproduction is attained. It is the period which links childhood with adulthood. Normal pubertal development occurs in a predictable, orderly sequence over a definite time frame.

Physical Changes

In girls pubertal development typically takes place over 4–5 years. The most common order is:
- Beginning of growth spurt
- Breast budding (thelarche)
- Pubic and axillary hair growth (adrenarche)
- Growth in height
- Menstruation (menarche).

Changes are usually completed between the age of 10 and 16 years. In male, pubertal sexual maturation is based on genital size and pubic hair development. The changes are:
- Testicular enlargement
- Increase in length and diameter of penis
- Growth of curly hair around the base of penis and over the genital area

- Symmetric or asymmetric gynecomastia
- Appearance of mature sperm in microscopic urinalysis.

Hormonal Changes

Hypothalamopituitary gonadal axis:
- Increase in luteinizing hormone (LH) and follicle-stimulating hormone (FSH) secretion. In boys, nocturnal increase in gonadotropins accompanied by simultaneous increase in testosterone
- Increase in adrenal androgen secretion that causes increased sebum formation, pubic and axillary hair growth and change in voice
- Increased secretion of estradiol by ovaries in girls
- Increased testosterone secretion from testes in boys
- Growth hormone secretion increases along with gonadotropins at the onset of puberty.

Stages of Pubertal Development in Girls (Tanner Stages)

Stage 1

Prepubertal stage: No palpable breast tissue, with the areola generally less than 2 cm in diameter. Nipples may be inverted, flat or raised. No pubic hair.

Stage 2

Breast budding occurs with a visible and palpable mound of breast tissue. The areola begins to enlarge and nipples develop to varying degree. Sparse, long hair on either side of labia majora.

Stage 3

Further growth of entire breast tissue, darker coarser and early hair over the mons pubis.

Stage 4

Secondary mound of areola and papillae appear projecting over the general breast tissue. Adult type hair covers the mons pubis.

Stage 5

Areola recessed to general contour of breast. Adult hair with an inverse triangle distribution is seen over the mons pubis.

Menarche

The onset of first menstruation in life is called menarche. It may occur any time between 10 and 16 years, the average time being 13 years. There is endometrial proliferation due to ovarian estrogen and when the level drops temporarily the endometrium sheds and bleeding occurs. The first period is usually anovular. Ovulation may be irregular for a variable period following menarche. It may take about 2 years for regular ovulation to occur. The menses may be irregular to start with and it may take about 2 years for regular ovulation to occur.

Growth

Growth in height in an adolescent girl occurs mainly due to hormones. The important hormones are growth hormone, estrogen and insulinlike growth factor.

Genital Organ Changes

Ovaries: Shape changes from elongated to avoid and becomes bulky due to follicular enlargement and proliferation of stromal cells.

Uterus

Enlargement of the body of uterus occurs, uterine body to cervix ratio becomes 1:1 when menarche occurs and thereafter rapid enlargement of the body occurs so that the ratio becomes 2:1.

Vagina

The epithelium becomes thick with many layers. The cells become rich with glycogen due to increased estrogen. Doderlein's bacilli appear, which convert glycogen into lactic acid. The vaginal pH becomes acidic ranging between 4 and 5.

Vulva

- Vulva becomes more reactive to steroid hormones
- Mons pubis and labia minora—increase in size.

Breast Changes

Marked proliferation of duct systems and deposition of fat occurs under the influence of estrogen. Breasts become prominent and round. Under the influence of progesterone, the development of acini increases considerably.

Common Disorders of Puberty

- Precocious puberty
- Delayed puberty
- Menstrual abnormalities (amenorrhea, menorrhagia, dysmenorrhea)
- Others (infection, neoplasm, hirsutism, etc.).

121. PUERPERAL SEPSIS

Definition

Puerperal sepsis or postpartum infection is an infection of the genital tract, which occurs as a complication of delivery.

Incidence

Puerperal sepsis affects 2–10% of patients. It is 5–10 times higher following cesarean section.

Common Infections (Table 121.1)

- Pelvic infections:
  - Endometritis
  - Pelvic cellulitis
  - Pelvic abscess

Table 121.1: Common postpartum infections.

Infection	Clinical findings	Management and teaching
Wound site infection (Cesarean wound, episiotomy wound and lacerations)	Edema Skin discoloraton, redness Warmth Tenderness Seropurulent discharge Wound edge weparation Fever Lochia color change Pain	Antibiotics Comfort measures such as frequent perineal care, sitz bths and warm compress Open and drain abdominal wound Teaching: • Frequent pad changes • Good handwashing technique
		• Wipe front to back Adequate diet and fluids
Endometritis	Uterine distention and tenderness Abdominal pain Malaise, lethargy Nausea and vomiting Anorexia Foul-smelling lochia Fever, chills Tachycardia Anemia Increased leukocytes Increased erythrocyte sedimentation rate (ESR)	Broad-spectrum antibiotics Rest Hydration
Mastitis	Sudden onset of flu like symptoms Chills, fever Tachycardia Headache, malaise Nausea, vomiting Unilateral breast pain Warmth, swelling and redness Axillary adenopathy Red, inflamed,	Analgesics Antibiotics Complete emptying of breasts Moist heat or ice to local area Hydration Analgesics Teaching on preventive measures: • Proper infant postition for correct latch on and sucking
	v-shaped area on breasts Leukocytosis	• Breastfeed every 2–3 hours • Avoid tight clothing

Contd...

Contd...

Infection	Clinical findings	Management and teaching
		• Avoid practices that put pressure on breasts, e.g. sleeping on stomach, resting infant on stomach while supine, stopping milk flow while pressing on areola • Empty breasts completely (avoid stasis) • Manually express milk, if duct is blocked • Avoid cracked nipples • Use larger bra for comfort
Thrombo-phlebitis deep vein thrombosis (DVT)	Rapid onset Severe pain and swelling Redness, warmth and tenderness in calves or legs Hardness or nodules along vein Varicosities Positive Homans' sign	Anticoagulation therapy with heparin Antibiotics Rest Hydration Analgesia Monitoring coagulation profile, prothrombin time (PT) and partial thromboplastin time (PTT) Evaluation of respiratory status q2-4 h
Urinary tract infection (UTI)	Manifestations of lower UTI: • Dysuria • Frequency • Urgency • Low grade fever • Bladder overdistension Suprapubic pain Urinary retention Hematuria Pyuria Manifestations of upper UTI: • Flank pain • Costovertebral tenderness • Bacteriuria > 100,000/mL	Antibiotic therapy Analgesics Hydration Teaching • Hygienic measures • Avoid carbonated drinks (increases alkalinity) • Wipe from front to back • Urinate frequently • Increase fluid intake

- Hematomas
- Septic pelvic thrombophlebitis.
- Extra pelvic infections:
  - Urinary tract infections
  - Episiotomy site infection
  - Mastitis
  - Thrombophlebitis (legs)
  - Peritonitis
  - Septicemia.

Predisposing Factors

- Cesarean delivery (20 times greater than vaginal delivery)
- Prolonged rupture of membranes (> 24 h)
- Prolonged labor with frequent vaginal examinations
- Internal fetal monitoring (fetal scalp electrodes, intrauterine pressure catheter)
- Dehydration and ketoacidosis during labor
- Traumatic operative delivery
- Hemorrhage (antepartum or postpartum)
- Retained bits of placental tissue or membranes
- Placenta previa: Placental site lying close to the internal os.

122. RECTOVAGINAL FISTULA

Definition

An abnormal communication between the rectum and vagina with involuntary escape of flatus and/or feces into the vagina is called rectovaginal fistula.

Causes

- Incomplete healing or unrepaired complete perineal tear
- Pressure necrosis, infection and sloughing following obstructed labor
- Instrumental injury following destructive operation

- Unrecognized trauma following surgeries such as perineorrhaphy, vaginal tubectomy, posterior colpotomy and reconstruction of vagina
- Fall on sharp pointed object
- Diseases affecting vagina, rectum and nearby structures such as:
  - Lymphogranuloma venereum of vagina
  - Tuberculosis of vagina
  - Diverticulitis of sigmoid colon; abscess bursts into the vagina
  - Crohn's disease involving the anal canal or lower rectum.
- Congenital defect; anal canal opens in the vagina.

Diagnosis

- Involuntary escape of flatus and/or faces in to the vagina
- Clinical examination of vagina and rectum
- Dye examination: Methylene blue dye introduced in the rectum escapes out through fistula into the vagina.

Treatment

Prevention
- Good intranatal care
- Identification of complete perineal tear (CPT) and timely repair.

Definitive
- Repair of the fistula: Depending on the location of the fistula, repair may done in one, two or three stages.

Nursing Implications

- Care to provide adequate perineal support while delivering the baby
- Thorough examination of the perineum and vagina following delivery and repair of episiotomy or laceration
- Support and encouragement to patient who has an embarrassing problem
- Instructions to client and spouse regarding the surgery and care to be taken following surgery.

123. RESPIRATORY DISTRESS IN NEWBORNS

Definition

Respiratory distress is defined as a respiratory rate of more than 60 per minute and it is usually associated with accessory muscle use, intercostal and subcostal indrawing, and an expiratory grunt. Imperfect aeration of the lung leads to the condition.

Causes of Respiratory Distress

1. Airway disease:
   - Respiratory distress syndrome
   - Pneumonia
   - Meconium aspiration syndrome
   - Transient tachypnea of the newborn
   - Lung hypoplasia
   - Tracheoesophageal fistula.
2. Airway obstruction:
   - Choanal atresia
   - Pierre Robin syndrome.
3. Space-occupying lesions:
   - Diaphragmatic hernia
   - Congenital emphysema, pulmonary edema
   - Pneumothorax.
4. Others:
   - Congenital heart failure
   - Metabolic acidosis, hypoglycemia.

Assessment of the Neonate

History

- Gestational age
- Risk factors for sepsis
- Presence of meconium in liquor at the time of delivery
- Use of positive pressure ventilation during resuscitation.

Nursing Implications

- Respiratory rates in newborns between 60 and 70 breaths per minute require continuous observation by the nurse

- The infant breaths faster when moving, irritated or crying and hence respiratory rate should be taken when the infant is calm or quiet
- A rapid respiratory rate in a quiet infant may be a temporary adjustment to extrauterine life. However, the nurse must be alert to the development of additional symptoms such as nasal flaring, grunting or intercostal retractions that would indicate development of a more serious condition
- The nurse should monitor skin color and capillary refill of both upper and lower extremities to complete the nursing assessment of the efficiency of the respiratory system
- The nurse must determine whether the absence of additional symptoms indicates that the infant is approaching respiratory stability.

124. RESPIRATORY DISTRESS SYNDROME

Definition

Respiratory distress syndrome (RDS) is a condition that is predominantly due to lung surfactant deficiency characterized by collapsed alveoli and low lung volume. The disease process worsens with decreasing gestational age.

Incidence

About 0.5% of all newborns are affected by RDS.

Pathogenesis

The lack of surfactant results in high surface tension, reduced lung compliance, atelectasis and impaired gaseous exchange in the alveoli. As the condition progresses, cyanosis and right-to-left shunt through ductus arteriosus develop.

Clinical Presentation

- Respiratory distress occurs within the first few hours of life
- Respiratory rate more than 60/minute
- Rib retraction

- Expiratory grunt
- Cyanosis.

Investigations

- Chest X-ray:
  - Fine mottling of the lungs due to the collapsed areas
  - Ground grass appearance of the lung fields.

Prevention

- Administration of betamethasone to patients anticipating preterm delivery before 34 weeks
- Assessment of lung maturity before premature induction of labor
- Prevention of fetal hypoxia in diabetic mothers.

Treatment

- Baby to be placed in intensive neonatal care unit (NICU) and nursed in warm incubator with high humidity
- Periodical endotracheal suctioning, minimum disturbance and handling
- Adequate warmed, humidified oxygen in concentration of 35–40% under positive pressure
- Continuous positive airway pressure (CPAP) if the oxygen tension (pO_2) cannot be maintained above 50 mm Hg
- Prevention and treatment of infection
- Correction of hypovolemia with albumin or other colloid solution
- Correction of anemia and electrolyte imbalance if present.
- Frequent monitoring of pO_2, partial pressure of carbon dioxide (pCO_2) and pH; correction of acidosis with sodium bicarbonate
- Surfactant therapy: Direct tracheal instillation
- Maintenance of adequate nutrition by intravenous (IV) route or intragastric feeding.

Complications

- Intraventricular hemorrhage
- Bronchopulmonary dysplasia
- Pulmonary hemorrhage
- Pneumothorax

- Retrolental fibroplasia
- Neurological abnormalities.

125. RESUSCITATION OF THE NEWBORNS

Resuscitation is a procedure done in delivery room for newborns who fail to undergo normal process of transition. If the newborn does not establish spontaneous respirations within 60 seconds, appropriate resuscitation must not be delayed.

AIMS OF RESUSCITATION

- To establish and maintain clear airway, ventilation and oxygenation
- To ensure effective circulation
- To correct acidosis
- To prevent hypothermia, hypoglycemia and hemorrhage.

Degrees of Resuscitation

1. Apgar score 7–10, blood pH 7.20–7.40:
   - Suction oropharynx, then nose to clear airway and provide tactile stimulation
   - Dry infant and provide warmth using warm blanket, on mother's abdomen or radiant warmer.
2. Apgar score 4–6, blood pH 7.09–7.19 (moderate acidosis):
   - Dry infant
   - Place under radiant warmer
   - Suction oropharynx and nose, provide tactile stimulation and freeflow oxygen by mask
   - If heart rate is below 100, begin positive pressure ventilation by face mask attached to an anesthesia bag or self-inflating bag, and provide 100% oxygen
   - Continue free-flow oxygen, after infant has established good respiratory effort.
3. Apgar score 0–3 and blood pH 7.0 or below (severe acidosis):
   - Suction and clear the airway
   - Dry the infant

- Place under radiant warmer
- Begin positive pressure ventilation
- Perform endotracheal intubation if positive pressure ventilation (PPV) does not establish respirations or prove successful
- Begin cardiac massage if heart rate is less than 60 after 30 seconds.

Resuscitation Equipment and Articles

It is essential that resuscitation equipment is always available and is in good working order and that personnel in attendance at delivery of a baby are familiar with the equipment and resuscitation techniques.

Suctioning Articles

- Bulb syringe
- DeLee mucus trap with #10 Fr catheter or mechanical suction
- Suction catheters # 6, 8 and 10.

Bag and Mask Equipment (Fig. 125.1)

- Infant resuscitation bag with pressure release valve or pressure gauge with a reservoir to deliver 90–100% oxygen
- Face mask with cushioned rims
- Oral airways: newborn and premature sizes
- Oxygen with flow meter and tubing.

Intubation Equipment (Fig. 125.2)

- Laryngoscope with straight blades No. '0' and No. '1'
- Endotracheal tubes sizes 2.5, 3.0, 3.5 and 4 mm internal diameter
- Stylet
- Scissors.

Medications

- Epinephrine 1:10,000 ampoules.
- Naloxone hydrochloride.

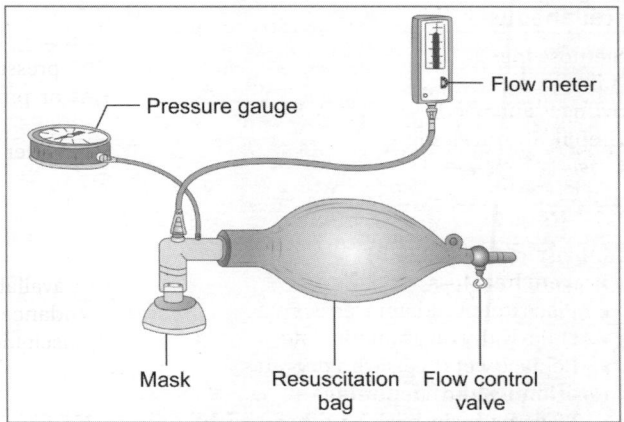

Fig. 125.1: Bag and mask equipment for ventilation.

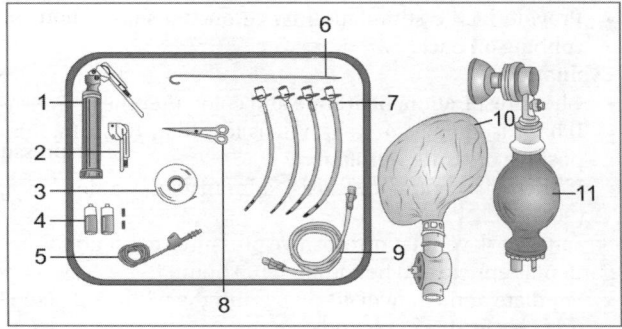

Fig. 125.2: Intubation equipment. **1.** Laryngoscope with blade; **2.** Laryngoscope blade; **3.** Roll of adhesive tape; **4.** Batteries for laryngoscope; **5.** Suction catheter; **6.** Stylet; **7.** Endotracheal tubes; **8.** Scissors; **9.** Oxygen tubing; **10.** Oxygen reservoir; **11.** Oxygen bag and mask.

- Volume expander; 5% albumin, normal saline, Ringer's lactate.
- Sodium bicarbonate 4.2%.
- Dextrose 10%.
- Sterile water.

Miscellaneous

- Stethoscope
- Adhesive tape
- Syringes and needles
- Umbilical cord clamp
- Gloves.

Procedure

1. Initial steps **(Fig. 125.3)**
   Prevent heat loss
   - Place under radiant warmer
   - Quickly dry off amniotic fluid
   - Replace wet sheets with dry ones.

   Positioning and suctioning
   - Place baby on back with head slightly down (15° tilt) and neck slightly extended
   - Suction mouth, then nose
   - Provide tactile stimulation twice on the sole of foot or by rubbing on back.

   Evaluation
   - Check respiration, heart rate and color after the above steps
   - If baby is apnoeic or heart rate is less than 100/min, initiate positive pressure ventilation
   - If there is central cyanosis, administer free-flow oxygen (90%).

2. Bag and mask ventilation/positive pressure ventilation.
   If infant is apneic and heart rate < 100 bpm:
   - Ventilate at the rate of 40–50 per minute with 20–25 cm H_2O pressure for 15–20 seconds
   - Have an assistant to evaluate heart rate.

   Evaluation
   - Heart rate > 100/minute and spontaneous breathing, discontinue bagging
   - Heart rate 60–100 and not increasing continue ventilation
   - Heart rate below 80 per minute, start chest compressions
   - Heart rate below 60 per minute, start intubation and medication, in addition to bagging and chest compressions.

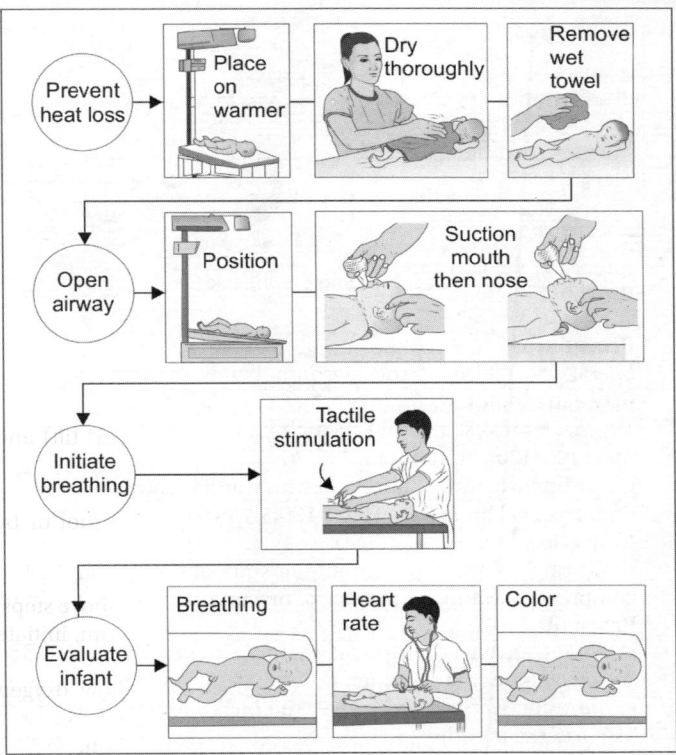

Fig. 125.3: Newborn resuscitation (initial steps).

3. Chest compressions **(Figs. 125.4A and B)**.

    Rhythmic compressions of the sternum that compresses the heart against the spine to increase the intrathoracic pressure and circulation of blood to vital organs. Chest compressions must always be accompanied by ventilation with 100% oxygen.

    Indication

    Heart rate less than 60 per minute or 60–80 and not increasing after bagging with 100% oxygen for 15–30 seconds.

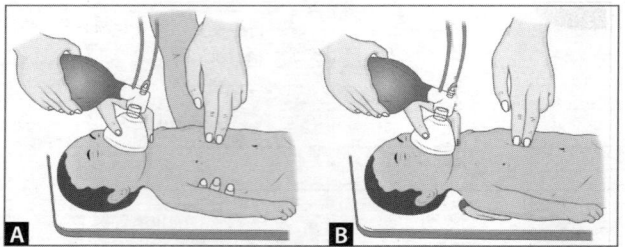

Figs. 125.4A and B: Chest compressions, two finger method.

Procedure

Site: Lower third of the sternum below an imaginary line between nipples.

Depth: Depress sternum ½–¾ inch.

Rate: 100–120 per minute.

Co-ordinate heart compression with ventilation.

4. Endotracheal intubation **(Figs. 125.5A and B)**.

   Indication

   Heart rate below 60 per minute in spite of bagging and chest compressions and/or presence of meconium in amniotic fluid.

   Procedure

   - Infant on back with head slightly extended with a rolled towel under the shoulder
   - Introduce laryngoscope over the baby's tongue at the right corner of mouth
   - Advance 2–3 cm until the epiglottis is seen and elevate epiglottis to view vocal cords
   - Suction secretions if needed
   - Pass endotracheal tube 1.5–2 cm into the trachea, hold it firmly and withdraw the laryngoscope gently
   - Attach endotracheal tube to bag and mask, and begin ventilation with oxygen.

5. Medications.

   Medications should be administered, if despite adequate ventilation with 100% oxygen and chest compressions, the heart rate does not increase above 80 bpm:

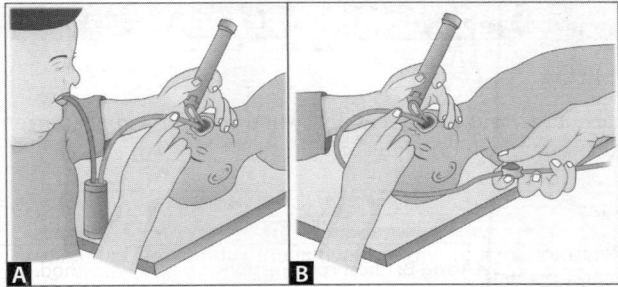

Figs. 125.5A and B: Endotracheal suctioning. **A.** Laryngoscope and DeLee mucus trap in place; **B.** Laryngoscope and suction catheter in place.

- Epinephrine or adrenaline: 0.1–0.3 mL/kg [intravenous (IV) or intratracheal (IT)]
- Volume expanders (whole blood, 5% albumin, normal saline, Ringer's lactate): 10 mL/kg (IV)
- Sodium bicarbonate: 2 mEq/kg (IV)
- Naloxone (Narcan): 0.25 mL/kg [IV/intramuscular (IM)/ subcutaneous (SQ) or IT]
- Dopamine: 5–20 mcg/kg/minute (IV).

6. Follow up care.
   - After stopping ventilation, place the baby gently between the mother's breasts with skin-to-skin contact so that he stays warm
   - Monitor the baby every 15 minutes. Reassure the mother that the baby will probably be well
   - Encourage mother to breast feed her baby as soon as they are ready, to prevent hypoglycemia.
   - Record the events/procedures performed in the labor record and baby's notes.

If the neonate continues to deteriorate despite effective resuscitation efforts, other possible causes that should be considered include depressed airways drive, airway malformations and congenital heart disease, and lung problems such as pneumothorax or diaphragmatic hernia.

126. RETAINED PLACENTA

Definition

A placenta is said to be retained when it is not expelled even 30 minutes after the birth of the baby.

Causes

- Retention of the separated placenta following exhaustive and prolonged labor
- Non-separation of the placenta due to atonicity of the uterus, e.g. over distension of uterus, bigger placental site, malformation of uterus
- Incarceration of separated placenta due to hour-glass contraction (constriction ring)
- Morbid adherence of placenta or placenta accreta (placenta is directly anchored to the myometrium).

Dangers

- Hemorrhage
- Shock due to blood loss and manipulation
- Puerperal sepsis.

Management

- During the 30 minutes following birth of baby, patient should be watched carefully for evidence of bleeding, either revealed or concealed, to note the signs of separation
- Expression and controlled traction if the placenta is separated and retained
- Unseparated retained placenta, which is uncomplicated, requires manual removal under general anesthesia:
  - General anesthesia would relax the constriction ring
  - During the attempt for manual removal, if placenta accreta is diagnosed management would be one of the following:
  - Hysterectomy in parous women.

- For women desiring to have another baby, treatment consists of cutting the umbilical cord as high as possible and leaving behind the placenta, which is expected to be autolyzed in due course of time.

127. RETROVERSION OF UTERUS

Definition

Retroversion is defined as a turning backward of the uterus with the long axes of the corpus and cervix in line in relation to the long axis of the birth canal. Retroflexion is a bending backwards of the corpus on the cervix at the level of internal os. The two conditions are usually present together and are referred to as retroversion-flexion or retrodisplacement.

Degrees

First degree: The fundus is vertical and pointing towards the sacral promontory.

Second degree: The fundus lies in the sacral hollow, but not below the internal os.

Third degree: The fundus lies below the level of internal os.

Causes

- Developmental defect
- Puerperal, due to stretched ligaments that fail to return to normal
- Prolapse, caused by traction following cystocele
- Fibroid in the uterine wall
- Pelvic adhesions.

Incidence

The condition is seen in 15–20% of normal women.

Signs and Symptoms

- Chronic premenstrual pelvic pain due to varicosities in broad ligament produced by the kinks

- Dyspareunia due to direct thrust by the penis against the retroflexed uterus or prolapsed ovaries lying in the pouch of Douglas
- Infertility as the external os is away from the seminal pool at the posterior fornix during coitus or it may be occluded by the anterior vaginal wall (in third-degree retroversion)
- Body of the uterus felt in the posterior fornix and cervix directed upwards and forwards on bimanual examination
- On speculum examination, the cervix is viewed easily and external os points forwards.

Prevention

- To empty the bladder regularly
- To increase the tone of pelvic muscles by regular exercise in postpartum period
- To encourage lying in prone position for 30–60 minutes twice daily in 2nd to 4th weeks postpartum.

Treatment

- Hodge-Smith pessary
- Surgical correction (ventrosuspension).

128. RHESUS INCOMPATIBILITY

Rhesus or Rh(D) incompatibility can occur when a woman with an Rh(D)-negative blood type carries a baby with Rh(D)-positive blood type.

Rhesus isoimmunization (production of immune antibodies in an individual in response to an antigen derived from another individual of the same species) can occur in the first pregnancy, but usually sensitization occurs in the first pregnancy and in subsequent pregnancies, isoimmunization causes destruction of fetal blood cells.

Mechanism of Isoimmunization

- Small amounts of the fetal Rh-positive blood may cross the placenta into the maternal circulation, this is treated as a foreign

body by the mother's immune system and antibodies are produced
- In subsequent pregnancies, these maternal immunoglobulin (IgG) antibodies may cross the placenta and destroy the erythrocytes of the fetus
- Sensitization may also occur following amniocentesis, abortion, antepartum hemorrhage and external cephalic version.

Effects on the Fetus

- Antibodies will not have any effect on Rh-negative fetus
- Lesser degree of destruction leads to hemolytic anemia
- Extensive destruction of red blood cells (RBCs) causes fetal death in utero.

Manifestations of Hemolytic Disease

1. Congenital anemia of the newborn: This is the mildest form of the disease. Anemia develops slowly as red cell destruction continues upto 6 weeks after which antibodies are not available.
2. Icterus gravis neonatorum: The baby is born alive without evidence of jaundice, but soon develops it within 24 hours of birth.
3. Hydrops fetalis: Extensive destruction of the fetal cells leads to severe anemia, tissue anoxemia and metabolic acidosis. Fetus develops generalized edema (hydrops fetalis), ascites and hydrothorax. Fetal death occurs sooner or later due to cardiac failure. The baby is either stillborn or macerated and even if born alive, dies soon after.

Prevention of Rh Isoimmunization

- Administration of Rh anti-D immunoglobulin (IgG) intramuscularly to the mother within 72 hours following childbirth and abortion
- Administration during pregnancy to mothers at risk, at 28 weeks and 34 weeks and again within 72 hours of birth of a Rh-negative baby.

129. RUPTURE OF UTERUS

Definition

Dissolution in the continuity of the uterine wall any time beyond 28 weeks of pregnancy is called rupture of the uterus.

Incidence

The incidence depends on the standards of obstetric care and varies from 1:500 to 1:4,000 with majority occurring in multiparae.

Classification

- Spontaneous rupture of intact uterus during pregnancy. Majority occur due to weakening of the uterine wall by previous operation such as myomectomy or cesarean section, or an old perforation, i.e. medical termination of pregnancy (MTP).
- Traumatic rupture: A rare occurrence from a fall, crushing accident or a blow on abdomen.
- Rupture during labor: Spontaneous rupture may be due to:
  - Overstretching of the lower uterine segment in obstructed labor
  - Defects such as weak uterine wall by scars of previous surgeries, e.g. cesarean section, myomectomy
  - Injudicious use of oxytocic drugs during labor.
- Rupture due to obstetric trauma: Obstetric interventions when the uterus has a scar from previous operation:
  - Internal version
  - Breech extraction
  - Difficult destructive operation
  - Difficult forceps, e.g. Kielland's rotation
  - Forceps before full dilatation of the cervix
  - Manual removal of placenta.

Causes of Rupture of Uterus

Spontaneous rupture of the uterus can be precipitated in the following circumstances:
- High parity
- Injudicious use of oxytocin particularly to mother of high parity

- Obstructed labor; owing to excessive thinning of the lower uterine segment
- Neglected labor; where there is history of previous cesarean section
- Extension of severe cervical laceration upwards into the lower uterine segment
- Trauma due to accident.

Pathology of Rupture

- Complete rupture: All coats including the peritoneum are torn
- Incomplete rupture: Rupture in which the peritoneal coat remains intact.

Spontaneous rupture is usually complete and is usually followed by the escape of the uterine contents (fetus or placenta, or both). In majority of cases, rupture begins in the lower uterine segment as this part is thinnest and is most liable to overdistension. The fetus generally dies because of the effect of uterine retraction upon the uteroplacental circulation.

Rupture of Cesarean Scar

A classical scar may rupture more frequently in a subsequent pregnancy (about 2%). A classical scar is more vulnerable because of the following reasons:
- Defective healing due to contractions in puerperium.
- Improper approximation, due to premature digestion of catgut sutures.
- Placenta situated over the existing scar.
- Infection during healing.
- Several previous cesarean sections.
- Overdistension of the uterus by large baby or multiple pregnancy.

Diagnosis of Rupture During Pregnancy

Complete
- Acute abdominal pain with features of shock and intra-abdominal hemorrhage
- Contracted uterus as seen after third stage of labor

- Easily palpable fetus
- Absent fetal heart

Incomplete
- Localized abdominal pain and tenderness
- Signs of frank hemorrhage and shock develop slowly.

Diagnosis of Rupture in Labor

- Premonitory signs of a long difficult labor, tonic contractions and overstretching of the lower uterine segment
- Sudden acute pain in the lower abdomen and previous labor pains appear to stop altogether
- Sudden collapse of the mother who complained of severe abdominal pain
- Maternal pulse rate increases with variation (late decelerations) of fetal heart
- Signs of internal hemorrhage depending on severity
- On palpation, fetal parts are easily palpable through abdominal wall, together with hard, retracted fundus
- On vaginal examination:
  - Hemorrhage through cervical os
  - Recession of the presenting part in complete rupture
  - Hematuria
  - Cervix hangs loose like a curtain.

Management

- Resuscitation of the mother
- Immediate cesarean section if the baby is still alive
- Repair of the rupture if it is small and if there is strong reason to preserve reproductive function
- Blood transfusion
- Hysterectomy.

Prognosis

The prognosis is dependent on the following factors:
- Promptness in diagnosis and efficiency of definitive management
- Amount of hemorrhage and extent of the tear, and whether the placenta is situated over the ruptured area

- The presence or absence of infection
- Ruptured lower segment cesarean section (LSCS) scar has the lowest mortality and morbidity.

130. SHOCK IN OBSTETRICS

Definition

Shock is a clinical condition arising out of an inability of the circulatory system to provide adequate tissue perfusion with resulting dysfunction of organs or cells.

Classification

- Peripheral circulatory failure:
    - Hypovolemic due to blood loss, plasma loss or fluid loss
    - Normovolemic.
- Cardiogenic: Impaired ability of the heart to pump blood
- Bactermic/Septic
- Anaphylactic
- Neurogenic.

Hypovolemic Shock

In most cases in obstetrics this is due to blood loss. Fluid and electrolyte loss due to postoperative intestinal obstruction or vomiting and plasma loss due to peritonitis may also present this picture.

Clinical Manifestations

- Pallor and coldness of skin due to peripheral vasoconstriction
- Sweating due to sympathetic overactivity
- Tachycardia, muscular vasodilation and increased myocardial contractility
- Hyperventilation due to hypoxia
- Raised blood glucose, and sodium and water retention
- Metabolic acidosis due to severely reduced perfusion
- Irreversible shock in severely reduced tissue perfusion.

Effects on Organs and Systems

- Brain: Level of consciousness deteriorates as cerebral blood flow reduces
- Lungs: Gas exchange is impaired leading to respiratory failure
- Kidneys: Urine output falls to less than 20 mL per hour
- Gastrointestinal tract: Bacteremia as the gut becomes ischemic and looses its ability to function as a barrier against infection
- Liver: Drug and hormone metabolism ceases due to death of hepatic cells.

Management

- Replacement of fluids:
  - Ringers lactate as rapid infusion
  - Blood.
- Oxygen administration for raising oxygen content of blood
- Positioning in Trendelenburg tilt
- Morphine to relieve pain and fear
- Maintain the airway
- Avoid warmth (covering with blanket, etc.).

Important Observations and Monitoring

- Level of consciousness, signs of restlessness or confusion
- Blood pressure every 30 minutes
- Urine output hourly using indwelling catheter
- Skin color, core and peripheral body temperature hourly
- Central venous pressure
- Occurrence of further bleeding including oozing from wound or puncture sites.

Cardiogenic Shock

Failure of left ventricular ejection. The failing heart does not cope with the venous return and thus the central venous pressure becomes elevated. The events lead to cardiac arrest (asystole or ventricular fibrillation) or myocardial infarction.

Bacteremic or Septic Shock

A state of shock associated with bacteria or bacterial products in the bloodstream.

Common Pathogens

Klebsiella, *Proteus* and *Pseudomonas pyocyanea*, which have endotoxins in their cells. Placental site is the point of entry for infection and infection may occur in following conditions:
- Septic abortion
- Prolonged rupture of fetal membranes
- Obstetric trauma
- Presence of retained placental tissue.

Pathology

- Peripheral vasodilation and increased capillary permeability
- Reduced venous return which leads to diminished cardiac output.

Clinical Features

- Pyrexia with or without rigors
- Tachycardia and tachypnea
- Hypotension with peripheral cyanosis
- Hemorrhage if patient develops disseminated intravascular coagulation (DIC)
- Oliguria, if kidney damage occurs (reduced glomerular filtration and tissue necrosis)
- Respiratory distress
- Multisystem failure as a result of continued hypotension and myocardial depression.

Anaphylactic Shock

Anaphylactic shock happens following the injection of a substance that causes an antigen-antibody reaction. The pathology is associated with the release of:
- Histamine and serotonin, which cause smooth muscle contraction and increased capillary permeability
- Plasma kinins, which cause vasodilation.

Etiology

Almost any drug could cause anaphylactic shock and among the most likely are:

- Antisera and toxoids
- Penicillin and streptomycin
- Intravenous iron
- Local anesthetics.

Neurogenic Shock

Neurogenic shock is similar to hemorrhagic shock except for the fact that it initially is normovolemic and becomes hypovolemic in the later phase due to pooling and stagnation of blood in the microvascular capillaries.

Associated Conditions

- Vasovagal stimulation, emotion and fear associated with trauma
- Uterine inversion
- Rapid cervical dilation (traumatic or during abortion)
- Supine hypotensive syndrome and pulmonary embolism (venacaval occlusion)
- Spinal anesthetic.

Common Causes of Shock in Obstetrics

In clinical practice, especially in obstetrics, the cause of shock is often multifactorial and the most common are those due to blood loss and trauma:

- Blood loss associated with antepartum and postpartum bleeding (hypovolemic)
- Trauma and operative delivery
- Uterine rupture
- Uterine inversion
- Hypovolaemic and neurogenic
- General anesthetic accidents
- Drug anaphylaxis
- Septic abortion
- Embolism: Air embolism, amniotic fluid embolism
- Cardiac failure: Rheumatic heart disease, eclampsia
- Others: Spinal anesthesia, postoperative ileus.

Management of Shock in Obstetrics

Diagnosis

Antenatal
- Blood loss: Antepartum hemorrhage, abortion
- Any evidence of unsafe abortion
- Pulmonary embolism.

Labor and immediate postpartum period
- Blood loss: Postpartum hemorrhage (PPH), difficult operative delivery, uterine rupture, uterine inversion and hematoma
- Drug-related anaphylaxis
- Embolism: Air embolism, amniotic fluid embolism
- Bacteremia and prolonged rupture of membranes
- Spinal or epidural anesthesia.

Puerperium
- Hemorrhage
- Pulmonary embolism
- Bacteremic puerperal infection
- Postoperative intestinal obstruction.

General Management of Obstetric Shock

Quick examination, accurate diagnosis and emergency treatment are essential:
- Set up intravenous drip with Ringer's lactate or isotonic solution
- Cross-match blood and give fresh blood as soon as possible in adequate amount and monitor central venous pressure (CVP)
- Oxygenation and/or artificial ventilation if indicated
- Identify specific cause and treat accordingly
- Hemostasis if bleeding
- Treat coagulation disorder if indicated
- Close observation to prevent, diagnose or treat acute renal failure, anterior pituitary necrosis and anemia.

131. SHOULDER DYSTOCIA

Shoulder dystocia occurs when the fetal shoulder width is so large that it is not deliverable beneath the maternal symphysis pubis without additional delivery intervention or fetal injury.

Predisposing Factors

- Fetal macrosomia: Weight 4 kg and above
- Obesity and excessive weight gain during pregnancy
- Anencephaly
- Fetal ascites
- Short cord or cord tightly round the neck
- Maternal diabetes
- Short maternal stature.

Diagnosis

- Upon diagnosis of shoulder dystocia, summon help immediately; an obstetrician and a neonatologist should be called
- Clear the baby's mouth and nose
- Abduct the maternal thighs and sharply flex them on to the abdomen
- McRoberts maneuver: Perform a wide mediolateral episiotomy. The obstetrician may attempt the following steps:
    - Head and neck grasped and taken posteriorly, while suprapubic pressure is applied by an assistant slightly towards the chest
    - This may help to abduct the shoulders and rotate the anterior shoulder towards the oblique diameter.
- Wood's maneuver: Under general anesthesia, the posterior shoulder is rotated to anterior position and with simultaneous suprapubic pressure in the opposite direction, delivery of shoulders is attempted
- Zavanelli maneuver: The fetal head is flexed and the fetus is replaced within the uterus; thereafter the baby is delivered by cesarean section
- Cleidotomy: One or both clavicles may be cut with scissors to reduce the shoulder girth.

Complications

Fetal: Brachial plexus injury, birth asphyxia and fetal death.

Maternal: Increased operative delivery and morbidity.

132. SEXUALLY TRANSMITTED DISEASES

A variety of organisms are capable of being transmitted sexually. Transmission is incidental in some infections, while in others sexual contact is the primary mode of transmission.

LOCAL AND SYSTEMIC INFECTIONS

Bacterial Vaginosis

This condition affects about 15–20% of all pregnancies.

Clinical Features

- Thin watery vaginal discharge
- Increased odor for the discharge (fishy smell) after intercourse
- Alkaline pH
- Vaginal itching, burning or dysuria.

Diagnosis

- Gram stain for increased clue cells
- Vaginal pH of greater than or equal to 4.5.

Management

- Metronidazole 400 mg orally, twice daily for 7 days
- Clindamycin 300 mg orally twice daily for 7 days after first trimester.

Effects on Pregnancy

- Increased risk of premature rupture of membranes (PROM) and preterm labor
- Increased risk of postpartum endometritis
- May rarely causes neonatal septicemia.

Candidiasis

Candidiasis is a fungal (yeast) infection caused by *Candida albicans* and *Candida tropicalis*.

Clinical Features

- Vaginal irritation and pruritus
- White, thin vaginal discharge
- Dysuria.

Management

Clotrimazole (antifungal agent) as vaginal tablet or cream for 7 days.

Effects on Pregnancy

Apart from local discomfort, candidiasis does not have any effect on the pregnancy outcome.

Gonorrhea

The organism responsible for gonorrhea infection is *Neisseria gonorrhoeae*.

Clinical Features

- Profuse and purulent vaginal discharge
- Itching of vulva
- Painful urination
- The infection is asymptomatic in 50% of cases.

Management

Single dose of ceftriaxone 250 mg intramuscular (IM) or procaine penicillin 4.8 million units, combined with probenecid 1 g orally.

Alternatively amoxicillin 3 g and probenecid 1 g orally.

For disseminated infection, injection ceftriaxone 750 mg, three doses 8 hourly is given.

Effects on Pregnancy

- Spontaneous abortion in first trimester
- Preterm delivery or preterm rupture of membranes

- At the time of delivery if infection is present it can cause gonococcal ophthalmia for the neonate resulting in blindness. All neonates are treated with erythromycin ophthalmic ointment or tetracycline ophthalmic eye ointment to prevent neonatal infection
- Untreated gonorrhea can cause postpartum endometritis.

Chlamydiosis

Chlamydia trachomatis, an intracellular, bacteria-like parasite is the organism responsible for infection.

Clinical Features

- Increased yellowish vaginal discharge
- Painful, frequent urination
- Mucopurulent cervicitis.

Diagnosis

- Tissue culture
- Direct fluorescent antibody test (DFA)
- Enzyme immunoassay.

Treatment

Erythromycin 500 mg tid for 10–14 days.

Effects on Pregnancy

- Pelvic inflammatory disease, which can lead to infertility and ectopic pregnancy
- Increased risk of PROM, prematurity, low birth weight and perinatal mortality
- Delayed endometritis
- Conjunctivitis or pneumonitis for neonate if present at the time of delivery.

Syphilis

Causative organism is *Treponema pallidum*. Infection occurs either before pregnancy or during pregnancy. The symptoms are suppressed or appear in milder form during pregnancy.

Effects on Pregnancy

No adverse effect on mother during pregnancy.

Effects on Fetus (Baby)

- The placenta becomes bulky, heavy, greasy and pale
- Abortion
- Intrauterine death leading to either a macerated or a fresh stillbirth
- Birth of highly infected baby with early neonatal death
- Survival with congenital syphilis.

Diagnosis

- Serological test venereal disease research laboratory (VDRL)
- Fluorescent treponemal antibody test (FTA) for confirmation if VDRL is positive
- Detection of spirochetes from cutaneous lesion if any by dark field examination
- Detection of *Treponema pallidum* in amniotic fluid in case of fetal infection.

Presentation of infected baby

- May appear normal at birth, signs of infection appear within 1 or 2 weeks
- Purulent nasal discharge, hoarse cry, maculopapular rash and pemphigus, on soles and palms
- Late features:
  - Eighth nerve deafness
  - Saddle nose
  - Intestinal keratitis
  - Frontal bossing.

- VDRL positive
- Spirochetes may be detected from maculopapular rash
- If still born, spirochetes may be detected from liver or spleen.

Treatment

For mother:
- Benzathine penicillin 2.4 million units as a single dose as soon as diagnosis is made when the duration of illness is < 1 year. For duration > 1 year, Benzathine penicillin 2.4 million units weekly for 3 doses. If patient is allergic to penicillin, oral erythromycin 2 mg daily for 15 days
- Treatment should be repeated in subsequent pregnancies, irrespective of serological report.

For baby:
- Infected baby:
    - Isolation with mother
    - Aqueous penicillin G 50,000 units per kg body weight qd for 10 days.
- Positive serum reaction without clinical signs
- Penicillin G 50,000 units per kg, single dose
- Healthy baby of a syphilitic mother:
    - Serum test weekly for 1 month, then monthly for 6 months.

Human Papilloma Virus

Caused by human wart virus.

Clinical Features

- Warty growth in and around vulva
- Itching and vaginal discharge
- Vulval pain.

Diagnosis

- Visualization
- Tissue biopsy
- Cytology smear for koilocytes.

Treatment

- Topical application of bichloroacetic acid (BCA) or trichloroacetic acid (TCA); three times per week
- Cryotherapy in 2nd and 3rd trimesters
- Electrocautery on small lesions
- Laser treatment.

Effects on Pregnancy Outcome

- Condylomata accuminata (genital warts) have insignificant effects on pregnancy
- Pelvic outlet obstruction and severe hemorrhage related to lacerations of the friable condylomatous tissue
- High-risk of causing dysplacia and squamous cell genital carcinoma.

Trichomoniasis

Responsible organism is *Trichomonas vaginalis,* a flagellated protozoan.

Clinical Features

- Frothy, gray-green foul discharge
- Constant itching
- Erythema (strawberry spots)
- Vaginal pH alkaline.

Diagnosis

- Presence of motile trichomonas on wet slide.

Treatment

- Metronidazole 400 mg, two tablets at bedtime and two in the morning or metronidazole 200 mg tid for 7 days
- No alcoholic beverages for 48 hours after therapy to avoid nausea, vomiting and headache.

Effect on Pregnancy

No known fetal risks.

Herpes Simplex

Caused by herpes simplex virus [a deoxyribonucleic acid (DNA) virus].

Clinical Features

Symptoms appear 3–7 days following exposure:
- Mild paresthesia and burning.
- Low grade fever, malaise and inguinal lymphadenopathy.
- Clear, painful, tender vesicles on the labia and perineum.
- Vesicles rupture in 1–7 days leaving behind shallow, painful raised edge ulcers that heal within 10 days.
- Dysuria and retention of urine if urinary tract is involved.
- The virus lies dormant until reactivated by stress, respiratory infection or menses.

Diagnosis

- Virus culture of fluid aspirate from vesicles or debrided ulcer
- Cytology test.

Effects on Pregnancy

- Spontaneous abortion
- Intrauterine growth retardation
- Fetal death
- Preterm labor
- Neonatal infection.

Neonatal Herpes

- Symptoms appear in 2–3 days
- Almost 60% of affected infants die
- About 40% suffer from permanent sequelae such as microcephalus, mental retardation, seizures, etc.

Management

- No effective cure
- Sitz bath for symptomatic relief
- Administration of acyclovir 200 mg, qid for 14 days
- Topical application of acyclovir cream
- Abstinence when active lesions are present
- Vaginal delivery if there are no vaginal lesions
- Cesarean section to avert neonatal exposure to infection.

Human Immunodeficiency Virus

The human immunodeficiency virus (HIV), I and II are retroviruses, which infect human cells with the glycoprotein CD4 surface marker. The virus causes alteration in the immune system that characterizes acquired immune deficency syndrome (AIDS). After entering the cell, the virus follows a unique reproductive cycle that involves reverse transcription of their ribonucleic acid (RNA) followed by incorporation of the newly synthesized DNA into a host cell DNA and their subsequent translation into viral components. The viral DNA remains incorporated into the host cell DNA for prolonged latent periods until viral synthesis is activated.

Susceptible cells with the glycoprotein CD4 are T4-helper-inducer T-lymphocytes. Invasion and eventual destruction of these cells by the HIV-1 virus causes alteration in the immune system that characterizes AIDS.

Diagnosis

- Initial screening test for specific antibodies using enzyme-linked immunosorbent assay (ELISA)
- Positive tests are confirmed by western blot
- The median time between HIV infection and full blown AIDS is about 10 years
- Clinical progression of the disease is monitored by evaluating the CD4 cell counts:
  - CD4 counts > 500/mL, need no medical intervention as there is no clinical evidence of immunosuppression

- CD4 counts of 200–500/mL, patients suffer from infections such as persistent thrush, fever and increased risk of complications (opportunistic infections).

Management

- Prenatal HIV counseling to all pregnant women
- Prophylaxis of opportunistic infections
- Assessment for presence of other STDs
- Aerosolized pentamidine spray prophylaxis for Pneumocystis carinii pneumonia (PCP)
- Trimethoprim-sulfamethoxazole double strength for PCP
- Reducing the viral load with antiviral drugs such as zidovudine (AZT)
- Cleansing the vagina with antiviral chemical preparations to reduce the risk of infection from maternal secretions.

Obstetric Precautions

- Limit vaginal examinations to a minimum during intrapartum period
- Avoid using scalp electrodes or intrauterine monitoring catheters
- All soiled linen should be collected in a vessel containing hypochlorite solution
- All cotton swabs, dressing/perineal pads, mops, etc. must be discarded in container with hypochlorite solution
- All needles, syringes and sharp blades must be collected in puncture-proof containers and disposed of with due precautions
- After delivery the floor must be cleaned with antiseptic solution
- Fumigate the labor room/operating room
- Autoclave all instruments after proper cleaning
- Patient should be explained the need for protection of staff
- Zidovudine 2 mg/kg intravenous (IV) during the 1st hour of labor and 1.0 mg/kg throughout the rest of labor
- After birth, newborns are treated with zidovudine oral syrup 2 mg/kg for 6 weeks (most newborns become seronegative by the end of six months)
- Barrier contraception to be recommended to the couple.

133. SEXUAL VIOLENCE

INTRODUCTION

Sexual violence is any sexual act or attempt to obtain a sexual act by violence or coercion, acts to traffic a person or acts directed against a person's sexuality, regardless of the relationship to the victim. It is considered to be one of the most traumatic, pervasive and most common human rights violation. Sexual violence remains highly stigmatized in all settings, thus levels of disclosure of the assault vary between regions and societies. It is widely an underreported phenomenon. Sexual violence is also called rape, sexual abuse or sexual assault – is any sexual contact or behavior that happens without a person's consent.

Types of Sexual Assault

Sexual assault can take many different forms and be defined in different ways, however it is over the victim's fault.

- **Child sexual abuse**
  When perpetrator intentionally harms a minor physically, psychologically, or by acts of neglect, the crime is known as child abuse.
- **Sexual assault on men and boys**
  Men and boys who have been sexually assaulted or abused may also face some additional challenges because of social attitudes and stereo types about men and masculinity.
- **Intimate partner sexual violence**
  A perpetrator can have any relationship to a victim, and that includes the role of an intimate partner.
- **Incest**
  Unwanted sexual contact from a family member can have a lasting effect on the survivor.
- **Dug facilitated sexual assault**
  In these cases, survivors often blame themselves. Using drugs or alcohol is never an excuse for assault and does not mean that it was your fault.

- **Sexual harassment**
  This happens in a person's place of work or school and make one uncomfortable.
- **Stalking**
  Unwanted or repeated surveillance by an individual or group. This can be reported to police.
- **Using technology**
  To hurt others such as digital photos, videos, apps and social media to engage in harassing.
  - Social abuse by medical professionals.
  - Sexual exploitation by helping professionals.
  - Multiple-perpetrator sexual assault or gang rape.
  - Elder abuse.
  - Sexual abuse of people with disabilities.
  - Prison rape.
  - Military sexual trauma.

Commonly Occurring Sexual Violence

- **Conflict related and domestic sexual violence**
  These are sexual violence perpetrated by combatants, including rebels, militants and government forces. Various forms of sexual violence can be used systematically in conflicts to torture, injure, extract information, degrade, threaten, intimidate or punish.
- **Domestic sexual violence**
  The type of sexual violence perpetrated by intimate partners and by other family or household members, and is often termed as intimate partners and by other family/household members and is often termed intimate partner violence.
- **Possible victims**
  A spectrum of people can fall victim to sexual violence. This includes women, men children and also people who define themselves as transgender individuals.

Effects of Sexual Assault

- Sexual violence is a serious public health problem and has profound short and long term impact on physical and mental

health such as increased risk of sexual and reproductive health problems as increased risk of suicide or HIV infection.
- Murder occurring either during a sexual assault or a result of an honor killing.
- Sexual violence can occur to anybody at any age; it is an act of violence that can be perpetrated by parents, caregivers, acquaintances and strangers, as well as intimate partners.
- It is rarely a crime of passion and is rater an aggressive act that frequently aims to express power and dominance over the victim.
- Intimate partner violence is an individual person forcing sex on another person.

Risk Factors

The following are the individual risk factors:
- Alcohol and drug use.
- Delinquency.
- Empathetic deficits.
- General aggressiveness and acceptance of violence.
- Early sexual intimation.
- Coercive sexual fantasies.
- Preference for impersonal sex and sexual-risk taking.
- Exposure to sexually explicit media.
- Hostility towards women.
- Adherence to traditional gender role norms.
- Hyper-masculinity.
- Suicidal behavior.
- Prior sexual victimization.
- Family environment characterized by physical violence and conflict.
- Childhood history of physical, sexual or emotional abuse.
- Emotionally unsupportive family environment.
- Poor parent-child relationship particularly.

What a Victim Needs to do

- **Self-care after trauma**
  Whether it happened recently or years ago, self-care can help one cope with the short-term and long-term effects of a trauma like sexual assault.

- **Reporting to law enforcement**
  Understanding how to report and learning more about the experience can take away some of the unknowns and help you feel more prepared.
- **Receiving medical attention**
  After sexual assault, a medical exam can check for help, check for injuries even those one may not be able to see.

Helplines

- All India Women's Conference 10921/011.
- National Commission for Women Helpline 7827 170 170.
- Recovering and Healing from Incest (RAHI).
  A support center for women survivors of child sexual abuse (011) 2523 8466/2622 4042

134. SINGLE PARENT

A single parent is a person who lives with a child or children and who does not have a spouse or live-in-partner. Reasons for becoming single parent include divorce, break-up, abandonment, domestic violence and rape, death of the other parent, childbirth by a single person or single person adoption.

SINGLE PARENT CHALLENGES

Child rearing can be difficult under any circumstances. Without a partner, the stakes are higher. A single parent has the sole responsibility for all aspects for day-to-day child care. Being a single parent can result in added pressure, stress and fatigue. If the parent is too tired or distracted, to be emotionally supportive or needs to consistently discipline the child/children behavioral problems might arise.

If it is a low income family and has less access to health care, struggle may be more as work and child care can be financially difficult and socially isolating. They might also worry about the lack of a female or male parental role model for the child.

POSITIVE STRATEGIES

To reduce stress of a single parent family:

- **Show love to the child:**
  Remember to praise the child and give him or her unconditional love and support. Set aside time each day to play, read or simply sit with the child.
- **Create a routine:**
  Structure time such as regularly scheduled meal times and bed times as this would help the child know what to expect.
- **Find quality child care:**
  If you need regular child care, look for a qualified care giver who can provide care and attention in a safe environment. Do not rely on older child as the only baby sitter. Be very careful about asking a new friend or partner to watch your child.
- **Set limits:**
  Explain house rule and expectations to the child – such as speaking respectfully and enforce them. Work with other caregivers in your child's life to provide consistent discipline. Identify the times when the child shows the ability to accept more responsibilities.
- **Do not feel guilty:**
  Do not blame yourself or spoil your child to make up for being a single parent.
- **Take care of yourself:**
  Include physical activity in your daily routine, eat a healthy diet and get adequate sleep. Arrange time to do activities you enjoy alone or with friends. Call your loved ones, friends and neighbors for help when requires.
- **Stay positive:**
  It is OK to be honest with your child if you are having a difficult time, but remind him or her that things will get better. Give your child appropriate level of responsibility rather than expecting him or her to behave like a little adult. Keep your sense of humor when dealing with everyday challenges.

Talking to your Child about Separation or Divorce

If separation or divorce is the case in your family, talk to your child about the changes you are facing. Listen to your child's feelings and try to answer his or her questions honestly – avoiding unnecessary details or negativity about the other parent. Remind the child that he or she did nothing to cause the divorce or separation and that you will always love him or her.

If the other parent is alive or around communicate with your child's other parent about your child's care and well-being. Children who fare best in divorce have parents who communicate on co-parenting issues, placing their children's needs above their own desire to avoid the ex-spouse.

Positive Outcomes of Single Parenting

- Children do well when they have nurturing, warm, sensitive, responsive and flexible parenting.
- Strong relationships with children are built on everyday moments, positive attention, praise and more.
- Clear rule encourage good behavior and help children feel secure.
- Parents become confident about parenting.
- Often have support from family and friends.

Single Parenting Advantages

On the bright side, there are some advantages of single parenting:
- **Undivided attention:**
  Children of a single parent usually get their parent's undivided attention. Love and attention will be reserved just for the child or children.
- **Freedom to make decisions:**
  Single parents have the freedom to make all the decisions that can affect their children, such as food they eat, places to eat, rules and restrictions.
- **Fewer arguments:**
  A single parent family will have fewer arguments. This can make the home environment less stressful. Children will feel safer and more secure in such a house.
- **Good role model:**
  Children will look at the parent who is his/her role model and also realize the importance independence and how life can be managed without a partner.

- **Independence and responsibility:**
  Single parents can get busy with juggling work and family. Children of single parents often take responsibility for manageable home chores. They also learn how to be independent.

135. STILLBIRTH

DEFINITION

Birth of a fetus after 28th completed week with no sign of life and weighing 1000 grams or more. Fetal death may occur during labor, resulting in a fresh stillbirth or before the onset of labor as intrauterine fetal death (IUFD/IUD).

Causes of Stillbirth

A number of different disorders can cause stillbirth. These include:
- Pregnancy complications
  - Preeclampsia and eclampsia causing placental insufficiency.
  - Antepartum hemorrhage; both placenta previa and abruptio placentae; due to acute placental insufficiency.
- Maternal illness during pregnancy
  - Chronic hypertension
  - Diabetes
  - Thyroid disorders
  - Cytomegalovirus infection
  - Malaria
  - Severe anemia
  - Preterm premature rupture of membranes
- Fetal causes
  - Abnormalities in the fetus caused by infectious diseases including syphilis, toxoplasmosis and cytomegalovirus infection
  - Congenital malformations
  - Rh incompatibility
  - Postmaturity where pregnancy has lasted 42 weeks or more
- Iatrogenic causes
  - Administration of quinine group of drugs
  - External version

- Intrapartum causes
  - Acute fetal distress
  - Traumatic vaginal delivery leading to intracranial injury
  - Short umbilical cord and true knots in the cord.

Symptoms

In most cases the only symptom is that the baby has stopped moving. In some cases the sign of fetal death is occurrence of premature labor.

Diagnosis

When the mother notices that fetal movement has stopped, several techniques can be used to evaluate whether the baby has died. These include:
- Listening to the fetal heartbeat with a stethoscope
- Use of Doppler ultrasound to detect the heartbeats
- Give the mother an electronic fetal non-stress test.

Treatment

- Induction of labor
  In most cases of intrauterine fetal death the mother will go into labor within two weeks of the baby's death. If spontaneous labor does not begin, labor usually is induced using oxytocin.

Care of Mothers who Lost their Babies

Emotional support to mother from staff, family members and counseling by a professional can help bereaved parents cope with their loss. Following delivery of a dead fetus:
- Ensure that the mother is not left alone. Arrange for the spouse, a family member or a close friend to be present with her.
- Convey an attitude of understanding and empathy that the fetus or infant is special and significant to the mother.
- Help to validate the loss by providing an opportunity to grieve and verbalize their feelings.
- Convey a feeling of caring by touching and holding the mother when she cries.

- Give some mementos for the mother to keep, such as a crib card with information of the baby, a lock of hair or a certificate of life or death.
- Prepare parents for what they will see if they choose to see and hold the dead baby.
- Wrap the baby in a clean and warm blanket or towel and show care and respect to the dead baby.
- Share medical findings and autopsy result (if done) in a frank and sensitive manner.

Prevention

The risk of stillbirth can be lowered to some extent by good prenatal care and avoiding mother's exposure to infectious diseases, smoking, alcohol abuse and illicit drug consumption. Antepartum testing such as ultrasound examination, alpha-fetoprotein and other genetic tests in selected cases, and electronic fetal non-stress test can be used to evaluate the health of the fetus before there is an intrauterine death or stillbirth. Most stillbirths happen before a women goes into labor, but a small number happen during labor and birth. Screening and antenatal care to women who are more likely than others to have stillbirth include:

- Those who are obese with body mass index (BMI) 30 or higher.
- Pregnancy with multiples (twins, triplets or more)
- Age 35 or older for first pregnancy.
- Medical conditions like diabetes and hypertension.
- History of miscarriage or stillbirth in a previous pregnancy.
- Complications in past pregnancy such as premature delivery, preeclampsia or fetal growth restriction.
- Use of alcohol, illicit drugs and pain killers.

Prognosis

With good management of medical conditions, avoidance of harmful substances like drugs and alcohol and adequate prenatal care, women who had stillbirth can have a good chance of carrying a future pregnancy to term as a woman pregnant for the first time.

136. TEENAGE PREGNANCY AND ADOLESCENT PREGNANCY

DESCRIPTION

Teenage pregnancy is formally defined as a pregnancy in a young woman who has not reached her 20th birthday when the pregnancy ends, regardless of whether the woman is married or legally an adult (age 14 to 21, depending on the country). Usually this refers to unmarried minors who become pregnant unintentionally.

Adolescent pregnancy is pregnancy in girls age 19 or younger. Adolescent pregnancy is a complex issue with many reasons for concern. Younger adolescents (12–14 years old) are more likely to have unplanned sexual intercourse and more likely to be coerced into sex. Adolescents 18 to 19 years old are technically adults, and about half of adolescent pregnancies occur in this age group.

CAUSES OF TEENAGE PREGNANCY

Teenage pregnancy is defined as an unintended pregnancy during adolescence. Many teenagers do not believe that they will get pregnant if they engage in sexual activity and it happens because of peer pressure, absent parents, lack of knowledge, sexual abuse or rape and teenage drinking.

RISK FACTORS FOR ADOLESCENT PREGNANCY

- Younger age.
- Poor school performance.
- Economic disadvantage.
- Single or teen parents.

DIAGNOSIS

The adolescent may or may not admit to being involved sexually. If the teen is pregnant, there are usually weight changes (usually a gain, but there may be a loss if nausea and vomiting are significant).

Examination may show increased abdominal girth and the health care provider may be able to feel the fundus. Pelvic examination may reveal bluish or purple discoloration of vaginal walls, bluish or purple discoloration and softening of the cervix, and softening and enlargement of uterus. Pregnancy test of urine and/or serum hCG are usually positive. An ultrasound examination may be done to confirm or check for accurate dates for pregnancy.

MANAGEMENT

All options available to the pregnant teen should be considered carefully, including abortion, adoption and raising the child with family support.

- Pregnant teens should be assessed for smoking, alcohol use and drug use and they should be offered support to help them quit.
- Adequate nutrition should be encouraged through education and family/community support. Adequate exercise and sleep should also be emphasized.
- Contraceptive information and services are important after delivery to prevent them becoming pregnant again.

Teen mothers should be encouraged and helped to remain in school or re-enter educational programs that give them skills to be better parents and provide for the child financially and emotionally.

PROGNOSIS

- Teen mothers are about two years behind their age group in completing their education or may even discontinue their education.
- Teen mothers who have history of substance abuse may start abusing by about 6 months after delivery.
- Ten mothers who have history of substance abuse may start abusing substances by about 6 months after delivery.
- They are more likely than older mothers to have a second child within two years of their first child.
- Infants born to teenage mothers are at greater risk for developmental problems. Girls born to teen mothers are more likely to become teen mothers themselves, and boys born to teen mothers have a higher than average rate of becoming criminals.

COMPLICATIONS

- Pregnant teens are at much higher risk of having serious medical complications such as placenta previa, pregnancy, induced hypertension, premature delivery and significant anemia.
- Infants born to teens are 2 to 6 times more likely to have low birth weight than those born to mothers age 20 or older.
- Prematurity and resultant low birth weight and intrauterine growth retardation (IUGR) are also import problems.
- Infants are at greater risk for inadequate growth, infection or chemical dependence as mothers are more likely to have unhealthy habits. It is important for pregnant teens to have early and adequate prenatal care, and counseling regarding birth control methods, prevention of sexually transmitted diseases (STD) and pregnancy risks.

PREVENTION

Programs for teen pregnancy prevention include:
- Knowledge-based programs that focus on teaching adolescents about their bodies and their normal functions as well as providing detailed information about contraception, and preventing STDs.
- Abstinence education programs to encourage young people to postpone sexual activity until marriage or until they are mature enough to handle sexual activity and a potential pregnancy in a responsible manner.
- Clinic focused programs to provide easier access to information, counseling by health care providers and contraceptive services. These programs are offered through school-based clinics.
- Peer counseling programs which typically involve older teens to encourage adolescents to resist peer and social pressures to become sexually involved. These programs tend to use a personal approach, helping teens understand their own risks.

137. ULTRASONICS IN OBSTETRICS

Ultrasound is a sound wave beyond the audible range of frequency greater than 2 MHz (cycles per second). The commonly used

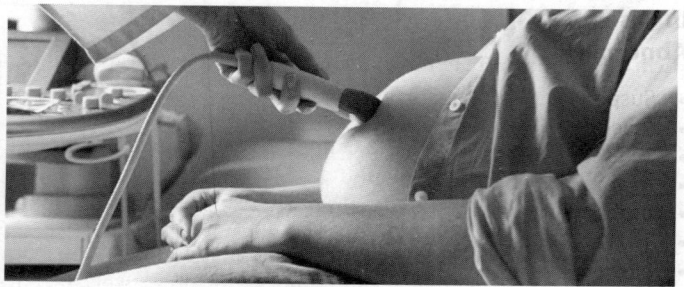

Fig. 137.1: Ultrasound examination in pregnancy.

frequency range in obstetrics is 3.5–5 MHz, the sound, navigation and ranging (SONAR).

Ultrasonography equipment consist of two major components: The transducer, which emits and receives the reflected sound wave energy and the video display terminal, which converts the reflected waves into a visual image on screen **(Fig. 137.1)**.

The real-time equipment produces moving pictures. Transabdominal scanning is most common, but the selector probe used vaginally is especially useful in early pregnancy. As the transducer is more closer to the object, the images are of enhanced quality.

PATIENT PREPARATION

- No special preparation is required
- A full bladder is required in non-pregnant patients and patients in first trimester of pregnancy.

INDICATIONS OF SELECTIVE SONOGRAPHY IN CLINICAL PRACTICE

To Determine the Maturity of the Fetus

- Uncertain gestational age
- Discrepancy between amenorrhea and uterine size
- Prior to elective induction of postmaturity or elective cesarean section.

In Cases of Suspicion of Fetal and/or Placental Abnormalities

- Suspected ectopic pregnancy
- Bleeding in early months
- To ascertain localization of placenta
- In abruptio placentae
- Intrauterine growth restriction
- To confirm intrauterine death of fetus
- High-risk pregnancies such as Rh-incompatibility, diabetes and pregnancy induced hypertension (PIH)
- Malpresentations such as breech, transverse or face
- Twins
- To exclude congenital malformations
- Polyhydramnios.

Other Indications

- Prior to invasive diagnostic procedures
- For antepartum fetal surveillance such as biophysical profile
- To check the integrity of previous cesarean scar
- In postpartum period: secondary postpartum hemorrhage (PPH), retained bits of placenta, subinvolution
- For neonatal head scanning.

ULTRASONOGRAPHY FINDINGS

First Trimester Scanning

Fetus

They can generally be visualized satisfactorily after 7 completed weeks of gestation. The scan could reveal the following:

- Regular fetal heart pulsations
- Measurement of crown-rump length (CRL)
- Fetal activity
- Biparietal diameter, femur, humerus and abdomen after 10 weeks
- Fetal anencephaly after 12 weeks.

Placenta

The site where the trophoblast seems to be localizing to form the placenta can be visualized

Pelvic Adnexae and Abnormalities

- Ovarian neoplasms
- Ectopic pregnancy
- Blighted ovum
- Missed abortion
- Incomplete abortion
- Hydatidiform mole
- Threatened abortion
- Myomas in the uterine wall.

Second and Third Trimester Scanning

Pelvic Anatomy

- Uterine size, any fibroids
- Length of cervix, any incompetence of os
- Any solid or cystic mass.

Amniotic Fluid

- Oligohydramnios
- Polyhydramnios.

Fetus

- Size, growth pattern, serial biparietal diameter, femoral length and abdominal circumference
- Estimation of fetal weight
- Multifetal pregnancy
- Malpresentations
- Malformations.

Viability of Fetus

- Heart pulsations
- Fetal limb movements.

Placenta

- Location
- Abruption, presence of retroplacental clot.

Valuable Information Based on Scans at Different Gestational Age

- Normal growth and well-being, if all data fall within normal range
- First trimester scan at 7–8 weeks provides reasonably accurate data about gestational maturity at expected date of delivery (EDD)
- Scanning between 16 and 20 weeks of gestation helps to detect fetal malformations
- Serial measurements of fetal diameters (biometry) to assess fetal growth pattern
- Placental grading prior to considering elective labor induction or cesarean section.

RISK OF ULTRASONICS

Diagnostic ultrasound does not have any significant biologic effects in human tissue as opposed to radiography.

138. UNWED MOTHER

INTRODUCTION

An unwed mother is a girl or woman, 13–35 years who is not legally married to a man by whom who has conceived a child. In India, a child to an unwed mother is taken as a social stigma of a serious nature and she does not want to carry such stigma for her entire life. The tragedy of unwed motherhood in India goes back to Hindu mythology with the legend of Kunti, who was made pregnant by the Sun God, ultimately had to abandon her firstborn, Karna. For modern day Kunti's fate is not different, if anything, it is even more cruel.

CAUSES OF UNWED MOTHER

- Broken homes either by death or divorce.
- Psychiatric illness or mental retardation.

- Necessity for both parents to work causing lack of parental supervision.
- Lack of parental devotion.
- Loss of security for the girl.
- Rebellion of the girl against parents, particularly against mother.
- Fantasies of the girl.
- Rape.
- Lack of proper sex education.
- Poor economic status.

UNWED MOTHER IN INDIAN TRIBAL SOCIETIES

Sexual exploitation of the poor in tribal communities continues unabated in India. Men use tribal women and girls to satisfy their lust and abandon them mercilessly. South Indian governments announce rehabilitation projects periodically, aimed at providing land for the landless, monthly aid, free residential education for their children. But the projects failed as numerous other tribal schemes.

This problem leads rise of suicide among tribes and mysterious infant deaths. There are hardly any attempt to trace the biological fathers of the children of these unwed mothers and to establish their legal rights.

AGE AND EDUCATION-WISE DISTRIBUTION

Study findings show that:
- 49% of unwed mothers were teenage girls.
- 68% were uneducated or had only primary education and
- 58.9% had some pre-disposing factors.

CONSEQUENCES

- Out-of-wedlock child bearing often sets teenagers on an unfortunate life course, one that places them theirs at greater risk of additional unintended child rearing, diminished economic opportunities and unstable and unhealthy marriages.
- Women who have children outside marriage are less likely to marry, stay married or marry well. Out of wedlock childbearing reduces women's attractiveness in the marriage market.

- 40–50% of non-marital births are cohabiting couples. Evidence suggests that the bonds between cohabiting couples are much less stable than those between married couples, especially among poor cohabiting couples with children.

THE ROLE OF SINGLE MOTHER

This is a challenging one especially when the family is headed by a woman. Problems of single mothers are linked with the upbringing of children, their future and settling down in life. Till the time children get married and or get jobs, they are dependents on the single parent. After that, problems are considerably reduced.

Results of related studies reveal that

- Financial problem was the main stressor for majority of single mothers.
- Emotional health of a single mother was also affected by their single status.
- Majority of single mothers reported that they felt lonely, helpless, hopeless, lack of identity and lack of confidence.
- Regarding social life, majority of the single mothers found it hard to maintain discipline among the children due to absence of male members.
- Mothers explained about loneliness, traumatic experiences and depression found it difficult to handle the responsibility of childcare and to establish a routine for her children.

CARE OF UNMARRIED MOTHER

The problems presented by unwed mothers are that they are mostly psychological. These girls present many special problem which are important for social workers, obstetricians and nurses when an unwed girl or woman become pregnant, it is a crisis in her life.

- It is a time of great physical and physiological changes and also a time of great emotional stress.
- Apprehension, fear, pleasurable expectations, pride in physical achievement and a deep sense of wonder about the mystery of reproduction etc., fill her mind.
- The unmarried girl usually comes from an emotionally disturbed background.

- Because of the mores of our civilization she has a tremendous sense of guilt and shame.
- Her fears are magnified far beyond those of the ordinary patients because she does not know where to turn to. In order to help these girls, nursing and medical personnel as well as social workers can do much to ease their pains of labor, then turn them loose when they have been healed physically.
- These girls must be helped to work through their guilt complexes and be made to feel that although they have committed the original sin/mistake, they have fulfilled an obligation the child they have borne and given it a start in life to the best of ability. Every girl coming to the health facility needs to be carefully studied by a social worker so that there is knowledge her particular problems.

PREVENTIVE MEASURES

- To establish the right sex morality through the education in families.
- The society's role is to share the responsibilities and care to single parent homes.
- The 'right sex education' in schools and society must be encouraged and enforced.
- Governmental aids for unwed mothers in financial and nutritional aspects must be made available to every single parent.

Support to Unwed Mothers and Single Parents in Tribal Communities in Order to Clarify the Government Programme to Help Tribal People

Sexual exploitation of the poor in tribal communities continue unabated in India. Men use tribal women and girls to satisfy their sexual lust and abandon them mercilessly. Governments announce rehabilitation projects periodically, aimed at providing land for the landless, monthly financial aid and free residential education for their children such as tribal hostels attached to schools for tribal children. But the problem continues and lands in suicides among tribal women and mysterious infant deaths. There are hardly any attempt to trace the biological fathers of the children of these unwed mothers and to establish their legal rights.

Several state governments provide supplemental nutrition programs for women, infants and children. There are single mother grants. Young mothers mostly rely on close family members.

139. UTERINE PROLAPSE

The uterus descends down from its normal position due to weakness of the structures supporting it.

POSITION AND SUPPORTS OF UTERUS

Position

- Anteverted and anteflexed
- Lies between the bladder and rectum
- The external os lies at the level of the ischial spines.

Supporting Structures

- Endopelvic fascia covering the uterus
- Round ligaments
- Broad ligaments
- Fibromuscular tissues surrounding the cervix
- Pelvic cellular tissue
- Pelvic floor at the lower end.

CAUSES OF PROLAPSE

Vaginal delivery with consequent injury to the supporting structures.

Factors Leading to Injury

- Overstretching of the Mackenrod's and uterosacral ligaments
- Overstretching of the endopelvic fascial sheath of the vagina
- Overstretching of the perineum
- Subinvolution of the supporting structures
- Early resumption of activities, which greatly increase intra-abdominal pressure before the tissues regain their tone
- Repeated childbirths at frequent intervals

- Persistent overfilling of the uterus at frequent intervals
- Congenital weakness of the supporting structures.

Aggravating Factors

- Postmenopausal atrophy
- Increased intra-abdominal pressure as in chronic cough and constipation
- Increased weight of the uterus as in fibroid or myohyperplasia
- Asthenia or undernutrition
- Traction by the anterior vaginal wall or cervical polyp.

Degrees of Prolapse

- **First degree:** The cervix descends down from its normal position into the vagina. The external os reaches below the level of ischial spines
- **Second degree:** The cervix reaches to the level of vulva
- **Third degree:** The cervix protrudes outside the vagina
- **Fourth degree or complete procidentia:** The whole uterus protrudes outside the vulva bringing with it both vaginal walls **(Fig. 139.1)**.

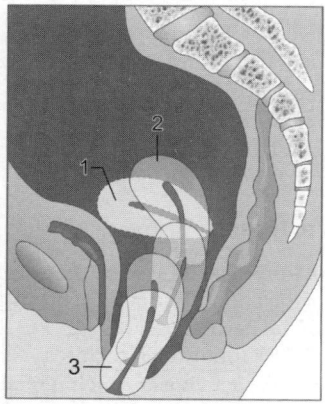

Fig. 139.1: Uterine prolapse. **1.** Normal position; **2.** Slight prolapse; **3.** Marked prolapse (procidentia)

ASSOCIATED SYMPTOMS

- Feeling of something coming down per vagina specially, while she is moving about
- Backache or dragging pain in the pelvis
- Urinary symptoms such as:
  - Difficulty in passing urine. Patient will have to elevate the anterior vaginal wall to empty the bladder
  - Frequent desire to pass urine
  - Urgency and frequency of micturition due to cystitis
  - Painful micturition due to infection
  - Stress incontinence due to associated urethrocele
  - Retention of urine.
- Bowel symptom (in presence of rectocele):
  - Difficulty in passing stool. Patient may have to push back the posterior vaginal wall in position to complete the evacuation of feces.
- Excessive white or blood stained discharge per vagina due to vaginitis or ulcers on the dependant part of the prolapsed mass.

CLINICAL EXAMINATION AND DIAGNOSIS

The findings on examination depend on the type or degree of prolapse:
- Inspection of vagina, rectum and perineal region
- Examination in squatting position as the patient strains, if inspection findings are negative
- Assessment of the involvement of adjacent organs.

TREATMENT

Preventive

Effective Antenatal Care

- Nutritional supplements
- Antenatal hygiene
- Relaxation exercises.

Adequate Intranatal Care

- Preventing premature bearing down efforts
- Preventing premature application of forceps, before the cervix is fully dilated
- Avoiding too much fundal pushing to expel the placenta
- Performing timely and adequate episiotomy
- Repairing perineal lacerations immediately and accurately.

Adequate Postnatal Care

- Preventing undue distension of bladder
- Encouraging early ambulation
- Encouraging pelvic floor exercises.

General Measures

- Avoiding strenuous activities for at least 6 weeks following delivery
- Avoiding future pregnancy too soon.

Conservative

Conservative treatment is recommend only for first degree uterine descend occurring within 6 months of delivery. These measures include:

- Assurance
- Improvement of nutritional status
- Pelvic floor exercises to strengthen the muscles.

Ring Pessary

It is used in selected cases such as in:

- Early pregnancy, i.e. up to 18 weeks when the uterus becomes enlarged to sit on the brim of pelvis
- Puerperium to facilitate involution
- Patients unfit for surgery especially with short life expectancy
- Patients waiting for surgery.

Surgery

Surgical correction to place the herniated mass in position.

Types of Operation

- Anterior colporrhaphy
- Colpoperineorrhaphy
- Repair of enterocele
- Pelvic floor repair
- Fothergill's operation
- Vaginal hysterectomy
- Repair of vault prolapse
- Cervicopexy or sling operation.

Complications of Pelvic Floor Repair

- Hemorrhage
- Trauma to bladder with anterior colporrhaphy or to rectum
- Retention of urine
- Sepsis
- Rectovaginal fistula (RVF) and vesicovaginal fistula (VVF).

140. URINARY TRACT INFECTIONS

Urinary tract infections (UTI) result from bacterial invasion or from congenital anomaly that obstructs urine flow. The changes that occur in the urinary tract during pregnancy make the woman more susceptible to infection.

Causative Organisms

- *Escherichia coli (E. coli)*
- Other gram-negative aerobic bacilli
- Group B streptococcus.

Predisposing Factors

- Extrapelvic infection (most common)
- Risk factors:
  - Bladder hypotonia
  - Urinary stasis
  - Intermittent catheterization
  - Epidural anesthesia.

- High number of pelvic examinations
- History of UTI
- Bacteriuria
- Operative delivery
- Anatomic disorders
- Impaired bladder function; bacteria ascends from perineal or vaginal site into urethra.

Signs and Symptoms

- Manifestations of lower UTI:
  - Dysuria
  - Frequency
  - Urgency
  - Low grade fever.
- Suprapubic pain
- Urinary retention
- Hematuria
- Pyuria
- Manifestations of upper UTI:
  - Flank pain
  - Costovertebral tenderness
  - Insufficient urination
  - Foul smelling urine.

Investigations

- Urinalysis
- Culture and sensitivity
- Ultrasound examination.

Management

- Antibiotic therapy for 10 days
  - Ampicillin
  - Cephalosporin.
- Analgesia
- Hydration
- Monitor temperature, pulse, bladder function, urine appearance.

Teaching

- Self-care measures
- Reporting complications
- Preventive measures
- Avoiding carbonated drinks (increases alkalinity)
- Drinking acidic fluids (fruit juice)
- Wipe from front to back
- Increase fluid intake
- Urinate frequently.

Complications

- Pyelonephritis
- Premature labor.

PYELONEPHRITIS IN PREGNANCY

Infection of the kidney substance occurs in about 1–2% of all pregnancies:
- The causative organism is often *E. coli*
- Bacteriuria in early pregnancy is a predisposing factor.

Signs and Symptoms

- Pyrexia, which may reach up to 40°C and rigor
- Acceleration of maternal pulse and fetal heart rate
- Nausea, vomiting and dehydration
- Pain and tenderness over the loins
- Pain along the path of ureters radiating to the suprapubic region
- Burning on micturition and desire to pass urine even when bladder is empty
- Cloudy urine
- Urine pH acidic if infecting organism is *E. coli*.

Management

- Admission in hospital
- Antibiotic intravenously based on culture and sensitivity report. In severe infection, antibiotics may be continued for six weeks

- Urine culture to be repeated at intervals even after resolution to ensure there is no recurrence
- Intravenous fluids to correct dehydration with accurate record of intake and output
- Monitoring uterine activity as there is risk of labor commencing when temperature rises
- Antipyretics and tepid sponging when the temperature rises
- Monitoring temperature, pulse and respirations 4-hourly
- Analgesics and antiemetics as prescribed for back pain and vomiting.

Complications

- Recurrence of infection if there is abnormality of the renal tract
- Intrauterine growth retardation
- Preterm labor
- Congenital anomalies of the fetus
- Increased perinatal mortality.

URINARY TRACT INFECTION IN EARLY PUERPERIUM

Bacterial infection of the kidney substance in the early puerperium.

Causes

- Stasis of urine, which occurs during pregnancy
- Trauma during labor.
- Inadequate vulvar hygiene leading to an ascending infection.

Signs and Symptoms

- Malaise
- Aches and pains in the back and loins
- Pain and burning on micturition with cystitis
- Pyrexia, hematuria and pain over kidney region if there is pyelonephritis.

Investigation

Midstream urine for urinalysis and culture and sensitivity.

Management

- Appropriate antibiotics
- Increased fluid intake
- Analgesics
- Urinate frequently
- Self-care measures.

141. VASA PREVIA

Vasa previa refers to the cord vessels crossing the cervical os. It is associated with velamentous insertion of the cord where the junction of the cord is at the edge of the placenta. The vessels separate and traverse through the membranes overlying the internal os; in front of the presenting part. Rupture of the membranes involving the overlying vessels leads to vaginal bleeding.

ASSOCIATED CONDITIONS

- Placental abnormalities such as placenta previa or irregularly developed placenta
- Multiple pregnancies
- Pregnancies that result from in vitro fertilisation.

EFFECTS

Bleeding from a cord vessel is entirely fetal blood and causes the following problems:
- Hypoxia
- Hypovolemia
- Fetal exsanguination
- Fetal death.

MANAGEMENT

- Early detection by ultrasonography and planning for alternative form of delivery prevents fetal problems
- If detected during labor, urgent delivery either by cesarean section or vaginally may be done
- If the baby is dead, vaginal delivery is awaited.

142. VASECTOMY OPERATION/MALE STERILIZATION

Vasectomy is the permanent method of sterilization operation done in the male where a segment of vas deferens on both sides is resected about 1 cm and the cut ends are ligated. **(Figs. 142.1A and B)**. The ligated ends are then folded back on them and sutured into position so that the cut ends face away from each other. This will reduce the risk of recanalization later.

Following vasectomy, sperm production and hormone output are not affected. The sperm produced are destroyed intraluminally by phagocytosis. This is a normal process in the male genital tract, but the rate is increased after vasectomy. The vasectomized person is not immediately sterile after operation, usually until after 30 ejaculations have taken place, as the semen is stored in the distal part of the vas deferens for about two to three months. During this period, another contraceptive method must be used.

ADVANTAGES AND DISADVANTAGES OF VASECTOMY

Advantages

- The vasectomy operation is simple and can be performed as an outpatient or outdoor procedure
- Complications; immediate or later are few

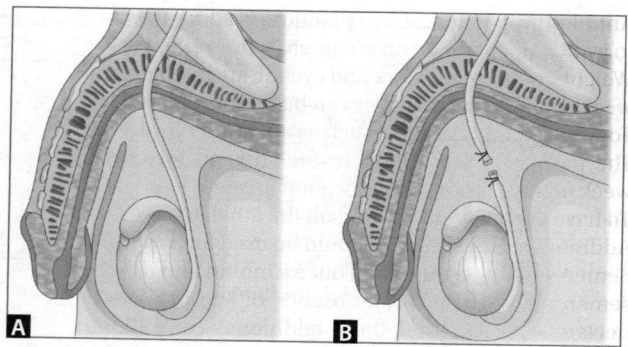

Figs. 142.1A and B: Vasectomy. **A.** Vas deferens before surgery; **B.** Vas deferens after surgery.

- Failure rate is about 0.15% and there is a fair chance of success of reversal anastomosis (recanalization) operation (50%).
- The overall expenditure is minimal in terms of equipment and hospital stay. Cost-wise the ratio is about five vasectomies to one tubal ligation.

Disadvantages

- Additional contraception is needed for about two to three months following vasectomy, i.e. until the semen becomes free of sperm
- Frigidity or impotence if occurs, is mostly psychological.

SELECTION OF CANDIDATES

Sexually active and psychologically adjusted husband having the desired number of children is an ideal candidate. Any misconception about fear of castration, loss of hormones and impotence are to be removed by explanation. Eczema or scabies in the scrotal region is a temporary contraindication. In the presence of hydrocele or inguinal hernia, vasectomy can be done only along with the operative correction of these conditions.

POSTOPERATIVE INSTRUCTIONS

- Antibiotic injection such as penidure is administered as a routine to avoid infection and an analgesic is prescribed to reduce pain
- Weight lifting, heavy work and cycling are restricted for about two weeks while usual activities can be performed forthwith
- To wear a scrotal support such as a T-binder for 15 days
- The patient should report to the surgeon for check-up after 1 week or earlier if any complication arises
- To have the stitches removed on the 5th day
- Additional contraceptive should be used for 3 months
- Semen should be examined once a month and if two consecutive semen analyzes show an absence of spermatozoa, the man is declared sterile. Until then, additional contraceptive such as condom should be advised.

COMPLICATIONS

Immediate

- Wound sepsis, which may lead to scrotal cellulitis or abscess
- Scrotal hematoma.

Remote

1. Some men complain of diminution of sexual vigor, impotence, headache or fatigue and these are mostly psychological in origin
2. Sperm granuloma or sperm granules caused by accumulation of sperm. These appear in 0–14 days after the operation. The most frequent symptoms are pain, swelling and a hard mass. The mass may be about 7 mm, which will eventually subside. This problem can be prevented by cauterization or fulguration of the cut ends.
3. **Autoimmune response:** Vasectomy is said to cause an autoimmune response to sperm. Blocking of the vas causes re-absorption of spermatozoa and subsequent development of antibodies against sperm in blood. Normally about 2% of men have circulating antibodies which are harmless to physical health. In vasectomized men the percentage is about 54. It is likely that they can cause a reductions in fertility, despite successful reanastomosis of the vas deferens.
4. **Spontaneous recanalization:** The incidence of recanalization varies from 0–6%. Its occurrence is serious and therefore the surgeon should explain the possiblity of this complication to every acceptor, prior to the operation and have written consent acknowledging the possibility. Regular follow up for about 3 years is recommended to avoid this possiblity.

OTHER TYPES OF VASECTOMY

No-scalpel Vasectomy

No-scalpel vasectomy is a new technique that is safe, convenient and acceptable to males. This new method is now being canvassed for men as a special project, on a voluntary basis under the family welfare program in India. This method is performed under local anesthetic. The stretched skin over the vas is punctured with one blade of a sharp pointed dissecting scissors, instead of using a scalpel. The hole is then increased and the vas is dissected out by using the tip of the scissors.

The testicular end is dropped back into the scrotum and the upper end is cauterized. The procedure is repeated for the second vas through the same incision. The rest of the steps are same as for the regular vasectomy procedure.

Open-ended Vasectomy

In open-ended vasectomy procedure the abdominal end of the resected vas is coagulated. The testicular end is left open. This is to prevent congestive epididymitis.

143. VESICOVAGINAL FISTULA

DEFINITION

An abnormal communication between the bladder and the vagina, and urine escapes into the vagina causing incontinence.

CAUSES

1. Obstructed labor causing ischemic necrosis, infection, sloughing and fistula formation.
2. Instrumental vaginal delivery such as destructive operations.
3. Abdominal operations such as hysterectomy for rupture of uterus, or repeat cesarean section.
4. Gynecologic surgeries such as anterior colporrhaphy, and abdominal hysterectomy for removal of malignant lesions.
5. Trauma due to fall on pointed objects, criminal abortion or fracture of pelvic bones.
6. Malignancy: Advanced carcinoma of the cervix, vagina or bladder.
7. Infective lesions such as tuberculosis, lymphogranuloma venerium or actinomycosis.

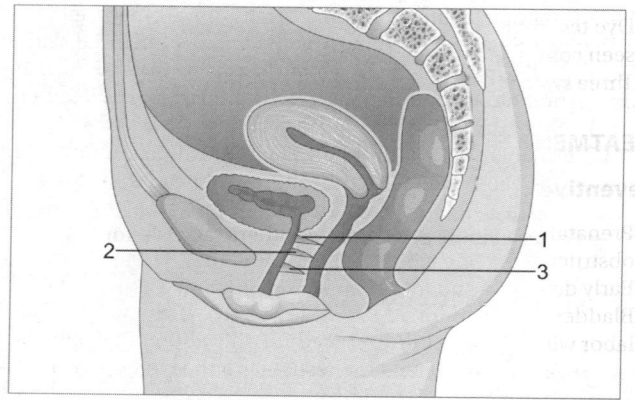

Fig. 143.1: Sites of vesicovaginal fistula. **1.** Juxtacervical; **2.** Midvaginal; **3.** Juxtaurethral.

SITES OF VESICOVAGINAL FISTULA (Fig.143.1)

- Juxtacervical (close to the cervix)
- Midvaginal (between the base of the bladder and vagina)
- Juxtaurethral (between neck of the bladder and vagina).

CLINICAL FEATURES

- Continuous escape of urine per vagina (true incontinence) with ammoniacal smell
- Pruritus vulvae and excoriation of skin
- Varying degrees of perineal tear
- Prolapse of bladder mucosa through the fistula seen on speculum examination
- Associated complete perineal tear or rectovaginal fistula (RVF).

DIAGNOSIS

- Examination under anesthesia
- Examination in Sim's or knee-chest position to check if bubbles of air are seen through the anterior vaginal wall, when the woman coughs

Vesicovaginal Fistula

- Dye test: Methylene blue dye introduced into the bladder will be seen coming out through the fistula
- Three swab test to locate the level of fistula.

TREATMENT

Preventive

- Prenatal screening to detect mothers at risk for developing obstruction during labor
- Early detection and ideal management to relieve obstruction
- Bladder drainage for 5–7 days following prolonged obstructed labor with cephalic presentation.

Surgery

Local repair of the fistula.

Preoperative Preparation

- General health status to be improved
- Any local infection present should be treated
- Urinary infection if any should be treated.

Postoperative Care

- Retention catheter for 10–14 days.
- Periodic clamping to see for leakage prior to removal
- Removal of catheter only after confirming that there is no leakage
- Urinary antiseptic to be administered
- Bladder wash with lotion acriflavine 1 in 10,000 once daily beginning 48 hours after the surgery and not exceeding 30 mL at a time
- Patient to be instructed to pass urine every 2 hours following removal of the catheter and the interval to be increased gradually.

Instructions for Care After Discharge

- To pass urine more frequently
- To avoid intercourse for at least 3 months

144. VENTOUSE DELIVERY (VACUUM-ASSISTED BIRTH)

Delivering a baby using a ventouse/vacuum extractor. The procedure involves placing a cup connected to suction over the occiput on the fetal head and after negative pressure (suction) is attained, applying traction downward and outward during contractions to deliver the fetal head. Traction should be sustained during contractions and the direction of the pull should correspond to the axis of the birth canal.

DESIGN OF THE INSTRUMENT

The vacuum extractor has the following components:
- Specially designed metal cups, a means of creating a chignon, which can be firmly gripped within the cup. The cups are available in three sizes of 40 mm, 50 mm and 60 mm
- A hollow tubing
- A glass trap bottle with manometer
- A chain attached to the cup, which passes through the tubing and attaches to a cross and handle used for traction.
- A suction hand pump.

INDICATIONS/CONTRAINDICATIONS FOR USE OF VENTOUSE

Indications

- Occipitolateral and occipitoposterior positions
- Delay in late first stage or second stage of labor
- Maternal exhaustion
- Maternal medical disorders such as heart disease, hypertensive disorders and moderate to severe anemia.

Contraindications

- Fetal distress where fast delivery is indicated
- Face presentation
- Prematurity
- Suspected fetal coagulopathy
- Earlier use of scalp electrode.

CONDITIONS TO BE FULFILLED

- Ensure that there is no bony resistance below the head
- Head of a singleton baby should be engaged
- Cervix should be at least 6 cm dilated.

PROCEDURE

- Patient is placed in lithotomy position
- Ensure that bladder is empty
- Clean the perineum with antiseptic lotion and drape with sterile sheets
- A thorough internal examination is done to determine station of fetal head, position of occiput and suture lines, adequacy of pelvis and cervical dilatation
- Pudendal block anesthesia is given
- The largest size cup that can be introduced comfortably is applied over the fetal scalp taking care that maternal soft parts are not included in the cap
- Suction is applied and gradually increased at the rate of 0.2 kg/cm every two minutes up to 0.8 kg/cm
- Traction is made intermittently coinciding with the uterine contractions and supplemented by maternal bearing down efforts. Direction of the pull should correspond to the axis of the birth canal.
- Delivery is usually effected with 4–6 pulls given over a period of 15–20 minutes. Once the head is delivered, suction is released, the cup slips off and delivery completed in the usual manner.

COMPLICATIONS

Maternal

- Soft tissue injuries such as cervical tears, vaginal tears, perineal lacerations and extension of episiotomy
- Traumatic postpartum hemorrhage
- Infection.

Fetal

- Sloughing of the scalp
- Cephalhematoma
- Subaponeurotic hemorrhage (not limited to suture line)
- Neonatal jaundice
- Chignon: This is an area of edema and bruising where the cup was applied. All babies delivered by ventouse will have a '.chignon'. Normally it subsides eventually, but may occasionally become infected.

145. VOMITING IN NEWBORNS

In the newborn period vomiting is a common manifestation. Regurgitation or possetting that occurs after feeding due to swallowed air or over handling should not be confused with vomiting. Vomiting with or without other signs may be a manifestation of gastrointestinal problems.

CAUSES OF VOMITING

Intracranial Injuries

Raised intracranial tension due to hemorrhage or depressed skull fracture.

Infections

Gastroenteritis, meningitis, septicemia, etc.

Obstructive

Gastrointestinal obstruction due to congenital problems such as:
- Esophageal atresia
- Cardiospasm
- Chalasia (relaxation of esophageal-gastric sphincter)
- Pyloric stenosis
- Duodenal atresia
- Diaphragmatic hernia or hiatus hernia.
- Meconium ileus
- Late case of imperforate anus
- Hirschsprung's disease
- Malrotation of the gut.

Associated Manifestations

Gastrointestinal problems often present with additional manifestations which include:
- Abdominal distension
- Failure to pass stools
- Diarrhea with or without blood in stools
- Temperature instability
- Poor feeding.

Other Causes

- Irritation of the gastric mucosa by swallowed materials such as meconium or maternal blood during birth
- Overfeeding or qualitative change in feed or excessive air swallowing.

MANAGEMENT

- Gastric lavage for vomiting due swallowed substances
- Education of mother about avoiding overfeeding and burping after feeding
- Correction of fluid imbalance and appropriate medical or surgical therapy for any underlying pathology.

STUDY QUESTIONS

1. **When performing pelvic palpation, the hands converge around the presenting part if the head is:**
   a. Fixed
   b. Not engaged
   c. Engaged
   d. Floating

2. **The total duration of labor is less than 2 hours in:**
   a. Preterm labor
   b. Post-term labor
   c. Precipitate labor
   d. Obstructed labor

3. **Inadequate food intake is the most common cause for:**
   a. Gestational diabetes
   b. Iron deficiency anemia
   c. Urinary infection
   d. Morning sickness

4. **The placenta covers the internal os when it is closed, in:**
   a. Type I placenta previa
   b. Type II placenta previa
   c. Type III placenta previa
   d. Type IV placenta previa

5. **The factor most associated with the increased risk for perinatal complications is:**
   a. Heredity
   b. Extremes in maternal age
   c. Geographic location
   d. Multiparity

6. **The most serious complication to affect newborns in developing countries is:**
   a. Low birth weight
   b. Macrosomia
   c. Hyperbilirubinemia
   d. Postmaturity

7. **A recent technological advance that has affected maternal-newborn nursing is:**
   a. Forceps for delivering babies
   b. Intravenous infusion pump
   c. Electronic fetal monitoring
   d. Radiant warmer

8. **A presumptive sign of pregnancy is:**
   a. Fetal outline
   b. Amenorrhea
   c. Fetal heart sounds
   d. Abdominal enlargement

9. **Mrs John's 1st day of her last menstrual period was 2nd January. Using Naegele's rule, her expected date delivery is:**
   a. October 9
   b. October 20
   c. September 9
   d. November 2

10. **The greatest degree of change during pregnancy occurs in which system?**
    a. Musculoskeletal
    b. Urinary
    c. Cardiovascular
    d. Reproductive

11. **A warning sign of a complication developing during pregnancy is:**
    a. Weight gain of 1/2 kg a week in the second or third trimester
    b. Braxton-Hicks contractions
    c. Nausea and vomiting during the first trimester
    d. Sudden increase in facial, hand/feet edema

12. **An effusion of blood under the periosteum is:**
    a. Cephalohematoma
    b. Caput succedaneum
    c. Subdural hemorrhage
    d. Subaponeurotic hemorrhage

13. **One of the four forces of labor is:**
    a. Position
    b. Pitocin
    c. Passenger
    d. Placenta

14. **The term for a breach presentation in which the fetal hips and thighs are flexed and the buttocks present towards the maternal pelvis is:**
    a. Frank breech
    b. Complete breech
    c. Footing breech
    d. Knee breech

15. **The fetal position that is usually the most uncomfortable for a laboring woman is:**
    a. Sacroanterior position
    b. Right sacrum transverse
    c. Occiput posterior
    d. Occiput anterior

16. **Biparietal diameter of the fetal skull measures:**
    a. 9.0 cm
    b. 9.5 cm
    c. 10.0 cm
    d. 8.5 cm

17. **The diameter of the fetal skull that measures from the point where the chain joins the neck to the center of bregma is:**
    a. Submentobregmatic
    b. Mentobregmatic
    c. Submentovertical
    d. Mentovertical

18. **The region of fetal skull that is bounded by the anterior fontanel, the two parietal eminences and the posterior fontanel is the:**
    a. Sinciput
    b. Occiput
    c. Face
    d. Vertex

19. The suture on the fetal skull that lies between the two frontal bones extending from bregma to the glabella is:
    a. Sagittal suture
    b. Coronal suture
    c. Frontal suture
    d. Lambdoidal suture

20. An abnormal or difficult labor due to mechanical factors or inadequate muscular activity is called:
    a. Dysfunctional labor
    b. Dystocia
    c. Hypertonic labor
    d. Prolonged labor

21. The most common cause of preterm labor is:
    a. Premature rupture of membranes
    b. Having a stressful lifestyle
    c. Cervical incompetence
    d. Eating fatty meals

22. The nursing intervention that is crucial in caring for the preterm labor patient on magnesium sulfate is:
    a. Monitoring patent's respiratory rate
    b. Padding the side rails of bed
    c. Having the antidote inderal on hand
    d. Forcing fluids

23. The most common cause of intrapartum hemorrhage is:
    a. Placenta accreta
    b. Placenta previa
    c. Abruptio planceta
    d. Uterine atony

24. The greatest risk of abruption of placenta to the fetus is:
    a. Rhesus incompatibility
    b. Severe hypoxia
    c. Coagulopathy
    d. Chest infection

25. Women who are at greatest risk for developing pregnancy-induced hypertension are:
    a. Pregnant women having blood group 'O'
    b. Pregnant women who are anemic

c. Primigravida under 19 and over 35 years of age
d. Multigravida

26. **Pain during labor and childbirth is primarily caused by:**
    a. Dilatation of cervix and uterine cell hypoxia
    b. Pressure on the urinary bladder
    c. Stretching of the pelvis
    d. Increased levels of endorphin

27. **Before administering a narcotic analgesic to a woman in labor, the nurse should:**
    a. Discourage the patient from taking it
    b. Verify that the patient is soon to deliver
    c. Assess maternal respirations, fetal heart rate and labor progress
    d. Notify the head nurse

28. **Maternal side effects from intravenous meperidine hydrochloride (Demerol) include:**
    a. Respiratory depression and tachycardia
    b. Hypertension an decreased pulse rate
    c. Agitation and hypertension
    d. Dehydration and muscle cramps

29. **The major side effects of epidural anesthesia are:**
    a. Hypertonus and fetal bradycardia
    b. Hypertension and increased placental blood flow
    c. Dehydration and rapid delivery
    d. Hypotension and urinary retention

30. **The fetal circulation consists of three circuits, the systemic, pulmonary, and:**
    a. Cardiac
    b. Renal
    c. Placental
    d. Mesenteric

31. **The part of fetal circulation that directs most blood flow to bypass the lungs is the:**
    a. Aortic valve
    b. Ductus arteriosus
    c. Ductus venosus
    d. Hypogastric arteries

32. **The most common cause of fetal hypoxia is an alteration in:**
    a. Maternal position
    b. Fetal position
    c. Maternal glucose levels
    d. Uteroplacental blood flow

33. **In beats per minute, the normal fetal heart rate is:**
    a. 80–120
    b. 100–120
    c. 140–180
    d. 120–160

34. **Abdominal pain and vaginal bleeding in the pregnant patient may indicate:**
    a. Abruptio placentae
    b. Nuchal cord
    c. Uteroplacental insufficiency
    d. Placenta previa

35. **Metabolic derangement in response to fetal asphyxia includes:**
    a. Acidosis
    b. Alkalosis
    c. Hypomagnesemia
    d. Hperglycemia

36. **A test of fetal well-being that involves evaluating movement and change in fetal heart rate in response to that movement is the:**
    a. Oxytocin challenge test
    b. Non-stress test
    c. Contraction stress test
    d. Nipple stimulation test

37. **The initial fetal response to hypoxia generally is:**
    a. A decreased heart rate
    b. An increased heart rate
    c. An increase in movement
    d. A decrease in movement

38. **A test for fetal well-being that involves the intravenous administration of a uterine stimulant is the:**
    a. Nipple stimulation test
    b. Non-stress rest

c. Fetal scalp pH test
d. Contraction stress test

39. **A fetal heart tracing associated with compression of the fetal head during a contraction is:**
    a. Late decelerations
    b. Early decelerations
    c. Early accelerations
    d. Variable decelerations

40. **A fetal heart tracing seen commonly during labor is:**
    a. Late decelerations
    b. Variable decelerations
    c. Early decelerations
    d. Early accelerations

41. **Lake decelerations noted on the fetal heart monitor requires:**
    a. Immediate and further assessment of fetal well-being
    b. No intervention
    c. Turning the mother on her back
    d. Putting the mother in a semi-Fowler's position

42. **The absence of variability in a fetal heart rate generally indicates that the fetus is:**
    a. In good condition
    b. Suffering distress
    c. Dead
    d. Not ready to be delivered

43. **You are caring for a labor patient when fetal bradycardia suddenly develops. What should you do?**
    a. Sit the mother up in bed, ask her to pant and reassure her that baby is surviving.
    b. Turn the mother on her right side and perform a pelvic examination
    c. Sit her up and give her a drink
    d. Turn the mother on her left side, apply an oxygen mask and call for assistance

44. **The cardinal movement of labor, which occurs when the fetal chin rests against the chest is called:**
    a. Expulsion
    b. Descend

c. Internal rotation
d. Flexion

45. The type of forceps that is used when the fetal head is visible on the perineum is called:
   a. Mid forceps
   b. Low forceps
   c. High forceps
   d. Axis traction forceps

46. An indication for cesarean delivery is:
   a. Pregnancy-induced hypertension
   b. Diabetes
   c. Dystocia
   d. Vertex presentation

47. One of the most important nursing interventions to assist the neonate in adapting to extrauterine life is to:
   a. Maintain a stable body temperature for the infant
   b. Initiate breastfeeding immediately
   c. Perform a heel stick to assess for hypoglycemia
   d. Transfer the baby to nursery as soon as possible

48. An Apgar score of 5–7 at 1 minute of life indicates the neonate has:
   a. No apparent distress
   b. Good cardiorespiratory rate, vigorous cry and pink skin color
   c. Mild respiratory, metabolic or neurologic depression
   d. Severe depression requiring resuscitation

49. In neonatal resuscitation, the neonate is given positive pressure ventilation if:
   a. Apgar score is less than 6 at 5 minutes
   b. Heart rate is less than 100 beats per minute
   c. Color is acrocyanotic
   d. Meconium is present in amniotic fluid

50. During neonatal resuscitation, chest compressions are to be initiated when the heart rate is below:
   a. 120 beats per minute
   b. 80 beats per minute and not increasing
   c. 80 beats per minute and increasing
   d. 100 beats per minute

51. The average birth weight for newborns is approximately:
    a. 1.5–2 kg
    b. 2.5–3 kg
    c. 2–2.5 kg
    d. 3–3.5 kg

52. The most common benign transient lesion in a newborn is:
    a. Lanugo
    b. Mongolian spot
    c. Milia
    d. Erythema toxicum

53. A condition in the newborn in which a collection of blood develops between a skull bone and periosteum without crossing suture lines is called:
    a. Caput succedaneum
    b. Intraventricular hemorrage
    c. Bulging fontanel
    d. Cephalhematoma

54. A sign of respiratory distress in the newborn is:
    a. Heart rate 120 per minute
    b. Grunting
    c. Acrocyanosis
    d. Respirations greater than 30 per minute

55. The umbilical cord lies alongside or in front of the presenting part with the fetal membranes intact, in which of following situations?
    a. Cord prolapsed
    b. Cord around the baby's neck
    c. Cord presentation
    d. Short umbilical cord

56. The postpartum period generally is considered to end how long after delivery of the baby?
    a. 2 weeks
    b. 4 weeks
    c. 6 weeks
    d. 8 weeks

57. The initial maternal genital discharge after childbirth is normally:
    a. Red
    b. Brown
    c. Pink
    d. Yellow

58. The discharge after childbirth is initially termed lochia rubra, which then becomes:
    a. Lochia alba
    b. Lochia sanguina
    c. Lochia sebaceous
    d. Lochia serosa

59. About how much blood is generally lost during a routine vaginal delivery?
    a. 500 mL
    b. 1,000 mL
    c. 200 mL
    d. 50 mL

60. In premature newborns, respiratory distress syndrome (RDS) occur due to:
    a. Oligohydramnios in pregnancy
    b. Neural tube defects in fetus
    c. Deficiency of surfactant in fetal lungs
    d. Polyhydramnios in pregnancy

61. About how much blood loss would the nurse expect in a patient undergoing cesarean section:
    a. 500 mL
    b. 2,500 mL
    c. 250 mL
    d. 1,000 mL

62. A common complaint of postpartum patient is:
    a. Cracked nipples
    b. Back pain
    c. Chest pain
    d. Constipation

63. **In a woman who does not breastfeed, the menstrual cycle usually resumes in about:**
    a. 1–2 weeks
    b. 2–4 weeks
    c. 3–5 weeks
    d. 7–9 weeks

64. **The primary cause of postpartum hemorrhage is:**
    a. Retained placental fragments
    b. Uterine atony
    c. Genital tract lacerations
    d. Perineal hematoma

65. **Common organisms causing mastitis are:**
    a. *Escherichia coli* and *Serratia*
    b. *Haemophilus* and gonorrhea
    c. Staphylococci and streptococci
    d. *Trichomonas* and *Candida*

66. **A nursing action when caring for the postpartum patient, who complains of pain in the leg is to:**
    a. Massage the leg
    b. Call the nursing supervisor
    c. Ask the patient to perform range of motion exercises
    d. Assess the leg for swelling and discoloration

67. **A positive Homan's sign may indicate:**
    a. Endometritis
    b. Thrombophlebitis
    c. Mastitis
    d. Cervicitis

68. **The part of pelvis lying below the pelvic brim is:**
    a. True pelvis
    b. False pelvis
    c. Gynecoid pelvis
    d. Android pelvis

69. **Anteroposterior edge of the first sacral vertebra is termed:**
    a. Sacral foramina
    b. Sacroiliac joint
    c. Sacral promontory
    d. Sacrococcygeal joint

70. **Frank breech is also termed as:**
    a. Footling presentation
    b. Knee presentation
    c. Complete breech
    d. Breech with extended legs

71. **The female breast is partly formed from which type of tissue?**
    a. Glandular
    b. Nervous
    c. Muscle
    d. Granular

72. **The hormone primarily responsible for lactation is:**
    a. Estradiol
    b. Progesterone
    c. Estrogen
    d. Prolactin

73. **How many lobes are generally found in a breast?**
    a. 20
    b. 10
    c. 30
    d. 40

74. **The sucking of the infant causes the pituitary to release which hormone?**
    a. Follicle-stimulating hormone
    b. Oxytocin hormone
    c. Gonadotrophin hormone
    d. Prolactin hormone

75. **Face presentation occurs when the attitude of the fetal head is:**
    a. Complete flexion
    b. Complete extension
    c. Incomplete flexion
    d. Incomplete extension

76. **The diameter of the fetal skull, which measure 13.5 cm is the:**
    a. Occipitofrontal
    b. Suboccipitobregmatic

c. Submentobregmatic
d. Mentovertical

77. **Measures to reduce the incidence of uterine atony following delivery include:**
    a. Diuretic administration and breastfeeding
    b. Oxytocin administration and oral fluids
    c. Fundal message and breastfeeding
    d. Application of tight abdominal binder and oxytocin administration

78. **Lactation is effectively suppressed by:**
    a. Binding the breasts
    b. Avoidance of sucking
    c. Application of ice
    d. Injection of prolactin

79. **Lactation is the result of complex neurohormonal events, but is primarily mediated by which gland?**
    a. Mammary
    b. Ovary
    c. Pituitary
    d. Salivary

80. **The newborn period refers to the first:**
    a. 2 hours of life
    b. 28 days of life
    c. Year of life
    d. 7 days of life

81. **The downy hair that covers the body of the fetus is called:**
    a. Lanugo
    b. Surfactant
    c. Meconium
    d. Vernix caseosa

82. **The bones of the newborn's head are joined by connective tissue called:**
    a. Fontanels
    b. Sutures
    c. Ligaments
    d. Surfactant

83. Tiny projections on the hard palate of the newborn are usually:
   a. Thrush
   b. Milia
   c. *Escherichia coli*
   d. Epstein's pearls

84. A bluish, cyanotic tinge of the lips of newborn baby is called:
   a. Circumoral cyanosis
   b. Acrocyanosis
   c. Hypoxic cyanosis
   d. Oral cyanosis

85. The condition in which the infant's sternum appears to pull back toward the spine is:
   a. Grunting
   b. Flaring
   c. Retraction
   d. Hypoxia

86. An infant with a 1 minute Apgar score of 9, requires:
   a. Immediate resuscitation
   b. No intervention
   c. Intubation
   d. Suctioning

87. The Apgar scoring system rates the infant's heart rate, respiratory effort, muscle tone, reflex irritability and:
   a. Cry
   b. Color
   c. Eyes
   d. Kick

88. A condition where bowel sounds can be heard in the chest of a newborn is:
   a. Omphalocele
   b. Cystic fibrosis
   c. Diaphragmatic hernia
   d. Esophageal atreia

89. **The condition in pregnancy where the volume of amniotic fluid is 500 mL or less between 32 and 34 weeks is:**
    a. Polihydramnios
    b. Oligohydramnios
    c. Hydatidiform mole
    d. Fetal ascites

90. **A thick, sticky, green or black substance found in the large intestine of a full-term neonate is:**
    a. Surfactant
    b. Vernix caseosa
    c. Lanugo
    d. Meconium

91. **The first action when caring for a baby, born with meconium staining is:**
    a. Suctioning
    b. Giving oxygen
    c. Ventilating the lungs with positive pressure
    d. Drying

92. **Hyline membrane disease of the newborn involves a deficiency of:**
    a. Meconium
    b. Vernix caseosa
    c. Surfactant
    d. Lanugo

93. **The first treatment for hyperbilirubinemia is often:**
    a. Exchange transfusion
    b. Oxygen therapy
    c. Phototherapy
    d. Isolation

94. **Hyperbilirubinemia can lead to:**
    a. Respiratory distress
    b. Kernicterus
    c. Meconium aspiration
    d. Hypothermia

95. **Hypoglycemia in the newborn can lead to:**
    a. Seizures
    b. Aspiration
    c. Kernicterus
    d. Phenylketonuria

96. **For a patient on induction of labor with oxytocin, an indication to stop the infusion is:**
    a. Mild uterine contractions
    b. Mother complaining of headache
    c. Any evidence of fetal distress
    d. Urine output above 30 mL per minute

97. **The most appropriate time to make an episiotomy incision is:**
    a. At the time of crowing
    b. When the mother relaxes after a strong uterine contraction
    c. When the cervix is dilated about 6 cm
    d. Soon after the rupture of membranes

98. **In the labor mechanism of left mentoanterior position, attitude of the fetus is:**
    a. Flexion of body and extension of head
    b. Flexion of both body and head
    c. Extension of limbs and flexion of head
    d. Extension of head and back

99. **The structure in fetal circulation that carries oxygenated blood to the fetus is:**
    a. Umbilical arteries
    b. Umbilical vein
    c. Ductus venosus
    d. Ductus arteriosus

100. **In X-linked gene disorders, the affected gene is carried by:**
    a. Females and males
    b. Females or males
    c. Females
    d. Males

Answers

1. b	2. c	3. b	4. c	5. b	6. a
7. c	8. b	9. a	10. d	11. d	12. a
13. c	14. b	15. c	16. b	17. a	18. d
19. c	20. b	21. a	22. a	23. b	24. b
25. c	26. a	27. c	28. a	29. d	30. c
31. b	32. d	33. d	34. a	35. a	36. b
37. b	38. d	39. b	40. b	41. a	42. b
43. d	44. d	45. b	46. c	47. a	48. c
49. b	50. b	51. b	52. d	53. d	54. b
55. c	56. c	57. a	58. d	59. a	60. c
61. d	62. d	63. d	64. b	65. c	66. d
67. b	68. a	69. c	70. d	71. a	72. d
73. a	74. b	75. b	76. d	77. c	78. b
79. c	80. b	81. a	82. b	83. d	84. a
85. c	86. b	87. b	88. c	89. b	90. d
91. a	92. c	93. c	94. b	95. a	96. c
97. a	98. d	99. b	100. c		

Bibliography

1. American Society of Reproductive Medicine. 209 Montgomery Highway. Birmingham. AL: 35216 (205) 975–1000: Available from: http:/www.asrm.
2. Bhaskar Nima. Midwifery and Obstetrical Nursing, 2nd edition. Bangalore: EMMES Medical Publishers; 2015.
3. Bonnar J, McNicol GP, Douglas AS. Coagulation and fibrinolytic mechanisms during and after a normal childbirth. British Medical Journal. 1970;25:200-3.
4. Duftary SN, Chakravarti S. Manual of Obstetrics, 2nd edition. New Delhi: Elsevier; 2700.
5. Dutta DC. Textbook of Gynecology, 5th edition. Kolkata: New Central Book Company; 2008.
6. Dutta DC. Textbook of Gynecology including Contraception, 3rd edition. Calcutta: New Central Book Agency; 2001.
7. Dutta DC. Textbook of Obstetrics, 5th edition. Kolkata: New Central Book Company; 2001.
8. Dutta DC. Textbook of Obstetrics including Perinatology and Contraception, 6th edition. Calcutta: New Central Book Agency; 2004.
9. Frazer DM, Cooper MA. Myles Textbook for Midwives, 14th edition. Edinburgh: Churchill Livingstone Publications; 2003.
10. Freudnlich Madelyn. Adoption and Assisted Reproduction. Child Welfare League of America. Washington D. C; 2001.
11. Government of India. Ministry of Health and Family Welfare. Annual Report. 2005–2006, New Delhi: 2006.
12. Government of India. Rural Health Division, Bulletin for Health Statistics in India. New Delhi: March 2002.
13. Grotevant D. Harold, Dunbar Nora, Kohler, L. Julie, Lash Esau Any. Handbook of Adoption: Implications for Researchers, Practitioners, and Families. Thousand Oaks, Cage Publications; 2007.
14. Gupta S. The Short Textbook of Pediatrics, 9th edition. New Delhi: Jaypee Brothers Medical Publishers (P) Ltd; 2001.
15. Halliday HL. Handbook of Neonatal Intensive Care. London. Balliere Tindal; 1989.
16. Indrani TK. Domiciliary Care in Midwifery. New Delhi: Jaypee Brothers Medical Publishers (P) Ltd; 2004.

17. Jacob A, Rekha R, Jadhav S. Clinical Nursing Procedures. The Art of Nursing, 3rd edition. New Delhi: Jaypee Brothers Medical Publishers (P) Ltd; 2014.
18. Jacob A. A Comprehensive Textbook of Midwifery and Gynecological Nursing, 4th edition. New Delhi: Jaypee Brothers Medical Publishers (P) Ltd; 2014.
19. James DK, Steer PJ, Weiner CP, et al. High Risk Pregnancy: Management Options, 3rd edition. New Delhi; Elsevier India (Pvt) Ltd; 2006.
20. Kattiwinkel J. University of Virginia .1995; Newborn assessment and resuscitation. Virginia. www.vital.com
21. Kattwinkel J, Perlman JM, Aziz K, et al. Neonatal resuscitation: 2010 American Heart Association Guidelines for Cardiopulmonary Resuscitation and Emergency Cardiovascular Care. Pediatrics. 2010;126(5):1400.
22. Kattwinkel J, Short J, Niermeyer S, et al. Textbook of Neonatal Resuscitation, 4th edition. Elk Grove Village, IL: American Academy of Pediatrics and American Heart Association; 2000.
23. Kozier R, Erb G, Berman A, et al. Fundamentals of Nursing, 3rd edition. New Delhi: Dorling Kindersley (India) Pvt. Ltd; 2007. p. 1010-20.
24. Littleton LY, Engebretson JC. Maternity Nursing Care. Thomson Delmar Learning. Australia: 1st Indian reprint, Haryana: Sanat Printers: 2007. P. 191–238.
25. Manning FA. Dynamic Ultrasound-based fetal assessment: The fetal biophysical profile score. Clinical Obstetrics and Gynecology. 1995;38:26-34.
26. May AK, Mahlmeister LR. Maternal and Neonatal Nursing: Family Centered Care, 3rd edition. Philadelphia: JB Lippincott Company; 1994.
27. Menon KMK, Palaniappan B, Shastri K, et al. Clinical Obstetrics, 9th edition. Chennai: Orient Longman (Pvt) Ltd; 2002.
28. Mitchell H. Vaginal discharge—causes, diagnosis, and treatment. British Medical Journal. 2004;328(7451);1306-8.
29. Neonatal Intensive Care Unit (NICU) https:/www.cimarindindia.com.
30. Padubidri VG, Daftary SN. Howkins and Bourne Shaw's Textbook of Gynecology, 13th edition. New Delhi: Elsevier Publications; 2004.

31. Padubidri VG. Obstetrics, 2nd edition New Delhi: Elsevier India (Pvt) Ltd; 2004.
32. Park K. Park's Textbook of Preventive and Social Medicine, 21st edition. Jabalpur: M/S Banarasidas Bhanot Publishers; 2011. pp. 408-526.
33. Pillitteri A. Maternal and Child Health Nursing: Care of the Childbearing and Childrearing, 5th edition. Philadelphia: Lippincott Williams and Wlkins; 2007.
34. Rampaga Cheryl, Eovaldi Marina, Ma Cassandsra, Weigel Catherine. Normal Family Processes: Growing Diversity and Complexity, 3rd edition. New York: Guilford Press; 2003.
35. Rao KS. Textbook of an Introduction to Community Health Nursing, 4th edition. New Delhi: BI Publications(P) Ltd; 2004.
36. Robertson NRC. Disorders of Respiratory Tract. A Manual of Neonatal Intensive Care, 3rd edition. Edward Arnold; 1993.
37. Sharma KN, Gupta PA. Textbook of Midwifery and Gynecological Nursing. Jalandhar City: S Vikas and Company; 2010.
38. Sharma MP. Selected Health Statistics of India. October 2012. Available from: http:/www.ucms.in.
39. Sheth SS. Essentials of Gynecology. New Delhi: Jaypee Brothers Medical Publishers (P) Ltd; 2005.
40. Skidmore RL. Mosby's 2009 Nursing Drug Reference. Noida: Reed Elsevier India Private Limited; 2009.
41. Smeltzer SC, Bare BG, Hinkle LJ, et al. Textbook of Medical-Surgical Nursing, 11th edition. Philadelphia: Lippincott Williams and Wilkins; 2008. pp. 1610-98.
42. The newborn intensive care unit (NICU)-March of Dimes. https://www.marchofdimes.com
43. The newborn intensive care unit. https://www.stanfordchildrens.org
44. Varney H, Kriebs JM, Gegor LC. Varney's Textbook of Midwifery, 4th edition. New Delhi: All India Publishers and Distributors; 2005.
45. Vashishtha VM, Kalra A, Bose A, et al. Indian Academy of Pediatrics (IAP) recommended immunization schedule for children aged 0 through 18 years. India, 2013 and updates on immunization. Indian Pediatrics. 2013;50(12):549-64.
46. Yadav A, Arora VS. Synopsis of Medical Instruments and Procedures. New Delhi: BI Publications (Pvt) Ltd; 2003.

Index

Page numbers followed by *b* refer to box, *f* refer to figure and *t* refer to table.

A

Abdomen 79
    enlargement of 260
    inspection of 412
Abdominal distension 440, 444, 781, 207
Abdominal examination 1, 216, 261, 325, 625
Abdominal tightness 559
Ablation 291
    endometrial 15, 275
Abnormal uterine action 5
    types of 5
ABO incompatibility 4, 500
Abortion 19, 31, 48, 394, 405, 445, 732, 733
    classification of 19*b*
    clinical types of 19*b*
    complete 22, 22*f*
    criminal 28
    habitual 28
    illegal 28
    incomplete 23, 24*f*, 551, 758
    induced 26
    induction of 309
    inevitable 21, 21*f*
    isolated 20
    legal 26
    medical method of 570
    mid-trimester 554, 557
    missed 25, 309, 758
    recurrent 28
    septic 27, 299, 420, 731, 732
    spontaneous 20, 245, 741
    threatened 20, 20*f*, 758
    tubal 323, 324*f*
    unsafe 28
Abruptio placentae 65, 66, 75, 75*t*, 299
Acardiac formation 560
Accredited Social Health Activist 569
    responsibilities of 572
    selection of 572
Acetone, urine for 184
Achondroplasia 379, 382
Acidosis, metabolic 712
Acquired immunodeficiency syndrome 40, 447, 742
Activated partial thromboplastin time 79
Acute pelvic inflammatory disease 271, 310
Adenocarcinoma 331
Adenomyosis 13, 33
Adhesiolysis 332, 333
Adhesions 16, 294
Adhesive tape 718
    roll of 717*f*
Adjuvant therapy 454
Adnexal mass, presence of 422
Adoption Laws in India 35
Adoption procedure 40
Adrenaline 721
Adriamycin 124
Agglutination test 453
Air embolism 732
Airborne infection isolation room 581
Airway 89, 91, 92*f*, 730
    disease 712
    obstruction 712
Alanine transaminase 682
Alcohol 315, 746
    abuse 577
    based hand rubs, use of 583
Allergy 493
Allis tissue forceps 462*f*, 462*f*

Alpha-fetoprotein 250
    maternal serum 389
Amenorrhea 21, 233, 260, 287, 707
    lactational 220
    secondary 552
American Cancer Society 127
American Joint Committee on
    Cancer 111
Ammonium dermatitis 546
Amniocentesis 47, 79, 250, 389
    mid-trimester 391
    risks of 48
Amniotic fluid 758
    embolism 49, 299, 732
    leakage 48
    volume 93
        index 94
Amniotomy 78, 435
    benefits of 78
Amphetamines 315
Ampicillin 768
Analeptic drugs 237
Analgesia 313768
    patient controlled 313
    regional 313, 314
Analgesics 313, 771
Anaphylaxis 306
Anemia 50, 60, 369, 559, 691
    aplastic 50
    classification of 50b
    congenital 725
    nutritional 50
    rare forms of 54
    severe 750
Anencephaly 196, 197f, 734
Anesthesia 555
    epidural 767
    spinal 732
Anesthetic 315
    complications 157
    gel 273
    local 732
    spray 273

Angel kisses 545
Ankle clonus 320
Anovular bleeding 17
Anovulation 453
Antacid therapy 157
Antenatal 147, 437, 561
    hygiene 765
    management 148
Antepartum hemorrhage 48, 65,
    66, 733
    classification of 65b
    general management of 66
Anterior vaginal wall retractor 467,
    467f
Anteroposterior diameter 359,
    531
Antibiotics 299
Anticonvulsants 315, 679
    drugs 310
Antidepressant therapy 700
Antifibrinolytics 365
    agents 15
Antihypertensives 307t, 680
    drugs 307
Antimetabolites 315
Antisera 732
Antisperm antibodies 454
Antithyroid drugs 315
Anus 595
Anxiety 32, 544
    disorder 697, 699, 701
Aorta, coarctation of 155, 169, 174,
    176
Aortic stenosis 169, 174
Apert's syndrome 215
APGAR score 93, 424, 715
Apnea 440
Appendicitis, acute 288
Apresoline 307, 308
Arm
    circle exercise 140, 141f
    lift exercise 133, 134f
    swinging 139, 140f

Arrhythmia 306
    cardiac 172, 175, 306
Arterial blood gases, maternal 177
Artery forceps 457, 458f
Artificial insemination 84, 85, 455
Artificial reproductive methods, prognosis of 88
Asherman's syndrome 275
Aspartate transaminase 682
Asphyxia 251
Aspirate sample tissue 272
Aspiration 157
Assisted breech delivery 146, 150
Assisted reproductive technology 83, 455
    techniques of 83b
Asthma 310
Atresia, vaginal 284
Atrial septal defect 169, 174, 204
Atrophic vulvovaginitis 442
Atrophy
    vaginal 319, 442
    vulvar 442
Attitude 360
Auscultation 4, 147, 261, 412
Automated external defibrillator 92
Autosome, numerical abnormalities of 378, 380
Auvard's weighted vaginal speculum 470, 470f
Axillary lymph node 109
    dissection 129
Axis traction devices 375, 478, 478f
Ayer spatula 265f
AYUSH 573
Azoospermia 85, 454

B

Babcock tissue forceps 487, 488f
Baby, care of 423, 562
Baby-Friendly Hospital Initiative 107
Bacillus Calmette-Guérin 566
Backache 542
Bacteremia 733
Bacteremic puerperal infection 733
Bacteriuria 768
Bag and mask equipment 716, 717f, 718
Bakri balloon 491, 492f, 494f
    parts of 492f
    placement of 493
Ball squeezing exercise 134, 135f
Balloon, mechanism of action of 493
Barrier methods 219, 221
Bartholin gland cysts 318
Barton's forceps 375
Basic life support 88
    sequence of 89, 89b
Bednar's aphthae 545
Below poverty line 573
Beta-thalassemia major 56
Bichloroacetic acid 740
Biophysical profile 93, 94t, 250
Biopsy
    catheter 274f
    percutaneous 117
    surgical 117
    wedge 553
Biparietal diameter 359, 669
Bipolar disorder 699, 701
Birnberg bow 224
Birth
    asphyxia 157, 577
    injuries 95, 95b, 157, 246
Bishop score
    predictive value of 432t
    system 432t
Bitemporal diameter 359
Bladder 330, 405, 655, 671
    changes 405
    extrophy of 211, 211f
    function 201
    hypotonia 767

Bleeding 31, 79, 577
   antepartum 732
   character of 68
   control of 493
   excessive 14
   heavy 276
   idiopathic 65
   intermenstrual 226
   irregular 13
   nature of 75
   postmenopausal 19, 275, 281, 550
   postmenstrual 271
   postpartum 732
   severe 157
   time 300
   types of 13*b*
   vaginal 21, 229, 268, 408, 544
Bleomycin 166
Blighted ovum 758
Blink reflex 646
Bloating 228
Blood 237
   borne spread 167
   character of 75
   coagulation studies 50
   glucose 65
      fasting 247
      values 247*t*
   group 22
   hemoglobin 69
   loss 50, 519, 732, 733
   oxygen content of 730
   pressure 71, 79, 184, 252, 418, 639, 671
      diastolic 677
      systolic 677
   sugar, fasting 248
   tests 444, 453
   transfusion 578
   urea nitrogen 61, 665
   volume 640

Body
   delivery of 511
   external rotation of 150
   fibroids 363
   temperature 594
Bone
   marrow
      aspiration 58
      insufficiency 50
   metabolism 537
   parietal 357
Bowel 656
   movement 444
   obstruction 288
Brachial palsy 101
Brachy technique 165
Brain 730
Brandt-Andrew method 517*f*
Breast 537, 642, 654
   antenatal care of 144
   cancer 108, 112, 119*f*, 125, 229
      diagnosis of 112
      invasive 110
      metastatic 111
      risks factors of 110
      staging of 111
      surgical management of 120
      types of 118
   care of 104, 104
   changes 257, 707
   conditions, malignant 110
   feeding positions 106*f*
   infection 143
   inspection of 115
   lymphatic system of 109
   magnetic resonance imaging of 117*f*
   malignancy 533
   milk, composition of 522*t*
   normal 109
   Paget disease of 120
   palpation patterns 114*f*

reconstruction after surgery 126
self-examination 108, 112, 113f
tenderness 228
Breastfeeding 104, 522, 523, 663
benefits of 524
Breath, shortness of 41, 559
Breathing 89, 92
Breech delivery 577
hazards of 152
spontaneous 146, 149
Breech extraction 146, 152
principles of 152
Breech hook and crochet 482, 482f
Breech presentation 4, 145
causes of 146
types of 145, 146f
Broad ligament cyst 288
Bromocriptine 689
Brow presentation 153
Bruise 99
Bulb syringe 475, 475f
Burning 442
vaginal 735
Buttocks
internal rotation of 149
restitution of 150

C

Cachexia 41, 165
Caffeine 316
Calendar method 220
Cancer
antigen, serum marker 125 330
cervix 158, 402
invasive 402
diagnosis of 128
invasive 119
pre-invasive 402
uterus 166
Candida
albicans 143, 437, 735
infection 144
tropicalis 735
Candidiasis 735
Cannula 289f
Caput succedaneum 99
Carbamazepine 316
Carbohydrate
excessive 298
metabolism 244
Carcinoma
advanced 164
breast 120
cervix 163
early 163
endometrial 550
medullary 119
mucinous 119
ovary 419
varieties of 163
Cardiac arrest 157
Cardiac decompensation, severe 533
Cardiac disease 169, 304
classification of 169b
Cardiac failure 52, 732
congestive 13, 175
Cardiomyopathy 169
Cardiopulmonary disease, severe 333
Cardiorespiratory disease, severe 288
Cardiospasm 781
Cardiotocography 348
Cardiovascular disease 310
Cardiovascular system 169, 537, 594, 639
anomalies 203
Carotid pulse 90f
Carpal tunnel syndrome 543
Cat's cry syndrome 187, 379
Catheter, insertion of 493
Causative organisms 438, 441, 443, 767
Central Adoption Resource Authority 34, 37

Central nervous system 93, 595, 683
  anomalies 195
Central venous pressure 71
Cephalhematoma 95, 96f
Cephalic presentation 4
Cephalopelvic disproportion 96, 181, 156
  diagnosis of 181
  risks of 182
Cephalosporin 768
Cephalotribe 483, 484f
Cerebral malformation 237
Cerebrospinal fluid 198, 237
Cervical
  biopsy 553
    types of 553
  brush 269f
  canal 293
  cancer 272, 275, 493
  carcinoma 65
  dilatation 502
  dilation 10, 21, 184
  dilator 272, 272f
  dysplasia 293
  dystocia 9, 557
  effacement 502
  erosions 65
  fibroid 368
  hostility 86
  incompetence 29, 295, 552, 554, 557
  infection 272, 275
  intraepithelial neoplasia 292, 402, 419, 555
  malignancy 533
  mucus
    method 219
    test 452
  polyps 65
  rigidity 156
  scraping 266
  smear 263
  stenosis 295, 554, 557
    severe 272
  tear 420
  tissue, condyloma of 293
Cervicitis 284, 442
Cervicopexy 767
Cervix 22, 272, 419, 638
  amputation of 556
  congenital elongation of 556
  dilation of 550
  incomplete dilatation of 151
  purulent infection of 493
  ripening of 502
  structural problems of 450
  surface of 293
Cesarean
  birth 160
  delivery 577
  hysterectomy 158
  scar, rupture of 727
  section 78, 155, 243, 299, 425, 561, 627
    complications of 157
    elective 182
    indications for 155
    previous 304, 377
  wound 708
Chadwick's sign 258
Chalasia 781
Chemical contraceptives 219, 223
Chemoprevention 127
Chemotherapy 124, 165, 166, 168
Chest
  compressions 89, 90, 91f, 719, 720f
  pain 41
  X-ray 714
Chickenpox 447
Child Adoption in India 34
Child sexual abuse 744
Child Welfare Committee 38

Chills 444
Chlamydia 268, 450
 trachomatis 443
Chlamydiosis 737
Chloramphenicol 315
Chloroquine 315
Chlorpromide 315
Chlorthiazide 316
Choanal atresia 202, 712
Chocolate cyst
 infections of 331
 rupture of 331
Chorioamnionitis 299
Choriocarcinoma 419
Chorion epithelioma 550
Chorionic villi
 biopsy 389
 sampling 392
Chromosomal disorders 378, 379
Chromosome abnormalities 184
Chromosome instability syndrome 188, 378, 380
Circulation 89, 90
Circulatory collapse
 signs of 69
 symptoms of 69
Circulatory fibrinolysis test 300
Circulatory system 542
Cisplatin 166
Clammy extremities 21
Clavicle 103
Cleft
 lip 205, 205f, 206, 206f, 315
  bilateral 205f
  unilateral 205
 palate 205, 206, 206f, 315
Cleidotomy 734
Clomiphene citrate 86, 455
Clonic phase 320, 681
Clonus 158
Clot
 observation test 300
 passage of 14

Clotting disorder 272
Club foot 212, 212f
CO_2 laser machine 293f
Coagulation
 correction of 71
 detection of 71
 profile 69, 70
 time 300
Coagulopathy 65, 239, 272
 conditions of 299
Cocaine 316
Coccyx 528
Coitus interruptus 220
Cold 21
Colicky pain 369
Collar bones 109
Color coded bins 586t
Colostrum 521
 composition of 522t
Colpoperineorrhaphy 767
Colporrhaphy, anterior 767
Colposcopy 292
Coma 320
 stages of 681
Combination therapy 165, 166
Combined oral contraceptives 227
Compaction 149
Complete abortion 22, 22f
Complete blood count 29, 58, 159, 237, 256, 444
Complete breech 145
Compressions, cardiac 91f
Computed tomography 370, 444
Conception, retained products of 275
Condom 221
 distribution 566
 female 222
 male 221f
Cone biopsy 553
Confusion 306, 312
Congenital anomalies 190, 195
Congenital defects 315

Conizely 291, 553
Conjoined twins 558, 560
Conjunctivitis 438, 546
Constipation 444, 541
Constriction ring 7
Continuous positive airway pressure 714
Contraception 31, 56, 173, 219
  barrier method of 56
  emergency 230
  permanent methods of 234
  surgical methods of 234
Contraceptive
  injectable 231
  methods 219b
Contraction
  premature onset of 544
  stress test 217, 254, 606
Controlled cord traction 517f
Cord
  clamp 476
  presentation 240, 241f
  prolapse 241, 242f, 344
Cordocentesis 238, 239
Core needle biopsy 117
Corneal reflex 646
Coronal suture 358
Coronary artery disease 229, 379
Corporeal fibroids 363
Corpus
  cancer syndrome 166
  luteum hematoma 288
Costovertebral tenderness 768
Cough 41
Couvelaire uterus 68
Cramp 542
Cranioclast 481, 481f, 483, 484f
Cri-du-chat syndrome 187, 378, 379
Criminal abortion 28
Crohn's disease 711

Cross contamination, prevention of 585
Crown-rump length 669
Cryosurgery 555
Cu T 200 224, 225
Cu T 380 A 224, 225
Culdocentesis 326
Culdoscope 284, 285f
Curved artery forceps 458
Cusco's bivalved speculum 469, 469f
Cyanosis 207, 714
Cystic fibrosis 379, 384
Cystic glandular hyperplasia 17
Cysts 294
Cytology test 741
Cytomegalovirus 41, 237
  infection 447, 750

D

Danazol 15, 365
Das's cervical dilators 471, 471f
Das's forceps 375, 477
Death 48
  causes of 164
  prevention of 567
Deep breathing 660
Deep tendon reflexes 657
  hyperactivity of 320
Deep vein thrombosis 709
Dehydration 158
DeLee mucus trap 721f
Delinquency 746
Delivery 694, 511
  expected date of 62
  spontaneous 344, 626
  vaginal 72, 251
Denominator 361
Deoxyribonucleic acid 40
Depot medroxyprogesterone acetate 231

Depression
  major 697, 700
  maternal 699
  postpartum 702
  respiratory 306, 312
Dermatitis
  forms of 42
  perianal 546
Dexamethasone 455
Dextran infusion 299
Diabetes mellitus 155, 229, 243, 248, 379, 412, 533, 577, 750
  insulin-dependent 245
Diaphragm 222
  fitting of 222
Diarrhea 297
  diseases 567
  feeding related 298
  infective 298
Diazepam 310, 311, 313, 314
Diet 249
Diethylstilbestrol exposure, assessment of 284
Digestive system 540, 642
Digits 595
Diminished cervical mucus 554
Dinoprostone 309
Diphtheria 566
Direct agglutination test 259
Direct fluorescent antibody test 737
Directly observed treatment short-course 573
Disposable cord clamp 476f
Disseminated intravascular coagulation 25, 157, 299, 300, 679, 731
Distress, abdominal 306
Dizziness 228, 306, 312
Doderlein's bacillus 536, 706
Doppler
  studies 355
  ultrasound 280

Down syndrome 185, 378, 380, 489
Doyen's retractor 466, 466f
Doyen's towel clip 466, 466f
Drew-Smythe catheter 473, 473f
Drowsiness 312
Drug
  abuse 577
  anaphylaxis 732
  toxicity 237
  withdrawal 237
Duchenne's muscular dystrophy 379, 385
Ductal carcinoma 118
Ductal carcinoma
  in situ 118
  infiltrating 119
Ductus arteriosus 345
Ductus venosus 345
Duodenal atresia 412, 781
Dysfunctional contractile pattern 158
Dysfunctional uterine bleeding 13, 14, 16, 369, 419, 550, 551
  types of 16
Dysmaturity 525
Dysmenorrhea 195, 226, 317, 329, 707
  pathologic 550
  primary 317
  secondary 318
Dyspareunia 318, 329, 369, 442, 724
Dysplasia, bronchopulmonary 408, 714
Dyspnea 41, 170, 559
  paroxysmal nocturnal 170
Dysrhythmia 176
Dystocia 158
Dysuria 330, 735, 768

E

Ear deficits 202
Early icon II test 259

Echocardiogram 171
Eclampsia 158, 299, 319, 377, 732
    complications of 322
    management of 677
    treatment of 680
Ectocervical scraping 266
Ectopic pregnancy 284, 288, 322, 332, 757, 758
    sites of 322
Ectopic rupture, acute 325
Eczema 42
Edema 228, 691
    generalized 158, 683
    peripheral 170
    pulmonary 172, 306, 712
    sudden development of 544
Edward's syndrome 185, 378, 381, 489
Egg donor 85
Ehlers-Danlos syndrome 379, 383
Eisenmenger's syndrome 169, 174, 175
Ejaculation, premature 318
Elbow spread exercise 136, 137f
Electrocardiogram 248
    maternal 177
Electrocardiography 171
Electrolytes, serum 418
Embolism 732
Embryo
    biopsy 389
    transfer 83, 86, 87
Embryotomy scissors 482, 482f
Emergency
    obstetric care 568
    surgery, indications of 367
Empathetic deficits 746
Emphysema, congenital 712
Encephalocele 195, 196f
Endocarditis, vascular 175
Endocervical smear 266
Endocrine glands, disorder of 331
Endocrinopathy 331

Endometrial biopsy 271
    instruments for 272f
    sites of 274f
Endometrial cavity, fiberoptic viewing of 370
Endometrial sampling 370
Endometrial suction catheter 272
Endometrioma, drainage of 333
Endometriosis 86, 288, 294, 318, 327, 329, 332, 419, 454
    complications of 331
    sites of 328f
Endometritis 443, 707, 708
Endometrium 275, 328, 419
Endotoxemia 299
Endotracheal tubes 717f
Enterocele, repair of 767
Enzyme-linked immunosorbent assay 42, 259, 448, 742
Epimenorrhea 13, 14, 319
Epinephrine 721
Episiotomy 335, 336, 656
    repair of 336
    scissors 474f
    site infection 710
    types of 335f
    wound 337, 708
Epispadias 210, 210f
Epstein pearls 545, 549f
Erb's palsy 101, 102f
Erectile dysfunction 455
Ergometrine 305
Ergot derivatives 302, 304
Erythema toxicum 544
    neonatorum 547f
Erythroblastosis fetalis 500
Erythrocyte
    count 58
    sedimentation rate 58, 177, 444, 635
Erythroplasia 294
Escherichia coli 298, 438, 443
Esophageal atresia 207, 412, 781

Esophageal gastric sphincter,
relaxation of 781
Estrogen 14, 166, 228, 316
dependant neoplasia 229
excess 228
stimulation 166
Ethamsylate 15
Euglobulin clot lysis time 301
Exchange transfusion 501
Excision biopsy 118
Exercise 132, 135, 249, 659
postpartum 660*f*
side bends 139, 139*f*
Extension 343
External cephalic version 148, 338
External genitalia
benign lesions of 294
malignant lesions of 294
Extremities 657
Eye
abnormalities 315
coloboma of 202

F

Face presentation 340, 627, 779
primary 340
reversal of 344
secondary 340
six positions of 342*f*
types of 340
Facial
bruising 344
clefts 412
expressions 674
nerve, damage of 100
palsy 100, 101*f*
Failed ovulation induction 86
Fainting 542
Fallopian tube 235, 235*f*
X-ray image of 279*f*
Fallot tetralogy 169, 174, 175
Falope ring 235*f*
Family planning services 566

Fat, excessive 298
Fatigue 170, 258
Feed, regurgitation of 207
Femilon 227
Femur 103
length 669
Fern test 686
Fertilization 87
Fetal 48, 154, 156, 157, 340, 430, 687, 780
abnormalities 560, 757
ascitis 413, 734
bradycardia 79
breathing movements 93, 94
circulation 345, 346*f*
characteristics of 345
complications 559, 668
compromise 251
condition 514, 622
death 307, 741, 771
distress 158, 347, 577, 779
acute 751
reducing risk of 161
effects 246
exsanguination 157, 771
factors 489
growth restriction 525
head 241*f*
descend of 632
heart rate 10, 11, 177, 184, 503, 630, 669
monitoring 348, 349, 349*f*, 350
reactivity 93
heart sound 6, 76
heart tones 69
location of 64*t*
maximum intensity of 4
hydantoin syndrome 25
hyperinsulinemia 246
imaging 353
indications 376
kick count 250, 490

limb movements 758
macrosomia 246, 734
malpresentation 251
membranes, prolonged rupture of 731
monitoring
  external 351f
  internal 349, 352f
morbidity 562
movements, reduced 544
parts 69
presentations 558
skull 356
  diameters of 359, 359f
  regions of 357
  sutures of 357
surveillance 250
tachycardia 79
tone 93, 94
vital centers, depressed 315
Feto-maternal hemorrhage 48
Fetoscope 389, 484, 485f
Fetus 182, 757, 758
  determine maturity of 756
  effects on 725, 738
  hydrocephalic 149
  hyperactive 79
  papyraceous 557
  viability of 758
Fetus-in-fetu 560
Fever 41, 276, 444
  high 237
  low grade 768
Fibrin degradation products 301
Fibrinogen 640
  estimation 301
Fibroid 278, 367
  effects of 394
  polyp 368
  submucous 363
  tumors 363
  types of 363
  uterus 13, 392, 419

Figure W exercise 142, 142f
Filshie clip 235f
Fine needle aspiration 117
Fingers, abnormalities of 315
First response pregnancy test kit 260
Flaccid paralysis 306
Flank pain 768
Flexion 343
  lateral 150, 343
Flow, long duration of 14
Fluid
  balance 12, 80, 184
  intake 418
  replacement of 730
Fluorescent treponemal antibody test 738
Fluorouracil 124
Flushing 306
  curette 472, 472f
Foam 223
Folate 53
  deficiency 50
Follicle-stimulating hormone 17, 536, 651, 705
Follicular growth, monitoring of 86
Folliculitis 42
Fontanelle, anterior 358
Footling presentation 145
Foramen ovale 345
Forceps
  application, prerequisites for 377
  delivery 374, 577, 627
  design of 374
  use of 375, 376
Formalin solution 273
Fothergill's operation 767
Foul odor 444
Foul-smelling
  discharge 369
  urine 768
Fracture 103
  skull 99

Fragile X syndrome 188, 378, 380
Fundal
    dominance 502
    height 63
        measurement of 63*t*
    palpation 1*f*, 2
    pressure 517
Fundus, height of 64*f*, 75

G

Galactokinesis 521
Gallbladder disease 229
Gallstones, presence of 229
Gamete intrafallopian transfer 83, 87
Gastric emptying, delayed 314
Gastroenteritis 298
Gastrointestinal function 608
Gastrointestinal reflux 202
Gastrointestinal system 656
    anomalies 204
Gastrointestinal tract 205, 730
Gastroschisis 208
Gene disorders 378
    autosomal
        dominant 379, 382, 384
        recessive 379
General anesthetic accidents 732
Genetic counseling 189, 378, 389
    prenatal diagnosis for 391
Genetic screening 188, 378, 387
    purposes of 388
    timings of 388
Genital crisis 547
Genital herpes 155
Genital organ changes 706
Genital tract, diseases of 452
Genitalia 595
    ambiguous 211
Genitourinary anomalies 210
Genitourinary system 536, 542
German measles 446

Gestation, multiple 690
Gestational age 712
    large for 252
    small for 525, 526
Gestations, ectopic 325
Glomerulonephritis, chronic 533
Glucocorticoids 316
Glucose tolerance test 248
Glucose-6-phosphate dehydrogenase deficiency 57, 379, 385, 386
Glycosuria 247
Gonadotropin-releasing hormone 536
    agonists 15, 689
    analogues 331, 365
Gonorrhea 268, 736
Goodell's sign 258
Gräfenberg's ring 224
Grand multipara 304
Grasp reflex 647, 648*f*
Gravid uterus 403
Gravindex test 259
Great vessels, transposition of 204
Greater sciatic notch 529
Green armytage forceps 461, 461*f*
Grief 47
Gross body movement 93, 94
Growth 202, 363, 619, 706
    retardation 315
Guaiac test 58
Guardian and Wards Act 35
Gut, malrotation of 781
Gynecological disorders 392
Gynecology, instruments in 456

H

Habitual abortion 28
Haig Ferguson's forceps 375
Hand hygiene 582
Hands behind head exercise 141, 141*f*

Handwashing
    station 582
    steps 582*f*
Hazards 687
Head
    birth of 150, 509
    descent of 151
    external rotation of 343, 511
    internal rotation of 150, 343, 509
    lag reflex 647
    tilt-chin lift maneuver 91, 92*f*
Headaches 228, 306
    cyclic 228
    frontal 544
    recurring 544
Health
    education 65, 144
    promotion 607, 610
Heart 639
    defects 202
        congenital 315
    disease 377
        congenital 169, 174
    failure 170
        congenital 712
        congestive 172
    pulsations 758
    rate 671
Heartburn 541
Heavy discharge 276
Hegar's sign 258
Hematocrit 58, 177, 640
    levels 79
Hematologic system 639
Hematoma 48, 710
    epidural 98*f*
    formation 157
    subdural 98*f*
Hematometra 195
Hematuria 330, 768
Hemoglobin 22, 29, 58, 70, 177, 640
    electrophoresis 58
    estimation 20
    glycosylated 248
Hemoglobinopathies 50, 239
Hemolysis 50
Hemolysis, elevated liver enzymes and low platelets 299
    syndrome 299, 679, 681
Hemolytic disease, manifestations of 725
Hemoperitoneum 333
Hemophilia 379, 386
Hemorrhage 52, 68, 157, 164, 307, 557, 722, 731, 733, 767
    accidental 65, 66, 68, 559
    antepartum 48, 65, 66, 733
    atonic postpartum 420
    causes of 75
    cerebral 344
    classification of 67
    external 67
    intraventricular 408, 714
    mixed type of 68
    postpartum 72, 195, 345, 491, 733, 757
    pulmonary 408, 714
    secondary 554
    subaponeurotic 96, 97*f*
    subdural 97
Hemorrhoids 559
Hemostat 457
Hepatitis 229, 310
Hernia
    abdominal 288
    diaphragmatic 202, 288, 712, 781
    hiatus 781
Herpes
    neonatal 741
    simplex 42, 268, 741
        virus 447
    zoster 42
High-resolution ultrasonography 389

Hindu Adoption and Maintenance
　　　Act 35, 36
Hindwater rupture 436
Hip, developmental dysplasia of 212
Hirschsprung's disease 781
Hirsutism 234
Hodge-Smith pessary 487, 487f
Homan's sign 657
Home pregnancy test kits 260f
Hookworm infestation 50
Hormonal contraception 219, 227
Hormonal implants 232
Hormonal therapy 124
Hormonal treatment 331
Hormone 14, 689
　　replacement therapy 373, 539
Huge ovarian cyst 413
Human chorionic gonadotropin 20,
　　　85, 389, 455, 540
Human immunodeficiency virus
　　　41, 223, 447, 742
　　tests 65
Human milk, composition of 525
Human papilloma virus 268, 739
Humerus 103
Hyaline membrane disease 406
Hydatidiform mole 299, 408, 420,
　　　758
　　entities of 410
　　partial 410
Hydralazine 307, 308
Hydramnios 411
Hydration 768
　　adequate 505
Hydrocehalus 199f
Hydrocele, congenital 546
Hydrocephaly 147, 198
Hydrocortisone 50
Hydrops fetalis 412, 725
Hydrosalpinx 287
　　presence of 422
Hyperbilirubinemia 246
Hypercalcemia 236

Hypercholesterolemia, familial
　　　379, 382
Hyperemesis 559
　　gravidarum 416
　　　　intractable 533
Hyperglycemia 236
Hyperlipoproteinemia 382
Hypermenorrhea 13
Hypernatremia 236
Hyperplasia, endometrial 166, 419
Hyperreflexia 158
Hypersensitivity 310
Hypertension 158, 228, 229, 247,
　　　306, 310, 340, 379, 577
　　chronic 155, 247, 750
　　pregnancy-induced 79, 245,
　　　355, 559, 602, 676, 757
　　severe 13
　　uncontrolled 533
Hyperthermia 237
Hypertonic solutions, intrauterine
　　　instillation of 534
Hypertrophied cervix following
　　　chronic cervicitis 556
Hypocalcemia 236, 246, 306
Hypogastric arteries 346
Hypoglycemia 236, 246, 251, 306,
　　　712
Hypogonadism 450
Hypomagnesemia 236
Hypomenorrhea 13, 16
Hyponatremia 236
Hypospadias 210, 210f
Hypotension 22, 157, 306, 312, 731
Hypothermia 690
Hypothyroidism 13
Hypotonia 7
Hypovolemia 771
Hypovolemic state 304
Hypoxanthine-guanine
　　　phosphoribosyl transferase
　　　387
Hypoxia 578, 771

Hysterectomy 15, 367, 419
 advantages of 367
 extended 419
 indications for 367
 radical 419
 subtotal 419
 total 419
 types of 419
 vaginal 367, 767
Hysterosalpingography 277, 421
Hysteroscope 275f
Hysteroscopy 274, 332, 334, 370
 laser machine 292
 operative 334
Hysterotomy 304, 535

I

I-can pregnancy test kit 259, 260f
Icterus gravis neonatorum 725
Idiopathic thrombocytopenic purpura 14
Ileopectineal eminence 530
Ileopectineal line 530
Ileus 288
Ilium 528
Illegal abortion 28
Immunization 425, 566
Immunoglobulin
 G 4
 M 4
Immunological tests 259
Imperforate anus 209, 318, 781
Imperforation, types of 209
Impotence 318
In vitro fertilization 83, 86
Incest 744
Incision 293, 335
 biopsy 118
 extension of 157
Incomplete abortion 23, 24f, 551, 758
Incomplete breech 145
Induced abortion 26

Induction
 drugs used for 435
 indications for 430
 methods of 432
Inevitable abortion 21, 21f
Infections 48, 143, 157, 158, 268, 437, 446, 551, 690, 780
 bacterial 179, 441
 control 580
  protocols 587
 extra-pelvic 710
 intrauterine 239, 307
 local 735
 neonatal 344, 741
 postpartum 708t
 reducing risk of 59
 severe 50
 signs of 201
 staying free of 513
 symptoms of 201
 systemic 439, 735
 vaginal 275
 viral 442, 446
 vulval 318
Infective diarrhea 298
 treatment of 298
Infertile couple, assessment of 451
Infertility 226, 277, 287, 329, 369, 445, 449, 550, 554, 724
 male factor 86
 management of 453
 unexpected 451
 unexplained 86, 455
Inflammatory carcinoma 120
Influenza 446
Infraclavicular nodes 109
Infusion intravenous 157
Inhalation agents 313
Injury
 intracranial 236, 780
 minor 99
 vaginal 268
Insomnia 544

Instant pregnancy test kit 260f
Institutional delivery 567
Insufflation cannula 289f
Insulin 249
   use of 249
Integrated Child Development
   Scheme 564, 574
   team 576
Integumentary system 642, 658
Intensive care 691
   unit 251
Interconceptional period 29
Interpersonal therapy 700
Interstitial fibroids 363
Intestinal obstruction 331, 333
Intra-amniotic hypertonic saline,
   instillation of 299
Intracranial pressure 200
Intracytoplasmic sperm injection
   83, 88
Intramural fibroids 363
Intrapartum therapy 44
Intrauterine adhesions 275
Intrauterine balloon tamponade
   491
Intrauterine contraceptive devices
   13, 173, 219, 224, 225f, 281,
   454, 550, 566
   removal of 551
   services 566
Intrauterine death 315
Intrauterine device 56, 225, 445
Intrauterine fetal death 246, 750
Intrauterine growth restriction 175,
   183, 355, 488, 525
   severe 307
Intrauterine growth retardation
   488, 741, 755
   asymmetric 489
Intrauterine insemination 83, 84
Intrauterine tamponade 491
Intubation equipment 716, 717f
Invasive carcinoma 402
   cervix, effects of 402
Iron
   deficiency 50
      anemia 51
   intravenous 732
Irritability 228
Irritation 442
Ischemic injury 236
Ischium 528
Isoimmune diseases 239
Isoimmunization, mechanism of
   724
Isolated abortion 20
Isoxsuprine 306
Itching 442
   generalized 543
   vaginal 735

J

Jacob's syndrome 186, 378, 381
Jacquemier's sign 258
Janani Suraksha Yojana 564, 569
   salient features of 569
Jardine's decapitation hook 483
Jaundice 57, 498, 691
   mechanism of 498
   pathological 499
   physiological 498
Jaw thrust maneuver 91, 92f
Jewelry and fingernails policy
   584
Joints 529
Jugular venous pressure 170
Juvenile Justice Act 35, 36

K

Kaposi's sarcoma 42
Kegel exercise 659, 661
Kelly's deep retractor 467, 468f
Keratitis, intestinal 738
Kernicterus 236, 500
Kidneys 730

Kielland's forceps 375, 479, 479f
Klinefelter syndrome 186, 378, 381
Klumpke's palsy 102
Knee
   flexes 660
   presentation 145
   reflexes, depressed 306
Kocher's forceps 457, 457f

L

Labetalol 307, 308
Labor 52, 195, 394, 395, 397, 399-402, 559, 694
   course of 622
   disorders 156
   first stage of 172, 502
   induction of 303, 309, 429
   management of 561
   mechanism of 154, 509, 510f
   nonprogress of 156
   obstructed 195, 304, 344, 621
   outcome of 343, 626
   premature 195, 769
      induction of 182
   progress of 184
   prostaglandins induction of 434
   second stage of 173
   third stage of 173, 516
Lacerations 708
Lactation 520
   physiology of 520
Lactogenesis 520
Lambdoidal suture 358
Laminaria tent 463, 464, 464f
Laparoscopic assisted vaginal hysterectomy 332, 333
Laparoscopic method 235
Laparoscopy 292, 326, 330, 370, 652
   complications of 333
   diagnostic 287
   procedure 291f

Laryngoscope 721f
   batteries for 717f
   blade 717f
Laser
   instruments 293f
   procedures 291
   surgery 291
      advantages of 294
      disadvantages of 294
      indications for 292
   vaporization 291
   wave guides 292
Last menstrual period 669
   date of 62
Leg cramps 228
Legal abortion 26
Legionella 41
Legs
   edema of 559
   raises 660, 661
Leiomyomas 493
Leopold's maneuvers 1f, 11
Lesch-Nyhan syndrome 379, 385, 387
Lethargy 440
Leukemia 14
Leukocyte count 640
Leukoplakia 293
Leukorrhea 542
Levonorgesterel 331
   intrauterine device 224
Ligaments 529
Light Amplification by Stimulated Emission of Radiation 291
Limbs 595
Lithium 316
Liver 730
Lobular carcinoma, infiltrating 119
Localized breast cancer 110
Lochia 656, 670
Long curved forceps 477f, 478f
Lower segment cesarean section 251

Lung 730
  hypoplasia 712
Luteinizing hormone 17, 453, 536, 651, 705
Lymph node 109*f*, 122
Lymphatic spread 167
Lymphogranuloma venereum 711

M

Macrosomia 251
Magnesium sulfate 306, 310, 321, 679
Magnetic resonance imaging 116, 117*f*, 295, 353
  scanner 296*f*
Mala D 227
Mala N 227
Malaise 444
Malaria 50, 750
Malformations, congenital 246, 251, 750
Malnutrition 16
Malpresentation 76, 183, 195, 304, 560
Mammogenesis 520
Mammography 115
  examination 116*f*
Manual vacuum aspiration 571
Marfan syndrome 379, 382
Mastalgia 233
Mastectomy 121
  procedures, types of 121
  prophylactic 127
  risks of 121
Mastitis 144, 708, 710
Maternal injury, reducing risk of 162
Maternal vital signs 513
Matthew's Duncan method 516, 516*f*
Mayo scissors, straight 474*f*
McRoberts maneuver 734

Mean arterial pressure 677
Measles 446
  mumps-rubella vaccine 447
Meconium
  aspiration syndrome 531, 712
  ileus 781
  stained amniotic fluid 577
Medical Termination of Pregnancy
  Act 533
    provisions of 533
  complications of 535
Membranes
  artificial rupture of 78, 435
  delivery of 517
  examination of 518
  high rupture of 436
  perforator 473
  premature rupture of 48, 686, 690
  preterm
    prelabor rupture of 686
    premature rupture of 750
  rupture of 149, 339, 340, 544
Menarche 706
Meningitis 237
Menopause 535, 536
  abnormal 539
  age of 535
  artificial 539
  delayed 539
  diagnosis of 538
  late 166
  management of 538
  premature 539
Menorrhagia 13, 17, 226, 319, 707
  functional 16
Menses, irregular 233
Menstrual abnormalities 707
Menstrual flow
  amount of 13
  shorter duration of 13
Menstrual regulation 534

Menstruation
- abnormal 329
- abrupt cessation of 537
- cessation of 257, 538
- pattern 537
- scanty 13

Mental retardation 202
Mentovertical diameter 360
Metabolism, inborn errors of 236
Metal
- catheter, female 486, 486*f*
- chain 480*f*
- suction cups 480*f*

Metastasis 165
Methergine 305, 655
Methotrexate 327, 534
Methyldopa 307, 308
Metronidazole 316, 740
Metropathia hemorrhagica 17
Metrorrhagia 13, 15
Microbes
- prevent entry of 581
- prevent proliferation of 585

Microbiology 634
Microcephaly 198, 198*f*
Microsurgical epididymal sperm aspiration 88
Micturition, frequency of 258, 542
Midazolam 313, 314
Mid-trimester abortion 554, 557
Mifepristone 15, 534
Migraine headaches 229
Milia 545
Milk ejection 521
Milne Murray's forceps 375
Minilaparotomy 235
Minor disorders, causes of 540
Miscarriage, late 195
Missed abortion 25, 309, 758
Mitral regurgitation 169, 173
Mitral stenosis 169, 170
Molar pregnancy 416
- termination of 309

Molding 362
Mongolian spots 545, 548*f*
Monilial infection 247, 442
Monitor blood pressure 255
Monitoring fetal heart rate 696
Mood disorders 697
Morbid adherent placenta 420
Moro reflex 647, 649*f*
Morphine 730
Mouth to mouth
- maneuver 91
- respiration 92*f*

Mucopolysaccharidosis 379, 384
Mucus sucker 475, 476*f*
Mullerian agenesis 287
Mullerian duct 190
Multifactorial disorders 379, 387
Multifetal pregnancy 557, 562
- types of 557

Multiload 250 224
Multiload 350 224, 225
Multiparity 147
Muscle
- relax, abdominal 659
- weakness 306

Musculoskeletal system 211, 542, 659
- formation of 211

Mycobacterium 450
Mycoplasma 450
Myocardial infarction 228
Myomas 294, 758
- multiple 158

Myomectomy 333, 366, 368
- hysteroscopic 332
- vaginal 366

N

Naloxone 721
Napkin rash 546
Narrow introitus 318
National Family Welfare Programs 563

National Immunization Schedule 426*t*
National Rural Health Mission 564, 571
Natural methods 219
Nausea 158, 228, 258, 260, 306, 314, 540
    feeling of 325
Neck masses 412
Needle holder 485, 485*f*
Neisseria gonorrhea 450
Neonatal grey baby 315
Neonatal intensive care unit 250, 576, 580, 587, 604
    goals of 579
    housekeeping measures for 584*t*
    levels of 578
    records, types of 589
Nephropathy, complications of 533
Nerve
    deafness 738
    injuries 100
Nervous system 543, 643
Neurobehavioral sequelae 700
Neurofibromatosis 379, 383
Neuropathy, peripheral 312
Neville Barnes forceps 375
Nevus flammeus 545, 548*f*
New York Heart Association 170
Newborn care 566, 596
Nifedipine 307, 308
Nipple
    care of 104
    squeezing 114
Non-steroidal anti-inflammatory drugs 317
Non-stress test 81, 94, 217, 250, 254, 605
Non-toothed dissecting forceps 465*f*
Norethindrone 231
Noristerat 231

North American Nursing Diagnosis Association 607
    nursing diagnosis 609, 610
No-scalpel vasectomy 774
Nosocomial infection 583
Novethindrone enanthate 231
Nuchal cord 577
Nuchal translucency 391
Nursing care 199, 675, 692
    plans 653
Nursing management 303, 441
Nutrition 607, 610
Nutritional supplements 765

O

Obesity 247, 379, 734
    extreme 333
    morbid 272
Oblique diameter 530, 531
Obstetrics 729
    forceps
        types of 375*f*
        varieties of 374
    instruments in 456
    shock, general management of 733
    trauma 731
Occipital bone 357
Occipitofrontal diameter 359
Oligohydramnios 147, 149, 340, 414, 690, 758
    diagnosis of 415
Oligomenorrhea 13, 15, 16
Oliguria 320
Omphalitis 438
Omphalocele 208, 208*f*
Operative delivery 732, 768
Ophthalmia neonatorum 438
Opioid analgesics 313
Optimal urinary output 665
Oral contraceptive 173, 227
    advantages of 228
    dispensing 566

pills 689
    types of 227
use of 16
Oral rehydration solution 298, 573
Oral thrush 546, 549f
Organ
    changes 536
    effects on 730
Organisms 143
Orthopnea 170
Osiander's sign 258
Osteogenesis imperfecta 379, 383
Osteoporosis 538
Ovarian
    abnormalities 450
    biopsy 332
    cystectomy 333
    cysts 262, 288, 318
    neoplasms 758
    tumor 400
        benign 419
        effects of 401
Ovary 332, 706
    granulosa cell tumor of 13
Ovral L 227
Ovular bleeding 16, 17
Ovulation
    prediction kit 453
    problems of 450
Ovum
    forceps 459, 459f
    retrieval 87
Oxygen
    administration 730
    bag and mask 717
    reservoir 717
    tubing 717f
Oxygenation 50
Oxytocin 302, 633
    challenge test 254, 303, 627
        advantages of 628
        disadvantages of 628
    dangers of 433

    effectiveness of 302
    induction 433
    infusion 535
    sensitivity test 303
Oyosalpinx 287

P

Paget disease 120
Pain 21, 79, 161, 519, 672
    abdominal 68, 329
    cramping 226
    epigastric 158, 320, 544
    lower abdominal 408, 444
    relief 71
        methods of 313
    severe abdominal 276
    suprapubic 768
Pallor 14, 21, 68, 440
Palmar reflex 647, 648f
Palmer's sign 258
Palpation 2, 115, 147
    abdominal 1f, 154
Palpitation 170, 176, 306
Pan hysterectomy 419
Pap smear 370
    abnormal 268, 271
    sampling device 265f
Pap test 263
    abnormal 275
Parameters 93
Paresthesia 312
Parity 166
Partial thromboplastin time 79, 300
Partograph 628
    components of 630
Parvovirus B19 237
Patau syndrome 186, 378, 381, 489
Patent ductus arteriosus 169, 174, 175, 203
Pawlik's grip 1f, 3, 339
Pelvic
    abscess 707

adnexae 758
anatomy 758
brim, diameters of 531*f*
cavity 531
cellulitis 707
congestion syndrome 288
endometriosis 13
endometritis 287
examination 64, 444
floor repair 767
    complications of 767
infection 226, 422, 707
    signs of 369
inflammation, acute 284
inflammatory disease 275, 281, 284, 288, 318, 323, 443, 633
joints 529
ligaments 529, 530*f*
organs 441
outlet 531
pain 276, 329, 444
    acute 288
    chronic 288, 723
palpation 1*f*, 3
pathology 13
peritonitis 445
shapes, variations of 532*t*
thrombophlebitis, septic 710
tilt 660
tumors 147, 333
ultrasound 280, 281, 370
    examination 281*f*
    procedure of 283
    reasons for 281
    risks of 282
Pelvimeter 484, 484*f*
Pelvis
    assessment of 216
    bones of 527
    classification of 531, 532*t*
    contracted 215, 304
    divisions of 529
    false 529
    female 527*f*
    functions of 527
    maternal 526
    true 529
Pendulum exercise 139, 140*f*
Penicillin 732
Penis, congenital anatomic defect of 318
Pentozocin 313
Peptic ulcer 310
Percutaneous umbilical blood sampling 238, 239, 354
Peres reflex 651
Perinatal mortality 246
Perineal body 556
Perineal tear, complete 711
Perineal tissue, condyloma of 293
Perineoplasty 556
Perineum 151, 671
    care of 337
Peripheral smear 300
Peritoneal adhesion, extensive 333
Peritoneum, parietal 157
Peritonitis 710
    generalized 288, 333
Peritubal adhesions 287
Pertussis 566
Pethidine 313
Phenobarbitone 310, 312, 316
Phenylephrine 455
Phenylketonuria 379, 384
Phenytoin 310, 312, 316
Phototherapy 500
Pica 541
Pierre Robin syndrome 712
Pigmentation 543
Pinard's stethoscope 484
Piper's forceps 375
Piskacek's sign 258
Placenta 758, 759
    accreta 158
    cornual implantation of 147

delivery of 517
descend of 515
examination of 518
expulsion of 516
previa 65, 72, 73f, 74f, 75, 147, 157, 559
  central 74
  features of 75t
  incomplete central 74
  lateral 74
  marginal 74
retained 195, 722
separation of 339, 515
Placental abruption 679
  complications of 72
Placental expulsion
  Duncan mechanism of 516
  methods of 516f
  Schultz mechanism of 516
Placental separation 515
Placental site bleeding 65
Placental tissue 731
Plantar reflex 647, 649f
Plasma volume 640
Platelet
  count 300
  disorders 239
Plygenic disorders 379
Pneumocystis carinii pneumonia 41, 448, 743
Pneumonia 567, 712
Pneumothorax 408, 712, 714
Polarity 502
Polycystic kidney disease 379, 383
Polycystic ovarian
  disease 29, 287, 453
  syndrome 651
Polydactyly 213, 214f
Polygenic disorders 387
Polyhydramnios 147, 241, 247, 411, 559, 690, 757, 758
  acute 414
  complications of 413

Polymenorrhea 13, 14, 16, 319
Polyp, endometrial 275, 550, 551
Pontazocin 314
Port-wine stain 545, 548f
Positive pressure ventilation 716, 718
Postcoital test 453
Postoperative intestinal obstruction 733
Postpartum care 449, 654
Post-prandial blood
  glucose 247
  sugar 250
Post-term gestation, types of 668
Potassium chloride 327
Povidone iodine solution 272
Prednisolone 316
Pre-eclampsia 68, 307, 340, 676, 690
  management of 677
  mild 677
  severe 299, 677
Pregcolor card test 259
Pregcolor test kit 259
Pregnancy 29, 40, 50, 52, 169, 229, 243, 244, 248, 271, 299, 307, 307t, 333, 392, 394, 397, 399, 401, 402, 413, 446, 559, 637, 697, 769
  adolescent 690, 753
  complications 750
  diagnosis of 257, 260, 262
  differential diagnosis of 262
  disorders 156
  early 402
  ectopic 284, 288, 322, 332, 757, 758
  effects of 55, 245, 395, 398, 402, 405, 735-738, 740, 741
  factors 692
  late 155, 403
  management of 250
  medical termination of 26, 234, 533, 566, 726

minor disorders of 540
multiple 149, 340, 412, 413, 416, 577
normal 640*t*
postdated 355, 667
post-term 667
post-tubal 278
second trimester 288
termination of 678
test kits 259
third trimester 288
unplanned 416
unwanted 226
Premenstrual syndrome 687
Pressure symptoms 394
Preterm labor 48, 554, 692, 741
Primigravid status 416
Procidentia 764
complete 764
Progestasert 224
Progesterone deficiency 29
Progestin 14
deficiency 228
excess 228
Progestogen 15, 316, 365, 689
Prolapse 369, 398
causes of 763
cord 158
degrees of 764
effects of 399
Prolonged labor 343, 695
causes of 695
Prophylactic forceps 377
Propranolol 307, 308
Prostaglandins 302, 309, 327, 434, 534
synthetase inhibitors 365
use of 434
Prosthetics 127
Protein
excess 298
urine for 70
Prothrombin time 300, 321

Pseudocyesis 263
Pseudomonas pyocyanea 731
Psoriasis 42
Psychiatric disorders 533, 697, 701
treatment of 700
Psychiatric illnesses 379
Psychoprophylaxis 313
Psychosexual therapy 455
Psychosis, postpartum 703
Psychotherapies 700
Psychotic disorders 700, 701
Ptyalism 541
Pubertal development, stages of 705
Puberty 704
delayed 707
disorders of 707
precocious 707
Pubic bone
body of 530
superior ramus of 530
Pubis 528
Puerperium 52, 143, 173, 394, 395, 399, 400, 403, 559, 701
early 770
management of 251, 562
Pulmonary disease 307
Pulmonary embolism 732, 733
Pulse, maternal 184
Pump 132*f*
Punch biopsy 553
Pyelonephritis 769
Pyloric stenosis 781
Pyrexia 731
Pyridoxine dependence 236
Pyuria 768

R

Radiant warmer 423*f*
Radiation 50
therapy 123
combined 168
intraoperative 123

Radical mastectomy, modified 122*f*
Radioimmunoassay 259
Radiotherapy 165, 168
   primary 165
Random blood glucose 247
Rapid cervical dilation 732
Rash 306, 544
Rectal injury 268
Rectouterine pouch 285*f*
Rectovaginal fistula 710, 767
Recurrent abortion 28
Red blood cell 498
   character of 54
   disorders 239
Red cell volume 640
Reflex, embracing 647
Regurgitation, aortic 169
Relaxation exercises 765
Renal anomalies 202
Renal disease 307
Renal failure
   acute 679
   prevention of 71
Renal function 248
Reproductive
   and Child Health Program 564
   period 19
   system 637
   tract infections, management of 564
Respiratory distress 48, 440, 712
   causes of 712
   syndrome 157, 246, 406, 712, 713
Respiratory function 608
Respiratory system 594, 641
   anomalies 201
   malformation of 201
Resuscitation 71, 715
   aims of 715
   articles 716
   cardiopulmonary 88
   degrees of 715
   equipment 716
   newborn 719*f*
Reticulocyte count 58
Retinopathy, complications of 533
Retrolental fibroplasia 408
Retroversion 403, 723
Rhesus
   disease 690
   incompatibility 412, 499, 724
   isoimmunization 48
      prevention of 725
   treatment of 694
Rheumatic heart disease 169, 170, 732
Rhythm method 219
Ribonucleic acid 40, 742
Rigid hymeneal ring 556
Ring pessary 486, 487*f*, 766
Ringer's lactate 721
Ritodrine 306
Rooting reflex 645, 645*f*
Rubella 446
   immune status 65
Rubin's cannula 289*f*

S

Sacrocotyloid 530
Sacroiliac joint 530
Sacrum 527
Saddle nose 738
Safe abortion services 564, 570
Sagittal suture 357
Salivation, excessive 541
Salpingectomy 332
Salpingitis 284
Salpingo-oophorectomy 332
Salpingo-oophoritis, acute 288
Salpingo-ovariolysis 333
Salpingostomy 332
Scalp
   edema of 99

hair, loss of 234
injuries 99
Schultz method 516*f*
Sciatic notch 529
Scissors 272, 474, 474*f*, 717*f*
Scope 189
Screening test 247
Sedatives 313
Segmental resection 332
Seizure
    activity 158
    eclamptic 680
Selective estrogen receptor modulators 124
Selective sonography, indications of 756
Semen analysis 453
Sepsis 164, 557, 767
    puerperal 52, 707, 722
    umbilical 438
Septic abortion 27, 299, 420, 731, 732
Septicemia 445, 710
Serum fibrin degradation products 25
Severe anemia 750
    complications of 52
Sex chromosomes, numerical abnormalities of 378, 381
Sexual assault 744
    effects of 745
    types of 744
Sexual dysfunction 615
Sexual harassment 745
Sexual violence 744, 745
    domestic 745
    intimate partner 744
Sexuality 614
Sexually transmitted disease 43, 221, 443, 452, 577, 735, 755
Shock 52, 157, 722, 729
    anaphylactic 731
    bacteremic 730
    cardiogenic 730
    causes of 732
    hypovolemic 729
    management of 733
    neurogenic 732
    obstetric 733
    septic 445, 730
Shoulder
    blade squeeze exercise 133, 134*f*
    circles 132, 133*f*
    dystocia 733
    internal rotation of 150, 343, 510
    rolls 132
        exercise 133*f*
Siamese twins 558
Sickle cell
    anemia 50
    disease 54, 229, 379, 384, 385
Sidewall stretch 138, 138*f*
Sigmoid colon, diverticulitis of 711
Silastic vacuum cup 480*f*
Silicone material 493
Sim's double bladed vaginal speculum 468, 468*f*
Sim's double ended uterine curette 470
Simple ovarian cysts, aspiration of 332
Simpson's forceps 375
    short 375
Simpson's perforator 481, 481*f*
Single gene disorders 379, 382
Single parent challenges 747
Skin 543
    assessment of 593
    care 620
    changes 260
    discoloration 658
    infections 439
    injuries 99
Skull bone fractures 103

Sling operation 767
Small pelvic masses 288
Smear brush 269
Sodium bicarbonate 721
Soft tissue dystocia 156
Sonography 341, 652
Sparse pubic hair 442
Spastic lower segment 7
Spermatogenesis 454
Spermicides 223
Spina bifida 200, 200f
    cystica 200
    occulta 200
Spine 595
Sponge 224
Sponge holding forceps 272, 272f, 456, 456f
Spontaneous abortion 20, 245, 741
Staphylococcus aureus 143, 438
Stepping reflex 650, 650f
Sterilization 56
    female 234, 235f
    male 235, 772
Sternomastoid hematoma 100
Steroids 316
Stethoscope 718
Sticky eyes 546
Stillbirth, causes of 750
Stork bite 545, 547f
Straighten legs 661
Strengthening referral system 569
Streptococcus 443
Streptomycin 316, 732
Stress 697
    emotional 416
    psychological 416, 559
    tolerance 615
Stuffy nose 546
Submentobregmatic diameter 360
Submentovertical diameter 360
Suboccipitobregmatic diameter 359

Suboccipitofrontal diameter 359
Sucking 646, 646f
Suction catheter 717f
Sulphonilamide 316
Super fecundation 558
Super numerary digits 213
Superficial tissues 99
Supine hypotensive syndrome 732
Supportive therapy 7
Supraclavicular nodes 109
Surgery 165, 168, 366, 766, 777
    endoscopic 332
    fear of 158
    laparoscopic 332
    methods of 235
    minor 550
    primary 165
    routes of 419
Swallowing reflex 646, 646f
Sweating 258, 306
Swelling, abdominal 444
Symphysis pubis 63
    upper inner boarder of 530
Syncope 228
    following vasovagal attack 226
Syndactyly 214, 214f
Syphilis 237, 268, 738

T

Tachycardia 21, 176, 306, 731
Tachypnea 731
    transient 712
Talipes 48
    calcaneovalgus 213, 213f
    equinovarus 212, 212f
Tamoxifen 118, 125
Tanner stages 705
Tay-Sachs disease 379, 384, 385
Teenage pregnancy 753
    causes of 753
Telangiectasia 547f
Telangiectic nevi 545

Telescope 289f
Temporary methods 219
Tenaculum forceps 463, 463f
Teratogenesis 700
Teratogenic drugs 533
Terbutaline 306
Testicular sperm extraction 88
Testosterone 455
Tetanus 237, 566
Tetracycline 316
Thalassemia 56
Thalidomide 316
Thermal cauterization 554
Thermoregulatory problems 312
Threatened abortion 20, 20f, 758
Thrombin time 300
Thromboembolism 157
Thrombophlebitis 229, 709, 710
Thyroid
  disorders 750
  dysfunction 16, 29
Tissue
  culture 737
  layer of 275
Tocolytic drugs 306, 306t
Toes, abnormalities of 315
Tolbutamide 316
Tonic neck reflex 646, 647f
Tonic uterine contraction 6
Torsion 395
Total brachial plexus palsy 102
Total iron binding capacity 58
Tough hymen 318
Toxoids 732
Toxoplasmosis 237
Toxoplasmosis, other (syphilis, varicella-zoster, parvovirus B19), rubella, cytomegalovirus and herpes infections 237
TPR, graphic charts of 589
Tracheoesophageal fistula 207, 712
Trachomatis 450

Traction device 479
Trail labor, conduct of 183
Tranexamic acid 15
Transabdominal placement postcesarean delivery 494
Transabdominal ultrasound 280
Transcutaneous electronic nerve stimulation 313
Transvaginal ultrasound examination 280, 281
Transverse diameter 359, 530, 531
Transverse lie 4
Trauma 65, 307, 732
  maternal serum 344
Trendelenburg tilt 730
Treponema pallidum 738
  detection of 738
Trichloroacetic acid 740
Trichomonas
  infection 268
  vaginalis 740
Trichomoniasis 740
Trimethoprim 316
Triple X syndrome 378
Trisomy 185, 186, 378, 380, 381, 489
  profile test 391
Trocar 289f
Trophoblastic disease, persistent 411
Truncus arteriosus 203
Tubal
  abortion 323, 324f
  adhesions 284
  block, sites of 287
  disease 86
  kinks 287
  ligation 219, 235f, 284, 332
  mole 324, 324f
    formation of 324
  pregnancy
    possible outcomes of 324f
    recurrence of 327
  rupture 324, 324f

Tubectomy 219, 235f
Tubercular endometritis 13
Tuberculosis 41, 711
    endometrial 16, 550
    genital 287
    peritonitis 288
Tubo-ovarian mass 13, 287, 288, 419
Tubular ductal carcinoma 120
Tumors 278, 288, 319
    growth of 363
Turner syndrome 187, 378, 381, 450
Twin fetus 558f
Twin pregnancy
    diagnosis of 560
    types of 557
Twisted ovarian cyst 288
Two finger method 720f

U

Ultrasonics, risks of 759
Ultrasonography 22, 70, 76, 116, 250, 259, 261, 279, 280, 326, 330, 353, 355, 412, 490
    intravaginal 391
    serial 177
Ultrasound
    application, types of 280
    examination 147, 354, 756f
        abdominal 282, 283f
    scan 561
Umbilical arteries 345
Umbilical cord 241, 241f
    clamp 718
    cutting scissors 474f
    knotting of 339
Umbilical vein 345
Umbilicus 63
Unsafe abortion 28
Uremia 164
Ureteral obstruction 331
Urethra 405
Urethral caruncle 293
Urethral pathology 318
Urgency 768
Urinary
    function 608
    retention 768
    stasis 767
    system 643
    tract 247
        infections 665, 692, 709, 710, 767, 770
Urination, insufficient 768
Urine 237
    culture 248
    output 69, 79
    pregnancy test 20
    retention of 767
Uterine
    abnormalities 147
    abscess formation 445
    action 304
    agenesis 193, 193f
    anomalies 195
        congenital 190, 493
        development of 190
        types of 190
    bleeding, abnormal 13, 271, 444
    cavity
        distorting pathology 493
        measure length of 272
    contractions 21, 184, 632
    curette 471f
    dehiscence 272
    dressing forceps 461
    feel 69
    fibroids 262, 364f
        location of 393f
        tumors 318
    fundal height 490
    fundus 79
    height 69
    inertia 52

inversion 732
malformations, congenital 275
packing forceps 461, 462f
perforation 226, 420, 551
polyps 278
prolapse 397, 763
rupture 195, 493, 732
sarcoma 419
scar 310
sound 272, 272f, 473, 473f
synechia 16, 552
tetany 8
tumors 294
wall 758
Uteroplacental apoplexy 68
Uteroplacental tissue perfusion 81, 179
Uterosalpingography 277
Uterus 284, 333, 363, 405, 494f, 637, 655, 670, 706
acute inversion of 497
arcuate 190, 191f
bicornuate 191, 192f
body of 724
chronic inversion of 496
congenital anomalies of 190
contracted 673
didelphis 190, 191f
enlargement of 369
feel of 76
inversion of 495
position of 763
purulent infection of 493
retroverted 13, 403
rupture of 158, 420, 726
septate 192, 193f
structural problems of 450
supports of 763
unicornuate 191, 192f
X-ray image of 279f

V

Vaccine 426
Vacuum
    assisted birth 778
    extractor, components of 480f
Vagina 272, 639, 706
    lymphogranuloma venereum of 711
    purulent infection of 493
    structural problems of 450
    tuberculosis of 711
Vaginal birth, normal 97
Vaginal discharge, abnormal 444
Vaginal dryness 442
Vaginal examination 70, 76, 78, 148, 154, 261, 325, 341, 409, 625
Vaginal infection 275
    active 268
    acute 272
Vaginal inspection 76
Vaginal lesions 294
Vaginal mucosa 442
Vaginal septum 319
Vaginal smear 267
Vaginal speculum 264f, 272, 272f
Vaginal ultrasound, procedure of 283
Vaginal wet mount 267
Vaginitis 268, 284, 319
Vaginosis, bacterial 268, 735
Valporic acid 316
Vandemataram Scheme 564, 570
Varicella zoster 237, 447
Varicose veins 559
Vas deferens 455, 772, 772f
Vasa previa 771
Vasculopathy, evidence of 247
Vasectomy 235, 772, 772f
    advantages of 772
    disadvantages of 772
    male 219

open-ended 775
operation 772
types of 774
Vasoepididymostomy 455
Vasovagal attack 422
Vasovagal stimulation 732
Vaso-vasoanastomosis 455
Vault
   bones of 357
   prolapse, repair of 767
Velocit eazy pregnancy test kit 260, 260f
Venacaval occlusion 732
Venereal Disease Research Laboratory test 65, 738
Ventilation 50
Ventouse cup 479
Ventouse delivery 778
Ventral suspension 650, 650f
Ventricular septal defect 169, 174, 203
Vertex, six positions of 362f
Vesicovaginal fistula 156, 767, 775
   sites of 776, 776f
Vesicular mole 408
Viagra 455
Vinblastin 166
Visual disturbances 228
Vitamin B12 58
   deficiency 50
Vomiting 158, 228, 260, 360, 314, 440, 540, 780
   causes of 780
   feeling of 325
von Willebrand's disease 14
Vulsellum forceps 460, 460f
Vulva 707
   care of 337
Vulval varicosities 65
Vulvar dystrophies 293
Vulvar tissue, condyloma of 293
Vulvar vaginal intraepithelial neoplasia 292
Vulvar vestibulitis syndrome 318
Vulvovaginitis 441

W

Walking reflex 650
Wall climbing
   exercise 138f
   facing wall 137f
Wall crawling 136
Wand exercise 135, 136f
Warfarin 316
Warmth, feeling of 258
Warts, genital 268
Waste segregation 585f, 586t
   Protocol Adopted in India 585
Wasting syndrome 41
Wedge pattern 114
Weight gain 233
   cyclic 228
White blood cell 10, 22, 58
   count 79, 177
WHO model partograph 631f
Withdrawal method 220
Wood's maneuver 734
Wound site infection 703
Wrigley's forceps 375, 477, 477f

X

X-linked disorders 379, 385
X-ray examination 147

Y

Yeast infection 268

Z

Zavanelli maneuver 734
Zidovudine 449, 743
Zygote intrafallopian transfer 83, 87